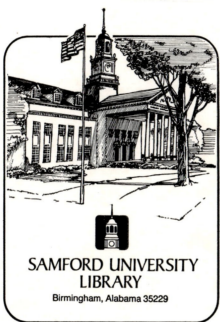

THE HEALTH OF THE REPUBLIC
Epidemics, Medicine, and Moralism
as Challenges to Democracy

HEALTH, SOCIETY,
and POLICY,
a series edited by
Sheryl Ruzek and
Irving Kenneth Zola

T H E

HEALTH
OF THE
REPUBLIC

Epidemics, Medicine, and

Moralism as Challenges

to Democracy

Dan E. Beauchamp

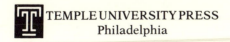 TEMPLE UNIVERSITY PRESS
Philadelphia

Temple University Press, Philadelphia 19122
Copyright © 1988 by Temple University. All rights reserved
Published 1988
Printed in the United States of America

Library of Congress Cataloging-in-Publication Data

Beauchamp, Dan E.
The health of the Republic / Dan E. Beauchamp.
p.   cm. — (Health, society, and policy)
Bibliography: p.
Includes index.
ISBN 0–87722–558–3 (alk. paper)
1. Public health—United States.   2. Medical policy—United
States.   3. Medicine, State—United States.   I. Title.   II. Series.
RA445.B39   1988
362.1'0973—dc 19   87-35335
                                                          CIP

To my mother and to the memory of my father

CONTENTS

Contents

PREFACE

This book didn't turn out the way I thought it would. I originally intended to write a book that brought the community perspectives of public health more into the mainstream of social and political philosophy, acquainting those outside public health with the power of the only nonindividualistic mode of thought flourishing in the field of health policy. I also hoped to impress those outside public health proper, especially philosophers and public policy experts in the health field, with the utility of a public health approach to health problems.

I began this task over a decade ago, seeking to translate the public health viewpoint into the language of social justice and equality, suggesting that "public health," and not "health care," should be the primary or basic good—to put the idea of community at the center rather than at the periphery of a scheme of distributive justice.

One stumbling block to my early attempts was the problem of "lifestyle" risks: personal behavior that resulted in a heavy toll on the public's health. Most egalitarians are committed in one way or another to a rather fundamental concept of individual autonomy and find restrictions on individual liberty to promote the good of individuals—paternalism—questionable, or at best acceptable only with special justification. In working with this problem I argued that we needed communal definitions of public health problems, even those that result largely from voluntary personal actions, because the point of restrictions was to promote a common, not a private, good. Thus, I saw such restrictions as not paternalistic in the traditional sense.

Most nonphilosophers working in public health dislike

being labeled paternalist. They prefer to justify their call for limits to such lifestyle risks as smoking and alcohol use on the grounds that smokers or drinkers impose burdens on society or on the grounds that these risks are so socially influenced that the issue of voluntariness is irrelevant. I kept looking for justifications for these limits that drew on our sense of community, at least in some respects—a set of reasons that rejected both paternalism and the "harms to others" framework.

I began to explore the roots of public health in constitutional law, and especially the development of the police power. Here I discovered an older, but still fresh, justification for public health—the republican tradition. Courts display a well-known deference to legislatures' wishes to restrict property rights and even personal liberty in order to promote the public's health. What is not so well known is that the police power, itself a restriction of personal liberty or property to promote public welfare, is firmly rooted in the republican soil of our political tradition.

In my other professional area of interest, alcohol policy, I came to appreciate the deep tangle of moralism in alcohol policy and in public health generally. Of course, most historians have long stressed the moralist argument in interpreting Prohibition; few, however, have noted that moralism and public health ideas were deeply intertwined in the Progressive era, a pattern that shapes our views of many public health problems to this day.

For a long time I tried to work all of this out within the framework of John Rawls's powerful work of 1971, *A Theory of Justice*. I modified his categories of the primary goods to give them a more communal dimension, seeking to show how persons in the original position—a position outside and prior to society where persons are kept ignorant of their fate in life and asked to draft principles governing the allocation of certain basic goods like liberty, fair equality of opportunity, and the like—would arrive at that view, rather than the more individualistic view that I found in Rawls's writings.

Somewhere along the way I began to sense that my resolution of republicanism, paternalism, equality, and community, all the while retaining liberalism's key idea of a fundamental autonomy in many spheres, could not easily be accommodated within some master theoretical framework based on a single or small set of abstract principles. It gradually became clear to me that the proper path lay along the lines advocated by Michael Walzer in his *Spheres of Justice*, published in 1983.

Walzer argues for a complex equality that construes society as a plurality of spheres, each allocating a different set of social goods according to its own logic or principles. What I found especially helpful about Walzer's argument is its primary reliance on history and the sense of community, distributive justice, and equality formed by that history. I had already found that, for public health, the historical record was crucial to understanding the key ideas.

Walzer's work helped me in three ways. First, it showed me that equality might, in a given society, require differing limitations on individual autonomy depending on the specific good being distributed and the sphere of its distribution. For example, autonomy might be fundamental in the sphere of democratic discussion and the private sphere but less fundamental in the spheres of the market and communal welfare.

Second, Walzer's theory helps get across a central point that most modern philosophers handle badly or not at all: the dominant role of the market over other spheres in capitalist societies. This point is central to understanding equality in health care. But the market is not the only sphere that tends to invade its neighbors; moralism—the deformed morality that reduces moral questions to adherence to a narrow behavioral code, and immorality to a species of moral pollution—has similar predatory tendencies. Many of our most pressing health issues, from AIDS to the commercialization of medicine, are understandable only in the context of the tendency of either the market or moralism to become tyrannical beyond its proper sphere of action.

Third, and perhaps most important, in Walzer's ideas I began to see that the idea of public health in a republic requires more than social organization to promote the people's health, a perspective I have long relied on. I have not abandoned that viewpoint here, but I have come to see that in many crucial areas, public health in a republic requires a retreat of government and a limit on the power of majorities to shape individual conduct. In other words, protecting the public health is often a matter of strengthening civil liberties.

Thus, as my research progressed, public health became a more complex issue for me, mirroring the way in which a modern democratic society is itself complex, based on distinctive spheres in which differing rules and logics apply. As I hope to show in this book, our health policy is part of our history of trying to untangle the various spheres of the republic: democratic discussion and free speech, communal provision, privacy, the market, and religion.

Finally, health policy is central to reclaiming our sense of a republic. An improved health policy can help restore to our common consciousness a lively awareness that we live together in order to accomplish things together, and that paradoxically the sense of a shared fate in a republic is also linked to the freedom of the individual, in basic and fundamental matters, to be left alone.

I have incurred many debts along my way. To my many colleagues in the field of alcohol and alcoholism studies, and in the larger domain of public health, I am grateful for encouragement to pursue these ideas. One of my great good fortunes was, after leaving graduate school, to have encountered difficulties in locating a position in an academic political science department, partly because political scientists seemed at that time (and still largely seem) to view health policy, and especially alcohol policy, as a quaint and marginal interest for and to a great discipline. So I found myself in a school of public health, and I am forever thankful for that happy accident.

If I name a few specific individuals who have helped me with this project I will unfortunately miss many others who have had a hand in improving it. But I owe a special debt to Kenneth Warner, John Romani, Toby Citrin, and other members of the faculty of the Department of Public Health Policy at the School of Public Health, University of Michigan, who gave me an office and a relatively light teaching load in 1983–1984. That year was a wonderful one for my wife and for me. The University of Michigan and Ann Arbor are tremendously exciting places to work. As a lifelong southerner who was shocked by the average winter temperature, I nevertheless came to understand why a Michigan faculty member once told me he was going to retire in Ann Arbor "in spite of the weather."

My largest debt is to my own University of North Carolina, to my colleagues in the School of Public Health and the Department of Health Policy and Administration, and especially to the steady stream of students over the years who have sensed that I needed encouragement and have given it freely. Considering all the current pressures to transform public health into just another wing of the health care industry, the support of my students and colleagues for an endeavor that departs from the stubborn empiricism that is the fundamental virtue of public health is deeply appreciated.

I owe a special debt to my research assistants over the past several years: Carolyn Cantlay, Sandra Robinson, Jan Kaplan, Darrel Cox, Mary Ella Payne, and Linda Shear. All have tolerated my maddening, incessant demands for material located all over the University of North Carolina campus with good grace and cheer, and this I deeply appreciate.

I owe a personal debt to David Galinsky, who helped me to understand that complexity is a virtue not only of societies but of human personality, and who probably is as responsible as anyone for my finishing this project in reasonably sound mind.

I would like to also remember Jean Yates, our departmental reference librarian for many years, who tirelessly read earlier versions of this manuscript, counteracting at least some of the most serious crimes I committed against the English language. Her death deprived us all of a good friend and colleague.

I want to thank Molly, our golden retriever, for coming along at the right time; she has been a faithful companion at the word processor for hours on end.

I also want to thank Janet Francendese and Mary Capouya of Temple University Press, and Sheryl Ruzek and Irving Zola, Coeditors of the Press's Health, Society, and Policy series, for many helpful suggestions in revising the manuscript. I also appreciate the comments of many reviewers, especially Patricia Barry, Larry Churchill, Jean Forster, Deborah Freund, David Jolly, Nancy Milio, David Musto, Thomas Ricketts, William Sullivan, Lawrence Wallack, Kenneth Warner, Kenneth Wing, and several anonymous reviewers. Also, Harry Scheiber, George Annas, and John Kaplan reviewed the chapter on constitutional law in a very early stage. Laurette de Veaux provided invaluable editorial assistance in the nick of time. All of these individuals gave me very sound advice, most of which I took. Still, I am sure they would want me to say that the faults of the book remain the responsibility of the author.

Finally, my wife Carole has borne the brunt of the time and energy this project has taken from our marriage. My debt to her is the largest of all—a debt I intend to repay.

THE HEALTH OF THE REPUBLIC
Epidemics, Medicine, and Moralism
as Challenges to Democracy

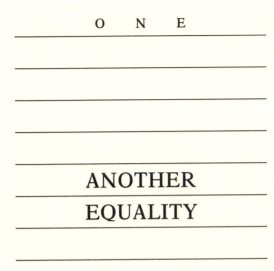

O N E

ANOTHER
EQUALITY

This book is about the link between equality and the health of the American republic—the health of its citizens and its democratic institutions.

Drawing on Michael Walzer's *Spheres of Justice*,[1] it focuses on the development of a more complex concept of equality in which the central issue is to discern the distinctive goods and values distributed by the several spheres of a democratic society and the conflicts that arise when one sphere dominates another. Throughout, I concentrate on how protection of the public's health requires the prevention of the market sphere or the sphere of a religiously inspired moralism from invading and dominating other spheres, such as those of privacy, the common provision of communal health protections, and democratic discussion. I explore

1

conflicts about ideas, particularly the constant battles over the meaning and application of equality in a democratic society. I discuss how differing ideas about equality, liberty, and community affect distribution in health policy and other areas of society. I describe attempts to suppress conflict, to ignore its existence, or to narrow its range of application. As it does in any conflict, the history of efforts to protect the public's health in our democracy remains part of the ongoing debate about health policy; this history is part of my book.

I use Walzer's basic perspective to construct a theory of republican equality whose overall task is to strengthen a sense of common membership in a republic of equals. Thus, this is a book on political philosophy and the structure of an egalitarian health policy, not a book on the ethics of health care. I have little to say about the many vexing issues we face today in health policy: how we ought to ration medical care, what the duties of doctors to patients ought to be in an age of soaring medical costs, or whether surrogate motherhood should be banned or regulated. My purpose is to demonstrate the ways in which a more complex, republican equality would help provide a political framework for a fairer and more expeditious settling of these specific conflicts.

Because my framework is political philosophy, not systematic moral theory or ethics, the reader will not find here several chapters discussing alternative theories of the right, the good, or justice as an ideal. Nor will the reader find extensive discussion of why health care or health protections as a good deserve honored places in such theories. I ignore these topics for a number of reasons, not the least of which is that these subjects are so expansive as to leave little time or space to treat issues that I believe to be far more relevant to today's health policy: the meaning of the democratic community, the links between community and equality, the structure of equality in health provision, the assurance of a stable scheme of health protections, and the like.

2

Thus, I start with the assumption that illness is the relevant reason for distributing medical care and health protections. To quote Bernard Williams, "Leaving aside preventive medicine, the proper ground of distribution of medical care is ill health: this is a necessary truth."[2] (Unlike Williams, I see little reason for treating preventive medicine any differently: the relevant reason for distributing preventive measures is to prevent illness and early death.)

Thus, I treat the principle of equality in health policy as given, turning to issues like the *structure* of equality for health policy and its implementation and social organization. The United States may finally reject equality for health. But, for me, the central question I address is not whether we ought to accept equality as a basis for distributing health care and health protections; the question is what pattern of organization of equality we ought to employ to make the equal distribution of medical care effective. That is, how can we make the principle that illness is the relevant reason for distributing medical care operative and stable?

Should equality mean equal access to health care, where equal access means that medical care should be organized in such a way that it is reasonably available and affordable to everyone alike? Or should the principle be equity—the notion that society has a responsibility to ensure that the poor and others without medical insurance still receive at least a decent minimum of medical care, leaving the rest of society to the market—or should it mean something else?

Republican Equality

My proposed answer to these questions rests in the concept of republican equality.[3] Republican equality would limit the power of money and moralism over health policy by constructing an autonomous and common health system, the American republic's own version of a national health program that both works to prevent disease and ministers to the suffering as a basic token of equal citizenship.

But a healthy republic is not solely the handiwork of a strong and autonomous sphere of communal welfare; it is also the result of a vigorous and expanded democratic discussion about the public's health, as well as a strengthened private realm where all citizens have the right to be left alone in matters of intimate decision, to shape their own particular lives. In other words, the task for equality in health policy is to meet the challenge of a modern, democratic republic with a complex structure for providing the goods critical to its common health and safety, enhancing the health not only of its people but of its rich heritage of democratic institutions and values.

While my interpretation of equality—with its somewhat unusual name of republican equality—differs from more widely discussed ideas like "equal access" and "equity," I argue that a complex and republican equality more adequately describes what is now occurring in health policy, especially in the broad range of political conflicts that have developed since World War II. Moreover, a republican equality more effectively both secures the public's health and solidifies and expands the sense that we are a commonwealth.

Republican equality is both conservative and radical. It is conservative because it saves the best of medicine from the market, preventing a corporate takeover of the health industry and the commodification of medical practice, protecting local communal institutions (like local hospitals) from disappearing into national chains and other destructive changes that follow from market competition. It is radical because it expands the sphere of individual rights and democratic discussion to protect the individual and the body politic from the moral crusades of majorities or well-organized minorities. It is radical also because it employs a system of communal provision of health protections—and the other facets of health policy—in ways that betoken to everyone their equal citizenship and individual dignity, assuring all that in matters of health we are equal rather than unequal.

Where We Stand: Domination by the Market Sphere

I am painfully aware that we now fall short of almost anyone's definition of equality in health provision. Despite the fact that medical inflation persists almost unchecked, our currently popular limited method for controlling inflation—the Diagnostic-Related Groups (DRGs), which fix prices for more than four hundred separate diagnostic categories under the Medicare program—has brought only an astonishing level of administrative interference by government and private insurance companies with the practice of medicine. Even though we spend over $500 billion annually on health care—more per capita than any other society—and though our health spending is likely to climb from 11 to 15 percent of our GNP in little more than a decade, today as many as 35 million Americans do not have adequate health insurance.

The commercialization of medicine grows as we struggle to mend the huge gaps of inequality in our social "safety net." Indeed, the simplistic way we pursue equality in medicine may be the principal cause of the commercialization of medicine, and may be permanently eroding our fragile ideal that illness is the relevant reason for distributing health care. Already, prestigious and influential groups advocate abandoning a more vigorous equality in distributing health care, substituting instead the principle of equity with its precarious dependence on motives of political altruism or charity.[4]

I believe that a major contributing factor in the commercialization of medicine, and in other issues such as medical inflation, is a theory of simple equality that myopically focuses on a shortage of money as the main problem, seeking to spread money around more equally to give the poor more purchasing power for medical care. This thoughtless preoccupation with money alone ignores the power of the larger market to absorb medicine, converting it into a commodity. More government subsidies simply place medicine more clearly in the market, driving its price upward and destabilizing existing arrangements for medicine for the poor. We may be approaching a time when doctors practice medicine mainly to make money rather than to heal the sick, practicing what Nozick calls "schmoctoring."[5]

The same process of market domination is also occurring in public health policy, from worker safety to environmental protection. The "deregulation" movement of the seventies was not simply the result of business mobilizing against the new agencies created during the Great Society; it was also the result of attempts to marry market incentives with communal health protections. The result has been a growing confusion of realms, with a republic's historic protection of the health and safety of its citizens potentially a permanent captive of the market.

Money is not the only good that republican equality seeks to limit to its proper sphere. From AIDS (acquired immunodeficiency syndrome) to abortion, a private and largely religious moralism distorts health policy, limiting the scope of preventive measures and determining who receives treatment and even whether needed medical procedures like abortion are available to poor women. As money and moralism spill over into the sphere of communal welfare, dividing citizens into creditors and debtors, saints and sinners, the meaning of equal citizenship is diluted.

Before going into more detail concerning the nature of republican equality, let me first take up five key issues in health policy today, showing how each involves the dominance of one good over another and the necessity for protecting the autonomy of the distinctive spheres of a democratic republic.

Whose Life Is It, Anyway?

Tom, a thirty-seven-year-old construction worker, has smoked since his early teens. Most of his friends smoke, although his children do not, and neither does his wife. Not that he hasn't tried to quit. Like almost three-fourths of all smokers, Tom has made many serious efforts to stop smoking. He knows there are serious health risks, and he could do without the expense of smoking. He predicts that someday he will finally kick the habit.

Nevertheless, Tom has little patience with current anti-smoking propaganda. He thinks that his union's health promotion program, which stresses nonsmoking, is okay because it is voluntary. But he doesn't believe in forcing people to stop smoking. Recently he worked on an inside job for a company that had rules against smoking. Tom had to smoke outside, on his breaks. He was surprised that he got used to the new rules, but nevertheless he believed them to be an unjust interference with his personal right to choose. And Tom definitely believes that the government should not try to stop people from taking risks that involve no one else.

A huge fraction of our death and disability tolls (perhaps half) stems from self-inflicted risks that are substantially voluntary, from smoking to driving without seat belts. What can government do about such risks, especially in a democratic society in which each is supposed to plan his or her own life?

Most Americans have mixed feelings about such questions of paternalism. Self-regarding risks don't seem to involve other people, at least not directly. Also, most people seem to fear health becoming part of a kind of religion, the religion advocated by Dr. Pickerbaugh, the Health Officer of Zenith in Sinclair Lewis's *Arrowsmith*—a religion made of "good health, good roads, good business, and the single standard of morality." Despite these reservations, most Americans regard protections against death and serious disability as central, if not preeminent, societal goods.

Such contradictions abound. Legislators increasingly embrace public health legislation limiting personal liberties, such as our laws for water fluoridation, helmets for motorcycle operators, and seat belts for drivers. Recently, and partly to avoid the backlash associated with paternalism, we legislated the creation of a whole new class of underage citizens who, by definition, were changed into legitimate targets for paternalistic legislation. The raising of the drinking age to twenty-one only a few years after many of these age limits were lowered to eighteen changed these people from autonomous adults to dependent children, at the mercy of paternalistic protective laws.

In an odd way, the extreme antipaternalism of our time, particularly among philosophers, exemplifies the dangers of too simplistic equality, basing it on an ideal of fundamental autonomy that moves beyond the sphere of privacy and free discussion to range over all of the distinctive spheres of a complex republic. The perspectives of republican equality would restore a more complex and balanced autonomy: a basic autonomy that nonetheless permits limited restrictions on liberty to protect the health and safety of citizens as a body, the *public health*—a central goal of all republican schemes of government. And as I argue in Chapter Four, this is precisely the republican rationale for such legislation in our constitutional tradition.

What Kind of Community Are We?

Sam is a thirty-five-year-old male homosexual who works as a bank executive in a large southwestern city. He has just learned that he has tested positive for HIV antibodies and so has his lover. While they have lived together for many years, neither has objected when the other visits a gay bar or bath occasionally for an anonymous sexual encounter with a stranger. Sam believes this is how they became infected with the AIDS virus, but he cannot be sure.

AIDS has claimed more than thirty-five thousand lives since it was first discovered in 1981; there are now more than sixty thousand diagnosed cases of AIDS.[6] In America, more than 90 percent of the victims are male homosexuals, bisexuals, or intravenous drug users. Battling AIDS raises basic questions about society's long-standing laws against homosexuality, and some groups are now calling for stricter measures against homosexuality.

This latter view is usually called "legal moralism."[7] Legal moralists believe that the purpose of the law is to punish vice and promote virtue, and that society is held together by a shared moral code based on a traditional morality. In the legal moralist's view, good health is a product of virtuous living, and suppressing the vice of homosexuality is a way of promoting the public health.

Moralism in our common life is dangerous precisely because it dominates distributive systems outside the private and the religious spheres. A simplistic equality responds to moralism by arguing that in all matters of private conduct the individual ought to be left alone. But republican equality moves in a more complex fashion; its radical side fights the moralism that sponsors a communal bigotry that leads society virtually to make a pact with the epidemic and attack its victims. More conservatively, a republican equality would seek, through education and democratic discussion, safer and more prudent sexual practices. But a republican equality would also depend on building trust with the epidemic's victims through guarantees of confidentiality and freedom from discrimination in medical treatment, work, education, and housing.

Medicine and Equality

Sarah is a professor of social policy in a leading university institute for public policy and public affairs, where she teaches the courses on health policy. A major theme of her courses is the idea of equality in medical care organization.

A decade ago her courses focused on the benefits and drawbacks of national health insurance; now she barely mentions the subject. "National health insurance is an idea whose time has come—and gone. Maybe forever. Americans don't want that kind of equality in health care services, or so it is believed," she says.

A recent report of the President's Commission for the Study of Ethical Problems in Medicine and Biomedical and Behavioral Research (created by Congress in 1978) reflected the ethical and philosophical issues in providing access to health care, confirming Sarah's point. Equity—patching up the failures of the market—not equality, should guide our health policy. Though weakened by Reagan appointees to the commission, the report still reflected the prevailing opinion that equality is too costly or will require too severe a restriction of individual freedom. The option of a shared equality achieved by providing an adequate level of health care for all—in other words, creating a common system with a ceiling on health care spending and requiring all to observe it—was rejected as too coercive to be consistent with American values.[8]

Thus, despite social reforms of the sixties and even earlier when a wide cross-section of Americans viewed equality in health care as a right, and universal health insurance as an inevitability, today equality and universal health insurance are regarded as utopian. The commission did not even consider the option of universal health insurance or a national health service, the approach of most other Western democracies.

Regulating Business

Michael Pertschuk, the former chairman of the Federal Trade Commission, in a recent book mourns the passing of the consumer "impulse."[9] Pertschuk laments the eclipse of the movements to control business through stringent public health, environmental, and consumer regulations that were started during the sixties and seventies. He believes that regulatory agencies started then, though less heralded than the antipoverty programs, the civil rights debates, or the antiwar protests, deserve recognition as equal to the other achievements of the period.

Pertschuk and others justify the agencies as exceptions to the normal rule of markets and self-interested politics. Agencies formed to combat threats to the public health now face formidable opposition because public health problems affect specific individuals only diffusely or rarely, and current antipaternalistic sentiment objects to protection against such small risks. Yet these problems accumulate over a broad public into significant numbers of premature deaths or injuries—that is, into significant public health problems.

Traffic safety is a good example. Though about forty-five thousand individuals lose their lives in highway crashes each year, at the individual level driving automobiles is extremely safe on a per trip basis—the chances of dying are less than one in one million. The protective measures government has tried to implement for the public—seat belt laws, lowered speed limits, stringent manufacturing requirements—add up to great political difficulty and require painful restrictions on powerful corporations.

Most political scientists treat the creation of these agencies as something of a political miracle, as an exception to the usual domination of public health policy by business interests. But in the strategy of republican equality, defending the public's health is not an exception to pluralist politics or a minor correction to market failures. Under republican equality, protection of the public health is a central task of government, one that symbolizes more than anything else that we are a republic and not simply a private society that operates at the pleasure of corporations or at the often conflicting convenience of millions of autonomous citizens.

Democratic Discussion

Ken is a Washington-based activist who first started with a Ralph Nader–like organization fighting unsafe corporate working conditions. Today he is involved in a campaign to combat the ceaseless promotion of alcohol on radio and television and advertising for cigarette smoking everywhere else.

Like most liberal activists, Ken sees such advertising as a sign of a reckless corporate irresponsibility that preys particularly on the nation's youth. Oddly, he is joined in his battles on Capitol Hill by some very conservative groups— parents' groups who also object to advertising and television programming that they believe promote drugs, alcohol, sex, and "loose living" generally.

Controlling television, and to a lesser extent radio, has become something of a separate agenda for many conservative and liberal groups. The liberals began with driving cigarette ads off television; the conservatives have tried to control pornography and the commercialization of sex.

Paradoxically, leading liberals on the Supreme Court have expressed a lack of enthusiasm for many of the attempts to control commercial advertising, constructing, at least for the time being, a measure of First Amendment protection for commercial advertising, usually termed the "commercial speech" doctrine. Whether the new doctrine of commercial speech would limit the ability of government to regulate advertising for cigarettes and for alcohol remains undetermined.

Ken is both angered by the sheer bulk of commercial advertising for beer and smoking and dismayed that attempts to counter these ads bring angry opposition from liberal groups such as the American Civil Liberties Union, which argues that his proposals constitute an abridgment of freedom of speech and are extremely paternalistic. He is also bothered by the fact that so many legislators who sponsor the bills for which he lobbies are highly visible conservatives like Senator Strom Thurmond from South Carolina and Senator Orrin Hatch from Utah.

The media, and in a much larger sense the public discussion that is essential to any democracy, have become a crucial battleground for health policy, from alcohol and AIDS to teenage pregnancy and abortion. In a liberal society, with its militant defense of freedom of expression, democratic discussion is a central part of public policy formation. A theory of republican equality, with its recognition that battles over public policy and equality are fought in many different distributive spheres, may be the only way to understand this aspect of health policy adequately.

Complex Equality

What Michael Walzer calls "complex equality," and I call republican equality, rejects the idea of pursuing equality as a general principle of distribution, whether it is equal opportunity or Rawls's theory of justice as fairness.[10] According to Walzer, "Every social good or set of goods constitutes a distributive sphere within which only certain criteria and arrangements are appropriate."[11] Complex equality seeks to protect the various realms of society from domination by other and more powerful realms, ensuring that equality is the principle of distribution where it is relevant and observing the particular form equality must take in each distinctive sphere. Medicine (at least ideally) is distributed to the sick; television sets to those with money; university admission to those with intellectual capacity. The

13

distinctive feature of complex equality—republican equality—is its acknowledgment of the plurality of social goods and their distinctive meanings, and its struggle to "vindicate the autonomy of the distributive spheres,"[12] attempting to reduce the dominance of powerful goods with an imperial nature.

Obviously, as Walzer notes, the distributive spheres for social goods are only relatively autonomous.[13] Medicine and university admission are available to those with money despite their needs or talents; indeed, in the United States, the market remorselessly invades other spheres, and money converts to advantage in many different realms.

Walzer argues that "simple equality" theories, which are usually based on single or uniform principles throughout capitalistic society,[14] seek to eliminate the domination of some powerful good, usually money (by radically redistributing the wealth) or political power (through a radical redistribution of the right to participate in democratic decision). Walzer's thesis can be applied to the field of health, where nearly every variation of equality is simple equality. Whether paraded under the banner of equity, equal access, or (sometimes) the equal right to health care, every theory of simple equality sees the principal problem in health care as the need to destroy the monopoly of money over health care. The standard suggested remedy is to have the government create "medical money" in many different forms to equalize access to medicine for all, or to establish a floor below which the very poorest in society would not be allowed to fall. Above this floor, these theories argue, the rest of the society and the organization of medicine itself should be left largely undisturbed. Paradoxically, the strategy of breaking money's monopoly by leaving medicine mostly in the market brings many unexpected results, such as medical inflation, isolated islands of charity medicine, and increasingly detailed and onerous regulatory mechanisms.

The trouble with simple equality in health policy, then, is

that it puts too much emphasis on government subsidies to expand the medical market and too little attention to the market's capacity to destroy medicine as an egalitarian good, converting it to an ordinary item in trade. Thus, simple equality, far from being a gradualist, conservative approach, actually works to transform medicine radically into a commodity and the health industry into yet another domain within the market sphere.

Republican Equality and Community

One distinctive feature of republican equality is its deliberate attempt to foster a sense of common membership and community, a root idea of a republic or commonwealth.

Community is an old political idea, actually the central political idea for the greatest part of the Western political tradition. Community, like friendship, family, kinship, fraternity, and patriotism, refers to shared sentiments and attachments that bind people or groups to one another. A republic, with its stress on virtue and a shared common life, is a species of political community. The democratic community of a republic is not only the whole citizenry considered as a body but also the consciousness of this common life and the obligations and willingness of citizens to subordinate themselves to the needs and good of the group.

For settlers in the New World, far from the traditional communal institutions of Europe, ideas of community were borrowed from the biblical tradition. Later, both the biblical and the civic republican traditions helped shape our revolutionary ideas.[15] Both these civic and religious traditions contained the idea that we are a people and a community as well as a collection of individuals and that we share common purposes and a common good. This theme was especially prominent in the republicanism of the most influential of the early state constitutions, that of Massachusetts.[16]

15

The idea of community has waxed and waned. Today it is enjoying a modest revival among social commentators, but already there is a growing controversy about the conflict of community and liberalism.[17] One group of philosophers argues that liberalism lacks the idea of community "whose primary bond is a shared understanding both of the good for man and the good for that community."[18] Modern society, at least after the Enlightenment, saw the shattering of community with the birth of the core idea of liberalism: Each individual is free to pursue his or her own interests and to select his or her own final ends. Critics of liberalism yearn for a return to the community of the past where the identity of the individual is shaped more decisively by communal understandings.

Unfortunately, the current debate usually frames the choice between liberalism, which denotes equality, and republicanism, which denotes community. But some ways of thinking about community and republican values incorporate equality as a central value. In this approach, which remains broadly liberal in spirit, individuals can disagree fundamentally about many things and still form a shared community. Community, and republican government, "regulates our social life, not our entire lives."[19]

In *Habits of the Heart*,[20] a recent critical reinterpretation of liberalism, Bellah and his coauthors note that individualism is the dominant language of American politics and culture.[21] America as a nation has been molded by a number of "individualisms": biblical, economic, and political. This individualism can cripple community. Indeed, our most honored critic, Alexis de Tocqueville, argued that equality dissolved the bonds of community: "Equality puts men side by side without a common link to hold them firm."[22] In fact, Tocqueville goes on, despots prefer equality because it "disposes [citizens] not to think of their fellows and turns indifference into a sort of public virtue."[23] According to Tocqueville, the despot "calls those who try to unite their efforts to create a general prosperity 'turbulent and restless spirits,' and twisting the natural meaning of words, he calls those 'good citizens' who care for none but themselves."[24]

But despite the dominance of individualism, there are "second languages" of republicanism and community in the United States that add an element of collective responsibility for our common welfare and soften and qualify, without eliminating, the tradition of individualism. These alternative languages provide a rich and neglected republican vocabulary for expanding our understanding of and responses to our shared problems.

The authors of *Habits of the Heart* make clear that they are not advocating a nostalgic resurrection of the local, traditional community.[25] Rather, for them community means something closer to the republican idea of public virtue and common possession. Republican equality seeks to foster a more spacious and generous sense of community, one in which common provision and common possession in the case of health protection, symbolizes a common membership in a republic of equals, and that in matters of health and safety we are a people as well as a collection of private citizens. Thus, community in republican equality is closer to the ideal of the Roman and republican idea of *communitas*; the cohesive spirit of a people produced by possessing something in common, such as goods or values distributed in a common sphere.[26]

As I will discuss more fully in Chapter Four, public health has always been one of the distinctive second languages of republicanism and community in the United States. Public health stands for collective control over conditions affecting the common health—a very sturdy republican idea. Yet most Americans—even many public health officials—either are ignorant of or choose to ignore the republican tradition behind public health; to them, the term *public health* calls up only the picture of a local health department office located downtown, filled with poor people.

It was not always this way. The opening of the twentieth century in the United States was the age of public health—a

17

period of progress based on organized group action to attack disease. By 1900 we had begun to make dramatic gains in controlling the most deadly infectious diseases—smallpox, cholera, typhus. Public health proponents used legislation, regulation, and education to make the water and milk supplies safer, to provide for sanitary waste disposal, and to immunize vulnerable populations in cities like New York, Milwaukee, and Providence.

The success of these methods lay as much in their evoking a republican and communal consciousness as in the new science of battling epidemics and infectious disease. Public health was a symbol of the Progressive Era, when the theme of republicanism and community dominated the writings of new liberals like Lippmann, Croly, Weyl, and later Dewey.[27] As Dewey put it, "Fraternity, liberty, and equality isolated from communal life are hopeless abstractions."[28]

Community was a core concept in American progressivism, as David Price has argued.[29] Though public health reformers have demanded a common health care system from the Progressive Era to the Great Society and even to the present, the language and ideals of public health have not been successful in helping forge a more communal American idea of equality. Public health has largely been considered a possible exception to standard liberal schemes for redistributing valued goods to overcome market inequities. The more communitarian and republican language of equality has definitely remained secondary.

John Rawls and Justice as Fairness

Today, those who write about equality mention republicanism and community only peripherally. Although the most eloquent restatement of liberal theory of our time, John Rawls's *A Theory of Justice*, clearly argues for a more extensive equality for our democratic republic, the dimension of community and the focus on preserving the autonomy of separate distributive spheres is strikingly absent.[30]

Rawls's theory of justice is based on the most extensive allocation of primary goods. Primary goods are goods that everyone would want no matter what else they would want.[31] Rawls's principles of justice are those that self-interested individuals would derive, given certain highly restrictive conditions—the procedural devices of the "original position" and the "veil of ignorance."[32] The original position is a position outside of and prior to society from which persons, acting as ideal legislators or representatives, view the world without knowing whether their constituents are male, female, white, black, poor, sick, healthy, and so on. The point is that radical ignorance forces the representatives in the original position to develop agreements for the provision of certain paradigmatic primary goods that are necessary if everyone's plan of life is to have a reasonable chance of completion. The primary goods are the basic liberties, fair equality of opportunity, powers and prerogatives, income and wealth, and the bases of self-respect.

Rawls's theory is striking because according to it the representatives, seeking to protect the interests of their constituents, would agree to a most extensive equality and social redistribution. This structure of justice embodying a "fair system of cooperation" would lead to a view of the political community as a kind of social union of social unions and might even encourage a limited spirit of fraternity.[33] Yet the very abstract quality of Rawls's method of ethical invention creates problems, problems that could be averted by a complex equality like republican equality.

I have already discussed the emphasis on building and strengthening the community in republican equality through the common provision of health protections. In Rawls's scheme this emphasis on common provision is absent. Rawls seeks to elaborate an abstract theory of justice and to identify in only a general way which goods are primary; health care is considered not a primary good but an important social good that advances the primary good of fair equality of opportunity. Rawls's theory would justify a far more equitable allocation of health care in the United States than now obtains, yet it ignores both whether a common health care system is crucial to stabilizing equality in the face of the dominance of markets and the need for defense measures to protect the primary goods from domination by other realms. This failure is significant because Rawls's theory is among the most influential philosophical works of our time. Its very influence in persuading a generation of moral philosophers that the task of moral philosophy lies in discovering the basic ethical principles that underlie such actual problems as the provision of health care may be helping to divert attention from the equally important task of protecting the primary goods from market engulfment.[34] Thus, Rawls's seeming indifference to the issue of common provision for at least some goods in society leaves this issue to the contingencies of particular societies and historical precedent. One of Rawls's most sympathetic interpreters, Norman Daniels, in his *Just Health Care*,[35] argues for a vastly more fair distribution of medical care but says almost nothing about whether common provision is the only way a more fair distribution could survive. Nor does Daniels devote much attention to how the absence of a common framework, and of common provision, undermines the special character of medicine.

Furthermore, in Rawls's scheme, primary goods sound suspiciously like another kind of "good," economic commodities that can be appropriated by individuals separately, for their personal use. Rawls's theory of justice is tinted with the normal commodity bias that characterizes liberal thought influenced by market ideals; indeed, his cursory treatment of public goods (as distinct from the primary goods) implies that primary goods are largely similar to other economic commodities in society, differing only in their rules of distribution. The idea of prevention, and the collective character of provision that it demands, thus plays almost no role in Rawls's theory; nonetheless, Daniels argues that the Rawlsian approach would give priority to prevention, for only when we prevent serious disease and disability can we assure the greatest number of "active, able, fully cooperating members of a society over the course of a life."[36]

I believe that prevention does enjoy a kind of moral priority over treatment for the simple reason that prevention, at least ideally, can avert far more suffering and illness than cure can. But the relationship between prevention and treatment is complex. Even in the sphere of communal health protections, where persons are necessarily treated as members of a public and as a group, republican equality does not lose sight of the individual person and his or her suffering and needs for treatment. Although prevention is more effective in avoiding suffering, the manifest sufferings of specific persons often help widen and strengthen the solidarity within the community for more prevention in health policy.

But equally important, as I argue in Chapter Three, is that the logic of distribution behind the prevention of disease and premature death in modern developed societies makes the communal dimension crucial. Alleviation of modern public health problems requires the reduction of risks that are faced by the community considered as a whole. Moreover, the preventive measures taken to reduce risks provide benefits that seem marginal when viewed from the standpoint of individuals considered privately; they are group or community gains. Seatbelt laws are an excellent example of this distinction.

The group or republican character of common protections through prevention forces us to alter our thinking about the role of government in lifestyle, as well as to temper our dogmatic antipaternalism with a more complex political philosophy. Rawls, like most of us, is ambivalent about paternalism. According to Rawls, the representatives in the original position would agree to a scheme of penalties to discourage foolish or irrational actions, but he makes this point tentative because the representatives would also want to guarantee, for their principals, "the integrity of their person and their final ends and beliefs whatever they are."[37] Rawls concludes that the representatives would agree on some limited forms of paternalism—weak paternalism—when the evidence suggests that there is a "failure of reason and will."[38]

Daniels disagrees with even these mild permissions for lifestyle limits on Rawls's part. Daniels writes that

> health may be special or important from the perspective of a theory of justice because of its impact on opportunity, and this importance may give rise to social obligations to protect health. But nothing in this view makes health protection *so* overriding a concern that we may deny individuals the autonomy to take risks that endanger life, liver, and lungs.[39]

I disagree, but my disagreement is a complex one. Health in a republican scheme of equal provision would permit some restrictions on voluntary and personal risks, but the reasons would not be particularly paternalistic. As a society, the most serious risks we face, those resulting in the greatest loss of life in the aggregate, are risks more to the community than personal ones. This suggests that limiting the liberty of individuals to promote the public health is to promote a common good and not a private or paternalistic one.

Making Equality Stable

Rawls is one of the few contemporary philosophers who have addressed the issue of the stability of justice. Rawls argues that the representatives in the original position would recognize that the principles of justice and equality need to be stable and enduring over time. Stability, as I am using the term, is an attribute of the social organization of health care and prevention policy, one that guides, holds constant, and even enlarges the dominant loyalties of the citizenry and their representatives for equality in health provision. Properly designed, the Health Insurance Fund discussed later would make the loyalties of the citizenry to universal health insurance more enduring and stable. A stable form of common provision is one that does not rely upon shifting, shaky, and precarious motives of altruism or benevolence for the poor or for the needs of the community, but through a common structure relieves citizens, in the words of Oscar Wilde, "from that sordid necessity of living for others which, in the present condition of things, presses so hardly upon almost everybody." For Rawls, justice and equality will only "cohere together into a workable and stable basic structure as a framework of social cooperation over a complete life" when the ties of justice are strengthened by feelings of benevolence and loyalty to those principles.[40]

Rawls develops a complex and interesting social psychology of justice, explaining how justice as fairness would encourage cooperation and the internalization of the principles of just treatment. In Rawls's scheme, justice becomes psychologically stable over the lifetimes of the individual members of society, moving from childhood experiences of authority, through the experience of associational cooperation, to the experience of just social institutions. Cooperation is strengthened among the members because of the perceived fairness of the principles behind the major institutions of society.

But it seems to me that those in the original position would be poorly situated to understand, much less to develop, a stable and operative scheme of justice. As Michael Walzer notes, it is not only that people distribute goods; the patterns of distribution that people create influence the specific identities of the participants.[41] Thus, the logic of common provision, whether for health care or for retirement, is to forge a set of loyalties not simply to the good in question, but to the pattern of common distribution itself, so as to prevent its being undercut by alternative schemes, which might encourage abandonment of the poor and like threats.

Thus, republican equality would seek to anchor justice not on an abstract psychology of justice as fairness but on the particular and shared loyalties to common institutions. This would create popular solidarity based on political and communal loyalties stemming from the experience of common possession of shared institutions.

Thus, particular societies—for example, many contemporary democratic societies—turn to communal provision of health and safety as especially strategic for anchoring equality in a liberal democracy: communal solidarity in the face of death has strong historic and religious significance; it is one of the central ways in which we show ourselves to be a community and to have a common life. The central institution of medicine—the hospital—with its historical meanings, is one of the few places left in the American republic where an open dependence on others is permitted and even encouraged.[42]

If, as Michael Walzer argues, "political community [is] for the sake of provision, provision for the sake of community,"[43] then political community stands for protecting life and limb, and protecting life and limb stands for the political community. As Walzer notes, "the process works both ways, and that is perhaps its crucial feature."[44] In a republican equality, health and safety strengthen both the health of the citizenry and their shared consciousness that they are a people who live together in order to accomplish things together. This shared consciousness in turn promotes loyalty among the citizenry for the common provision of health and safety.

In health policy, the strategy of republican equality would be to protect the autonomy of medicine and the larger sphere of health and safety by shifting the loyalties of citizens, public officials, and the political parties to a common system and policy for health care, one that guarantees equality through common provision. This sounds more radical and complicated than it really is.

Shifting to a Common System

The common provision of medical care can take many forms; the national health service of England, the national health insurance scheme of Canada, and the mixed national plans of continental Europe could be used as models for developing a workable American system. At a minimum, a common system should provide for universal coverage with comprehensive and standard benefits for all citizens. The plan should be publicly administered so that hospitals, nursing homes, and physicians all operate within a common policy and set of public incentives; the plan would act as society's agent having the authority to set the terms and conditions for affordable and accessible medical and hospital practice.

In the past common systems were financed by the government, with only a minimal role played by commercial insurance. Today, a publicly financed plan would require nearly two hundred billion dollars in new taxes and seems wildly utopian. But total governmental financing may not be necessary or even desirable. A Health Insurance Fund that would combine public support and private health insurance is one way to shift from a market-centered to a government-centered system.

A Health Insurance Fund could work along the following lines. The fund would issue all citizens of the United States a health security card that would entitle them to a comprehensive range of medical care services at any health facility or from any provider entitled to participate in the scheme. Although patients' choices would be limited by the capacities and locations of providers, the card would symbolize that the health care system is a common one, shaped by a public policy rather than by market forces.

In order to become members of the overall plan established by the fund, hospitals, long-term care facilities, physicians, and third party insurers would have to meet certain conditions of participation. For example, hospitals would operate as nonprofit institutions; depreciation schedules for facilities and equipment would be developed based on resources and needs of communities and society, not to fuel a constant and wasteful modernization of hospital facilities. Hospitals and other health care facilities would operate within annual budgets and statewide plans that would require approval from the plan authorities. Expansion of medical facilities, or major equipment acquisition, would also require prior approval by plan authorities. Physicians would have to accept fees set by negotiated fee schedules as total payment for covered services. Similarly, insurance plans would conform to certain standards of minimum and maximum service coverage. Hospitals or physicians would be free to opt out of the system, but opting out would mean their relying entirely on private funding.

Such a plan would alter the current private insurance system for both collecting premiums and paying the bills; insurance companies would function mainly to collect premiums that would be deposited in the Health Insurance Fund, which would pay hospitals, nursing homes, and physicians. If patients were required to pay a small part of their bill at the outset (called deductibles) or to pay a portion of their overall bill (called copayment), they would pay the fund directly.

This common structure, although it would sharply curtail the freedom of physicians and hospitals to determine their charges, would still entrust them with the daily operation of the health care system. In many ways the fund would simplify hospitals' and physicians' paperwork, eliminating the bewildering array of forms from myriad private and public insurance sources. Providers would face new government-imposed limits on their annual expenditures, their fees, and greater supervision by committees of peers over their practice. Most important, providers would no longer have any incentive to throw back the "economically unattractive patient."

Paying for the Common System

Because so many persons in the United States lack health insurance, operating the fund would require additional taxes. The tax burden could be limited if all employers were required to pay for expanded standard insurance coverage as part of employee wages. Such coverage would also provide catastrophic benefits as well as more extensive health care during unemployment. The costs of such health insurance to very small businesses could be subsidized by government. State and local governments would be required to contribute to the fund, depending on their ability, wealth, needs, and so forth.

Creating a common policy and framework for medicine along the lines of a Health Insurance Fund creates something quite different from a "floor" for the poor; it would set the standard for health care for the whole society. It would also provide the overarching framework in which physicians and hospitals operate, preserving them as communal institutions and protecting them from the commercializing pull of the marketplace. The fund would diminish wasteful, destructive competition between hospitals and other health care organizations, providing stability and order in local communities where commercial pressures are destroying local institutions. The fund would set a ceiling each year for total expenditures for medical care. New technologies like the artificial heart or transplant technology would be evaluated, not as new ways for hospitals to make money or as opportunities for further medical specialization, but against the need for basic medical care of everyone in society, and the republic's resources to meet those societal needs.

A common system, designed along the lines of the fund, beyond controlling medical inflation and ensuring universal coverage, would also shift and shape the loyalties and even the identities of the members of society who share in its benefits.[45] If carefully designed, common provision, unlike a "safety net," fosters a sense of shared dependency, cooperation, and a common fate, using the experience of common possession to deepen the sense among all citizens that we are a republic of equals and that we live together to accomplish certain things together.

The existence of a plan for common health care could ease tremendously the task of reacting to new challenges such as AIDS, providing badly needed federal leadership and helping the states and localities meet the new demands for medical care in those areas hardest hit. Another achievement of the fund would be to dramatize the links between health insurance and the other spheres of health policy. For example, taxes on alcohol and tobacco (discussed in later chapters) could be powerful revenue sources for the fund, while simultaneously dramatizing the link between alcohol and tobacco prices and consumption. Finally, the fund and its management, annual budget, and policies could quickly become an important part of the national political agenda, making the links between health policy and the good of the republic as a whole a critical part of the ongoing process of public deliberation, rather than the private discussion among economists, industry representatives, and other specialists that it is now.

At the heart of the idea of republican equality is the tension between the individual citizen and the citizenry as a body. A republican equality seeks to manage rather than eliminate that paradox, rejecting democratic collectivism or individualism. Joseph Tussman expresses this ambiguity in a different way:

> Familiar as it is, there is something fundamentally misleading about the slogan that the aim of government is "the welfare of the individual." . . . It is hard to quarrel with the demand that the body politic provide or safeguard the conditions necessary for the fullest development of each of its citizens. . . . But I do not think we can escape the distinction between the demands or interests of a particular individual and the demands of the system of interests of which any individual's is only a part. Government, that is to say, serves the welfare of the community.[46]

TWO

MEDICINE AND THE
MARKET PRISON

In this chapter, I examine why our prevailing conceptions of equity and equal access for health care are politically unstable, leaving medicine vulnerable to commercialization and supporting its conversion to a commodity and its absorption into the larger market system. Republican equality, on the other hand, would use a common framework and policy to promote universal coverage and to make health care for the poor stable and complete, holding off the market and its commercializing tendencies, and fostering a sense of community and loyalty to the principle that the ways in which individuals are equal are more fundamental than the ways they are unequal.[1]

Charles Lindblom has argued that the market is unique as a social institution; its radical instability (at the level of individuals and firms) makes it as a structure extraordinarily stable and difficult to change or control.[2] The market is the constantly shifting sum of myriad individual decisions to seek gain and avoid loss in changing circumstances, and businesspeople and consumers alike are prisoners to its logic.

But Lindblom's point is larger; in time politicians too become captive to the market. Deliberate attempts to channel the market are often met with unanticipated and unpleasant results. When government regulates the market it often raises costs, and businesspeople have little choice but to respond by reflecting these high costs in higher prices or reduced output or by curtailing their work force. Politicians try to avoid this punishment by avoiding controlling the market, and policy itself thus becomes prisoner to the market.

The market is also a magnet, drawing to itself all activities and goods. It rewards not just those who offer goods and services at the lowest price but also those who successfully convert goods or services offered outside the market into market commodities. The pulling power of the market serves as a potent destabilizing force on communal and political institutions.

Today, the market is destabilizing justice and equality in health care and medicine generally, leading to commercialization or monetarization. Hospital chains, overspecialization, commercial blood banks, the marketing of hospital services—all are signs of the power of the market to undercut other spheres, drawing ever larger parts of the health care system into itself.

Most democratic societies use public power to counter the market's subverting force in the sphere of health care through some form of national health service or insurance. Common health care provision, combined with other entitlements of the welfare state, is treated as central to the strategy of democratic equality, creating a stable majority for the popular parties and deterring business from driving a wedge between the middle class and the poor.

But this has not happened in the United States, and in this chapter we consider why. Because the United States has passed over the strategy of common provision and its political and moral logic, it has set in place forces that are permanently altering not only the nature of medicine and health care but also the pattern of politics that frames our health policy. Although organized medicine, the absence of socialism, and other factors have played a major role in the unfolding story, an inadequate and simplistic account of equality is the major villain. The idea of equality in the United States—whether it is called equal opportunity or, in the case of health care, equal access or equity—is based on unstable political and ethical values like benevolence and altruism or charity, or (in the case of equal access) unrealistic expectations about the ability of the health care system to reorganize itself without a framework of centralized public policy. This chapter attempts to demonstrate that the current conception of "equity" or "equal access" for health care creates the conditions for abandoning equality as a hope for health care and for the absorption of medicine into the market system. It also shows how a republican theory of equality would create the political and moral conditions for sustaining and strengthening a just and equal health care system.

Equity Versus Republican Equality

Imagine two modern democratic societies with very different ways of providing medical care to their citizens. In Society A, with what might be called the equitable health care system, health care is provided by several different groups: the government, voluntary and nonprofit organizations, and profit-making businesses. There are national for-profit chains of hospitals as well as chains that are run by church and nonprofit organizations. All levels of government have a hand in delivering health care, principally to the poor and elderly.

Society A spends almost 11 percent of its gross national product (GNP) on medical care, and there is persistent medical inflation. The method of payment is a mixture of government, private, and not-for-profit insurance schemes. Despite Society A's marked pluralism, everyone in the society receives a decent and adequate level of health care; no one is turned away from a hospital for lack of funds. There are differences in the level and quality of care available to urban and rural residents, and there are discrepancies in medical care along class lines. The more affluent can and do purchase more medical care than the poor, and though the rich can assure themselves a place in the front of the line for the latest in medical technology, for the most part a decent level of modern medical care is provided to everyone alike.

Society B has a common health care system, perhaps patterned along the lines of the Health Insurance Fund discussed in Chapter One. Health care is organized and provided through governmental auspices, as part of a universal health insurance scheme. All citizens carry insurance cards entitling them to service anywhere. While the federal and state levels of government share responsibility for this system, citizens are entitled to medical care no matter where they reside, and all rightly see themselves as participating in a common and universal health system. Except for a few minor charges, all medicine is provided without direct expense to the patient. The government negotiates a fee schedule on a national basis, but physicians still retain the principal elements of a fee-for-service system. Hospitals prepare annual budgets each year, and capital expansion is funded by the government; the costs of the system are financed through a mixture of premiums, employer taxes, employee payroll taxes, and general state and federal taxes. As in Society A there are differences in the quality of health care for rural and urban people as well as differences in terms of class, but rough equality is achieved in medical care throughout society. Society B spends roughly 8 percent of its GNP on medical care; everyone, except for a few wealthy individuals who opt out of the system, receives roughly the same level of adequate medical care.

Now a question: Which of the two societies ought to be regarded as providing the more just level of health care? Does the fact that everyone in Society B receives a roughly equal and adequate level of care under a common system make that system more just?

Society A: Equity

Many commentators in the United States would argue, especially today, that neither system is more *just* than the other; if anything, the "pluralism" of Society A—the equitable health care system—makes it more just because it provides all with an adequate level of medical care "without . . . excessive burdens."[3] The fact that Society B provides health care through a common and public system would be considered more a matter of history and national tradition than of justice.

Even among philosophers, the distinction seems unimportant. Rawls sees no necessary connection between justice and the provision of public goods on the one hand and the public ownership of the means of production on the other.

A private-property economy may allocate a large fraction of national income to these purposes, a socialist society a small one, and vice versa. There are public goods of many kinds, ranging from military equipment to health services. Having agreed politically to allocate and to finance these items, the government may purchase them from the private sector or from publicly owned firms.[4]

Walzer makes much the same point.

> It might be argued . . . that the refusal thus far to
> finance a national health service constitutes a political
> decision by the American people about the level of
> communal care (and about the relative importance of
> other goods): a minimal standard for everyone . . . ; and
> free enterprise beyond that. That would seem to me to
> be an inadequate standard, but it would not necessarily
> be an unjust decision.[5]

In my view, Society A is rooted in the myth that we can
leave unchanged most of the features of our present system,
permitting the market to undercut communal institutions,
drawing medicine and even the politics of medicine into its
sphere, while piously hoping that, despite these defections,
we can mobilize the political will and benevolence to provide a decent and equitable level of care for the poor.

A good example is the President's Commission for the
Study of Ethical Problems in Medicine and Biomedical and
Behavioral Research, which in 1983 issued a report on
increasing access to medical services, *Securing Access to
Health Care*.[6] Charged with looking at the differing availability of medicine to various groups in the United States,
the commission completed the report at a time when universal health insurance had disappeared from the national
agenda.

Noting that in 1952 another presidential commission had
viewed access to medical services as a basic right for each
citizen,[7] the later presidential commission dismissed talk of
rights, preferring to use terms like "ethical obligations."
"Society has a moral obligation to ensure that everyone has
access to adequate health care without being subject to
excessive burdens."[8] Here we see justice divorced from the
political and institutional conditions that make justice
stable and self-sustaining. The commission made society,
not government, the source of our shared obligations to

36

ensure that everyone has access to adequate health care, preferring pluralism to government responsibility even though government bears the ultimate financial responsibility for providing health care.

As a goal for health care the commission urged "equity" over equality, which could lead to two evils.[9] Equality, the commission claimed, could require that everyone have the same very high level of medical care, providing to all every conceivable benefit, or providing to each the level of medical care that the most affluent could afford. Either standard would lead to astronomical increases in public spending. A second option, a common system, would provide everyone with roughly the same, and adequate, level of health care, but it would mean an unacceptable abuse of the liberty of those who might want and be able to spend more.

Although the commission embraced solidarity in the face of death as an abstract principle—"the depth of a society's concern about health care can be seen as a measure of its sense of solidarity in the face of suffering and death"[10]— the commission rejected the practical political solidarity achieved through universal health insurance without even declaring it an option.

The goal of republican equality is to make justice operative and stable through common and equal provision. This stability occurs at three levels: individual, institutional, and political. Justice in the equitable health care system consists of setting a decent minimum, below which no one is allowed to fall. But in a stable system of justice, one that is designed along the lines of the Health Insurance Fund outlined previously coexisting with the market, it is necessary not only to determine what level of care is adequate for all, but also how much of its resources the larger society ought to devote to medical care in the aggregate. Also, how the system can be protected against the power of the market to undermine it by enticing citizens or providers to undercut the just structure of common provision must be taken into account.

Justice and equality, properly conceived, imply not only a

pattern or state of affairs in a society but also a realistic chance for that state of affairs to exist and support itself over time in the face of the temptations of the market. Amy Gutmann is one of the few philosophers to make this point for health policy, arguing for a common, one-class system.[11] Rawls argues that theories of justice that ignore the issue of stability are seriously defective and claims that when we consider the stability of justice, we must consider whether a given pattern encourages a "strong and normally effective desire to act as the principles of justice require," and whether, at a number of levels, "the sense of justice that a [pattern] cultivates and the aims that it encourages . . . normally win out against propensities toward injustice."[12]

As Rawls notes, the stability of a scheme of justice rests on a foundation of motives; and in a democratic and capitalist society, these motives must show a balance between self-interest and cooperation and justice. The stability of a democratic society that gives considerable scope to the private market depends directly on whether there are realms in which the motives of community predominate, where citizens of capitalist societies experience institutions that take into account the good of the whole community.

Republican equality does not necessarily mean complete equality, such as equal incomes; it is rather a device for limiting money and the market to their proper spheres. T. H. Marshall addressed this point over thirty years ago:

> The extension of the social services is not primarily a means of equalizing incomes. In some cases it may, in others it may not. . . . What matters is that there is a general enrichment of the concrete substance of civilized life, a general reduction of risk and insecurity, an equalization between the more and the less fortunate at all levels—between the healthy and the sick, the employed and the unemployed, the old and the active. . . . Equalization is not so much between

classes as between individuals within a population which is now treated . . . as though it were one class.[13]

Most theories of distributive justice and health care first take up the question of what principle—desert, need, free exchange, and so forth—should guide health policy, and the implications that choice has for the reform of the health care system.

Among those who respond that health protection and health care are basic needs for all alike, Norman Daniels provides the best recent discussion of justice and health care,[14] and I can offer little improvement. Using a broadly Rawlsian approach, Daniels argues that in the full and equal distribution of primary goods (consisting of basic liberties, a range of opportunities, income, powers and prerogatives of office, etc.) there is a special place for health protections. Health and safety are central to the completion of everyone's plan of life, no matter what that plan might be; ill health constitutes a serious impediment to exploiting the existing range of opportunities for each individual. And because the needs for health and education, unlike other needs—food or shelter, for example—are unequally distributed in the population, health and education take special priority. What Daniels is arguing is that because of the unpredictable and unequal distribution of needs for education and health care and their centrality to the completion of life plans, these goods cannot be included in the budget that each citizen gets in his fair income account.

Daniels quotes John Rawls in arguing that a just health care system should be configured to best meet the needs of the citizenry, with "need" suggesting those conditions that, if prevented or treated, are likely to restore individuals to or maintain them at the status of " 'normal, active, and fully-cooperating members of society.' "[15]

While Daniels argues that his scheme would not neces-sarily be inconsistent with a multitiered scheme, he is clearly arguing for reorganizing medical care in a way that provides equal access to health care for all and against guaranteeing a decent minimum of health care and leaving the rest of the system to the vagaries of the market and consumer choices. Daniels's just health care system would look very different from our current system and would require major government intervention, though he has little to say about just how much government control would be needed, and why.

Society B: Republican Equality

In my view, the case for a common health care system rests squarely on the need for a stable equality or justice. Society B, with its common framework, is based on a much more robust and complex theory of equality than Daniels's system, one that takes into account the fragile nature of altruism in politics and markets' power to subvert and transform the nature of medicine and to make justice unstable. Justice, in my account, is based not only on considerations for what each citizen needs but also on considerations for what everyone needs together. The common system stabilizes the politics of equality, setting up an alternative source of attraction for citizens' loyalty beyond the market, forging an enduring majority of the middle and lower income groups, and strengthening the ties of a common justice and community.

Giving everyone roughly the same level of care based on their need makes all people aware that they are equals. The very obviousness of a common and shared equality is the political glue for equality and justice in health, making it more difficult to island the poor, commercialize medicine, or allow an uncontrolled and expensive medical technology to erode further the society's commitment to equality in health.

Republican equality in health care does not mean an

absolutely equal provision for each citizen no matter where he or she may reside—it means that equality in treatment is the ideal. A common system affords a democratic sovereignty over the health care system, and an ethical and political framework for continual democratic discussion about disparities in the allocation of health resources.

The pattern of "simple equality" in the equitable health system contains within it the very logic of its own subversion. The principle of equal opportunity undercuts the political principle of the solidarity of the majority for equality. That is, it encourages individuals to try to obtain more than just equal provision, offering individuals the chance to compete for the prizes of capitalism even in health care and to distance one's self from one's inferiors. As John Schaar puts it, "When it is understood that the principle of equal opportunity is in our time an expression of the competitive, capitalistic spirit, and not of the democratic spirit, then the boundaries of its applicability begin to emerge."[16]

Republican equality does not reject the principle of equal opportunity, it merely limits its range of application. Equal opportunity in our current form of democratic capitalism is a key principle of our common life, operative in more realms than the market. Yet at the same time, a robust and complex theory of equality would require, alongside the spheres governed by equal opportunity, other spheres where cooperation, shared dependency, and solidarity are the dominant logic. The logic of shared equality in those areas—such as common schooling, common military service, Social Security, and a common health care system—help to hold together a society in which equal opportunity exerts such a strong centrifugal force, threatening to isolate the most vulnerable from the rest of society. The late Olaf Palme put it this way a few years back: "Weak members of society are best protected not by being given special treatment but by being included in programs that extend to all members of society."[17] Democratic equality promotes popular solidarity, which becomes political muscle at the polls; and popular muscle at the polls is the foundation of the welfare state.

The Great Society Experiment

Egalitarians believe that equal opportunity or equity, by neglecting the destabilizing effects of the market on communal institutions, sows the seeds of injustice and drives a wedge between community and democratic sovereignty over medicine. But conservatives and an increasing number of American liberals argue that universal programs actually discriminate against the poor, because they spend money on the well-to-do who don't need it, money that could better be spent on the poor. To determine who is right we need not rely solely on abstract arguments by philosophers or the experience of other countries. We might examine our own recent experience, beginning in 1965 to determine whether simple equality is adequate as a scheme of justice.

In 1965, with the inception of Medicare and Medicaid, as well as other federal and state health programs, the United States embarked on something of a national experiment to test the political possibility of the equitable health care system (Society A), trying to ensure health care for all without universal health insurance. The result of this grand experiment has been that, in aggregate, the amount the nation spends on medical care has increased dramatically. In 1965 we spent 6 percent of the GNP on medical care; today we spend almost 11 percent of GNP—roughly $500 billion—annually for health care. Private and public insurance covers up to 85 or 90 percent of the population,[18] and the nation is far healthier than it was during the sixties: Heart disease and stroke rates are down by roughly one-third, and infant mortality rates have fallen sharply (though they are starting to rise again in some parts of the country). These gains are not all, or perhaps even mostly, due to increased spending on medicine, but some are.[19]

The poor have far better access to health care today than in 1965. In 1965 the poor were far less likely to receive hospital care than the middle class; today, many Medicaid patients receive more hospital care than the middle class (of course, they usually need more). Almost all of the elderly are covered by Medicare, and even though that coverage is far less than comprehensive, this is an impressive accomplishment.

Nevertheless, there are dramatic gaps in this picture. What seems at first a triumph for pluralism and for the equitable health care system turns out to be a patchwork.[20] Today, twenty years after the start of Medicare and Medicaid, at any given point in a year, 35 million Americans have no health insurance. Roughly 10 percent of the population has no insurance for the entire year, and another 10 percent of Americans will be uninsured for at least part of that year. These gaps in insurance are not evenly distributed in the population; beyond the poor generally, the uninsured tend to be found in far greater numbers in the South and the West, among blacks, and among the young.

For example, Medicaid covers roughly one-third of the poor and near poor.[21] The poor often do have other sources of insurance (none so good as Medicaid, however), but roughly 5 million have no insurance of any kind. Eighteen percent of persons under the age of sixty-five are without health insurance at least part of the year (only 2 percent of the aged are without Medicare).[22] Twenty-five percent of blacks under sixty-five are without health insurance at least part of the year. Twenty percent of individuals living in the South and West are without insurance at least part of the time, a rate double that of the Northeast and the North Central United States.

Lack of insurance is linked to dramatically lower utilization of medical care services, both for physician visits and for hospital care. The rates of hospital and ambulatory health care were measured in a 1977 national survey that was repeated over an eighteen-month period and is considered our most authoritative account. This survey was an improved version of surveys of earlier years. Uninsured blacks and other minorities have on average 1.5 physician visits per year, compared with 3.7 yearly visits for insured whites. (Insured blacks in the South average 2.5 visits.) The insured receive 90 percent more hospital care than the uninsured except in the South, where the insured receive three times more hospital care than the uninsured.[23]

More to the point, since 1977, the number of people who are poor or near poor has increased by 13.5 percent, and the number of uninsured has grown by 7 percent.[24] Medicaid funds have been sharply cut; Medicaid may now cover only 31 percent of the poor. Infant mortality rates have begun to rise again, especially in the South and in large cities. By contrast, the rate of charity care by private hospitals has not increased appreciably, and care at public hospitals has even declined in some areas, especially where they were suffering financial difficulties brought on by the recession of the early eighties and a heavy burden of nonpaying patients.

Conditions have been getting worse, not better, since the initial gains of the Great Society experiments. The average state eligibility thresholds used for determining Medicaid fell from 71 percent of the official poverty level in 1975 to 48 percent in 1986. That is, in 1986, as a national average, families who qualified for Medicaid were those whose incomes fell below 48 percent of the official poverty level. New York's eligibility level fell from 99 percent to 67 percent for the same period. California has abandoned "MediCal," its extensive medical care program for the medically indigent; however, it still maintains 80 percent coverage for those below the official poverty level.

The worsening condition of Medicaid is due to many factors. The states have not raised their Aid to Families with Dependent Children (AFDC) poverty levels to reflect the impact of inflation over the years. Also, the federal government in 1981 made major changes when the Reagan administration and Congress cut taxes and spending across the board with the 1981 Omnibus Budget and Reconciliation Act.

This act reduced the federal government's share of the costs of the Medicaid program and limited the ability of poor or indigent people to deduct expenses from their annual incomes, thus making fewer people eligible for coverage. The budget cuts of 1981 resulted in federal Medicaid cuts of roughly $1 billion, and as many as 700,000 children lost Medicaid coverage. In the 1981 legislation, the federal government also permitted the states to abandon the principle of allowing the Medicaid patients to seek medical care anywhere they might be accepted. The states, if they choose, can require Medicaid patients to patronize "preferred providers," thus abandoning the principle of statewide coverage that was an original cornerstone of the Medicaid program.

Recently, with the sixth Omnibus Budget and Reconciliation Act of 1986, Congress permitted the states to "decouple" Medicaid and welfare assistance eligibility. This means that states can expand their coverage for children under five, pregnant women, and elderly and disabled persons with income below the poverty level, regardless of state levels for receiving welfare assistance. Later legislation extended Medicaid to the homeless and others not receiving welfare assistance. A number of states are beginning to expand their coverage for several groups, especially children and pregnant women and the disabled elderly. But before we conclude that we are entering a new era of state responsibility for the health care of the poor, we should recall that the state and local share of total spending for health care has remained at roughly 12 percent since 1950, dipping to lower levels in the early eighties with the recession and the 1981 Budget Act. What we are probably seeing is a return to the spending levels prior to 1981, with spending expanding for groups perceived to be more deserving, like women, children, and the elderly. Congress originally intended Medicaid to provide comprehensive coverage for all the nation's poor;

indeed, the states in the original legislation were required to move toward this goal. But Congress first delayed this requirement in 1969 and finally removed it in 1972.[25]

The growing competition, cost control, and commercialization of the health industry will make the problem of medicine for the poor worse in the future, not better. There is a growing shortage of paying patients; hospital censuses are down, and the pressure is on to fill the empty beds with paying patients and to eliminate those without funds. And the data here do not even begin to address the issue of the difference in quality of care the poor or the uninsured receive, especially in the shrinking number of crowded, understaffed public hospitals, or in the rural South. Nor does it reveal the increasing pressures on Medicaid for financing long-term care, the unwillingness of the Reagan administration to increase the federal role in Medicaid, and the incapacity of many states to increase their fiscal contributions to Medicaid substantially. The prospects for the poor are bleak indeed.

The data provide stark evidence that the United States has failed to provide a stable and equitable regard for the poor and the most vulnerable in our society. The poor have not achieved parity with the middle class in a pluralistic system; indeed, they have lost some of the ground they gained during the seventies. Many observers note that we are moving toward a permanently dual system of health care, one that creates two classes of citizenship.

Acknowledging the real gains of the Great Society should not prevent us from facing its central failure: The Great Society did not create the political conditions for a stable justice or equality. Providing medical care on a shared basis is a principal way in which democratic societies have shown their members that they are fundamentally more equal than unequal. The communal and solidaristic motive is fundamental to every political group, as Michael Walzer has argued:

Membership [in the democratic community] is important because of what the members of a political community owe to one another and to no one else, or to no one else in the same degree. And the first thing they owe is the communal provision of security and welfare. This claim might be reversed: communal provision is important because it teaches us the value of membership. If we did not provide for one another, if we recognized no distinction between members and strangers, we would have no reason to form and maintain political communities. "How shall men love their country," Rousseau asked, "if it is nothing more for them than for strangers, and bestows on them only that which it can refuse to none?" . . . Political community for the sake of provision, provision for the sake of community: the process works both ways, and that is perhaps its crucial feature.[26]

As medicine moves deeper into the stronghold of the market, justice for the poor and the vulnerable will be increasingly unstable, and the politics of a democratic majority moving to a common health care system may be permanently undermined. The health care system, far from serving as a symbol of shared equality, is rapidly becoming a symbol of inequality.

Destabilizing Majoritarian Politics

Republican equality is a strategy for making a shared equality stable in political institutions and in policies that offset the attractions of the market. The Democratic party is the logical party in the present period to pursue republican equality, and while at times it has moved in this direction, the post–World War II period has seen the party move more toward equality of opportunity and a market-dominated political pluralism. This strategy, while it has brought many short-term gains for the American people, is driving health policy and politics itself farther into the market and diminishing the prospects for justice.

In pluralist politics, organized groups and individual politicians compete for political support in a political marketplace, and many people assume that the " 'normal' American political process [is] one in which there is a high probability that an active and legitimate group in the population can make itself heard effectively at some crucial stage in the process of decision."[27]

But the American political system, with its loosely organized, decentralized parties and legislatures—made more so by social policies that weaken party structures and drive a wedge between the middle class and the poor—creates strong inducements for incumbents to defect from a majoritarian strategy and instead to maximize their personal electoral fortunes by promoting the good of their constituencies and those organized groups their legislative position can best help.

The Democratic party made some moves toward a more robust equality during the New Deal with the Work Projects Administration (WPA), Social Security, the beginnings of economic planning, and plans for future universal health insurance. But deep divisions within the party itself (especially separating Southern Democrats) and the opposition of organized medicine kept universal health insurance off Roosevelt's agenda.[28]

After World War II, President Truman was unsure about moving the Democratic party toward more emphasis on equality and majoritarian politics. Such a shift would mean exercising stronger controls over markets, providing basic securities in housing, education, health care, and the like as a way of expanding and solidifying the base of the Democratic party among the middle class and the poor. Truman did fight for universal health insurance, but he backed away from fundamental reforms in areas such as housing and education.

Instead, the country evolved a new style of politics: political pluralism, or the politics of distributing government's benefits to organized groups or interests. American parties have never functioned along the lines of European parties working within the context of parliamentary government. But American parties, and particularly the Democratic party in this century, could have evolved a strategy of interfering with the market to forge a welfare state with universal programs that would have won the loyalty of an enduring popular majority. In other words, the Democratic party could have expanded on Social Security and adopted policies that centralized and unified the party as a national institution, helping to counter the decentralizing and destabilizing effects of federalism on the welfare state and the party system. As Paul Starr notes, at the very moment that the Democratic party was rejecting Truman's entreaties for universal health insurance, it was strengthening and expanding Social Security.[29]

Instead of policies to strengthen the welfare state as a set of national policies, policies that would in turn help to make the parties themselves more national in character, what evolved was a form of politics that, like equality of opportunity, tried to marry distributive justice and the spirit of market competition. In this case it produced a competition of the legislative incumbents within the Democratic party for the support of organized interest groups. The result was a social policy that promised equity for the poor and a minimal interference with the dynamics of the market, using government programs to buy support from organized interest groups or "constituencies." Pluralism, like equality of opportunity, sacrifices the long-term goals of parties for an enduring popular majority for short-term success in building a coalition of organized interest groups.[30]

Housing offers an excellent example of the pluralist strategy tempting public officials to abandon the majority and mollify producer groups.[31] New Deal planners understood that the nation's housing shortage could be met only if the Democratic party prevailed over the powerful construction and real estate lobby. Facing severe housing shortages, the country needed an affirmative federal housing policy of slum clearance and the replacement of slum housing with adequate low-cost housing and price controls. The real estate lobby tagged this approach "European socialism" and the vanguard of communism. Southern Democratic leaders in Congress feared that blacks and poor whites would be prime beneficiaries of these policies, threatening local coalitions that were protective of their political incumbency. The result was not a national strategy but urban renewal, which destroyed slum housing without replacement; minimal and limited public housing for the poor; income tax subsidies for the housing industry and the middle class (only increasing the pull of the middle class to the suburbs); the abandonment of cities; and a vast overexpansion of privately owned homes. Today, housing costs rise endlessly, public housing is a scandal, housing policy for the poor has virtually disappeared, and millions of young Americans seem doomed never to own their own homes—unless they are located in a trailer park.

In the health field, the pattern of political pluralism began to take shape after World War II, as government gave tax breaks for individual and corporate contributions to private health insurance premiums.[32] Instead of universal health insurance, the Democratic party in Congress (in opposition to President Truman) moved to support the Hill–Burton program for hospital construction, to expand the Veterans Administration hospitals, and—during the fifties—to increase sharply the scope of the National Institutes of Health. Some of these moves, like the Hill–Burton program, were explicit strategies by the American Hospital Association, supported by the American Medical Association, to head off universal health insurance.[33]

The centerpiece of the pluralist strategy for expanding the

health care system, the private insurance system, shows how the market diminishes justice. The Blue Cross plans began in the thirties as a community-rated insurance scheme, offering the same premiums to the old and the young, the healthy and the unhealthy. But after World War II, competition from private health insurance schemes, which underwrote the plans for a younger and healthier blue-collar work force, caused the Blue Cross plans to abandon community rating schemes gradually.

Thus, the basic pattern emerged: the market looking for those who least need protection, destabilizing community organizations like the early Blue Cross plans that shared risks, leaving government responsible for those who most need protection. Medicare and Medicaid were developed during the sixties to provide insurance for those people left after the young, healthy, and employed sectors had abandoned them for cheaper rates. Special programs for those at very high risk, such as those with kidney disease, add yet another tier to our insurance system. The problem for government is that it must constantly follow the search of the market for the profitable risk, because, as one commentator says, "it is the ordinary and rational insurance practice to eliminate wherever possible from coverage the highest utilizers of care, that is, ironically, those who most need care."[34]

Medicare was a pivotal program in the pluralist strategy for health care. Originally seen as the opening wedge for universal health insurance, the program actually became a vehicle for appeasing the major organized interests in health. As Judith Feder argues, Medicare planners rejected a strategy of controlling costs and instead opted for "political balance," a term whose plain meaning came to be capitulating to the terms of the hospitals and physicians.[35] Doctors and hospitals were given extremely favorable reimbursement formulas, and hospitals were allowed generous write-offs for capital expenses and depreciation. The result was a sharp increase in what Wildavsky calls "medical money," which led to inflation in medical costs, increased incentives for medical specialization, overbedding in hospitals, and an extremely unwise increase in the number of physicians, producing not only an end to a putative doctor shortage but a new doctor surplus.

All told, the spate of Great Society health programs gave us redistribution without reorganization, to use Starr's terms. Hospitals and doctors got rich off Medicare, while the elderly today bear roughly the same out-of-pocket health care costs as before the passage of the bill. And as we have seen, Medicaid covers only a fraction of America's poor and near poor.

Even today, when we reflect on the situation, many still grasp the wrong point about the limits to Medicare. For example, one participant had this to say about Medicare as a political strategy to promote universal health insurance:

> If you stop and think about this, it was a crazy way to go about it, from a rational point of view. Here we took the one group in the population, the elderly, that was the *most* expensive, needed the *most* health care, for whom medical care would do the *least* amount of good, for whom there was the *least* payoff from a societal point of view. But we did it because that's politically what we could run with at the time. It didn't make rational sense to start a health insurance scheme with this sector of the population, but it's where we started anyway.[36]

But what caused the failure of Medicare is not that we started with the wrong (i.e., the most expensive) group; this belief is market logic applied to politics. The problem was that we thought we could start with only part of the population, leaving the market's undercutting influence on health care largely undisturbed, and unhurriedly move to increasingly larger segments of the population. No such incremental strategy for defending against the power of the market has yet been successful.

The Democrats' failure to pursue universal health insurance after nearly achieving their goal in 1974 is explained not just by the bad luck of Watergate and a worsening economic picture but also by the accelerating decline of interest among Democratic incumbents in pursuing a majoritarian strategy. This decline was hastened by the growing role of money and television in elections; both forced incumbent Democrats to placate business interests while merely giving lip service to equality as a political principle.

As Edsall documents, after Watergate, and as part of the growing monetarization of politics, congressional Democrats stressed the procedural rather than the substantive,[37] the presidential nominating process was democratized, campaign finance laws were reformed, and the power of seniority in Congress was loosened. Many of these reforms were undertaken for good reasons, but the result was a weakening of incentives for broad policies that forge a permanent majority for equality; the reforms also exposed the political process more and more to the influences of television and money, strengthening the position of business in national politics. Business cannot win in politics unless it can split the majority that normally favors equality, convincing the middle class that public programs benefit only the poor and that their future, like that of the wealthy, is made more secure by a rejuvenated market only loosely restricted by government.

Watergate only made matters worse, encouraging the Democrats to abandon social policy and focus on further procedural reforms. As Edsall has noted in his brilliant analysis of the politics of the seventies, Watergate also led to the election of new Democratic members from formerly Republican districts, but this brought in Democrats who represented suburban, upper-middle class districts with little interest in major new programs that might regain voter support among the middle and lower classes and that might expand the Democratic majority.[38] Meanwhile, as the Democrats more and more openly abandoned their interest in broad-gauged policies, voting rates declined precipitously, especially among the lower classes, where support for the Democratic party is typically higher. (As Edsall records, voting rates among blue-collar workers fell from 59 percent in 1968 to 44 percent in 1980; the differential between voting rates of blue- and white-collar workers grew from 24 percent in 1968 to 33 percent in 1980.)

The Carter administration reflected these growing contradictions within the Democratic party. Carter promised universal health insurance but gave greater attention to welfare reform. In time, hospital cost control became the dominant policy initiative; this was a gamble, and Carter lost. The 1980 Democratic platform hardly mentioned universal health insurance. The 1984 platform ignored it entirely; Walter Mondale effectively cut the Democratic party off from the New Deal tradition of spending to benefit middle-class and poor citizens together.

We are accustomed to thinking of politics as producing policies. But policies also produce their forms of politics, and a generation of pluralist policies has made the national Democratic party hostage to the short-run interests of Democratic incumbents.[39] Paradoxically, the decision of the Democrats to abandon majoritarian and egalitarian reforms has left them saddled with the responsibility of defending programs in the "second tier" of the welfare state, programs like AFDC. The fact that the Democratic party has, in recent years, accurately been labeled the party of minority groups and the poor indicates how narrow a strategy becomes that uncouples programs for the middle class and programs for the poor.

Commercialization and Instability

The rapid commercialization pulling medicine deeper into the market not only threatens the very character of medicine itself but represents another force undercutting the hopes for a democratic majority for equality. Medicine and the American hospital, rather than serving as symbols of equal citizenship in a republic, are being transformed into institutions for increasing inequality. Pluralist politics can be blamed for fostering this monetarization of medicine; but our failure to adopt universal health insurance itself intensified a pluralist politics of health.

Arthur Okun argued in the seventies that while markets have their place, they must be kept in their place.[40] (This could easily be the central slogan of republican equality.) Yet leading Democratic theorists have in recent years argued almost the opposite. For example, Charles L. Schultze, an economist and Democratic official in the Johnson and Carter administrations, in the seventies advocated the use of the market to "reduce the need for compassion, patriotism, brotherly love, and cultural solidarity."[41] But it is one thing to use taxes and other incentives for health; it is quite another to unleash market forces that convert nonprofit and communal institutions into competitive economic units and nonmarket goods into commodities. The principal threat is from the "commodity bias" found in the marketplace.[42]

Schultze notes that one of the most noteworthy features of markets is their tendency to "let the devil take the hindmost."[43] But this is precisely why markets are powerfully destabilizing to communal and governmental policies for justice and equality. Markets have their enormous vitality precisely because market competition abandons the "economically unattractive" participant. In health care, this translates into abandonment of the poor patient, the AIDS victim, or the elderly person with Alzheimer's disease. This ruthless drive for profits promotes economic efficiency in business but chaos in community and public institutions.

Thus, from the standpoint of market theory, the logical outgrowths of commercialization are such private market practices as "unbundling" (breaking up services and technology into smaller packages for more aggressive promotion and sales); advertising; skimming (trying to attract that patient who is most profitable); demarketing (trying to drive off the economically unattractive patient or unprofitable service); vertical integration (trying to tie together hospitals, physicians, suppliers, and the like to achieve economies of scale); and national chains. All are simply the result of a healthy and beneficial market competition for new commodity forms, or so the theory goes.

Markets in capitalist societies grow not only upward, through increased productivity, but also outward, capturing nonmarket institutions and practices and converting them into new fields for market competition.[44] Commercialization is one of the principal forces of capitalism. The market tends to engulf and privatize the realm of community and equality, converting goods such as medicine, sex, blood, body organs, and public lands into commodities and transforming communal institutions such as public schools, organized athletics, universities, hospitals, airlines, public utilities, public radio and television, and prisons into fields for more intensive economic competition and even new commodity forms.

Eli Ginzberg argues that monetarization has been occurring for a long time in health care, citing as evidence the decline of the role of philanthropy in financing health care after World War II.[45] Before that time interns, for example, were required to live in the hospital where they were training, were not permitted to marry, and were often not paid more than room and board. Care for the poor and capital construction were the work of charity. Since that time, with the introduction of private health insurance on a wide basis, the growth of real income in medicine, and the growing expansion of federal financing in the health field for capital construction and ultimately for services, health care has increasingly followed the dynamics of the money economy.

Thus, by ignoring universal health insurance, we left medicine more exposed to the money economy, and the governmental programs we adopted only accelerated market penetration. Specialization, for example, has developed in the United States to a degree not found anywhere else in modern medicine. While there are many reasons for American specialization, including public policy incentives, one of the major reasons is that specialization pays.[46] To specialize is to make more money, and making more money brings more specialization in its wake.

Another way markets encourage inequality is through social scarcity.[47] Socially scarce goods are goods that are made more valuable through some real or artificial crowding or increased use: The classic example is the status race for a house on the beach, which leads to high prices for beach property and its increasing rarity. Social scarcity in medicine occurs through the creation of tiers in medical care; highly exclusive and expensive settings for "gourmet" medicine, a standard and reliable form of "fast-food" medicine for the middle classes, and the government-issue basic diet of beans and rice for the poor. While the early forms of the new medical scarcity might bring more innocent forms of status competition in the settings for medical care, we can ultimately expect medical standards to decline if the market forces of competition are allowed full sway.

Markets also encourage social scarcity in the form of planned obsolescence. One of the main features of competition in the consumer goods industry is product redesign and change; producers constantly upgrade their product lines with the new and improved versions. As hospital and physician services are turned into commodities, the hospital will gradually change from the workplace of physicians into the product itself, and hospital owners will feel constant pressures to upgrade and change the product and its packaging.

This is already happening. Donald R. Cohodes notes that the expected life of hospitals has shortened considerably in recent years.

New technologies and medical breakthroughs have accelerated the demands of consumers for new services and treatments. These pressures are accompanied by the expectation that the latest facilities and equipment will be available for the consumer and the newly trained physician. As a partial result of these rising expectations, the perceived useful life of the physical assets of a hospital has shortened considerably. For accounting purposes, twenty-five years has frequently been considered the useful life of hospital plant, and seven years for equipment. Now it seems that rising expectations unrelated to useful life have lowered these figures to fifteen years for plant and four to five years for equipment.[48]

As Cohodes notes further, these rising expectations lead to greater demands for capital and increased competition among hospitals, which in turn intensifies the original pressures for plant modernization.[49]

Monetarization and commercialization create major pressures to push the poor out of mainstream medicine, abandoning them to the ghettos of public medicine. Hospitals competing for an increased market share are also anxious to "demarket" losing "product lines"—namely the poor patient. Several years ago, an official of the American Hospital Association, speaking to the American Health Planning Association, outlined stratagems for "demarketing" the emergency room service, which has been a source of many poor patients without insurance for many hospitals.[50] The official spoke of closing or reorganizing the emergency room (by such options as making the chairs less comfortable, making the lighting poor, taking out the candy machines) as one way hospitals could throw back the "too-small fish"—to use Brecht's term—limiting demand for service from people "considered relatively unprofitable in themselves or undesirable in terms of their effect on other valued segments of the market."[51]

Destructive competition is already changing the very face of hospitals. To maintain their financial position with a declining bed census, hospitals now make space for physicians' offices, pharmacies, long-term care facilities, substance abuse treatment centers, laboratories, fitness centers, freestanding emergency centers, and so forth. Hospitals are even seeking to expand beyond their walls, competing with other economic units in their local areas, such as parking facilities, gasoline stations, office buildings, hotels and motels, laundries, nursing homes, and apartments.

The latest entrants into this "medical arms race" are the new corporations in health—corporations building chains of hospitals, nursing homes, and even private practices. Chains now control roughly one-third of all hospital beds, with the for-profit industry holding one-tenth of all hospital beds.[52] The chains are still in the minority, but their influence may be far greater than their size because they are intensifying the pressures for harmful and wasteful competition while legitimating the unraveling of a social compact for medicine and health.

A recent report of the Institute of Medicine (an arm of the National Academy of Sciences), *For-Profit Enterprise in Health Care*,[53] expressed only mild concern over the growth of for-profit units in health care, despite the evidence that for-profit hospitals usually charge their patients more, treat fewer poor patients and others who cannot pay, and are slightly less efficient. Although the committee report stated that "we would have little to gain, and possibly much to lose, if for-profit corporations came to dominate our health care system,"[54] the committee still found no grounds to oppose or support the existence of for-profit organizations, at least at its present level in the United States. (The report includes a one-page supplementary statement by a minority of the committee, which sought to put more stress on the failings of for-profit chains and the dangers that this growth posed in a spreading commercialism and in exercising political influence against the social ends of medical care.)[55]

The authors of the report are right not to single out the for-profit corporations as the principal source of danger to health care. The rise of the for-profit companies and the spreading commercialization of health care are the price we pay for a decades-long refusal to undertake universal health insurance.

The principal weakness of the report is that it fails even to consider the possibility that the absence of universal health insurance is the cause of the spreading commercialization. One obvious reason for this is that the report reflects a distinctive industry bias. The chairperson was Walter McNerny, who served as head of Blue Cross–Blue Shield for many years; the committee included many other individuals, including members of the for-profit industry. Perhaps such a committee should not be expected to identify the failure to provide universal health insurance as the basic source of problems in the health care field, for this sort of analysis would take them far from the realm of economics or medical ethics and into the larger fields of equality and political philosophy.

The absence of a national health plan for health care is leading to rapid vertical and horizontal concentration in hospitals. The major changes are occurring at the vertical level—integration of hospitals into nationwide or regional chains—to provide hospitals with better access to capital and better managers and personnel, including physicians. The rationale is that large-scale operations should lead, at least in theory, to economies of scale and lower costs.

The evidence does not support this thesis. Several studies suggest that costs for the for-profit hospitals are in actuality higher.[56] This was also the conclusion of the Institute of Medicine report mentioned previously.[57] No studies suggest that the for-profit hospitals have substantially reduced the costs of treatment, which presumably would be their principal advantage. And as David Starkweather argues, the chains (not-for-profit and for-profit alike) actually make local coordination and planning much more difficult.[58]

The commercialization controversy was predicted many years ago, in the minority dissent to the report published by the Committee on the Costs of Medical Care (CCMC) in 1932.[59] The committee was assembled with the support of private foundations in 1927 and produced a series of reports, ending with the very influential *Medical Care for the American People* in 1932. The committee did not recommend a system of government-financed compulsory health insurance and took pains to put some distance between its own recommendations and what it called "state medicine." The committee stressed instead reforming the organization and structure of medicine with something like what came to be known as group practice.[60]

But the dissent to the final report by the economist Walton Hamilton was a prophetic commentary on the current state of the commercializing health field. Hamilton noted that in the early days of medicine there was a strong ethical bond between the patient and the physician: "The desertion [by a patient] to a fellow practitioner demanded an explanation." While money was paid for services rendered, the "ethics of the profession kept medicine rather free of commercialism."[61]

But physicians practice in an impersonal industrial civilization dominated by business, and business ideals have transformed medicine.

Doctors like others, must maintain standards of living, give opportunities to their children, and provide security for an old age. They must have money incomes, and incomes are to be had by securing and holding patients in rivalry with their fellows. . . . The result is that the pressure from the system within which [physicians] must live and work is slowly and insidiously, but rather surely, bringing to the physician a consciousness of his own pecuniary interests, making something more of a business man out of him, and converting the thing once called "private practice" into a system of individual business competition.[62]

Hamilton goes on to note that the ideal of personal choice is hardly operative in the medical world, where the consumer is not always the best judge of what is needed. In addition, the physician is forced to adapt his or her professionalism to the world of commercial struggle. The result is to make both physician and patient worse off.

Here is the heart of the problem of the organization of medicine. A profession has, quite by an historical accident which was not foreseen, fallen into a world of business and is making the adaptation which seems necessary to survival. . . . As a result the older order of "private practice" is being transformed into a system of competitive enterprise, which no one has consciously willed and which in insidious ways interferes with the great social task which medicine is to perform.[63]

Hamilton argued that only by sacrificing business enterprise can the public function of medicine be maintained. The development of a continental economy and division of labor has

bound the fortunes of each of us with the operation of an intricate industrial system and has made us inseparably "members one of another." This interdependence has made the maintenance of the "common health" a public necessity as well as a social duty. If we are to make the most of our human resources, for work and for life, it is necessary that our facilities for health shall be just as available for all who need them as are the schools and the churches.[64]

Are We Slouching Toward Universal Health Insurance?

While universal health insurance has all but vanished from the political agenda, it may well reappear. Some argue that the catastrophe of AIDS, with the tremendous strain that the probable hundreds of thousands of cases will place on the American health care system, may finally usher in universal health insurance. James Morone and Andrew Dunham offer a very interesting and provocative argument that cost-control efforts may bring universal health insurance to the American people, and that perhaps in the not-distant future.[65]

Morone and Dunham surveyed the cost-control history of the State of New Jersey. They note that, in the early seventies, when the state finally began to use its legislative authority to regulate Blue Cross rates and Medicaid reimbursement rates, "the results were widely compared to squeezing one end of a balloon—the air merely rushes to the other end."[66] The more the state clamped down on Blue Cross, the more hospitals shifted their costs to other, usually private, insurers. Five years after the program was implemented, private insurers were paying 30 percent more than Blue Cross.[67] And, as the authors note, urban hospitals were in a squeeze because they treated a "disproportionate number of patients who had Blue Cross and Medicaid, which paid less than commercial insurers. . . . Many other patients [who had no health insurance] paid nothing or only part of their bills."[68]

The authors noted that "this unstable policy environment, marked by large, attentive, well-organized, interdependent interests calling for action while checking one another, presented an opportunity for government entrepreneurs to restructure the hospital system."[69] The state shifted its rate setting to all (third-party) payers and implemented the now well-known Diagnostic-Related Groups (DRGs) system. The DRG system is based on fixed prices for more than four hundred diagnostic categories, paying efficient hospitals the full rate, even if they provide the service more cheaply, and penalizing inefficient hospitals for exceeding average prices.

Despite hospital opposition, the system was implemented, comprising one other important feature: The state provided, within the rates set for the DRGs, enough to compensate for the "uncompensated care" that the large, urban hospitals especially were experiencing.

The DRG system was adopted for the federal Medicare program in 1982, and Morone and Dunham argue that it will become the destabilizing force that brings about universal health insurance, or what the authors call "a government-centered hospital system providing universal coverage."[70]

The key to the authors' argument is that when we fix the prices for part of the system, we destabilize the rest of the system, producing insolvent urban hospitals, large-scale cost shifting, and unacceptable inflation in medical prices. Government will have to step in, as it did in New Jersey, and establish an all-payers (all third-party insurers) system with rates incorporating a subsidy for those urban hospitals that have a high mix of patients without insurance. As Morone and Dunham note,

In contrast to most quick solutions offered amidst cost crises, an all-payer DRG system which factors in the cost of uncompensated care combines an effort to reduce inflation with assistance to institutions that serve the poor. . . . For the first time, hospitals throughout the United States would be paid equally for all patients, regardless of wealth or insurance. For the poor, unsponsored patients and hospitals that treat them the provision would roughly approximate a universal national health insurance.[71]

To the authors, the appealing part of this scenario is that DRGs have been applauded as a device fostering competition; the new all-payers DRG system would not require major new funds, it would not be sold as a "big welfare proposal," and it would not require, as would the procompetition proposals of a few years back, major structural and organizational reforms of the health care system. The all-payers system would be an incremental step that ushered in nonincremental, large-scale change.[72]

Morone and Dunham ignore many objections to their prognosis. For example, the all-payers DRG system would put tremendous new pressures on government payers to cover the costs of uncompensated care, and state and local governments would be particularly hard hit. If the new system is to be a truly universal system, it is likely that Medicaid would have to be federalized, and this would represent a major shift toward the federal government.

Further, hiding the costs of treating the poor in the rates paid for each procedure might help to disguise what is going on, but government would still have to raise the revenues to help pay the bills for the poor and the uninsured if the rates for Blue Cross and Blue Shield and the private companies are to be kept from going through the roof.

The issue is whether the government will meet its responsibilities to the poor and others in a sufficiently just way. Federalizing Medicaid is only the beginning: there are the unemployed, the young, and those who live at or near the poverty line—all would sooner or later have to be incorporated into a uniform rate. The problem of what to do about physician visits is left out, creating incentives to overutilize the hospital, a problem that could be corrected by bringing physicians into the scheme.

It also seems at least plausible that the new all-payers

system would leave untouched the competition for the proper mix of profitable patients and diseases, especially by for-profit organizations. And there would still be competition and rivalry for the more attractive patients, leading to a two-tier system.

Perhaps the authors are correct that establishing an all-payers system would, at least for the long term, be a more stabilized system and create incentives for elected officials to move, if haltingly, toward a uniform, universal insurance scheme without, at least at first, a drastic new method of payment. But it would seem, at least to me, that we will not solve these problems by political sleight-of-hand. It is most likely that we will need to face frankly the need for an explicit policy and framework for the entire system, one, like the Health Insurance Fund, that includes doctors and hospitals and that addresses the needs of the republic as a whole. In such a system, the emphasis would shift from price controls to budgets and planning.

The most worrisome aspect of the Morone and Dunham scenario is their belief that, largely as a result of the work of policy analysts and economic advisors, we might stumble into universal health insurance without some rather fundamental political controversy and struggle. Politics is more than sound policy analysis or rigging a struggle between groups so that the public good is some happy accident. Politics is the public debate between the parties and interested groups about the good for society as a whole, a democratic conflict whose central virtue is publicity, disagreement, and a wide public awareness of the burdens and benefits of alternative schemes.

The central goal of universal health insurance is the stability of equality in health care and in the body politic generally. The plain reason Republicans have vigorously opposed universal health insurance is because of the fear that another major entitlement program would secure a permanent majority for the party of its opponents. And the Democratic party—the one that stands to benefit the most—has abandoned universal health insurance largely because the party has become a loose coalition of officeholders with ties to specific groups rather than to a permanent majority. Universal health insurance will come when the party that wants to use the strategy of equality to increase its hold on the democratic electorate decides to fight for it.

Many people find it hard to understand why the United States has for so long resisted a reform that most societies consider a matter of common decency. But this resistance surely cannot be blamed on the ordinary citizen; Americans are probably no more mean spirited than Europeans. The problem is that our ideas about equality are not complete; we wish to provide a welfare state without the inconvenience of limiting the market. We will have to decide soon, perhaps for all time, whether we want a just health care system or market institutions that spread to every corner of American life. Our choice will have profound consequences for health care, for equality, and for the American republic.

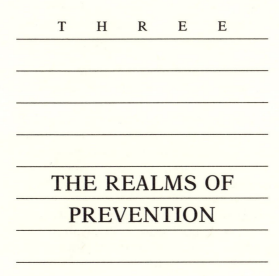

T H R E E

THE REALMS OF
PREVENTION

Ronald Bayer, in an important article on the AIDS epidemic, has this to say about the tension between public health and individual liberties:

> At the most fundamental level, the ethos of public health takes the well-being of the community as its highest good, and in the face of uncertainty, especially where the risks are high, would limit freedom or restrict, to the extent possible, the realm of privacy in order to prevent morbidity from taking its toll. . . . From the point of view of civil liberties the situation is quite the reverse. . . . [S]ince the freedom of the individual is viewed as the highest good of a liberal society, . . . measures designed to restrict personal freedom

must be justified by a strong showing that no other path exists to protect the public health. . . . These two great abstractions, liberty and communal welfare, are always in a state of tension in the realm of public health policy.[1]

While there is truth in what Bayer says, it is a truth limited to a single sphere of public health, and even there to a relatively small range of cases.

For example, in the last chapter I argued that equality in health provision is undercut by the competitiveness of the market. A common health care system, while limiting liberty, does so *primarily* to provide for a stable and more robust equality for everyone alike, not to promote the communal welfare.

In this chapter I consider the shift of the major responsibility for preventing disease and disability in the work place, the marketplace, and on the highways to the federal government during the Great Society. In that era, agencies like the Environmental Protection Agency (EPA), the Occupational Safety and Health Administration (OSHA), the Consumer Product Safety Commission (CPSC), and the National Highway Traffic Safety Administration (NHTSA) were created in only a ten-year interval.[2]

The primary goal of this shift was not to strengthen the communal welfare at the expense of civil liberties but to limit property rights (particularly of giant corporations) and bar unsafe or dangerous products or damages to the environment.

The regulatory successes of the Great Society ultimately led to policies like motorcycle helmet legislation, demands for higher cigarette and alcohol taxes, and seat belt laws, all of which limit personal liberties, and here Bayer is correct: the common good is valued over personal liberty. In this sphere, the language of prevention is based on a basic, rather than absolute, autonomy. But this is not the only realm of prevention in public health. In addition to the new health and safety agencies, there were other victories for public health and prevention during the Great Society that *expanded* the liberties of citizens.

In later chapters I consider in more detail the conflicts that emerged during the Great Society and earlier around the issues of birth control and abortion, conflicts that deeply affected unwanted pregnancies and the health of mothers and children. The victories of the groups fighting for birth control and abortion rights resulted in the establishment of family planning services in the federal antipoverty programs and foreign aid programs, in the repeal of the federal Comstock legislation that declared advertisement of contraceptives and abortion services "obscene," in the encouragement of a wider market for contraceptive devices, and in the series of Supreme Court decisions that established a right to privacy and limited the right of state legislatures to interfere with these activities.[3]

The struggle for birth control and abortion rights was conducted in the face of opposition by powerful religious groups; the result was the establishment of a sphere of sexual privacy in which all citizens might be free to make intimate decisions regarding themselves. In the private sphere, the language of prevention *is* absolute autonomy or liberty.

Similarly, during the Great Society period more than at any other time, the common health became the focal point of an expanded democratic discussion (the leading examples of which are automobile safety, pollution, smoking, and the labeling and advertising of cigarettes on television). This publicity helped initiate major changes in the health habits of the nation and helped put public health issues on the national agenda permanently. Here we discover another realm of prevention and public health: democratic discussion and deliberation, a realm where civil liberties are expanded, not diminished. Indeed, the case for an expanded democratic discussion rests on the fundamental right of every citizen to free speech and the common interest of all in promoting a vigorous self-government.[4]

Thus, the language of prevention and public health policy is complex, ranging across differing spheres, each containing somewhat differing conceptions of individual autonomy and individual and communal interests. Indeed, I argue in Chapters Five and Seven that in the AIDS epidemic, as with other health problems, the emphases in health policy on the role of education as democratic discussion unhampered by a narrow and often religious moralism, on laws limiting discrimination against at-risk groups, and on a more open and free discussion about safe and unsafe sex practices play an equally important role in fighting modern public health problems as regulations that limit personal liberty.

The Rise of the New Public Health

In this chapter I want to focus chiefly on a central sphere of prevention: public health regulations of industry, as well as the special occasions when public health regulations also affect individuals, limiting what have come to be called lifestyle risks.

The pace of federal regulation begun in the sixties has been slowed by a sluggish economy, a strong antiregulatory backlash from business and the Republican party, and a jittery Democratic party; however, public health remains firmly on the federal agenda.

Every night on network news some new danger to or hazard for public health is chronicled. Public health threats are no longer seen as arising "so naturally out of the environment that the population affected usually accepts them as inevitable and will even resist efforts to do anything about them."[5] Public health problems are preventable, and the public wants action. Despite a vigorous counterattack by business, the public still sees most public health problems as the dark side of the market and often as signs of corporate greed and irresponsibility. In the early days of the Great Society, most regulations were aimed at limiting what corporations did to the environment or to consumers, and so this form of governmental activity posed no difficulties for liberals. Limiting harms to others is the principal task of government in a society where the dominant language is individualism.

Nevertheless, most political scientists were puzzled by the political success of the new public health activists, a loose coalition composed of activist members of the Senate, public interest lobbyists, researchers, and crusading journalists. The main figure was Ralph Nader, who was viewed as single-handedly creating a new kind of institution, the public interest lobby.[6] Books like Nader's *Unsafe at Any Speed*[7] and Rachel Carson's *Silent Spring*[8] captured the public's imagination and helped launch the consumer and public health activists as well as the environmental movement.

The rapid growth of this side of the Great Society was thought to be unusual because of the peculiar character of public health problems. The most influential explanation of the burst of public health legislation during the Great Society is *The Politics of Regulation*,[9] in which James Q. Wilson develops a classification scheme for public policies based on the "perceived distribution of their costs and benefits." Wilson's scheme includes majoritarian politics, interest group politics, client politics, and entrepreneurial politics.[10]

Majoritarian politics arise when perceived benefits and costs are widely distributed throughout society: "All or most of society expects to gain; all or most of society expects to pay."[11] The Social Security Act of 1935 is an example of a majoritarian policy, as is collective defense. Interest group politics arise when two well-organized industries such as trucking and railroads try to get government to settle their disputes. Client politics are pork barrel politics, the politics of conferring valuable benefits on favored groups by using government power. This is the politics of rivers, harbors, and dams, as well as most occupational licensing.

In Wilson's scheme, all categories of action but public health and safety are governed by group and private interests rather than communal interests. Public health problems are spread diffusely through society, but the political task of solving these problems is extremely difficult because it pits a vast but weak and unorganized public against concentrated and powerful business interests. Only when political "entrepreneurs" become interested in these issues in cooperation with a crusading press and public interest advocates can these problems be overcome. Even in the case of public health, Wilson does not stray far from the language of private interests. Public health policies are a form of "entrepreneurial politics." Wilson puts it this way:

> Since the incentive to organize is strong for opponents of the policy but weak for the beneficiaries, and since the political system provides many points at which opposition can be registered, it may seem astonishing that regulatory legislation of this sort is ever passed. It is, and with growing frequency in recent years—but it requires the efforts of a skilled entrepreneur who can mobilize public sentiment . . . , put the opponents of the plan publicly on the defensive (by accusing them of deforming babies or killing motorists), and associate the legislation with widely shared values (clean air, pure water, health, and safety).[12]

Clearly Wilson sees prevention and public health legislation as the exception to the rule of a politics motivated largely by private, group interests. Interests that are public in character—loosely organized, diffuse, and pitted against entrenched private interests—are exceptions to the rule of "normal" politics, peddled by public interest advocates and activist senators who are not entirely devoid of their own, private motivations.[13]

However we characterize this phase of the Great Society, business fought back. Business formed political action committees along the lines by which labor groups had organized after World War II. New political entrepreneurs began to appear, this time fighting on the side of beleaguered business against government, trying to reverse regulation or safety legislation. Considerable deregulation legislation was passed, from airline and trucking deregulation to the repeal of measures requiring states to pass mandatory motorcycle helmet legislation. With the backlash came a whole new literature questioning the feasibility, or even desirability, of a "zero-risk" society.

Michael Pertschuk, a staff member of one of the key committees that created the new legislation during the sixties and later chairman of the Federal Trade Commission, recounted the history of this episode in his book, *Revolt Against Regulation*. He came to the bleak conclusion that, in normal times, public health and consumer legislation are prisoners to the market.[14] The trick is to find "windows of opportunity," when business's guard is down, to strike swiftly, and to hold on during the inevitable backlash. Pertschuk's argument supports Wilson's assumption that the provision of collective protections—collective goods, in the language of economists—is the exception to the normal rule of pluralist politics.

This idea depends on a conception of politics in which political action largely springs from private motivations of either individuals or groups. Politics in this view is simply a mechanism, a structure, a field of rules in which private interests compete for scarce resources: that is, politics is a market.

As William Sullivan points out, whether this conception of politics is adequate is one of the oldest issues in American politics—one we have yet to resolve.[15] At issue among merchants and artisans who formed the backbone of revolutionary committees in Philadelphia during the 1776–1779 period, Sullivan notes, were the huge profits made by some as a result of the war while others found themselves bypassed. Many of the committees urged that trade be subordinated to the common good, and that the market should be subordinate to the social compact. "The social compact or state of civil society, by which men are united and incorporated, requires that every right or power claimed or exercised by any man or set of men should be in subordination to the common good, and that whatever is incompatible therewith, must, by some rule or regulation be brought into subjection thereto."[16] Others argued that the common prosperity depended on unfettered trade and the freedom of the individual to dispose of his property as he pleased.

In general, those who argued for subordinating commerce to the social compact and to a civic republic lost the battle; as Sullivan notes, government was increasingly viewed as

> no longer a differentiated community but a mechanism, a collection of instruments for advancing interests. . . . The extraordinary achievement of the new Federalism was the creation of an instrumental structure at once expansive and stable. The key to success seemed to be the very lack of a unifying purpose in American political life.[17]

By "differentiated society," Sullivan is referring to John Adams's notion of a society made up of orders and a balanced hierarchy—the very order and balance that was being destroyed by the commercial changes sweeping over the new republic. But while I sympathize with Sullivan's critique of the commercial republic, I believe he overlooks the survival of the language of republicanism in differing spheres—including spheres like public health and the communal welfare—and the opportunity we have, as health policy looms larger in American life, to regain a better civic balance between the market sphere and the more communal and egalitarian spheres of the republic.

In the sphere of communal health protections—and for classic public health protections like vaccination or safe water—the nineteenth century never lost sight of the republican tradition, limiting both property and liberty in order to promote the common good. The health and safety legislation of the twentieth century in the sixties and seventies was not a marginal or exceptional deviation from the path of pluralist politics: This legislation like much of the rest of the Great Society legislation sprang from a politics founded more on public and common interests than analysts like Wilson allow. Indeed, as Robert Reich has argued:

> Consider the civil rights laws and regulations of the 1960s; the subsequent wave of laws and rules governing health, safety, and the environment; . . . These policies have not been motivated principally or even substantially by individuals seeking to satisfy selfish interests. To the contrary, they have been broadly understood as matters of public, rather than private, interest. And this perception has given them their unique authority. People supported these initiatives largely because they were thought to be good for *society*.[18]

The idea of a national community and a national citizenship was a common theme in the civil rights movement, the war on poverty, and in the health and safety legislation. In each of these strands of the Great Society, society was thought of as a great community bound up by an indivisible set of relations that govern the market and the larger society, a set of relations in which health and safety protections, like guarantees against racial discrimination, betoken a national citizenship. Far from being an exception to the normal rule of politics as private interests, health and safety legislation represented the most successful and popular phase of the Great Society, at a time when political leaders

redefined and enlarged the meaning of the political community and established these initiatives as a central federal
responsibility. Instead of Wilson's shrunken conception of
"entrepreneurial politics" as a stepchild of pluralist politics,
the legislative record of the Great Society in health and
safety reflected the republic's search for new meanings in
equality and community.

The Lifestyle Debate

One of the most vexing issues in the expansion of public
health activism during and after the Great Society was
the increasing attention paid to the role of individual behavior—the "lifestyle perspective." The document that
focused attention on this issue was *A New Perspective on
the Health of Canadians*, published in 1974.[19] Few policy
documents in the field of health have been as influential or
as widely quoted. *A New Perspective* noted that of the four
factors contributing to the health of a society or a people—
lifestyle, environment, human biology, and health services
organization—additional investments in health services
would bring the fewest gains in health status.

When *A New Perspective* first appeared in Canada, national budgets everywhere were beginning to strain under
the costs of health expenditure. A primary goal of *A New
Perspective* was to check government expenditure for health
care by channeling funds and effort toward prevention.
Instead of corporate greed, *A New Perspective* formulated a
new theory of the causes of public health problems. According to this account, at the turn of the century, when an
individual died or became seriously ill, chances were that
the death or disease was caused by typhus, cholera, pneumo-
nia, tuberculosis, or the many diseases of infants. Disease
came from the environment of early-twentieth-century
North America—poverty, poor nutrition, unclean food,

unsanitary hospitals, or unsafe water supplies. Today, when a person enters a hospital, chances are he or she does so because of lifestyle—ways of living that increase the chance of heart disease, cancer, stroke, serious injury from a highway crash, or liver cirrhosis.

This new pattern dampened the enthusiasm for a strong preventive role for government at any level, as limitations on lifestyle seemed to promise an ominous growth in big government. Aaron Wildavsky put it this way:

> We are not talking about peripheral or infrequent aspects of human behavior. We are talking about some of the most deeply rooted and often experienced aspects of human life—what one eats, how often and how much; . . . whether one smokes or drinks and how much; even the whole question of human personality. . . . To oversee these decisions would require a larger bureaucracy than anyone has yet conceived and methods of surveillance bigger than big brother.[20]

The lifestyle theory shifted attention from the misdeeds of corporations to the specter of governmental paternalism. To a democrat, the likely outcome of such a political philosophy would be, as Tocqueville feared, "an immense protective power . . . father-like . . . [keeping all] in perpetual childhood."[21]

During the second Nixon administration, officials of the U.S. Department of Health, Education and Welfare (now Health and Human Services) outlined, in two successive volumes of its *Forward Plan for Health,* ambitious plans for limiting hazardous lifestyle risks.[22] Whether the Nixon administration was serious or trying to undercut public support for regulation of corporations and divert attention from a gathering drive for universal health insurance, we cannot know. But the result was a new and increasingly accepted view of the public's health as a matter of personal responsibility. If individuals largely shape their own health, and if they accept risks far greater than those corporations place on them, why so much fuss about regulation?

As public awareness grew that personal health habits had more to do with health than medicine, the idea that medicine is a right was weakened. A president of the American Medical Association, writing in the *Newsweek* column "My Turn," argued that Americans do not have a right to health care precisely because lifestyle, not medicine, determines health.[23] Philosophers asked whether equal access to health care was a legitimate goal for society if personal habits play such a central role in the need for care. Do smokers, for example, have a right to health care equal to that of nonsmokers? Leon Kass argued that health is not a right but a product of living wisely—the reward of individual duty and virtue.[24]

The Prevention Paradox

During the height of the antiregulation backlash, a widely cited article by Chauncey Starr in *Science* tried to tie voluntary and involuntary risks together more directly, comparing the relative safety of largely voluntary activities and activities imposed on individuals.[25] Starr argued that the relative levels of safety (as measured by the expectation of fatalities per hour of exposure to the risk) reveal individual preferences for acceptable levels of risk. Starr found, among other things, that individuals found acceptable much higher levels of voluntary than involuntary risk—up to a thousand times higher. Flying by commercial airline is far safer than by private plane. Traveling by car is much riskier than by train. Starr emphasized the apparent paradox that we worry a great deal more about the smaller risks imposed on us than the risks we impose on ourselves. As he put it, we are "loathe to let others do unto us what we happily do to ourselves."[26]

Starr's paradox rests on a species of democratic individualism in which individual autonomy is the dominant value in all realms. If individuals freely choose a level of safety lower than that achieved through regulation, why shouldn't the lower standard become the general level of acceptable risk in society?

But Starr's paradox can be looked at another way. In a more complex society, one with differing distributive spheres, there is no one standard for safety—different spheres observe different standards. In such a society, we should expect that the level of safety we choose for ourselves privately is far different than the level we might choose for ourselves collectively.

The risks of fatal injury in an automobile accident provide an excellent example. Each year roughly forty-five thousand people lose their lives on the nation's highways or streets as a result of a crash in or with a personal vehicle. Further, proposals that would make wearing seat belts or making air bags compulsory would each save roughly ten thousand lives each year. Yet those forty-five thousand deaths, or the twenty thousand lives to be saved, are spread over 150 million drivers and 175 million vehicles. The level of safety for these millions of drivers, expressed on an annual basis, is approximately 2.7 deaths per 100 million vehicle miles. Furthermore, the rate of these deaths is falling.[27]

Thus, the paradox: At the individual level, highways are very safe and getting safer; at the community level, the level of safety could probably be doubled if everyone wore seat belts and air bags were installed in every car.

This way of looking at the problem suggests that many, if not most, modern risks to Americans are group rather than individual problems. We worry about problems at the collective level that we ignore or tend to neglect at the individual level. At the heart of prevention in modern society is Geoffrey Rose's *preventive paradox:* "A preventive measure which brings much benefit to the population offers little to each participating individual."

Rose goes on, "This has been the history of public health—of immunization, the wearing of seat belts and now the attempt to change various lifestyle characteristics. Of enormous potential importance to the population as a whole, these measures offer very little—particularly in the short term—to each individual."[28]

Rose is referring to what economists and political scientists call "collective goods," that is, goods that benefit a society or community but do not benefit any single individual—or group—sufficiently to make the individual wish to obtain it for him- or herself. In economic theory, markets exhibit two main kinds of failure: failures in which certain costs to third parties to a transaction (usually called "externalities") are not counted, and the failures in which markets do not provide goods that must be consumed jointly, called collective consumption goods.[29]

The classic example of externalities is pollution. Factory A produces goods for customers, but as a by-product produces waste that sullies the surrounding streams and air. Because these costs to society at large or the surrounding community are not included in the price of the goods (or are "external" to the market exchange), these costs are called externalities. Externalities could be benefits as well as costs; the important point is that in these cases the market price does not include them.

The standard examples of collective consumption goods are clean air, clean water, police protection, and a national defense. Because these have to be offered to the entire community or not at all, collective consumption goods must be provided governmentally. Collective goods also usually have another feature called "nonexhaustibility," which means that by using part of the good, a consumer does not reduce the amount available to others. Clean air is an example of this, and so is patriotism.

Economists have always recognized that many needed

collective goods can't be furnished by markets. Adam Smith admitted that there were

> public institutions and . . . public works, which, though they may be in the highest degree advantageous to a great society, are, however, of such a nature, that the profit could never repay the expence to any individual or small number of individuals . . . [to] erect or maintain.[30]

Now even liberals who make the autonomy of individuals their central value recognize that markets often ignore externalities or fail to provide certain classic kinds of collective consumption goods. Indeed, James Wilson describes entrepreneurial politics as simply a variant on the economists' notion of collective goods as a market failure: political markets, like ordinary markets, often fail to provide collective protections because they do not provide tangible benefits to organized groups.

I believe that the prevention paradox, in a republican scheme, rests on a different logic from this liberal "exceptionalism." In a republican order, we should *expect* the level of collective protections people want for society as a whole and protections individuals privately prefer to differ. To believe otherwise is to resort to what Brian Barry has called the "standard liberal fallacy, " or the view that what is in the interest of the private individual usually adds up to the good of the community.[31] The paradox has been expressed another way by the economist Thomas Schelling: "How well each [citizen] does for himself in adapting to his social environment is not the same thing as how satisfactory a social environment [citizens collectively] create for themselves."[32] The good of society and the sum of private goods of the individuals who make up society are not necessarily the same thing. And we may, and do, apply different standards to each.

In this way of looking at safety, the issue is not so much whether risks are imposed on me by others, or self-imposed (though this distinction is never lost), but *rather the scale or aggregate number of risks, both large and small,* that individuals impose on themselves or have imposed on them.[33]

There are myriad examples showing how the scale issue connects prevention policy to group rather than individual standards, at least in the sphere of communal provision. Let us take the case of heart disease. As Rose points out, the conventional wisdom is that we ought to worry most about those who are most at risk from heart disease; those who have very high cholesterol levels, or who smoke the most, or who completely ignore their physician's advice about exercise. And it is true that these individuals do have elevated risks for heart disease, suffering illness and premature death at a higher rate than their more moderate neighbors. But from the standpoint of the community or the population, a huge portion of the cases of heart disease and premature death comes from those who are, relatively speaking, at low risk from elevated cholesterol levels in the blood. In fact, those who are at low risk generate the most cases of heart disease.[34]

In drinking and driving, we find essentially the same phenomenon. As a report of the National Academy of Sciences found, the chronic recidivist turns up disproportionately in the statistics; yet the ordinary drinkers who occasionally drink too much cause the largest share of alcohol-related crashes simply because there are so many more ordinary than heavy drinkers.

> As we should expect, the fraction of people having [drinking] problems increases noticeably with given levels of consumption. But . . . people . . . in the highest consumption groups . . . account for only 24 percent of the population having problems. *The reason is that there*

are so many more people in the lower-consuming groups that even small proportions in trouble can swamp the larger fraction . . . from the higher-consuming group.[35]

The reason for these paradoxes of safety and health is that the risks we usually seek to control are so prevalent, shared by millions of individuals and encountered frequently. The large number of people who drink less than their fellow citizens, who eat less fat in their diets, and so forth, actually account for far more of the cases of avoidable disease and premature death than the much smaller number who are at much higher risk.

The paradox has its bleak side in changes in individual behavior. As Rose shows, using estimates of the risk of heart disease from Framingham data, the individual often gains little from many prevention interventions:

If we supposed that throughout their adult life, up to the age of 55, Framingham men were to modify their diet in such a way as to reduce their cholesterol levels by 10%, then among men of average coronary risk about one in 50 could expect that through this preventive precaution he would avoid a heart attack . . . : 49 out of 50 would eat differently every day for 40 years and perhaps get nothing from it.[36]

Examples of this ratio between the large numbers who must be encouraged to adopt a protective measure and the low numbers who actually benefit abound in the health field. Millions are immunized so that a few thousand might be saved. More than 150 million vehicles must have air bags installed so that ten thousand lives may be saved. At least 70 percent of those who drive—roughly 100 million individuals —must wear their seat belts each time they drive if we can expect a decline of ten thousand in highway deaths.

Now let's take the hard case: cigarette smoking. Cigarette smoking causes 350,000 premature deaths each year. It is our most deadly risk and it may well be the major exception to the paradox of prevention. But in an interesting recent article in *The American Journal of Public Health*, Mattson, Pollack, and Cullen note that the risk of dying prematurely from an automobile crash before age eighty-five is 1 in 100; the overall risk of dying from accidental injury is less than 3 in 100. On the other hand, the risk of dying prematurely before age eighty-five due to smoking is 1 in 3; the risk of dying prematurely before age sixty-five is 1 in 6.[37]

To teenagers, the group we should be most interested in preventing from smoking entirely, these dramatically higher risks for smoking pose threats decades in the future, a prospect that fills few young persons with terror. Moreover, there is some bad news for the current smoker. As the authors note, by quitting, the former smoker lowers his or her smoking-related risk of dying prematurely before age eighty-five from 33 to 11 percent. Still, even though they quit, ex-smokers are almost four times more likely to die prematurely before age eighty-five than those who never smoked—certainly not happy news for those seeking to motivate the public to quit smoking.

Thus, even for such a deadly lifestyle risk, the threat remains far in the distance and quitting brings rather slight shifts in the odds against a remote event. At least until middle age, dying from smoking remains more a communal threat than an imminent personal one. (The high percentage of smokers who repeatedly try to stop smoking is a sign that this threat is not altogether distant and that smoking carries as many present disadvantages as future perils. The cigarette industry is fortunate that its products are so highly addictive.)

One other aspect of the issue of scale deserves mention— one that draws the spheres of voluntary and involuntary risks even closer together. This is the commercialization process, or what Fred Hirsch calls "the commodity bias," the tendency for market societies to prefer goods in commodity form and to convert noncommodities to that form.[38] The commodity bias describes the way in which the market puts unrelenting commercial pressure on manufacturers to focus on individual transactions and ignore scale effects; in the case of pollution, to burden the environment with thousands of new and untested chemicals and toxic wastes and a flood of new, almost indestructible containers and wrappings. The commodity bias also pressures manufacturers to exploit relentlessly the commercial possibilities of our coastlines, natural forests, and mineral resources held in common. But this process of commercial exploitation courses beneath the markets for voluntary risks like cigarettes, guns, or alcohol. Thus, the smokestack and its spreading plume as the most familiar symbol of "harms to others" hardly captures the underlying and far more dangerous social process of commercialization, one that runs through the spheres of voluntary and involuntary risks alike.

An excellent example of how the commercialization process affects the issue of scale even for (more or less) voluntary risks is handguns. The slogan of the National Rifle Association is, "Guns don't kill people, people kill people." This is a perfect example of an ethic that ignores the effects of scale: handgun manufacturers work to sell a product that, although most sales may seem innocent or innocuous, will in the aggregate contribute to thousands of injuries and death.

There are approximately 100 to 150 million firearms in private hands in the United States; roughly 40 million of them are handguns.[39] The percentage of gun-owning households that holds handguns has risen from 25 percent to 50 percent since 1959; overall, one-quarter of all households own handguns. The total volume of manufacture or import of handguns in the last decade is larger than those of the preceding six decades combined. Roughly half of all homicides are committed with handguns. Gun ownership expanded sharply during the sixties and seventies, but sales have recently begun to level off and even slump, partly because of gun registration laws (though these were recently weakened) and partly because the market is becoming saturated.

One way manufacturers are trying to improve the stagnating market is by introducing the plastic handgun, a new product rapidly moving to our markets.[40] Plastic guns are cheap, accurate, and almost impossible to detect in airport metal detection systems, making the possibilities for escalating airline terrorism enormous. The gun's development is being fostered by military researchers who fear that the Soviets have perfected the technology, and by manufacturers who see in the new generation of light, superstrong plastics combined with ceramics the promise of lighter guns and cost savings.

The National Rifle Association, which backed the availability of submachine guns and high-velocity bullets that can penetrate armored vests worn by the nation's police, also backs the plastic handgun. The major reason, at least according to one author, is that the gun retailers and gun manufacturers that are big supporters of the gun lobby wish to make owners believe that those 150 million heavy long guns and handguns are obsolete.

The case for controlling handguns might seem fundamentally different from controlling alcohol. Yet the commercialization process works in exactly the same way for both products, leading the alcohol industries to introduce new alcoholic products, from alcohol in chocolate milk shakes to wine coolers; applying constant pressure to expand the hours and places of sale; and to escalate the promotion of alcoholic products through direct advertising and promotion of athletic events. This constant pressure seeks to expand steadily the occasions and forms in which alcohol is used, constantly threatening to efface and undermine communal traditions that seek to limit the availability of alcohol and the drinking of it.

Paternalism: Pro and Con

Clearly my argument is headed for the position that our objections to public health limits, based on a fundamental autonomy for citizens in every realm, need to be rethought. In the sphere of communal protections, even for some lifestyle risks, I believe that we must not permit a libertarian and absolute autonomy to be our reigning principle. Instead we must employ a standard of *basic* autonomy that permits reasonable, minimally intrusive restrictions that yield significant gains in the health and safety of the public.

This is a different argument from the "burdens on society" thesis, though it resembles this position. I argue that the justification for a more limited autonomy rests on the belief that reducing the level of risks that affect the community as a body, usually by reasonable (and long-debated) reductions in slight but widespread risks we all face, will cumulate in a large reduction in levels of preventable death, disease, and disability. This is different from the far more expansive thesis that we ought to limit an individual's action because it affects other individuals or poses some economic burden on society.

I am not advocating that we ignore the objections to paternalism or the difference between the risks to self and risks to others. I am arguing that we need to relax the rigid antipaternalism that results when we make the principle of absolute autonomy apply in all spheres of the republic.

Though I have discussed paternalism elsewhere, for the following discussion we should adopt a specific definition. According to Gerald Dworkin, paternalism is "the interference with a person's liberty of action justified by reasons referring exclusively to the welfare, good, happiness, needs, interests, or values of the person being coerced."[41] Dworkin's list of paternalistic policies includes requiring motorcycle helmet laws, laws forbidding swimming at a beach when lifeguards are not on duty, Social Security, laws forbidding suicide, laws regulating certain kinds of sexual conduct, and so forth.

Critics of paternalism argue that it leads to too large a government, and that, in the long run, individuals are better able than government to judge their own interests. But the central argument against paternalism is that the state acting as parent gives deep offense to the dignity of citizens. As Ronald Dworkin puts it, "laws that constrain one man, on the sole ground that he is incompetent to decide what is right for himself, are profoundly insulting to him."[42]

The most categorical case against paternalism is still that of Mill:

The only purpose for which power can be rightfully exercised over any member of a civilized community, against his will, is to prevent harm to others. His own good, either physical or moral, is not sufficient warrant. He cannot rightfully be compelled to do or forbear because it will be better for him to do so, because it will make him happier, because, in the opinions of others to do so would be wise or even right. These are good reasons for remonstrating with him, or reasoning with him, or persuading him, or entreating him, but not for compelling him, or visiting him with any evil, in case he do otherwise. To justify that, the conduct from which it is desired to deter him must be calculated to produce evil to some one else. The only part of the conduct of any one, for which he is amenable to society, is that which concerns others. In the part which merely concerns himself, his independence is, of right, absolute. Over himself, over his own body and mind, the individual is sovereign.[43]

The backbone of antipaternalism is Mill's harm principle. According to Mill, the state cannot legitimately require the individual to take care for his own safety. As Mill said elsewhere in *On Liberty*:

Self-regarding faults . . . are not properly immoralities,
. . . They may be proofs of any amount of folly, or want
of personal dignity and self-respect; but they are only a
subject of moral reprobation when they involve a
breach of duty to others, for whose sake the individual
is bound to have care for himself. What are called
duties to ourselves are not socially obligatory, unless
circumstances render them at the same time duties to
others.[44]

In Mill's scheme, regulating unhealthy or risky behavior
among autonomous adults can only be to prevent specific
wrongs that one group visits on another. In this view, drunk
driving would be a public problem; drunkenness pure and
simple is not. (Mill: "Drunkenness . . . in ordinary cases is
not a fit subject for legislative interference.")

The Rise of the "New Paternalism"

John Stuart Mill must be spinning in his grave. From seat
belt laws to antismoking regulations, public health restrictions on lifestyle, or what Richard Bonnie calls the "new
paternalism,"[45] is on the rise in the United States. One
reason for this is the momentum of the Great Society health
and safety legislation of the sixties and seventies; after two
decades of making the automobile safer, we shouldn't be
surprised that we are now passing seat belt legislation.
Another reason for the acceptance of the new public health
restrictions is that cases of "pure paternalism," when government limits purely voluntary risks and does so only for
the sake of the individual agent, are extremely rare. We raise
tobacco and alcohol taxes to raise revenues, and only partially to promote healthier behavior. Furthermore, regulating one industry often creates unexpected allies for new
regulation. The automobile industry has lobbied hard for

seat belt legislation, primarily to avoid government mandates for air bags in every car. And the furniture industry, faced with regulations to make fabrics more fire-retardant, eagerly supports measures to make cigarettes more firesafe. As Joel Feinberg argues, both tradition and common sense make us unwilling to reject all forms of paternalism. If we can save lives with "limited" or "weak" forms of paternalism, then our objections tend to fade away.[46] For Dennis Thompson, paternalism seems justified when the intervention is minimally restrictive, when the threatened harm is very great, or when the public's judgment seems genuinely impaired.[47] But Thompson's last point doesn't play a central role. Richard Bonnie is closer to the point when he argues that the new paternalism is justified precisely because it provides substantial aggregate savings in lives and serious disability through minimal restrictions on individual choice. Bonnie mentions four permissible forms of "weak paternalism": (a) altering the conditions of availability of harmful substances, (b) deterring harmful individual behavior through (mild) punishment (e.g., fines for smoking in public places), (c) symbolizing the posture of the government toward the behavior, and (d) influencing the content of messages in mass media.[48] Albert Weale sees a growing liberal justification for some forms of paternalism—those that save lives with minimal restrictions on goods or services.[49]

I believe that these public health restrictions are gaining acceptance among liberals because they increasingly recognize that a rigid distinction between voluntary and involuntary risks in public health can have ludicrous results. Something is fundamentally wrong when risks to the public health like alcohol and tobacco receive marginal attention in modern public health while air pollution is attacked with deadly earnestness. Does the fact that consumers buy cigarettes and take them home make them *completely* different from, say, the smokestack polluting the valley basin? Doesn't the fact that cigarette smoking probably kills a hundred times more citizens than smoking factories enter the equation of public health policy at all?

Most treatments of paternalism completely ignore these issues. For example, Feinberg argues that "if the state is to be given the right to prevent a person from risking harm to himself (and only himself), it must not be on the ground that the prohibited action is risky, or even extremely risky, but rather that the risk is extreme and . . . manifestly unreasonable."[50] If Feinberg is right, we should be far more concerned with legislating against jumping off cliffs than against driving without seat belts.

But we find just the opposite trends in our society. And I think the reason is that though few people jump off cliffs, millions drive their automobiles every day, facing very low risks but nonetheless generating aggregate levels of death and injury unacceptable in a great republic. Again, in Feinberg's world of individualist ethics the basic standard is an "absolute autonomy." But in a complex or republican scheme of equality, a different standard of autonomy is appropriate for the communal sphere. In my view, public health restrictions on lifestyle risks are not classically paternalistic; they are designed to promote a common, not a private good. We know from experience that these protections "are likely to benefit . . . a number of members of society, while not knowing which particular members will be affected on this or that occasion."[51]

In justifying his antipaternalism, Mill argued that only the individual can know his own particular good: "He is the person most interested in his own well-being: the interest which any other person, except in cases of strong personal attachment, can have in it, is trifling."[52] But when health and safety are viewed also as common interests, this is wrong. Governmental restrictions in regulating conditions of the common life are to promote the common good, not the good of any particular person. Again, as Richard Flathman notes, modern governments rarely paternalistically promote the good of particular persons.[53]

Like Feinberg, James Childress argues that, in a democracy, respect for persons implies a standard of absolute autonomy, to be overridden only in extreme circumstances.[54] Absolute autonomy means the freedom to choose the good for oneself in matters that pertain only to oneself. According to Ronald Dworkin, autonomy, not license, is the central point in Mill's *On Liberty*. But treating absolute autonomy as a general value that undergirds all the spheres of a democratic society would not only undercut attempts to reduce some of the most deadly threats to the public's health, threats like smoking, alcohol, and AIDS, but would pose dangers in other spheres as well. Because this position rests on a single and rather rigid standard of absolute autonomy, it threatens schemes of common provision like a common health care system or Social Security. While these liabilities can be overcome with unusual justifications, nevertheless the standard of absolute autonomy in the sphere of the community is a potent enemy of common schemes of action.

A single standard also threatens places where absolute autonomy ought to prevail, such as the sphere of privacy, or in doctor–patient and lawyer–client relations. A very common justification for requiring parental consent for teenage contraception or abortion is that we require teenagers to gain their parents' consent for other, less significant risks (like having their ears pierced, or obtaining a driver's license when underage), and so should permit teens to have an abortion or get contraceptives only under similar circumstances. In a differentiated and complex society, we would come to see that different spheres have different standards, and that limiting citizens' choices in relatively trivial matters while expanding their choices in fundamental matters makes perfect sense in a complex scheme of equality.

Ronald Dworkin argues that keeping absolute autonomy as the rule for the personal sphere actually handcuffs the government very little because the personal sphere is so small when compared to the rest of society.[55] But in

Dworkin's and Childress's world a near absolute autonomy dominates all realms, exonerating the alcohol and tobacco industry while exposing the smokestacks of the steel industry to stringent regulation. It also resurrects Chauncey Starr's paradox: If fundamental autonomy is the rule, and if we voluntarily select risks that are higher than the level of regulated safety, should we not lower the level of regulated safety to the standard we voluntarily choose?

Ronald Dworkin, in arguing for the limited impact of Mill's principle of autonomy, actually reveals the flaw in his own argument when he makes a basic distinction between common and individual interests.

> An individual's independence is threatened, not simply by a political process that denies him equal voice, but by political decisons that deny him equal respect. *Laws that recognize and protect common interests, like laws against violence and monopoly, offer no insult to any class or individual*, but laws that constrain one man, on the sole ground that he is incompetent to decide what is right for himself, are profoundly insulting to him.[56]

Dworkin here passes over the central justification for public health restrictions: promoting health and safety as common rather than private or narrowly paternalistic interests. Dworkin, a legal scholar, ignores the fact that the United States, in its constitutional tradition, treats health and safety as a compelling common interest in a republican scheme of government, and that the courts have almost always rejected absolute autonomy as the principle governing distribution in the sphere of communal welfare. In that sphere, as opposed to the realms of medicine and of the law, a democratically elected and publicly accountable legislature is responsible for determining what is in the interest of the people as a whole, and the individual's liberty and autonomy can be limited to promote that common good.

Further, the very development of the police power reveals

that judges increasingly permitted the expansion of the common law doctrine of "use your property in such a way as not to injure others" to become a community principle rather than merely an individual one.

In the classic case of *Commonwealth v. Alger*, Chief Justice of the Supreme Court of Massachusetts, Judge Shaw, argued that "things done may or may not be wrong in themselves, or necessarily injurious and punishable at common law, but laws are passed declaring them offenses, and making them punishable, because they tend to have injurious consequences."[57] This is a perfect summation of the paradox of prevention, and indeed, it has been linked explicitly by scholars to the need to prevent harms, and not necessarily to redress them. I discuss the constitutional tradition for public health at length in the next chapter.

Prevention and the Slippery Slope

In the balance of the chapter I address the issue of whether, by abandoning absolute autonomy in the communal sphere, we are placing the citizen at serious risk of the government becoming a "national nanny." In a complex society, especially one like the United States, based on a separated system of powers, each sphere has its special (but not sole) guardian. In the market and communal spheres, the legislative branch protects the liberties of the people. Should civil libertarians be wary of the increasing scope of communal life over individual choice?

Of course. Vigilance in any sphere for individual liberties is a primary element of a vigorous democracy. But as I see it, people who advocate communal restrictions over personal liberties face formidable obstacles in legislative bodies, with the burden on the advocates to prove that change would not only bring significant savings in lives and freedom from disease but would be accepted by the public, at least over the long term.

Currently, measures to restrict personal liberties in order to promote the public's health are few. Beyond limits on alcohol and tobacco through increased taxes and controls on availability, handgun controls, helmets for motorcyclists, and seat belts and air bags for cars, there are few remaining measures on the horizon available to a democratic government. Imaginative philosophers might still envision a time when American legislatures would dictate that citizens run three miles every day (or at least take long walks), eat more bran, eschew bacon, and so forth, but I see no prospect that we are slouching, even slowly, toward a vast paternal power exercised by our elected officials.

Of course, such restrictions cannot be ruled out in principle, and this bothers many philosophers. But this reflects the view that philosophy is a kind of superlegislative body overseeing democratic institutions and on which democratic officials rely. In my view, however, political philosophy can only demarcate the spheres of action and their basic logics, trusting that the institutions in question will use their powers in measured ways, if for no other reason than that they must face the electorate every few years and regular opposition from elected executives and the courts.

Indeed, we have seen how even successful safety regulations can be quickly repealed by "populist entrepreneurialism."[58] In the case of motorcycle helmets, a national law was passed requiring states to pass mandatory helmet legislation or face losses in federal highway transportation funds. All but California complied, and deaths from motorcycle crashes were cut almost in half in a few short years. But some biker organizations, coupled with liberal and Western opposition in the Senate and conservatives like Jesse Helms, joined to repeal this provision of the highway bill. Because few members of the Senate could envision themselves being punished for being "anti–public health" in

97

this instance, the deregulation movement was relatively painless. Now only about half of the states retain these laws, and the death rate has risen accordingly.[59]

Much more recently, Massachusetts and Nebraska had joined the almost thirty states who have passed mandatory seat belt laws, a movement begun in 1985. But very shortly after the passage of this legislation, opposition materialized with successful repeal referendums, and while the voting was close in both instances, the repeal efforts show how unstable some of these measures are. When motorists have spent a lifetime driving without seat belts, they perceive little danger in their actions and therefore are unlikely to be intensely interested, one way or the other, in such protective measures.[60]

Thus, I find the fear that permitting government to limit personal risks exposes the individual to unlimited and unchecked public health activism by democratic legislatures unfounded. Indeed, modern legislatures have been the most formidable opponents of personal restrictions, usually permitting them only after protracted debate. The fear of democratic government—especially the American democratic government—as the national nanny is, in the end, rather silly.[61]

It is usually at this point that the American experiment with Prohibition is brought up, a subject I address in a later chapter. Prohibition was primarily an episode in moralism, not paternalism; in fact, public health controls over alcohol should be treated as fundamentally different from state prohibition based on reforming the moral character of the nation.

Our principal need is to grasp that there are different realms and different languages of prevention, from privacy and its roots in a fundamental autonomy, to prevention in the market and the public spheres with public health measures based on a less restricted standard of autonomy, to prevention as moralism, carrying with it an utter disregard for autonomy. In a complex scheme of equality, we need to guard constantly against the confusion of realms and the danger of permitting simplistic and single standards of autonomy to dominate our discourse.

The American insistence on absolute autonomy has a kind of mythic quality that badly needs deflating. One of the most potent symbols of that independent spirit is Henry David Thoreau on Walden Pond. But most Americans are little aware that Thoreau lived only two miles from Concord and only a mile from his family home and that he visited his home and his mother, usually to take a meal, nearly every day of his two years on Walden Pond. He slept on sheets, and he could see the main road to Concord from his front door. Years earlier, when he graduated from Harvard, and when his mother suggested that he might leave home and travel around the world, he burst into tears, thinking he had been banished. Leon Edel, who recounts this story in his *Stuff of Sleep and Dreams*, notes that our idea of individualism has been inspired by an individual who was "dependent, insecure, mother-attached, and longing to be free."[62] His individualism was not a way of life, it was only a symbol and a gesture.

The answer is not to find new heroic individualists free from mother attachments but to espouse a mature freedom that acknowledges the complex meanings of autonomy in a democratic republic and of the need for many other goods besides autonomy in a mature and complex society. In truth, a stable and enduring republic needs both autonomy and dependence, self-reliance and common schemes, the right to be left alone to decide matters of life and death without coercion as well as communal solidarity in the face of death.

We saw in Chapter Two how a pattern of pluralist politics came to shape public policy for medical care during the Great Society and beyond, producing a decentralized, fragmented health care system, one rapidly being absorbed by the market. While health and safety legislation— the politics of prevention—exists under the shadow of deregulation and the market, the premise that this domain of policy is rooted in the good of society as a whole, and is not simply the sum of a myriad, private, particular interest, remains intact. The unanswered question is whether this basic split in health policy, a split we find in the American political tradition, can be resolved and the republican tradition emerge as the dominant one for all of health policy, for treatment and prevention alike.

THE CONSTITUTION
AND THE SPHERES
OF HEALTH POLICY

Robert Bellah and his coauthors, in *Habits of the Heart*, develop the idea of "languages" that shape the American political tradition.[1] The first language (or tradition of moral discourse) of American politics is individualism, whether biblical, economic, or political. This individualism has shaped our ideas about politics and public policy, stressing government as limited and liberty as private in nature. But as Bellah and his coauthors note, there are "second languages" of community rooted in the republican and biblical tradition that limit and qualify the scope and consequences of our individualism, stressing a public liberty and popular sovereignty, or the freedom of the people to shape the conditions of their common life.

If we are to move closer to a republican equality, we will

need to appreciate the second languages of republicanism and communal equality that already exist in our democratic tradition. It is not widely appreciated that the constitutional tradition for public health is one of the most striking examples of this communal liberty. We do not have to invent a new vocabulary of community and republicanism for the common health; we only have to renew and enlarge our understanding of the richness and complexity of our own constitutional tradition as the best record of our political journey and our political tradition.

One of the central themes of this tradition has been the struggle to use popular sovereignty to protect the public health. This struggle is usually discussed in terms of the struggle between judicial control and majority rule. As Henry Steele Commager has noted:

> What we have here are two fundamental . . . principles of American politics: the principle that men make government, and the principle that there are limits to the authority of government. The philosophical origins of the first principle may be found in the natural-rights philosophy of the seventeenth century—in the notion that all rights inhered originally in men, living in a state of nature, came together for mutual self-protection and set up government, and that the governments thus instituted derive all their just powers from the consent of the governed.[2]

Liberty in the United States has largely been treated as a private freedom from governmental restraint. But liberty can also be considered a public or common pursuit—the pursuit of the majority acting as a body or a group. As John H. Schaar has noted,

> Liberty [in the United States] was largely interpreted as private liberty, and equality soon came to mean equal opportunity to compete for the prizes of wealth

and power. There was little teaching of liberty as public liberty—the power of acting with others to shape the conditions of the common life.[3]

As we shall see, this overstates the case, at least for the public's health. The influence of the republican tradition, with its emphasis on popular or legislative sovereignty over the public health, goes back much farther than the Progressive era and can be traced to the non-Lockean and Puritan sources of the social compact in our democratic tradition.

But the republican tradition is not only popular sovereignty in conflict with the libertarian tradition of private rights; it is popular sovereignty *and* private rights—and more. The constitutional tradition, especially as it has developed around the public's health, is an excellent starting place to understand how our republicanism is less a matter of competing grand principles of government than a complex set of principles applied in distinctive ways to the separate spheres of the democratic polity—each with its own logic crafted over time and out of historical democratic controversy. Examination of the constitutional tradition reveals how we first struggled to clear the ground for a broad sphere of communal welfare and protection at the state level, how we have fashioned in this century a powerful role for the federal government in protecting the public's health, how we even more recently have constructed a sphere of free discussion as well as a sphere of privacy, and how each of these distinctive constituent spheres limits the reach of markets and moralism.

New England and Republicanism

Our constitutional tradition for health and safety is based on the state courts' fashioning of the sphere of the "police power," an unhappy term referring to the general powers of

103

the majority to promote their common health, safety, and morals by regulating private property and personal liberty. Given the structure of the nation in the nineteenth century, these powers were largely state and local in nature. Since these powers were nowhere discussed in the Constitution, the sphere of the police power was carved by the courts out of the colonial experience, the common law tradition, and the exigencies of a new nation.

The debate surrounding the regulatory power of the states helped answer fundamental questions about the relation of the citizen to the body politic and about the fundamental purposes of government. This is especially so because plaintiffs, whose property or liberty was limited by expanding state powers, could enter courts and complain that state actions exceeded their constitutional boundaries. Attorneys for the states and judges had to justify these expanding powers in the nature of the relation between the citizen and the state. Thus, the study of the evolution of this regulatory power is something of a mirror of our early thoughts about majority rule and the common life, at least at the state level.

The New England Puritan experience provides the first and longest-lasting influence in the evolution of state regulation. Puritans were not rugged individualists; they had a strong sense of community and the common life. The Puritans sought to check private interests in order to promote the common good, and their theory of policy and citizenship contained this view. New England Puritans were strongly influenced by the English Puritan tradition and by the radical republicanism of that period.[4] The Puritans, according to Roland Berthoff, shared a political philosophy that represented a balance between personal liberty and communal equality.[5] This theory of democracy as a complex and contradictory combination of personal liberty and property and democratic sovereignty was also present in our civic republican tradition with its ideas of public virtue and the common good. This republicanism carried over to the commonwealth tradition that shaped early New England state policy in the nineteenth century. The commonwealth tradition was the rationale for strong state powers to promote economic development ("internal improvements") and to protect the health, safety, and welfare of its citizens. (The rights side of the balance was more influential in shaping agrarian, laissez-faire ideas found in Jeffersonian theories of democracy.)

The Massachusetts Constitution of 1780 represents a synthesis between late Puritan and Congregationalist thought and democratic and republican ideology. This constitution contains two ideas that are at some tension: a very strong sense that the purpose of political association is the welfare of the community through popular sovereignty, and the protection of private rights. This constitution was perhaps the most influential of all those framed after the revolution on the development of the federal Constitution. The sense of this is captured in a decision of the U.S. Supreme Court dealing with a public health issue:

> In the Constitution of Massachusetts adopted in 1780 it was laid down as a fundamental principle of the social compact that the whole people covenants with each citizen, and each citizen with the whole people, that all shall be governed by certain laws for the "common good," and that government is instituted for the "common good," for the protection, safety, prosperity, and happiness of the people, and not for the profit, honor, or private interests of any one man, family, or class of men." The good and welfare of the commonwealth, of which the legislature is primarily the judge, is the basis on which the police power rests in Massachusetts.[6]

Ronald Peters, Jr., has detailed the political theory that stands behind this fundamental text of American constitutional government.[7] The Massachusetts Constitution contains both a recognition of the basic rights of citizens and a strong theory of majority rule: the individual citizen obligates himself to participate in authoritative schemes for the common benefit. This made sense because the New England states, like many of the original states, were strongly mercantilist, and the early state governments regulated prices, controlled interest rates, legislated consumption behavior, and so forth.

The strong sense of the community at the heart of the authority relationship shaping citizens' political obligations was formed in part by the Puritan interpretation of the social contract. The Puritan idea of community was also indebted to the notion of the "covenant," which comes from the religious tradition of Protestantism and earlier Jewish ideals of community. The covenant in Jewish tradition stood for a compact between God and each member of the Jewish community, reflecting reciprocal duties and obligations, one to the other. The individual was conceived of as voluntarily placing him or herself in a state of obligation to live according to the rules of God and do justice while on earth. The fact that each member of the community was conceived of as participating in this agreement is the reason for the strong emphasis on social justice and equality in this tradition.[8]

Throughout the nineteenth century, the concept of the political community as containing a large sphere where majority rule and the common good prevailed, limiting private desires and purposes, was challenged by an opposing idea: that private interests vigorously pursued produced the greatest social advantage. The republican concept of majority rule over the conditions of the common life remained alive and vigorous in the important area of public health, yet the competing idea of laissez-faire became increasingly lodged in a unique and powerful theory of the Supreme Court as constitutional tribunal, with the Court using the theory of contracts and later the Civil War amendments (especially the Fourteenth Amendment) to limit legislative majorities. Paradoxically, as the republicanism of an earlier era declined and laissez-faire ascended, the republican doctrine of popular sovereignty over the conditions of the common life flourished in public health, becoming the foundations of what legal scholars call the "police power."

The Development of the Regulatory Power

The principle of the power of the majority to shape the common life is a central idea behind public health, found everywhere in the nineteenth-century development of the state's power to protect the public's health and safety. Not coincidentally, Massachusetts was a key state in the development of this legal doctrine. In the founding document of American public health, the 1850 *Report of the Massachusetts Sanitary Commission*, Lemuel Shattuck, a member of the legislature, set out a definition of public health that stressed the idea of popular sovereignty over the conditions of the common health: "The condition of perfect *public health* requires such laws and regulations, as will secure to man associated in society, the same sanitary enjoyments that he would have as an isolated individual."[9]

The political theory behind Shattuck's definition of public health assumes that the citizen is a member of a democratic community joined together under a common authority for the explicit purposes of promoting the well-being of the body politic. As noted, the Massachusetts Constitution explicitly endorsed this conception: "The end of the institution, maintenance and administration of government, is to secure the existence of the body-politic."

Massachusetts was the site of major legal changes in favor of the use of state powers to promote economic growth while protecting citizens against the dangers of that growth. As a leading constitutional scholar, Leonard Levy, has argued,

> The police power may be regarded as the legal expression of the Commonwealth idea, for it signifies the supremacy of public over private rights. To call the

police power a Massachusetts doctrine would be an exaggeration, though not a great one. . . . [I]t is certainly no coincidence that in Massachusetts, with its Commonwealth tradition, the police power was first defined and carried to great extremes from the standpoint of vested interests.[10]

Apparently, Chief Justice John Marshall coined the term *police power* in referring to the powers of the states to regulate public health and safety matters in the classic *Gibbons v. Ogden* decision, in 1824, attempting to clarify the boundary between these powers and the powers of Congress over interstate commerce:

[Police powers] form a portion of that immense mass of legislation which embraces everything within the territory of the state, not surrendered to the general government: all which can be most advantageously exercised by the states themselves. Inspection laws, quarantine laws, health laws of every description . . . are component parts of this mass.[11]

The classic definition of the state's powers to regulate for health and welfare was established in *Commonwealth v. Alger* (1851), a decision written by Chief Justice Shaw of the Massachusetts Supreme Court, which established the basic premises of this power of the states.[12] Justice Shaw had a powerful influence on early constitutional history. Although he declined appointment to the U.S. Supreme Court, his decisions shaped legal opinion far beyond Massachusetts. His broad definition of the state's power to regulate for health and welfare remains the most influential to this date:

The power we allude to is . . . the police power, the power vested in the legislature by the constitution, to make, ordain and establish all manner of wholesome and reasonable laws, statutes and ordinances, either with penalties or without, not repugnant to the constitution, as they shall judge to be for the good and welfare of the commonwealth, and of the subjects of the same.[13]

In this decision Justice Shaw was ruling on what might seem a minor issue. The case involved a man who owned property on Boston Harbor and built a wharf that extended beyond a boundary to the public right of way established by the legislature. When the state ordered him to take it down, he went to court, arguing that the legislature had interfered with his property, and that it had not been demonstrated or even argued that his wharf constituted a nuisance or a harm to anyone.

As Levy notes, often in cases of little factual interest great principles are decided. Shaw set out the basic premise underlying state regulatory power:

> We think it is a settled principle, growing out of the nature of a well ordered civil society, that every holder of property, however absolute and unqualified may be his title, holds it under the implied liability that his use of it may be so regulated, that it shall not be injurious to the equal enjoyment of others having an equal right to the enjoyment of their property, *nor injurious to the rights of the community.* All property in this commonwealth . . . is derived directly or indirectly from the government, and held subject to those general regulations, which are necessary to the common good and general welfare.[14]

Justice Shaw was developing a republican and majoritarian justification for state regulatory power. To Shaw, the idea of the common good meant that the state, and the community or social compact on which it rested, took as one of its compelling interests the health, safety, or welfare of the citizens of Massachusetts. This treatment of health and safety as a common interest was not adequately protected by common law principles governing the use of property, and he believed health and safety could be adequately protected only through legislation and regulations affecting the whole people.

The common law doctrine regulating the use of property was *sic utere tuo ut alienum non laedas*, "Use your own property in such a manner as not to injure that of another."[15] In *Alger*, Shaw greatly broadened this principle from a case-by-case investigation of whether each citizen had harmed the interest of another to a broad instrument for the control of property potentially injurious to the interests of the Commonwealth of Massachusetts.

As Shaw argued, "Things done may or may not be wrong in themselves, or necessarily injurious and punishable as such at common law, but laws are passed declaring them offenses, and making them punishable, because they tend to injurious consequences."[16] Here Shaw is rejecting the harm principle in favor of the republican principle that aggregate consequences for the community must be taken into account if the community's health and safety is to be adequately protected. According to Levy, Shaw "believed that the general welfare required the anticipation and *prevention* of prospective wrongs from the use of private property."[17]

As the great Progressive legal scholar Ernest Freund argued decades later, the common law of nuisance could deal with evils only after they came into existence. But "the police power endeavors to prevent evil by checking the tendency toward it, and it seeks to place a margin of safety between that which is permitted and that which is sure to lead to injury or loss. This can be accomplished . . . by establishing positive standards and limitations which must be observed, although to step beyond them would not necessarily create a nuisance at law."[18]

The Supreme Court, in perhaps the second most influential police power decision of the nineteenth century, *Munn v. Illinois* (1877), affirmed the republican principle underlying state regulation in a case involving the State of Illinois and its regulation of grain operators' rates in Chicago.[19] Justice Field, arguing for the minority, stated that the market was essentially a private institution:

> The business of a warehouseman was, at common law, a private business, and is so in its nature. It has no special privileges connected with it, nor did the law ever extend to it any greater protection than it extended to all other private business.[20]

But Chief Justice Waite, arguing for the majority disagreed:

> Property does become clothed with a public interest when used in a manner to make it of public consequence, and affect the community at large. When, therefore, one devotes his property to a use in which the public has an interest, he, in effect, grants to the public an interest in that use, and must submit to be controlled by the public for the common good, to the extent of the interest he has thus created.[21]

Justice Waite is shifting the justification away from the harm principle and toward a majoritarian and republican justification. He does not argue that to be regulated the prices set by the grain operators must first injure some private interest; rather he argues that the public has the right to secure collective benefits by regulating commerce in the public interest.

While all authorities agree that the regulatory power of the states is extensive and is checked only by express grants of the Constitution to protect basic rights, some scholars still argue that the legal principle behind regulation is the harm principle, or *sic utere*.[22] But the leading scholars reject this view. For example, Ernest Freund, in the best study of the police power of any period, argues:

111

No community confines its care of the public welfare to the enforcement of the principles of the common law . . . it exercises its compulsory powers for the prevention . . . of wrong by narrowing common law rights . . . and [through] positive regulations which are not confined to wrongful acts. It is this latter kind of state control which constitutes the essence of the police power.[23]

This is a crucial issue because on it turns the relevance of the category of the community for public health and safety. If the regulatory power of government is simply the enforcement of the law that no one should use property in a way that directly harms another's interests, then the sphere of community is rendered meaningless. But as W. G. Hastings, a leading legal scholar writing early in this century, pointed out, a regulatory power limited to preventing harms to others does not explain the courts' uniform support of the drastic regulation of alcohol by the states.[24]

One of the confusing elements of this point is that judges and lawyers use both *sic utere* and the community principle to justify regulation. In *Crowley v. Christensen*, a well-known case of the nineteenth century, the Supreme Court affirmed the right of the state to regulate the alcohol trade completely, even to the point of abolishing it.[25] But though they based their decision on the community principle, the justices also took issue with the claim by the plaintiff that drinking was conduct in which individuals brought no substantial risk to third parties, noting the risks to the drinkers' families and to the community at large from their intemperance. Thus, adherents of both doctrines sometimes find solace in these early constitutional decisions.

Alcohol and the Constitution

The temperance and prohibition campaigns to control legally and even destroy the alcohol trade, first in the 1850s and later at the turn of the century, provided some of the strongest and clearest affirmations by the courts of the community principle justifying the state's regulatory powers.[26]

The Temperance movement first attempted to eliminate "grog shops" or saloons, which were often dirty, rowdy drinking halls that exploited the working class and the poor. Temperance strategy was to require that all distilled spirits be sold in very large quantities and for cash on delivery, which would eliminate the saloon. A number of these laws, passed throughout New England, were the subject of an early U.S. Supreme Court decision upholding them. Chief Justice Taney, in the *License Cases*, stated that he could see "nothing in the Constitution to prevent a state from regulating the liquor traffic or from prohibiting it altogether if it thinks proper."[27]

Corwin noted that no single measure constituted a more powerful attack on the power of vested property rights than did the state prohibition drives of the nineteenth century.[28] As Levy notes, "In the 1850's, state courts everywhere sustained prohibition laws, or intimated that they would do so if the legislation were properly drawn with procedural safeguards."[29] When the Massachusetts legislature outlawed the manufacture and sale of alcoholic beverages in 1852, the statute was declared unconstitutional only on procedural grounds; in the decision, Chief Justice Shaw upheld the right of the state to prohibit alcohol (*Fisher v. McGirr*, 1854).[30]

Perhaps the most significant case testing the constitutionality of state prohibition was *Mugler v. Kansas* (1887).[31]

Mugler concerned a brewery owner charged with making beer after the passage of a state constitutional amendment forbidding the manufacture, sale, and use of alcoholic beverages.

Plaintiff's counsel argued that the Kansas constitutional amendment was an attempt to regulate purely personal conduct not subject to a compelling state interest. Counsel quoted John Stuart Mill and the common law principle of *sic utere* as the basic founding principles of the English and American legal tradition. As counsel for the plaintiff argued, "If a state convention or legislature can punish a citizen for manufacturing beer . . . for his own use, then instead of civil liberty, we are living under the most unlimited and brutal despotism known in history. . . . Broad and comprehensive as this [police] power is, it cannot extend to the individual tastes and habits of the citizen, which are confined entirely to himself and have no effect upon others."[32]

The court held for the State of Kansas. Justice Harlan, writing for the majority, had this to say:

> There is no justification for holding that the State under the guise merely of police regulations, is here aiming to deprive the citizen of his constitutional rights; for we cannot shut out of view the fact, within the knowledge of all, that the public health, the public morals, and the public safety, may be endangered by the general use of intoxicating drinks; . . . So far from such a regulation having no relation to the general end sought to be accomplished, the entire scheme of prohibition, as embodied in the [state] constitution and laws of Kansas, might fail, if the right of each citizen to manufacture intoxicating liquors for his own use as a beverage were recognized. . . . Such a right does not inhere in citizenship. Nor can it be said that government interferes with or impairs any one's constitutional rights of liberty or of property, . . . Those rights are best secured in our government, by the observance,

upon the part of all, of such regulations as are established by competent authority, to promote the common good.[33]

Harlan was observing that an absolute autonomy did not inhere in citizenship where matters of the common good were at stake and that the legislature was competent to judge whether to abridge the basic—rather than absolute—autonomy of the citizens. The Court did not, and could not, pass judgement on the *wisdom* of the state prohibition measures. This judgement, in a republican scheme of government, rests with the legislative body. But the Court did affirm the basic political principles that empower the states to control and limit the market and private property to protect the health and safety of the citizenry.

Twentieth-Century Public Health

Even as the courts gave great latitude to the state legislatures in public health matters, they were showing in *Munn* and *Mugler* that citizens do have rights that state legislatures must respect. Clearly, the legal climate was shifting in the closing decades of the nineteenth century, and the Court increasingly was manned by judges receptive to protecting the rights of property against social experiments in the area of labor law and utility regulation. This was the period, stretching from roughly 1890 to 1937, of the doctrine of "due process of law," a term that connotes the transformation of due process from a requirement of fair procedures to substantive rights of persons to hold property and to be free from governmental interference.

The irony is that the new doctrine was almost exclusively developed to protect corporations from legislatures and to treat them as persons under the law. Using the Civil War amendments the courts set themselves up as almost a council of revision, a supreme tribunal that judged the handiwork of legislatures in all areas, but especially in limiting the scope of corporate discretion in dealing with consumers and labor. Once again, public health was spared, but it was spared only because the Court decided to spare it. As Leonard Glantz notes, while the courts, in the famous *Lochner* case, decided only two months after the *Jacobson* case, perhaps the most celebrated Supreme Court decision upholding broad public health authority, struck down limits on working hours for bakers, they pointedly noted that the case differed greatly from *Jacobson* and the earlier case limiting the working hours of miners, *Holden v. Hardy* (1898).[34]

Beginning with the Progressive era drive for pure food and drug legislation, but especially during the New Deal after 1937, the doctrine of "substantive due process" as it was applied to corporations passed from the scene. The courts increasingly refused to stand in the way of a sharp increase in the federal government's role in taxation and regulation of interstate commerce, and its ability to place conditions on federal grants to the states; the federal government used the courts' acquiescence to expand its dominance over the economy, health and safety, and other areas of social welfare. As Kenneth Wing argues,

> The explicit power of the federal government to regulate interstate commerce has been expanded to include not just the power literally to regulate commerce across state borders, but also to regulate goods after they have passed through interstate commerce as well as activities that are only indirectly related to people or goods that have previously been involved in interstate commerce. The courts have also interpreted the federal power to tax as including broad powers to regulate and control whatever federal tax revenues are spent for, the so-called power of "conditional spending."[35]

Paradoxically, as the courts permitted state legislatures great latitude over individual liberty and property in protecting the public's health, they gradually submitted that legislative power to stricter scrutiny, requiring medical and public health expertise to justify quarantine or other forms of isolation from the community. Thus, as the public power over the public's health was being upheld, courts more frequently signaled that they would submit these decisions to a closer scrutiny, a scrutiny that foreshadowed the modern Court's privacy decisions.[36]

One reason the republicanism behind the development of public health legislation is not more widely acknowledged is that the leading case of state regulation in the twentieth century dealt with contagious disease: the 1905 Supreme Court decision, *Jacobson v. Massachusetts*.[37] The Jacobson case dealt with a Cambridge, Massachusetts, ordinance requiring compulsory vaccination in the face of an outbreak of smallpox. The language of *Jacobson* contains an exemplary and classic defense of the police power, but the facts of the case focus on the control of infectious disease, and the overriding necessity for requiring compulsory vaccination to prevent the spread of infection. Because the facts of the case concern smallpox, many scholars have concluded that the principle of the regulatory power is to prevent harms to others. But this interpretation ignores the leading nineteenth-century cases of *Alger, Munn,* and *Mugler* and their stress on community harms as an aggregate or scale principle, and not simply as harms to others.

Justice Harlan, writing the opinion in the *Jacobson* case, had this to say:

> The liberty secured by the Constitution of the United States to every person within its jurisdiction does not import an absolute right in each person to be, at all times and in all circumstances, wholly freed from restraint. There are manifold restraints to which every

117

person is necessarily subject for the common good. On any other basis organized society could not exist with safety to its members. Society based on the rule that each one is a law unto himself would soon be confronted with disorder and anarchy. Real liberty for all could not exist under the operation of a principle which recognizes the right of each individual person to use his own, whether in respect of his person or his property, *regardless of the injury that may be done to others.*[38]

Now it would seem that the plain English of Harlan's opinion would support the view that the *Jacobson* case turns on the crucial point that vaccination is limiting the liberty of persons in order to protect the interests of others.

But it is interesting that in the actual opinion Harlan does not dwell to any considerable degree on the point that the unvaccinated person poses a threat to the rest of the community. Indeed, given the growing individualism that attends interpretations of the police power in our time, plaintiffs today might argue before judges that those who want to be protected can avail themselves of such protections.

I believe that a closer reading of the case suggests that what Harlan was most concerned with was the interest of the public in democratic sovereignty over the conditions of the public health, with its interest in problems of scale, or the republican principle that the legislature must supervise the welfare of the whole body. Elsewhere in the decision, Harlan had this to say:

We are not prepared to hold that a minority, residing or remaining in any city or town where smallpox is prevalent, and enjoying the general protection afforded by an organized local government, may thus defy the will of its constituted authorities, acting in good faith for all, under the legislative sanction of the state. If such be the privilege of a minority, then a like privilege would belong to each individual of the community, and the spectacle would be presented of the welfare and safety of an entire population being subordinated to the notions of a single individual who chooses to remain a part of that population. We are unwilling to hold it to be an element in the liberty secured by the Constitution of the United States that one person, or a minority of persons, residing in any community and enjoying the benefits of its local government, should have the power thus to dominate the majority when supported in their action by the authority of the state.[39]

What Harlan is affirming in this decision is not Mill's harm principle (although he surely would treat as significant the point that the unvaccinated might pose a threat to others) but rather that controlling the public health in a republican scheme requires that citizens submit to legislation designed to promote the common good, even when they might choose voluntarily to accept the risks of infection. This is because defections from such a common scheme would undermine its general effectiveness and the republican principle of legislative supervision of the public's health. Harlan is affirming the right of the legislature to promote the *public health* and to make all manner of laws pursuant to that objective, as well as the idea that no individual can withdraw from the compact of the community.

More recently, two constitutional controversies—the fluoridation and motorcycle helmet cases—have raised the same issues in our time as the earlier public health cases.[40] While the courts have generally affirmed the power of the states to protect the health and safety of the public in both of these controversies, in the case of the helmet decisions, the courts show many signs of increasingly blurring the distinction between the community and republican principle behind the police power and the "harms to others" principle, along with its close relative, the "burdens on society" argument.

119

The fluoridation cases are the best recent example of a majoritarian defense of public health regulation.[41] The Supreme Court has refused to review fluoridation cases, presumably because they pose no threats to constitutional rights. Plaintiffs have argued that fluoridation is an attempt to employ mass medication and constitutes a violation of individual autonomy in an area that is properly private. They have argued that the use of legislation checking private rights in order to protect the public health or safety was justified only in the past by the threat of contagious diseases.

A decision of the Washington Supreme Court is fairly typical of the courts' rejection of these arguments:

> Protection of public health includes protection from the introduction or spread of both contagious and noncontagious diseases. There is a direct and significant relationship between dental health and general bodily health. We find nothing in this jurisdiction which limits the police power, solely to the control of contagious diseases. . . . Further, under the police power, a health regulation may be an effective public measure, without the existence of some immediate public necessity.[42]

While fluoridation is not a measure to make water more safe, it is a measure designed to improve the health and safety of the public operating through a basic element of the common environment. Regarding the argument that fluoridation is "mass medication," the Illinois Supreme Court argued that "even if considered to be medication in the true sense of the word, [fluoridation] is so reasonably related to the common good that the right of the individual must give way."[43]

The courts might have pointed out that municipal water supplies became a major battleground for public health and other reform efforts of the nineteenth century; in these issues, control of private property rights was central because the waterworks were often operated as purely private companies.[44]

The courts have not been so consistent on the question of helmet laws for motorcyclists, discussed in Chapter Three. As noted there, forty-nine states adopted mandatory helmet laws after Congress made these regulations a condition of receiving federal highway funds. Although the overwhelming majority of the rulings have supported the states' power to require helmet usage, they have often done so because of the danger unhelmeted cyclists pose for others on the road or because unprotected cyclists may become wards of the state.[45] In 1968, a Michigan appellate court in *American Motorcycle Association v. Davids* overturned the Michigan helmet law.[46] Though the Michigan Supreme Court ultimately upheld the legislation, the appellate court decision in *Davids* is widely cited as containing the core of the argument limiting the police power in these cases. The court cited Mill and the common law principle *sic utere*. As Stone notes, "The court [in *Davids*] held that protection of the individual from himself did not bear a substantial relation to the public health or welfare. Therefore the statute was unconstitutional. The court rejected the argument that the state has an interest in the viability of its citizens, saying that such logic could lead to unlimited paternalism."[47]

The *Davids* decision is a serious departure from the community principle behind *Alger* and *Munn*. Most state courts that upheld the constitutionality of the helmet laws did so by invoking first the community principle, while also citing the principle of harms to others, construing the unhelmeted rider as a threat to others on the highway (because flying rocks or other objects might obstruct their vision) or as potential wards of the state if seriously injured.

These rulings were a response, in part, to the claims of cyclists that unhelmeted riders posed no threat to others. These courts have indicated in the overwhelming number of cases that this is not the legal issue in legislating for the public health and safety. The question was the power of the state to protect what is called here the common good by regulating the common environment. The judges could have noted that the motorcycle, like the automobile, is operated in the public and common world and represents a significant cause of death and disability in our society. Still, the helmet decisions, though upholding the constitutionality of this law, laid so much stress on the risks to others in these cases as to misconstrue the basis of the police power as the harm principle, perpetuating a misunderstanding of the community principle underlying the protection of health, safety, and welfare.

Public Health and the Private Sphere

The police power permitted states to regulate for public health, safety, welfare, and *morals*. In an important development (discussed briefly in Chapter Three), gradually the courts have begun to restrict and narrow the element of moralism in the police power, more narrowly restricting its application in the advancement of the public welfare, especially where these measures conflict with basic, if newly discovered, rights. Public health has added new weapons to its legal and constitutional arsenal—the spheres of privacy and of democratic discussion. These decisions illuminate how a theory of republican equality as it shapes the public's health requires more than a simple or single principle—in this case, popular sovereignty over the conditions of the common life. Such a theory also requires principles that limit popular sovereignty in specific realms of our common life.

The pioneer case in the "new privacies" is *Griswold v. Connecticut* (1965).[48] (I have relied in the following discussion on my colleague Kenneth Wing's excellent review of these cases.[49]) Connecticut law in 1965 made it a crime to

122

use contraceptives: "Any person who uses any drug, medicinal article or instrument for the purpose of preventing conception shall be fined not less than fifty dollars or imprisoned not less than sixty days nor more than one year or be both fined and imprisoned."[50]

Estelle Griswold, the executive director of Planned Parenthood in New Haven, opened a center for the distribution of birth control information, and Planned Parenthood was charged with "aiding and abetting" the commission of the crime of using contraceptives.

Justice William Douglas wrote the majority opinion, arguing that while the Constitution nowhere mentions privacy per se, the specific guarantees of the Bill of Rights have "penumbras, formed by emanation from those guarantees that help give them life and substance."[51] To accept otherwise would permit the government to invade the "sacred precincts of the marital bedroom."[52] In effect, Douglas's and the other opinions of the majority, and the decisions that followed this path-breaking case, created a form of analysis that argued that when fundamental rights like privacy exist (such as in the basic decision to control pregnancy), the legislature can limit that right only on a showing of a compelling state interest.

For Douglas and the other justices, health and safety would be a sufficient and compelling interest to permit regulating (or even banning) the sale and use of contraceptives. But the state had not made such a showing. Instead, the justices indicate that Connecticut was primarily interested in deterring immoral conduct: "The statute is said to serve the State's policy against all forms of promiscuous or illicit sexual relationships, be they premarital or extramarital."[53] While Justice White did not dispute the legitimacy of legislating to prevent promiscuous or illicit relationships (White termed this "concededly a permissible and legitimate legislative goal"), he argued that for the state to use the threat of pregnancy as a deterrence was not only illogical but confounded by the widespread availability—and legality—of contraceptives to "prevent disease."[54] The plain aim of the legislation, and especially the aiding and abetting section, was to control the opening of birth control clinics.

Massachusetts had a law similar to Connecticut's, which had been amended after *Griswold*, regulating the dissemination of contraceptive devices to individuals. (One reading of *Griswold* seemed to make the regulation of commerce in these devices legal but their use protected.) William Baird, a noted reformer and advocate in matters of birth control, gave a device to a single woman after a public lecture, whereupon he was arrested. The Supreme Court in *Eisenstadt v. Baird* found that the right to privacy included not simply the marriage relation but also the individuals involved in making certain basic decisions.

> It is true that in *Griswold* the right of privacy in question inhered in the marital relationship. Yet the marital couple is not an independent entity with a mind and heart of its own, but an association of two individuals each with a separate intellectual and emotional makeup. If the right of privacy means anything, it is the right of the *individual*, married or single, to be free from unwarranted governmental intrusion into matters so fundamentally affecting a person as the decision whether to bear or beget a child.[55]

The opinion of Justice Brennan reiterated Justices Goldberg and White's ridicule of the statute's attempt "to prescribe pregnancy and the birth of an unwanted child as punishment for fornication."[56] Because Massachusetts did not forbid contraceptives to married persons who had obtained them from physicians, such married persons would then be free to use the contraceptives in illicit sex with unmarried persons. And again, because condoms and the other nonmedical contraceptive devices were widely available to prevent disease, the impact of such legislation in deterring fornication was seen as minimal or nonexistent.[57]

(The aiding and abetting statute exposed the accused to up to twenty times the punishment for those convicted of simple fornication.) What is more, Massachusetts had amended its state statute after *Griswold* to protect morals exclusively: "A physician was forbidden to prescribe contraceptives even when needed for the protection of health."[58]

In *Carey v. Population Services International*, the court extended the right of privacy over the decision to bear a child to a minor, thereby committing itself against the theory that preventing the sale of condoms and other devices to minors would help discourage early sexual activity by those under age. Justice Brennan, writing the majority opinion, noted that even the state conceded that "there is no evidence that teenage extramarital sexual activity increases in proportion to the availability of contraceptives."[59]

The effect of these decisions, along with the abortion decisions I discuss next, was to limit the scope of the police power when its application fails to substantially advance a compelling state interest like health and safety. The justices showed a growing impatience with the lack of empirical evidence sustaining the claims of benefits to be gained through legislation forbidding contraceptives and were quick to note the difficulty of achieving the state's objective of preventing immoral conduct. The majority of justices clearly suspected that a central purpose of the legislation is to cast contraception as a moral evil and prevent it altogether. The corollary logic—using the threat of an unwanted pregnancy to prevent immorality—was held up to ridicule and as a threat to health and safety itself.

The implication in these decisions, including *Carey*, is that state protection of morals, though it masquerades as health and safety legislation, may actually threaten the public health. As Brennan notes in *Carey*, the condom and other articles for contraception pose no threat to health and safety, and devices that do are regulated by the Food and Drug Administration. Here the justices in the majority come close to suggesting that the right of privacy extends to all

125

sexual relations in private, even for minors. But not quite: "The Court has not definitely answered the difficult question whether and to what extent the Constitution prohibits state statutes regulating [private consensual behavior] among adults."[60]

In *Roe v. Wade*, the famous abortion decision, Justice Blackmun argues for a woman's right to an abortion on various grounds.[61] First of all, Blackmun notes "the wide divergence of thinking on this most sensitive and difficult question" and the great diversity of opinion on key issues among the churches, the law, philosophers, and medical experts. He notes that in "areas other than criminal abortion the law has been reluctant to endorse any theory that life, as we recognize it, begins before live birth."[62] Blackmun goes on to say that "in view of all of this, we do not agree that, by adopting one theory of life, Texas may override the rights of the pregnant woman that are at stake."[63]

In other words, Blackmun echoes the belief that in a liberal society, because there are many theories of life, none of which may be proven correct, the state may not enforce one of those theories on the citizenry even if that theory is held by a majority, because to do so would impermissibly invade the private sphere.[64]

At the same time, the state has an interest in protecting the health and safety of the pregnant mother and of fetal life. Blackmun goes on to argue that because maternal mortality from childbirth is higher than that from legal abortions, the state has no compelling interest to regulate abortion in the first trimester. The state's interest in regulating abortion in the remaining two trimesters is much greater, and limits the right to an abortion.

As I said previously, one interpretation of these decisions is that the Court has been engaged in renegotiating the bounds of community and majority rule, limiting the scope of state moralism when it reaches into the private sphere, yet affirming that we are, in matters of health and safety, one body and one community, subject to the protection of the legislature.[65] Indeed, the striking down of the majority's power to legislate morality in certain private arenas is not only legitimated by its protection of a basic right, but is also presented as an engine for the further advancement of the common health.

The logical extension of this thesis would have been for the Supreme Court to strike down the state sodomy statutes. A very good case can be made that laws proscribing homosexuality not only violate a basic privacy interest but also threaten the public health by discouraging homosexuals from seeking medical treatment necessitated by their illegal conduct. A few courts have taken this next step, but the Supreme Court in *Bowers v. Hardwick* (1986), in a narrow and very controversial 5–4 decision, upheld the right of the states to legislate against homosexuality.[66]

The Sphere of Democratic Discussion

In yet another path of decisions, the Court has been struggling with the relation between the sphere of free speech and discussion, and the role of market advertising and promotion in influencing the public's health and public information about health and safety. Here, we find the Court expanding the path for health policy in another direction, this time enlarging not the sphere of communal welfare or of privacy but of public discussion.

It has not been so easy to follow this logic in the separate decisions that have emerged, because, as in the privacy cases, what is at issue are often old tangles of moralism and the law and attempts by modern justices to restrict the scope of majority rule when fundamental interests—like freedom of speech—arise. I take up this issue in detail in Chapter Five, but it is important here to connect the various cases and issues.

The competing claims of legal moralism, advertising, and

the public welfare came up most recently in *Holiday Inn v. Tourism Company of Puerto Rico*.[67] The issue was a ban on casino advertising in Puerto Rico, but the public health issue that this case may ultimately determine is whether the federal government can, under the Constitution, ban the commercial advertising of beer and wine (distilled beverages are not advertised on the airwaves because of a self-imposed ban by the distilled beverage industry).

During the early seventies, the Court began to hammer out a doctrine of "commercial speech," eventually producing the decision in the 1979 *Central Hudson Gas and Electric Corp. v. Public Service Commission of New York*, where the majority argued that "it is well settled that the First Amendment protects commercial speech from unwarranted governmental regulation."[68] This doctrine held that advertising of legal products receives a certain amount of First Amendment protection because advertising is part of the political dialogue of democracy. In an earlier case, *Virginia Pharmacy Board v. Virginia Citizens' Consumer Council, Inc.*, this commercial speech doctrine was enunciated: "Commercial expression not only serves the economic interest of the speaker, but also assists consumers and furthers the societal interest in the fullest possible dissemination of information."[69] But because speech proposing a commercial transaction occurs in an area traditionally subject to governmental regulation, the Constitution "accords less protection to commercial speech than to other constitutionally safeguarded forms of expression."[70] Of course, commercial speech is not protected if it is false, misleading, or deceptive.

The controversy between moralism and the public health arose in the casino gambling case in an interesting way. The conservative majority on the Court upheld the right of Puerto Rico to ban casino advertising to its own citizens; the liberal minority dissented, presumably because no pressing welfare or health issues were involved.

The majority opinion applied the test developed in *Central Hudson Gas and Electric Corp.*[71] The criteria developed in that case concern whether the speech being regulated is deceptive or misleading, whether the regulation in question advances a compelling state interest, and whether the means chosen for regulation "fit" the ends in question. The majority found in *Holiday Inn* that reducing the demand for casino gambling was a compelling state interest and that the commonwealth reasonably believed that such gambling would "produce serious effects on the health, safety and welfare of the Puerto Rico citizens, such as the disruption of moral and cultural patterns, the increase in local crime, the fostering of prostitution, the development of corruption, and the infiltration of organized crime."[72] The majority went on to say that "these are the very same concerns, of course, that have motivated the vast majority of the 50 States to prohibit casino gambling."[73] The majority also found an immediate connection between advertising and the demand for casino gambling and that a total ban was not an unreasonable step to take, given that connection.

Justice Rehnquist, writing for the majority, takes note of the appellant's argument that the Court had struck down earlier attempts to limit the advertising of contraceptives and reversed a criminal conviction for advertising services at an abortion clinic.[74] How could the Court allow such advertising while restricting casino gambling advertising? Rehnquist argued that in the two earlier cases "the underlying conduct that was the subject of advertising restrictions was constitutionally protected and could not have been prohibited by the State. Here, on the other hand, the Puerto Rico Legislature surely could have prohibited casino gambling by the residents of Puerto Rico altogether. In our view, the greater power to completely ban casino gambling necessarily includes the lesser power to ban advertising of casino gambling."[75]

Rehnquist notes the related argument of the appellant that because Puerto Rico permits casino gambling for its residents it cannot then bar advertising of this legal activity. But this is, according to Rehnquist, to state the argument backwards. "It is precisely *because* the government could have enacted a wholesale prohibition of the underlying conduct that it is permissible for the government to take the less intrusive step of allowing the conduct, but reducing the demand through restrictions on advertising."[76]

The minority argued that neither "the statute on its face nor the legislative history indicates that the Puerto Rico legislature thought that serious harm would result if residents were allowed to engage in casino gambling; indeed, the available evidence suggest exactly the opposite."[77] After all, Puerto Rico legalized casino gambling and permitted its residents to patronize casinos. The minority believed that the main purpose of the act was to prevent other forms of gambling from declining, especially the Puerto Rico lottery.

In the dissent, Justice Brennan commented in a footnote that the majority

> seeks to buttress its holding by noting that some States have regulated other "harmful" products, such as cigarettes, alcoholic beverages, and legalized prostitution, by restricting advertising. While I believe that Puerto Rico may not prohibit all casino gambling directed to its residents, I reserve judgment as to the constitutionality of the variety of advertising restrictions adopted by other jurisdictions.[78]

The running battle between moralism and the public health reveals how central public health is to an emerging and more complex theory of equality being evolved by the Supreme Court and by our society as well. In my view of these developments, society is evolving a more complicated view of the meaning of equality and a more complex view of how to protect the public's health.

Laurence Tribe has offered a provocative theory of jurisprudence that has striking parallels with the idea of complex or republican equality developed by Michael Walzer and employed here.[79] According to Tribe, our society has moved through a succession of models of jurisprudence and constitutional theory, all concerned with ways

> of achieving substantive ends through various governmental structures and processes of choice. . . . Whether by separating and dividing these structures into mutually checking centers of power, by insisting that certain spheres of choice be placed beyond the reach of governmental authority, by demanding that certain problems be affirmatively addressed by governmental action, . . . each model has reflected a conception in which one or more features of the society's overall structure for making decision serves to implement, and at times to mirror, some set of social ideals or values.[80]

What is needed, according to Tribe, is a theory of jurisprudence which seeks to "achieve such ends as human freedom not through any *one* characteristic structure of choice but through that *combination* of structures that seems best suited to those ends *in a particular context.*"[81] Structural justice seeks "particular decision structures for particular substantive purposes in particular contexts, while avoiding generalizations about which decisional pattern is best suited, on the whole, to which substantive aims."[82]

In the oldest tradition, protecting the public health has meant enlarging the sphere of communal provision, often at the expense of private property and sometimes at the expense of individual liberty. Closer to our time, the Supreme Court and the Congress have enlarged the powers of the federal government to promote the general welfare and have staked out strengthened spheres of free discussion and of privacy for all citizens. These new structures of decision (to use Tribe's language) not only serve their own intrinsic ends, they help promote the public's health and safety. I will have much more to say about this in Chapter Five.

Equality and justice today are more complex and structurally differentiated than ever before, using different tools and different logics to dismantle the dominance of moralism or markets over individuals or majority rule. Rights and majority rule are often seen as pulling in opposite directions, but in a mature democracy the freedom to differ is a freedom that can strengthen union and advances our common life. Our common life is indeed not simply a common welfare but a common and continuous public discussion and conflict about the forms of life we all share, and this dialogue constantly, if subtly, serves as one continuous democratic experiment with the freedom to change and to conserve.

Thus, in matters that are most fundamental, a republican equality would permit us to be different and to disagree, and through this very freedom provide security for our common health and safety. In this body of law we see the truth that the good of each of us—the freedom to pursue our own ultimate good—is linked to the good of all of us together. In republican equality we promote our own good and our shared or common good within the same democratic scheme, replacing outmoded and harmful languages of traditional community with the new and more complex "second languages" of republicanism.[83] These languages of complex equality and justice bind the democratic community together with the inherent and healthy contradictions always present in democratic life: the tensions between the rules of the market and the common good, between individuals and the public health, between advertisers and public discussion, and between the majority's morality and privacy.

SPEECH, PRIVACY, AND THE PUBLIC'S HEALTH

In this chapter I explore more fully the realms of health policy beyond the sphere of communal provision. Beyond the domain of communal welfare where goods and protections are enjoyed in common, the health of the republic also depends on a wide and robust sphere of democratic speech and controversy, as well as a sphere where the right to individual dignity and privacy is carefully guarded.

This chapter is divided into two parts. In Part One, I explore the connection between free speech and democratic discussion and the public's health. I note the tendency of the market and moralism to limit the range of discussion and speech available to citizens and the need for governments to intervene, regulating advertising and limiting moralism to provide more controversy and speech. I end this section by returning to the Supreme Court's doctrine of "commercial speech" introduced in the last chapter. The rights to free speech and a free press are almost universally recognized as cornerstones of our democratic system. The media have been called the fourth branch of government, the fourth estate. The availability to the citizens of the widest possible divergence of views on any given topic in order to better govern the republic is axiomatic.

In Part Two, I examine the connection between the right to privacy and the health of the republic. The right to privacy is often thought of as the opposite to the publicity and controversy that are the lifeblood of democracy; privacy is seen as the right to be protected from unwarranted intrusion or to withhold from the world vital information about one's life and biography.[1] But as Gary Bostwick argues, privacy has another meaning: the right to intimate decision.[2] This side of privacy is rather a "freedom to" than a "freedom from"—the right to make certain fundamental decisions about one's present and future life.

Ironically, more privacy (as the right to intimate decision) usually implies more speech: that is, the right to pursue ends or ways of life that are out of the ordinary, even to the point where the majority might hear and see things that challenge traditional values.

Part One: PUBLIC HEALTH
AS MORE SPEECH

We have powerful evidence of the positive role that public controversy and democratic discussion play in improving the public health. By "more speech" here I do not mean what is typically viewed as health education: planned campaigns by government, schools, businesses, or voluntary agencies aimed at individuals, specific groups, or a mass audience to encourage voluntary changes in health behavior. Democratic controversy, or more speech, does not simply mean using mass communications or other means to better educate the public for health. More speech in a democracy means more of the collective but uncoordinated controversy and conflict within a democracy—democracy's talk. Democratic discussion, with its creation of conflict and mass publics around health and safety issues, often (but not always) plays a key role in improving the public's health, setting the stage for both planned health education campaigns, changes in mass behaviors, and policy development, encouraging differing conceptions of problems. As Nancy Milio argues (in discussing the relative contributions of the media and planned education campaigns in controlling smoking),

> In Finland, Australia, and the U.S., it was the long-term effect of health news punctuating the public mind and placing the smoking-health issue on the agenda of public discourse that defined it as a public problem about which people formed opinions. This then provided a social climate in which health instruction, intended to affect personal habits, was carried out. The news reports were not intended to lead to social changes or engender political action, but they did nonetheless tap and strengthen previously submerged antismoking sentiments and efforts. The resulting changes in law, regulation, and public opinion then made the difference in how effective health instruction could be in each of the countries.[3]

The instances where this has occurred are difficult to document with scientific precision, but the weight of evidence suggests a powerful link between democratic controversy and changing health patterns and public policy.

For example, the history of food and drug regulation in this century is as much a history of crusading journalism as it is of public health activism. It was muckraking journalism like Upton Sinclair's *The Jungle* and the series of articles in Edward Bok's *Ladies' Home Journal* exposing the worthlessness and hazards of patent medicine that prompted President Theodore Roosevelt to sponsor the Pure Food and Drugs Act passed in 1906.[4] It was the extensive coverage by the media of the 1937 scandal about sulfanilamide marketed by the Massengill Company (the prescription drug was found to contain diethylene glycol, or antifreeze) that finally broke through legislative roadblocks and drug industry opposition to creation of new standards requiring drug companies to test drugs for safety before trying them out on the public. And again, in the early sixties, the Senate hearings (conducted by Estes Kefauver) on drug prices and the lack of required testing for drug efficacy resulted in more stringent legislation—principally because of the scandal surrounding the sleeping pill thalidomide and the fetal defects this drug produced, publicity that paradoxically also helped open the early rounds of the abortion conflict.[5]

I mentioned in Chapter Three the power of the media in effecting the birth of the health and safety legislation in the Great Society; crusading media helped activists like Ralph Nader persuade Congress to pass health and safety regulations and helped make family planning, contraception, and world population growth national issues. The Great Society was the period in our history when the media's joint role, along with activists and public officials, in promoting public discussion and informing the public and the policymaking process with alternative conceptions of the good of society, became most explicit and self-conscious.

The role that democratic discussion now plays in health policy is perhaps best illustrated by the radical redefinition of the role of the U.S. Surgeon General from head of the rather obscure commissioned officer corps of the Public Health Service to our leading national spokesman on public health issues, from smoking to AIDS. Similarly, chief health officers like David Axelrod in New York State have made the media and democratic controversy a primary resource in mobilizing public support for aggressive public health action, from regulating hospitals to securing statewide antismoking initiatives.

This publicity has had direct effects on mass behavior. Since 1967, the American public has witnessed a decline in coronary heart disease and stroke rates of 33 percent, a drop of remarkable proportions.[6] The reasons for it are complex and still poorly understood; the decline in smoking likely is partly responsible, as is increased detection and treatment of hypertension. Changes in dietary practices to reduce blood fats and cholesterol, as well as increased exercise and weight loss, are probably important factors, too.

Promoting this sea change in mass behavior has been the volume of publicity devoted to heart disease, its causes, and the measures that might prevent it. As Linda Brewster and Michael Jacobson of the Center for Science in the Public Interest point out, there have been major shifts in our national diet since the fifties: Whole milk consumption has plummeted while low-fat milk sales have risen sharply; egg consumption has fallen by one-third; and butter consumption has fallen from 18 pounds per capita annually to less than 5 pounds.[7] The public commotion over diet and heart disease is not solely responsible for these changes, but it has been a material factor in making heart disease a matter of common concern, informing the public about diet and health, and providing a context for more explicit information, thus leading to a shift in dietary patterns.

Smoking is another example of the power of discussion in a democracy to promote the public's health. Kenneth Warner has provided some startling data showing the power of discussion in the antismoking controversy to shape policy and behavior. Warner, in a path-breaking analysis of the precipitous decline of levels of smoking in the United States since the early sixties, ties the fall in smoking levels from over 50 percent of all adults to roughly 30 percent to public controversy over and discussion of smoking.[8] Per capita consumption has declined in the United States in every year since 1973—an amazing reversal of previous trends. Warner's statistical analysis of these trends shows how the release of the Surgeon General's report on smoking in 1964, the debate over labeling cigarettes later in the sixties, the brief period of "equal time" when counteradvertising competed with cigarette ads in 1968–1970, and finally the removal of cigarette advertising from television and radio, after an initial surge in sales because counteradvertisements disappeared, contributed to sharp drops in the rates of smoking.

In another article, Warner and Hillary Murt estimate that this discussion has resulted in the savings of as many as 200,000 additional lives between 1964 and 1978, a remarkable achievement.[9] (Of course, as Warner and Murt point out, 4 million people died prematurely because of cigarette smoking during that same period.) Warner argues that

> while individual anti-smoking "events," such as the [1964] Surgeon General's Report, appear to have had a transitory and relatively small impact on cigarette smoking, the evidence . . . indicates that the *cumulative* effect of years of anti-smoking publicity [by 1975] has been substantial . . . [and] that per capita consumption would have been one-fifth to one-third larger than it actually is, had the years of anti-smoking never materialized.[10]

Warner and Murt note that studies of the impact of highway safety legislation estimate that setting new standards for highways and for automobiles saved 62,000 lives between 1966 and 1978. The number of lives saved by the anti-smoking campaign appears to be far greater than that.[11]

Indeed, this point suggests some limits to the power of discussion and health education. For risks like those of driving without a seat belt, mass education and public discussion have not appreciably caused Americans to buckle up—until laws were passed, seat belt use remained at roughly 15 percent. The "fallout" of public controversy seems mostly tied to the big diseases like heart disease, cancer, and stroke or to decisions to abandon using products like the pill (when it was suggested that for many women it might cause an increase in the risk of blood clots).

Warner argues that the antismoking publicity not only engendered declines in smoking and prevented disease and early death, he believes that this publicity also helped organize antismoking publics, which in turn became key groups pressing for increased state and local restrictions on where and when smoking was acceptable and even for higher levels of cigarette taxes.

The role of an expanded speech and discussion is far more than simply helping the public—as a series of individual citizens—live more healthfully. Public discussion and controversy help reshape the entire climate of public opinion, often changing the very definition of the problem under discussion, raising an issue to the status of a public agenda item. As Lawrence Wallack argues, democratic controversy and an expanded speech can help make health more a communal than an individual problem. Controversy focuses attention on the structural determinants of hazards like smoking or dietary practices, helping to recruit new publics to press for social change, and increasing awareness among the public that these are not merely individual problems— they are at the same time public problems, shaped and limited by corporations, advertising, and money.[12]

The AIDS epidemic may be shaping up as another instance where public controversy, discussion, and the media have helped shape important changes in sexual behavior.[13] Despite the media's initial reluctance to give as much attention to AIDS (acquired immune deficiency syndrome) as they did to the swine flu and Legionnaire's disease—primarily because AIDS affected special groups like homosexuals—the American media has devoted more and more

139

television and newspaper space to the details of the epidemic and to more and more explicit discussion of how AIDS is spread. In areas like San Francisco, the attention and controversy has been extensive and very frank, mainly due to the work of a gay reporter for the San Francisco *Chronicle*, Randy Shilts. It is in San Francisco and New York that we have the most extensive reports of changes in sexual activity. Again, we cannot conclusively attribute these changes solely to extensive media discussion, nor can we conclude that changes in sexual practices are sufficient to alter fundamentally the course of the AIDS epidemic. But in the absence of other evidence, we are entitled to presume that public discussion in general and specialized media have materially contributed to positive changes in sexual behavior, particularly among well-educated homosexual males living in New York and San Francisco.

One concrete way in which the media have helped inform the public is by making the deaths and suffering of AIDS victims more visible to the public. Obviously, the death of Rock Hudson triggered a turning point in media coverage of AIDS. But the media, by giving the disease a human face, help make the risks of AIDS, for groups like homosexuals and addicts as well as for others at lower risk, more credible and real. Those who study risk assessment by the public agree that either knowing someone who has suffered some serious disease or having tangible and visible evidence of the workings of the disease through extensive media coverage tends to increase not only awareness of danger but also a willingness to act in ways to avoid that danger.[14]

One special issue is the use of warning labels, from labels on cigarette packages and advertising to saccharin warning labels and labels on alcohol. Recently, in a report requested by Congress on the effects of warning labels, the Department of Health and Human Services reversed itself and supported a warning label policy for alcohol that took into account the tendency for labels, over time, to be ignored and that used imaginative designs and specific information to gain the attention of the public.[15] The report appropriately focuses significant attention on the task of informing the public in the context of larger public controversy, which is the primary aim of labeling policy, rather than focusing narrowly on trying to change dangerous health habits. The purpose of labeling is to promote and advance democratic discussion—discussion that advertising for alcohol undermines and suppresses. Labels properly considered are meant not to cause patrons to climb off bar stools but to promote a wider discussion and education about the role of alcohol and the public health and to oppose the tendency of advertising to undermine that end. This is what is usually meant by the consumers' right to accurate information.

Advertising as Limiting Speech

Despite the role of democratic controversy in promoting the public's health, we should not drift into the facile equation of a free media and an informed public with a constantly improving public health. In many ways the media seriously distort the information available to the public about the public's health. This is primarily due to the role of advertising and the market as they convert the mission of the nation's media from informing public discussion into means of delivering audiences to advertisers.

Perhaps the most notorious way advertising subverts free speech is by direct intimidation. A right to free speech helps assure that those who speak "shall not be questioned in any other place."[16] But this norm is sometimes cast aside in the market realm. For example, tobacco advertisers expect consideration for the revenues they provide magazines and other media, often withdrawing advertising from major

141

media that cover antismoking stories. Some magazines deliberately limit coverage of the hazards of smoking to protect their cigarette advertising revenues.

The cigarette companies have been able to use their advertising clout to buy silence on the hazards of smoking. Small and big magazines alike are involved in a sort of conspiracy of silence on the risks of smoking. *Mother Jones*, a small liberal political journal, lost all of its advertising revenues because of two stories on the risks of smoking. R. C. Smith, in an article in the *Columbia Journalism Review*, documented the link between advertising and coverage of cigarettes and disease.[17] For example, he noted that in a 1976 cover story on the causes of cancer run by *Newsweek*, cigarettes as a leading cause were given minor treatment.

According to Kenneth Warner, *Time, Parade, Newsweek*, and *U.S. News and World Report* derived, in 1981, 17.2, 25.4, 15.8, and 14.6 percent of their advertising revenues, respectively, from cigarette advertising.[18] Some magazines, like *The New Yorker* and *Readers Digest*, refuse cigarette ads.

As Warner documented in 1983, the American Medical Association, in collaboration with *Newsweek* magazine, ran a special supplement on health practices to protect and promote health.[19] Despite page after page of detailed health information, only a sentence or two was devoted to smoking, the leading health risk of our time. (The mention of alcohol was similarly negligible.) Something of the same series of events occurred the next year with *Time* magazine, collaborating with the American Academy of Family Physicians.

"In 1984 over \$2 billion was devoted to promoting the product, . . . over \$8 for every man, woman, and child . . . and \$35 for each of the nation's 56 million smokers."[20] (In 1970, the Public Health Cigarette Smoking Act excluded cigarette advertising from the airways, and the industry substantially increased its advertising in print media.)

The data do support one aspect of the "commercial speech" doctrine of the Supreme Court introduced in Chapter Four. The justices have argued that more speech may be better medicine than "enforced silence." In the case of cigarette advertising we have some evidence that this is true. Hamilton has analyzed the decline in smoking rates in the United States, and he argues that the most dramatic declines have occurred precisely when both advertising and counteradvertising and publicity are in force.[21]

George Seldes, in his autobiography, *Witness to a Century*, notes that Ralph Nader and his crusade against unsafe automobiles helped change a situation in which the press routinely ignored or gave scant attention to attempts by Congress to address the unsafe conditions of the nation's automobiles. The first congressional hearings on automotive safety were held in 1956, but until Nader was tailed by a private detective stupidly hired by General Motors a decade later, the press largely ignored the series of public conferences, studies, and data that called attention to the dangers of American automobiles. Many newspapers even refused to name the brands of automobiles believed to be most unsafe by public health researchers. And as Seldes points out, automobiles, alcohol, and cigarettes are the most heavily advertised commodities in America.[22]

It is the Supreme Court's thesis that more publicity prevents the "highly paternalistic" approach of government silencing advertisers to reduce consumption of legal products. The Court suggests that it would be more effective to shape that behavior directly.[23] Direct regulation makes the purposes of government visible, whereas silence hides those purposes. Yet advertising in many areas is little more than an economic means of "enforced silence" about the risks of commercial products.

Advertisers and corporations, for their part, frequently advance the thesis that advertising functions not to create new needs but to reinforce established ones and to switch users of one brand to another. Warner has some interesting data on this point. As he notes, the cigarette industry has a compelling interest in recruiting new smokers among the nation's youth:

Since 1964, the industry has lost an average of one and a half million smokers each year to quitting. If the industry now loses from 1 to 1.5 million smokers to quitting and perhaps a million to death (an estimate of the number of smokers dying annually from both smoking-related and other causes), approximately 2 to 2.5 million people must become new smokers each year simply to keep constant the total number of smokers. With about 90 percent of beginning smokers being children and teenagers, this means that at least 5000 children and teens have to start smoking each and every day.[24]

Warner doesn't argue that advertising causes those teens and children to start smoking; he simply points out the powerful interest the industry has in their starting, an interest the companies are nearly powerless to resist in a competitive marketplace.

The Commercial Speech Doctrine Revisited

In the next section I will review in somewhat more detail the major cases noted in the last chapter regarding commercial speech. I hope to show that these decisions err in destroying the commonsense distinction between commercial speech and other types of free speech. Given the evidence I have just reviewed, which demonstrates that more speech and democratic controversy help promote the public's health while advertising can limit that speech and controversy, the commercial speech doctrine needs serious rethinking.

Ironically, the "commercial speech" cases can be traced to a case involving advertising for abortion services, *Bigelow v. Virginia*.[25] On February 8, 1971, in the *Virginia Weekly*, an advertisement appeared stating in part:

144

UNWANTED PREGNANCY?—LET US HELP YOU
ABORTIONS ARE NOW LEGAL IN NEW YORK
THERE ARE NO RESIDENCY REQUIREMENTS
For Immediate Placement in Accredited
Hospitals and Clinics at Low Cost
Contact
WOMEN'S PAVILION

Women's Pavilion was a New York City referral service, helping women find abortion services for a fee. (Referral services often got a "kickback" of a portion of the fees charged by the clinic or hospital.)

The editor of the *Virginia Weekly* was convicted under a Virginia statute which stated that if any person, by "publication, lecture, advertisement, or by the sale or circulation of any publication . . . encourage or prompt the procuring of an abortion or miscarriage, he shall be guilty of a misdemeanor."[26]

Bigelow's conviction was twice upheld by the Virginia Supreme Court. After the first decision, the U.S. Supreme Court announced *Roe v. Wade*[27] and remanded *Bigelow* to Virginia in light of the decision protecting the right of women to obtain an abortion. But the Virginia court argued that its decision was about the legitimate state interest in regulating advertising, not abortion, and that *Roe* did not pertain to advertising.

The Virginia court was relying on the commonsense view that commercial advertising did not enjoy constitutional protection under the First Amendment, a view most sharply expressed in *Valentine v. Chrestensen* (1942), in which the court concluded that the First Amendment imposed "no . . . restraint on government as respects purely commercial advertising."[28] Yet the U.S. Supreme Court overturned Bigelow's conviction in 1972, and, according to Justice Blackmun later, "the notion of unprotected 'commercial speech' all but passed from the scene."[29] As Justice Blackmun stated for the majority in *Bigelow*, the "relationship of speech to the marketplace of products or of services does not make it valueless in the marketplace of ideas."[30]

In *Bigelow*, as Blackmun states, because the case "involved an activity [abortion] with which, at least in some respects the state could not interfere," and because it contained material of a clear "public interest," the case could have been decided without creating a new form of protected speech for advertisers.[31]

But in *Virginia State Board of Pharmacy*, the majority of the Supreme Court moved to establish a substantial degree of protection for commercial speech that involves little more than the proposal for a commercial transaction, in this case the advertising by a pharmacy of the prices of drugs.[32] The theory of the case was stated in the majority opinion:

> Advertising, however tasteless and excessive it sometimes may seem, is nonetheless dissemination of information as to who is producing and selling what product, for what reason, and at what price. . . . [T]he allocation of our resources in large measure will be made through numerous private economic decisions. It is a matter of public interest that those decisions, in the aggregate, be intelligent and well informed. To this end, the free flow of commercial information is indispensable. . . . [I]t is also indispensable to the formation of intelligent opinions as to how that system ought to be regulated or altered. Therefore, even if the First Amendment were thought to be primarily an instrument to enlighten public decisionmaking in a democracy, we could not say that the free flow of information does not serve that goal.[33]

Free Speech and Self-Government

In my view, the new doctrine of commercial speech hopelessly confuses the realms of democratic discourse and the

146

discourse of the market. In *Virginia State Board of Pharmacy* and subsequent decisions, the court has applied the doctrine of free speech to advertising in a way that, at least potentially, has ominous implications for the public's health and public discussion.

This has great bearing on the public's health and safety because the First Amendment promotes public discussion and public education and is as central to the public's health as to self-government. Indeed, self-government, properly understood, is what we mean by public health. To quote Alexander Meiklejohn in his classic *Free Speech and Its Relation to Self-Government*, "As interests, the integrity of public discussion and the care for the public safety, are identical."[34]

Meiklejohn argues that "the citizens of the United States will be fit to govern themselves under their own institutions only if they have faced squarely and fearlessly everything that can be said in favor of those institutions, everything that can be said against them."[35] This is true not just for political institutions but also for economic, social, and cultural arrangements and practices. Because many modern public health problems involve the dark side of the marketplace or call into question traditional values based on deeply rooted and unreflected fears—fears often stemming from ancient and discredited religious prejudices—discussion in a democracy is a principal way in which progress and change in the public health can occur peaceably.

Thus, freedom of speech and the public health are highly congruent interests. But the public and the market spheres are another matter; the task of the political sphere in a republican scheme is to oversee the market in order to protect the common welfare. Public health restrictions on liberty and property to limit the promotion of harmful or dangerous products, including restrictions on advertising, are a staple of public policy in a democratic republic.

But these restrictions should be granted not simply because the restricted activities pose a potential harm to the public but also because the advertising restricts and impedes speech in a democracy. In recent years national advertising, especially on television, has come under direct scrutiny by activists; there have been movements to control or eliminate cigarette ads, wine and beer ads, advertising aimed at children, and the use of sex to promote products. These movements should not focus only on the perils advertising might pose directly to audiences, whether children or adults, but also on ensuring that the government plays a role in affording more democratic speech.

As I suggested in Chapter Four, although a majority of the Supreme Court currently supports a sphere of "commercial speech," there are signs that the majority might not apply the doctrine to public health issues like smoking or alcohol use.[36] But the more important issue is to see the need not simply for government to regulate advertising as directly harmful but also for government to intervene in markets to provide more speech, through policies that limit advertising, that require warning labels, that provide equal time for opposing views, and the like.

As Justice Rehnquist argues,

> In the world of political advocacy and *its* marketplace of ideas, there is no such thing as a "fraudulent" idea: there may be useless proposals, totally unworkable schemes, as well as very sound proposals . . . the free flow of information is important in this context not because it will lead to the discovery of any objective "truth," but because it is essential to our system of self-government.[37]

The remedy for promoting the common good can never be found by requiring state legislatures to "hew to the teachings of Adam Smith in its legislative decisions regarding the pharmacy profession."[38]

Justice Rehnquist argues that the new commercial speech doctrine wrongly elevates commercial speech to the plane of the political. But the bigger danger is that it, along with the growing role of television in politics, *lowers* political and public speech to the plane of the commercial. In this new world, democratic discussion is shaped by the privatizing conventions of television as entertainment and advertising, forces I discuss more fully below. Although free speech has never been unregulated—we have laws against libel, slander, fighting words, obscenity, incitement—nevertheless there has always been something of a commonsense distinction between free speech and purely commercial speech, which Justice Rehnquist refers to as "a seller hawking his wares and a buyer seeking to strike a bargain."[39]

The doctrine that speech does not lose its protection simply because it contains an element of the commercial is sensible. In an earlier case involving a paid political advertisement run by several clergy in the *New York Times* attacking New York City police department's conduct in a civil rights demonstration dispute, the city successfully sued the clergy on the grounds of defamation and also because their speech appeared in a commercial format. The Court, in *New York Times Co. v. Sullivan*, reversed that conviction, arguing that simply because speech had a commercial aspect (appearing in an advertisement) did not invalidate the rights of the defendants to have their speech protected.[40] In *Bigelow* the Court could have reversed the Virginia Supreme Court on the same grounds, arguing that abortion was a protected activity and a matter of surpassing public interest, and therefore advertising for abortion could not be regulated in so blanket a fashion.

Yet as we shall see, the Court adopted a broader doctrine, creating a new realm of protected commercial speech, thereby entering new and dangerous territory. The Court advanced the thesis that advertising, like political speech, is "an instrument to enlighten public decisionmaking in a democracy."[41]

In taking this path, the Court has confused the spheres of the market and of free speech. The root of this confusion can be traced to Justice Holmes's famous dissent in the *Abrams* case, a classic case involving political dissent against American involvement in World War I, in which Justice Holmes argued that "the best test of truth is the power of thought to get itself accepted in the competition of the market."[42]

The majority has relied heavily on this thesis, citing Alexander Meiklejohn as support for the notion that self-government in a democracy is a struggle of opposing ideas to gain support, much like market competition. But Meiklejohn explicitly rejects Holmes's thesis in a way that illuminates the dangers lurking in the emerging commercial speech doctrine.

Meiklejohn argues that though it is true that discussion in a democracy is a struggle of ideas to gain acceptance in the public forum, this struggle is different from market competition. As Meiklejohn states, in the marketplace, "the truth is what a man or an interest or a nation can get away with. . . . [I]ntellectual laissez-faire . . . has destroyed the foundations of our national education."[43] The truth of the market rests on a private and *interested* view. The truth of the political sphere rests on a more general and *disinterested* view—what is good for the body politic and the community as a whole, not a truth limited to what is good for General Electric, or the tobacco farmer, or the automobile manufacturer, or physicians.

The new doctrine, at least potentially, poses a serious danger in those many instances where the domination by commercial interests of the media seriously impedes the public's access to available information about its common health.

The reasons the Court has taken this path are complex. First, the Court in interpreting the First Amendment, except for the broadcast media, has increasingly sought to limit the government's powers to regulate speech, often on the grounds of providing more speech. Thus, in the name of equality, the Courts have steadily curbed the government's powers to regulate all forms of speech—increasing access to speech in all its forms as a way of helping to promote the widest possible amount of information distributed among the citizenry. Because more speech is better than less, and because advertising is a kind of speech, then advertising should be accorded a certain level of constitutional protection.[44]

The Court could have taken a different path. The Court could have preserved the commonsense distinction between commercial and free speech, striking down those instances of regulation of commercial speech when the public interest was overriding. This was the line of argument developed in the *Bigelow* case, where the issue was advertising for abortion. The advantage of this path is that it would have permitted the Court to override commercial and moralizing suppression of speech, recognizing that private interests can suppress speech as effectively as governments.

Then the Court could have continued on its path of equating free speech with equal speech or more speech in the marketplace, seeing the need for government to intervene in the market to provide more factual speech to the public. In the market, the issue is what kind of toothpaste to buy, and the object is to persuade the citizen as an individual consumer or as part of the consuming public to purchase some item in trade. But in public discussion, the focus is not on consumption but on deliberation and resolution of issues dividing the common life, and the question of whether, and in what way, democratic opinion and decision ought to shift.

Thomas Scanlon has made the case for the Court another way, arguing that free speech is central in a democratic society that views the individual as sovereign "in deciding what to believe and in weighing competing reasons for action. . . . A person who acts on reasons he has acquired from another's act of expression acts on what *he* has come to believe and has judged to be a sufficient basis for action."[45]

In Scanlon's view, the state might well limit the liberty of citizens in drinking alcohol or smoking, while refusing to restrict advertising for these products, because the freedom

151

to decide what to believe and to weigh competing reasons for action is more basic. But Scanlon's view, even more than the Court's, moves the debate from the public spheres of the market and of public discussion to the largely private world of deciding and deliberating, making it impossible to make distinctions between the two spheres.

The argument for keeping the distinction between commercial speech and free speech does not necessarily rely on the view that advertising is pernicious in its influence. Much, perhaps most, advertising, is an innocent (if often irritating) diversion. Clearly, advertising also provides useful information to consumers who must make important choices. But to move from an appreciation of the positive functions of advertising to granting it constitutionally protected status is a very large step, one that prevents us from making the important political distinctions we need to make. The fact that advertising is not protected speech does not mean that legislatures should or will saddle it with meaningless or harmful regulations.

Scanlon's argument, like the Court's, is yet another variant on simple equality: More speech is the best way of breaking the monopoly of money and its speech. But this solution does not recognize those occasions when the power of money and money's speech mean *less* speech and threaten the public's health by seriously constraining the scope of public discussion. The Court's doctrine would obliterate the older and wiser view that money has its appropriate sphere and should be kept there, and that the legislature is the best place to lodge the power to safeguard the public's interest in fostering a wider public discussion about the public's health.

Here we see how the "market's truth" and "democracy's truth" can be at odds. As Hannah Arendt argues in her essay "Lying in Politics," there is a fundamental difference between the "defactualized speech" of advertising, with its interest in presenting an attractive image to the consumer, and the public controversy and discussion in a democracy for a decision by voters, which depends on at least some connection between claims made and the facts.[46]

Free speech and its public truth aim to promote the common interest of all in self-government, in discovering the facts of our common life and world, in learning about those conditions that advance or threaten both our republic's welfare and our private welfare. Commercial speech is interested and partial speech, seeking to convert public discussion with its emphasis on dialogue and conflict, to a species of salesmanship or entertainment.

Commercializing Speech

The potential for the commercial speech doctrine to undermine the historic function of public speech is especially grave in the American democracy. The electronic media have long operated under the Fairness Doctrine, the rule established shortly after the 1927 legislation creating the Federal Communications Commission (FCC). Because access to radio and television was limited to license holders, license holders therefore had an obligation to "afford reasonable opportunities for the discussion of conflicting views on issues of public importance."[47] Under the Reagan administration, the FCC dropped the Fairness Doctrine as an obligation on the electronic media. As Bagdikian notes, in most Western democracies, programmatic and centralized parties along with national and dominant media usually help simplify the choices of citizens. But because American parties are weak, because the media are almost exclusively in commercial hands, and because political philosophy is on the endangered species list, the burdens on citizens in making informed and general decisions are extremely heavy.[48]

Our media are almost strictly commercial, operating principally as businesses whose mission is to deliver an audience to advertisers. This doesn't mean that the media never enhance public discussion—that is obviously false. Rather it means we cannot assume that the media will not treat the news as a species of commodity and that there is a need to balance the daily "defactualized" diet fed to consumers and the tendency to make the news a step-child of sales.

Christopher Lasch argues that "the rise of mass media makes the categories of truth and falsehood irrelevant to an evaluation of their influence."[49] Neil Postman, in his *Amusing Ourselves to Death*, argues that Big Brother and the Ministry of Information are not our biggest danger, nor even censorship by the big corporations.[50] The big danger is that public discourse and even politics itself will be converted into a species of show business and entertainment—that public discourse will be trivialized by reducing the news to a species of entertainment.

Harry Frankfurt, in a wonderful 1986 article "On Bullshit," notes the pervasive existence of bullshitting as a form of deception quite different from lying.[51] The liar, as Frankfurt notes, honors the rational and the truthful by lying and deliberately misleading us on matters of fact. The bullshitter, on the other hand, deceives by drawing attention away from matters of truth and falsity altogether. The liar sells us a mink coat actually made of fake fur; the bullshitter sells us a coat, whether mink or not, draped on the shoulders of a nude woman.

Advertising contains, as Frankfurt notes, an inordinately high amount of bullshit: speech that contributes almost nothing to the questions about the actual properties, usefulness, or limitations of the products it promotes. Advertising like this severs the link between truth and the commodity, making the commodity itself little more than an object of fantasy, vague wishes, moods, or inchoate desires.

For this reason, advertising as bullshit is a more deadly enemy of the common life than is the deliberate lie. Advertising as bullshit is not just "defactualized speech," it is trivializing and diverting speech. Plainly, the advertising of automobiles, cigarettes, alcohol, and other products that cause disease or kill, requires a high level of bullshit—seeking not only to sell products but also to sell the idea that the truth about these products is not even pertinent.

Schudson argues that the ironic side of advertising may be its most important feature—that the consumer grasps that advertising need not be taken so seriously.[52] But the humor surrounding many forms of advertising may contain a more ominous message urging that we abandon any yardstick of truth for advertising.

Schudson refers to advertising as "capitalist realism."[53] Capitalist realism makes consumption the solution to life's problems, and by contrast undermines solutions that require public deliberation, common decision making, and concerted action. As Schudson notes, while public service announcements also invoke values that matter to people, "think how hollow public service announcements sound" when contrasted to the world portrayed in advertising. Advertisements ask for private, do-able consumption acts; public service ads ask for service and sacrifice. People are capable of both, as Schudson notes, but advertising makes acts of sacrifice seem "incongruous."[54]

All of this indicates that the doctrine of commercial speech weakens the power of government in drawing a line—not a bright line that absolutely separates the two spheres, but a line nonetheless—that restores the common-sense distinction between the different purposes of advertising and of free speech and public discussion in a democracy. The commercialization of public discourse makes all speech interested speech; even worse, it threatens to make all speech trivial speech, making truth and public utterances more like commodities or entertainment than democratic criticism and discussion.

What public policy implications flow from rejecting the "commercial speech" doctrine? First, we should recognize that there is a role for the Court in limiting the state's power to regulate advertising. Much commercial speech does serve a First Amendment function, especially when, as in the case of *Bigelow*, the interest in question—securing an abortion—was constitutionally protected.

Also, advertising can be harnessed to promote the public health. The National Cancer Institute endorsed a national advertising campaign by the Kellogg Corporation for high-fiber bran cereals, and research suggests that the campaign resulted in increased purchases of bran cereals.[55] There are many commodities and services in a capitalist society that promote health; more advertising here is to the good.

But generally speaking, in the "commercial speech" cases, the majority of the Court badly confuses the spheres of the political and the market, giving very powerful economic interests the mantle of First Amendment rights to contaminate, not liberate, our public discourse. Here, the Court ought to give way to the judgment of the legislative branch, especially because it cannot be argued that these interests are lacking in political influence and power.

The Court is correct in arguing that legislatures should consider more direct ways of regulating conduct than simply limiting advertising. Far too much of the current drive to control the media and their content, whether for public health purposes or for purposes of enforcing a public morality, is symbolic in nature, a search for painless but visible ways of seeming to act, all the while avoiding the more painful question of whether more direct limits over substances like tobacco or alcohol are needed.

Yet advertising can and ought to be limited and controlled, especially for commodities like alcohol and tobacco, to protect not only the public's health—the common good—but also the public's right to more speech and information. Limits on advertising, controls on its content, requirements for equal time, and even bans of many forms of advertising even for legal products like alcohol and tobacco should be vigorously pursued by state and federal legislators.

Part Two: PUBLIC HEALTH
AS MORE PRIVACY

The privacies of our republic, especially those concerned in the abortion, contraception, and AIDS debates, are often viewed as occupying the opposite shore of our moral continent from free speech, significantly expanding the domain in which we are free to escape the scrutiny of the community, to be left alone to pursue our own private ends.

This may well be true for privacy as repose (freedom from outside disturbances) or sanctuary (freedom to control information about one's person). But it seems far less true about privacy as the right to intimate decision. Here privac˘ suggests an expansion of discussion, speech, participation, and the right to live an autonomous if different life without fear of reprisal and discrimination from one's fellow citizens.

Indeed, in the abortion decisions, as Daniel Callahan argues, the expanding right of privacy has made what was previously private extremely public. These decisions, along with the quickening pace of technology and democratic discussion, have made the fetus more visible to us, even establishing the fetus as a moral claimant.[56] Just as women and men have gained greater rights over their reproductive processes, we have been forced to behold the fetus. And though, as I argued in Chapter Four, the right of women to have access to contraception devices and advice as well as abortion represented a major expansion of the right of privacy, the move is not so radical as it is sometimes represented. We have in earlier periods attempted to limit the reach of the law in matters of private (usually sexual) morality to reflect the evaporation of the moral consensus.

Abortion and Contraception in the Nineteenth Century

William E. Nelson has detailed the gradual decline in Massachusetts during and after the Revolutionary period of criminal prosecutions at common law for fornication, adultery, and failure to attend church.[57] Judges and prosecutors gradually stopped prosecuting these offenses, largely because the nation and the state had sharply changed, from a collection of communities held together by ethical and religious ends to a more pluralistic society. Given this pluralism, stability lay in loosening the claims of moralism, not tightening them; a loosening of the claims of moralism, and law to sanction that moralism, would promote more unity and harmony.

The withdrawal of the common law from areas of sexual morality was not followed by a tightening of the statute law until the later decades of the nineteenth century, when the nation was caught in an intense period of moralizing reforms. During this period, influential segments of society believed that moral decay was threatening society and that laws permitting abortion or contraception led to licentiousness and vice. Thus, the burst of legislation and Court decisions in the Great Society period expanding rights to abortion and family planning were something of a restoration of common law privileges enjoyed before the upsurge in moralizing of the late nineteenth century. Today courts, like the earlier common law judges, have been engaged in a project of rolling back moralistic legislation resting on extravagant claims linking sexual freedom with the moral decline of the republic. Again, the thesis is that the health and peace of the republic often depend on expanding, rather than limiting, the liberties of the citizenry.

As Kristen Luker argues in *Abortion and the Politics of Motherhood*[58] and James Mohr in *Abortion in America*,[59] the abortion controversy is relatively new. While there had been thousands of years of theological disputes about whether the fetus has a soul before quickening (the period when movement of the fetus begins to be detected, roughly four to five months), as a matter of law, in the nineteenth century women or doctors were free in the United States to attempt to abort the fetus before this time. As Mohr indicates, under the common law "the interruption of a suspected pregnancy prior to quickening was not a crime in itself."[60]

Mohr argues that

> the vast majority of American women during the middle decades of the nineteenth century, when contemplating the possibility of an abortion [before quickening], never had to face seriously the moral agonies so characteristic of the twentieth century's attitude toward . . . abortion. . . . In the minds of most Americans at the time, abortion was probably much closer morally to contraception.[61]

Abortion was clearly commercialized in the United States during the middle decades of the nineteenth century. Women had rather easy access to information on abortifacients as well as easy access to physicians and lay abortionists, and there was heavy advertising and promotion of abortion services and products. The abortion rate in the United States during these decades was around one abortion for every five or six live births, close to the present rate of one in four or five births. The birth rate in the United States fell precipitously over the century, and abortion played a role in this decline. Those who were obtaining abortions were predominantly white, middle-class, and Protestant.[62] Abortion and contraception were thus increasingly public matters in the United States.

A Century of Silence

This situation was changed in the period from 1860–1890, largely because of advocacy by doctors, by those fearing a falling birth rate (while immigrant birth rates remained very high), and by moralizers and purity crusaders like Anthony Comstock who spoke of a precipitous decline in American morals.

The work of the reformers began a hundred-year period in which silence about abortion and contraception became the rule, not the exception. The work of American physicians during the twenty years after the Civil War was decisive in enacting restrictive abortion laws, outlawing abortion *before* quickening. American physicians were still something of a motley collection of rival factions, many half-trained and most not trained at all. Those with some semblance of education, scientific training, and status were chagrined that so many of their untrained and illiterate competitors were taking business away from them, accepting the belief of their female clients that the fetus before quickening was not a living being or at least did not have a soul.

The better-trained physicians (called "regulars") recognized that the development of the fetus was a continuous process and that quickening was almost trivial in its scientific significance, and believed that to abort before quickening was to destroy a living being.

The regulars in time joined forces with those crusading against immorality, and abortion, as well as birth control, became associated in the public mind with obscenity and licentiousness, and laws against abortion and birth control were associated with campaigns to restore the republic to a higher standard of sexual purity.

Purity is fundamental in its importance to the individual, to the home and to the nation. There can be no true manhood, no true womanhood except as based upon the law of Purity. There can be no security for the home, there can be no home-life in its best sense, except as it is based upon the law of Purity. There can be no true prosperity, there can be no perpetuation of a nation except as its life is based upon the law of Purity. Impurity is destructive alike to the individual character, of the home, and of the nation.[63]

Physicians became successful advocates in gaining state legislation outlawing any abortion, save those to protect the life of the mother. A central theme of the doctors' campaigns was the dangerous nature of abortion as a procedure, which most now agree was grossly overstated.[64] Congress and state legislatures drastically curtailed not only the availability of abortion but also discussion and advertising about the procedure. Contraception was similarly treated. Abortion by the end of the nineteenth century had become largely illegal except in very specific circumstances; the issue of abortion entered a period of almost total silence and neglect.

From the turn of the century to the post–World War II period several reformers struggled to reverse the decisions, the most famous being Margaret Sanger. The abortion debate lay nearly dormant during this period; the main emphasis was on getting family planning into the public health clinics. This time, it was largely male philanthropists, progressive physicians, and public health leaders who advocated experiments in Appalachia, Puerto Rico, and North Carolina in family planning methods, seeking to compare the efficacy of foam and barrier methods. These various forces were often at odds with one another, but the American Family Planning Association, founded in the thirties, became a key group. After World War II with the successful development of the pill and the growth of concern about the world population explosion, contraception and family planning were successfully lodged on the national agenda during the Great Society.[65]

As these issues slowly moved to the public agenda the

ambiguous and differing meanings of the idea of privacy became clearer. At the end of the fifties, President Eisenhower scoffed at making family planning a political issue, arguing that this was a private matter best left to families (and to state legislation proscribing contraception and abortion). Clearly, by "private," Eisenhower meant that abortion was a topic which a democracy ought not even talk about, much less legislate about. This was a matter for religion and its friends in state capitals.

By the early seventies, this view of privacy was turned on its head, with courts and legislators using the term "right to privacy" to mean that individuals have a right to make autonomous decisions in such areas as sex education, family planning, and abortion without interference by the state, and that these topics were matters for public discussion. Such a right implied that citizens were entitled to know the facts about their reproductive processes and to have more control over their fertility. This right to privacy clearly implied the existence of private and even public agencies that would assure effective access by all in society to such knowledge and services, even if some in society found such knowledge and practices immoral or wrong. Thus privacy as the right to intimate decision clearly has its public side, implying an expansion of the freedom of speech, of assembly, and of public discussion and access to services that are fundamental to an individual's life.[66]

Abortion Today

Today, there are roughly 1.6 million abortions performed yearly in the United States.[67] This sounds like a lot of abortions, but it is likely that the abortion rate has not radically increased over earlier periods. To put things in perspective, a classic study of the number of abortions performed in the United States during the thirties, a time when almost all abortions were illegal, put the number of abortions somewhere between one-half million and one million.[68] It has been estimated that the Court decision itself likely increased the annual rate of abortion by 250,000 each year.[69] On the other hand, the decision probably decreased the number of later abortions. Roughly 90 percent of all abortions now occur within the first twelve weeks of gestation; in 1973 this figure was closer to 85 percent.

Roger Wertheimer, in a widely quoted article, "Understanding the Abortion Argument," argues that what has happened in the abortion debate is that the common understandings underlying what Wittgenstein called "forms of life" have suddenly shifted, and individuals and groups suddenly diverge in matters on which they had apparently agreed before.[70] But this overstates the case. How can we know what the "forms of life" were during a century when moralism suppressed not only abortion but public discussion and debate about abortion? The new "forms of life" behind the abortion decisions are the spreading consensus that democracy must protect the right of every individual to make certain intimate decisions that are fateful for his or her entire life without interference. The claim that the fetus is a person at any stage of its development is an attack on a basic foundation of the modern democratic republic, the rights of privacy and individuality, which, as Bostwick argues, have very old roots.[71]

Wertheimer's thesis was written without much historical perspective, and before the Supreme Court decision in *Roe v. Wade*. Indeed, the period from 1860 to 1960 was a century of massive silence about a topic that had enjoyed substantial publicity and discussion previously. If anything, the activity of the Great Society, both on the part of Congress (in repealing the Comstock legislation in 1970 and in providing for family planning in its community action programs) as well as state legislation liberalizing abortion laws were attempts to free the topics from a century of moralism.

Making the Private Public

Hixon argues that *Roe v. Wade* made the moral status of the fetus a private matter, a matter of mere opinion, a move that is roughly parallel to the Court declaring that the issue of freedom of speech is a matter of mere opinion.[72] But this is plainly wrong. *Roe* clearly establishes that the unborn are *not* persons and therefore are not entitled to the rights and immunities of those who are born. What *Roe* did was to decide that the view that the unborn *are* persons is a private and religious view, one the Court could not conceivably entertain.[73]

Again, *Roe* underscores the way privacy, as intimate decision, makes some private matters extremely public. The point seems to be that the right of privacy as it implies the right to contraceptive devices, abortion, sex education, and (perhaps eventually) homosexuality, is usefully ambiguous: It both places the intimate decision beyond the reach of government and publicly protects controversial intimate decisions. This has widespread public consequences in the way women, adolescents, and homosexuals are treated as well as in the general discussion of sexuality and reproduction in American life.

Indeed, perhaps the central feature of the right to intimate decision is that it nearly always touches deeply upon fundamental issues that are extraordinarily controversial. At the core is the democratic faith that conflict and diversity promote social order and cohesion, at least in the long run. As Justice Blackmun noted in *Bowers v. Hardwick* (quoting Justice Jackson):

> We apply the limitations of the Constitution with no fear that freedom to be intellectually and spiritually diverse or even contrary will disintegrate the social organization. . . . [F]reedom to differ is not limited to things that do not matter much. That would be a mere

164

shadow of freedom. The test of its substance is the right to differ as to things that touch the heart of the existing order.[74]

A good deal of our history has been devoted to moral crusades designed to protect society from deviations from some putative sexual or moral standard. The grip of moralism over public policy has produced in the United States the highest rate of teenage pregnancy in the developed world.[75] (The parallels between a moralizing approach to sex and such an approach to drugs are striking, as we see in the next chapter.) Because we refuse to accept the reality of sexually active teenagers, we enact legislation against family planning services like sex education and contraceptive services, as though such legislation would delay the age of onset of sexual activity. The attack by moralists on sex education, school-based clinics to provide contraceptives to sexually active teenagers, and free discussion of the risks of unsafe sex among homosexual lovers threatens the public health in direct and tangible ways. Instead of facing the sobering reality of a swelling population of poor, uneducated teenage mothers and the reality that one child in five is born into poverty, moralists focus on such issues as saving seriously ill newborns in expensive neonatal care centers.

The *Baby Doe* cases, concerning the right of seriously ill newborns to survive,[76] and the question of how and whether to care for seriously ill newborns, are not unimportant issues, but they clearly divert attention from the far greater tragedy of the epidemic of adolescent pregnancy, the growing numbers of children born out of wedlock, and the United States' rate of infant mortality—highest in the developed world. Some public officials are seemingly more worried about preventing the public from learning the facts of homosexual sex than combatting the epidemic of AIDS. The growing use of the fetus to dramatize consumer or voluntary risks (like smoking- or alcohol-related fetal anomalies) and work place risks to fetal and maternal health has further enhanced the moral claims of the fetus. Surrogate motherhood threatens to shift attention even further to the issue of the fetus and to treat the mother as simply a maternal environment or, as George Annas notes, a "fetal container."[77]

Privacy, Intimate Decisions, and Autonomy

Justice Stevens, in his dissent to *Bowers v. Hardwick*, the recent case about homosexuality, argues that rights to privacy represent something more fundamental than the right to

> unwarranted public attention, comment, or exploitation. They deal, rather, with the individual's right to make certain unusually important decisions that will affect his own, or his family's destiny. The Court has referred to such decisions as implicating "basic values," as being "fundamental," and as being dignified by history and tradition. The character of the Court's language in these cases brings to mind the origins of the American heritage of freedom—the abiding interest in individual liberty that makes certain state intrusions on the citizen's right to decide how he will live his own life intolerable.[78]

This right to intimate or fundamental decisions clearly means far more than withdrawing from the community; in the end it means freeing the community and the common life from a narrow moralism, broadening its foundations to support a republic of equals in which each is free to challenge traditional truths.

Blackmun, in his dissent to *Bowers*, argues that we protect privacy rights not because they contribute, in some direct and material way, to the general public welfare, but because they form so central a part of an individual's life. . . . "[T]he concept of privacy embodies the moral fact that a person belongs to himself and not others nor to society as a whole."[79]

As he further states, "We protect the decision whether to have a child because parenthood alters so dramatically an individual's self definition, not because of demographic considerations or the Bible's command to be fruitful and multiply."[80]

Further, Blackmun argues that the injunction that

"traditional Judeo-Christian values proscribe [homosexuality]" gives the State no license to impose their judgments on the entire citizenry. The legitimacy of secular legislation depends instead on whether the state can advance some justification for its law beyond its conformity to religious doctrine. . . . A state can no more punish private behavior for intolerance than it can punish behavior because of religious animus.[81]

The intense moralism that surrounds the abortion issue and all matters of sexuality weakens and effaces the complex idea that a republican equality requires a vigorous public discussion, popular sovereignty over the common welfare, and a strong private sphere. No one can say how, or whether, we can withstand these challenges, but it is clear that if we are to be a democratic republic of equals, we shall need ways to defend our common life from enemies and false ideals far more powerful than those inhabiting distant lands.

PROHIBITION
AND THE LEGACY
OF MORALISM

Alasdair MacIntyre, in a widely quoted passage, says that "modern politics cannot be a matter of genuine moral consensus. Modern politics is civil war carried on by other means."[1] I believe that MacIntyre is wrong about the demise of community in at least some of its forms, but his notion of modern politics containing long-standing civil wars over crucial issues is illuminating. Just as the Civil War lingers over black–white relations in the United States, so does the Prohibition experience overshadow alcohol and drug policy and public health generally.

The Prohibition experience and its legacy of moralism has been tremendously important in determining the bounds of our policy for alcohol and other drugs. And the moralism that was at the heart of Prohibition may well be on the

169

upswing again, threatening health policy for AIDS, drug treatment, teenage pregnancy, and even the prospects of a common health care system. We may never be able to remove moralism from American life—indeed, to seek its elimination would be a fateful mistake—but the central issue is to prevent moralism from dominating public policy outside its proper sphere, becoming a kind of civil religion that takes the place of genuine politics in a republic of equals.

What Was the Mistake of Prohibition?

A truism of our time is that everyone can recognize the awful political mistake of Prohibition. But knowing that Prohibition was objectionable and knowing precisely why are not the same thing. What precisely was the mistake of Prohibition?

For some, the mistake was Prohibition's making matters with alcohol worse. This is plainly wrong, as we shall see. To others, the mistake of Prohibition was its attempt to legislate private morality. Drugs, these people think, especially alcohol, should be matters of personal behavior, off limits to government except when harms to others are involved. As John Stuart Mill argued in *On Liberty*, drunkenness is not a fit subject for legislation.[2] But I stressed in Chapter Three that although Prohibition was politically unwise, surely it is just as unwise to declare drugs and drinking purely private matters, outside the reach of communal health protections.

The mistake of Prohibition was in letting concern about drunkenness and the saloon turn into a kind of mental medievalism, using the metaphor of the epidemic and claiming to purify society, purging it of threatening or alien elements. The idea that Prohibition was simply an outburst of the puritanical enthusiasm carried throughout America, in Richard Hofstadter's phrase, by the "rural-evangelical virus" is too general a characterization of the hundred-year experience of Temperance and Prohibition.[3] But it is accurate in describing the ultimate goal of Prohibitionists. Prohibition became a crusade against a moral virus, a crusade that sought to put the entire society into a permanent quarantine against the agents of alcohol problems, which were believed to be a predatory alcohol industry and the "vicious" elements of society: the poor, the laboring classes, Catholics, and immigrants. Prohibition became a kind of civil war inspired by the hope of resisting the advancing modern society by imposing a traditional moral order on the republic.

Today, America is in the midst of a new antialcohol movement. Researchers, newspaper writers, and television commentators speak of a new temperance movement. In a few short years, we have embraced twenty-one as the legal purchase age for alcohol nationally. After almost a generation of stability, taxes on distilled spirits were raised at the federal level, even if not for public health reasons. Sales of alcoholic beverages are either falling or not rising; millions are cutting back on their drinking or stopping for health reasons. Drunk driving legislation is being tightened everywhere, and local communities are legislating against "happy hours" in bars and lounges, or the practice of discounting drinking to increase sales.

The alcohol industry and its allies charge "neoprohibitionism." These groups argue that the new temperance falsely blames the substance of alcohol for what is at bottom a "people" problem. This $75 billion industry has mobilized to resist attacks on what it terms its constitutional rights to market and promote a legal product. In its view, law and policy never solve alcohol problems; the only successful movements to control alcohol have been religious in origin and have done their work outside of government: Government and alcohol don't mix.

While the reaction of the alcohol industry against regulation has a familiar ring, even outsiders must view the new temperance with a certain amount of uneasiness. Are we witnessing the unleashing, once again, of an unstable moral crusade that threatens the prospect of sensible and workable limits to drinking and drug taking? Could Prohibition happen again? Or is the new temperance the normal and long-overdue incorporation of alcohol into the sphere of communal health protections?

Alcohol and the Early American Republic

Most Americans would probably accept H. L. Mencken's indictment of Prohibition as evidence of a deep Puritanical flaw in the American character, a mean-spirited, haunting fear that "someone, somewhere, [may be] happy."[4]

But this familiar view of American Puritanism is seriously flawed.

In fact, alcohol was legitimate and widely used by the Puritans and throughout the American colonies. While drunkenness was condemned on occasion, the generous use of alcohol was part of daily life in the colonial order. Alcohol was regarded as a fortification against the ardors of hard work and as generally safer to drink than water. The tavern was a central part of colonial life. The assurance to travelers of a warm and hospitable inn with ample drink was a matter of public policy.[5] The tavern keeper in the seventeenth century was a person of some social standing, charged with serious community responsibilities.

This positive attitude toward alcohol began to shift gradually during the eighteenth century. Rorabaugh estimates that yearly per capita consumption of absolute alcohol (age fifteen and above) increased from 5.1 gallons to 6.8 gallons from 1710 to 1820.[6] (Current yearly per capita consumption stands at 2.65 gallons.) Most of this increase was in distilled beverages, with the sharpest increases occurring from 1770 to 1820.

The increases in the drinking of distilled beverages were due to a number of specific factors. Rum prices fell off during the last decade of the eighteenth century, and rum imports rose at the same time. Distilled whiskey also became an important farm product; there was an excess of grain, and small farmers could easily convert this grain into cheap whiskey and transport it over poor roads or by waterways without spoilage. At the same time, the tavern was changing to a "grog shop" and then a "saloon" where the "lower orders" drank. Tavern keepers began to lose their status. Further, as Rorabaugh notes, drunkenness was a badge of rough ,equality in America.[7] Drunkenness was a little like death—a rough leveler of all men.

These changes alarmed revolutionary leaders such as Benjamin Rush, John Adams, Alexander Hamilton, George Washington, and Thomas Jefferson. Benjamin Rush argued that ardent spirits are the "anti-Federal . . . companions of all those vices calculated to dishonor and enslave our country."[8] Rush advocated limiting the number of grog shops, raising taxes to make drink more expensive, and instigating a federal campaign equal to the public health campaigns against yellow fever of the late eighteenth century. Earlier, Hamilton, in *Federalist Number 12*, advocated the increase of excise taxes on alcohol to discourage intemperance and to raise revenues. "The single article of ardent spirits, under Federal regulation, might be made to furnish a considerable revenue. . . . [I]f it should tend to diminish the consumption of it, such an effect would be equally favorable to the agriculture, to the economy, to the morals, and to the health of society."[9]

The Congress passed such a measure in 1790, which resulted in the Whiskey Rebellion, the first serious challenge to the new federal government. The rebellion was really a local protest led by Pennsylvania farmers who felt singled out by the tax (while the Federalist leadership drank untaxed madeira). But the concern about drunkenness and the sharp increase in the use of spirits was felt in all quarters.

Jefferson, no friend of the Federalists, grew increasingly alarmed at the wide use of distilled spirits, especially rum and whiskey, and believed that the use of ardent spirits sapped civic virtue.[10] The use of ardent spirits encouraged "licentious" and "vicious" behavior, which in the high Federalist vocabulary meant disregard for order, lack of self-discipline, and contempt for authority. The Democrats (then called Republicans) were also deeply worried about the increase in drunkenness.

This concern with spirits can only be understood in the context of American democratic thought. American revolutionary leaders were almost morbidly preoccupied with the decay and decline of republics; this theme dominates the *Federalist*. The republic stood on the central pillar of *virtue*, which meant not private or ascetic denial but the preference for the good of the whole community rather than private selfish gain and the absence of *luxury*, an amount of wealth and ease that encouraged lack of civic concern.[11] This idea of virtue was essentially a public and political one. The rise of the Temperance movement in the 1820s and its succession by Prohibition can be traced in significant part to the element of democratic and republican theory that emphasized virtue in the citizenry as a pillar of the sound republic.

Prohibition and the Mischief of Faction

The course of the Temperance and Prohibition movements, from roughly 1820 to 1933, is not simple. The complexity of motives, groups, and goals of this protean social movement is only now becoming clear after a long period of neglect by scholars. (See Aaron and Musto for a good review of this literature.[12]) It comes as a surprise to most that Temperance and Prohibition stand squarely in the mainstream of the American reform tradition, drawing on many of the same ideals and remedies that motivated abolition, the

174

women's movement, prison reform, Populism, and the Progressive movement.[13]

As Daniel Bell has noted,

> The attack on the saloon allowed the Prohibition movement to bring together many diverse elements under one political banner. For the small-town native American Protestant, the saloon epitomized the social habits of the immigrant population. For the Progressive, the saloon was the source of the corruption he felt to be the bane of political life. For the Populist, it became the root of his antipathy to the debilitating effects of urban life.[14]

Bell could have added that for the feminists, the saloon represented oppression by besotted and violent spouses. Capitalists also joined the campaign against the saloon as a measure to increase the reliability of the working class.

But Prohibition in the end became moralism, and the highly individualistic vision of social change that was behind nearly all Temperance and Prohibition became a kind of civic moralism.

The individualism in Prohibition sprang from that side of Puritanism that stressed a militant religious appeal to individual conscience and called for individual moral reform as the road to societal reform. In this strain of Puritanism and evangelism, society was less a complex, interdependent order and more a battalion of true believers called to live up to a high standard of personal and visible piety. This ascetic and private standard for behavior became the central pillar of Prohibition, a civil religion that was to redeem the entire republic.

The current revisionist interpretation of Prohibition stresses the broad continuity between Prohibition and movements like Progressivism. Aaron and Musto note the emphasis in Prohibition on closing down the saloon and eliminating the "liquor traffic" as employing many of the ideas found in the public health movement in battling epidemic diseases.[15]

But as David Musto, writing elsewhere, has noted, public health has long been divided over the best means for battling an epidemic.[16] During the nineteenth century and earlier there was a keen debate over whether epidemics of yellow fever, typhus, or cholera were best controlled by quarantine and isolation or by sanitary improvement— clean streets, ventilated factories and housing, waste disposal systems, safe water, and a pure food supply. The more progressive elements of public health, following the lead of Edwin Chadwick in England and Benjamin Rush and Lemuel Shattuck of the United States, believed that lack of "domestic sanitation" was the root cause of epidemics, and that quarantine and isolation not only destroyed commerce but also disrupted the social fabric, turning entire communities into vast lazar houses, locked up against dangers from abroad or from outsiders.

Prohibitionists did come to embrace the metaphor of epidemics, but they strove to avoid blaming the victims for their problems. As Aaron and Musto note, "The liquor industry was perceived as quintessentially parasitic; the descriptive images of the prohibitionists were loaded with metaphors of cholera. Alcohol infiltrated the drunkard's body and the social body, breaking down self-control, and eventually resulting in a befouled and excruciating death."[17]

But metaphors of epidemics nearly always force a community to see both the purveyors and victims as morally contaminated. As Aaron and Musto note, the middle classes came to believe themselves to be immune to the avarice of the rich and especially the alcohol trusts on the one hand, and the addiction of the "vicious," now seen as the poor, an increasingly restless working class, the immigrants, and the uneducated, on the other. What was needed was national Prohibition to restore a coherent moral order destroyed by the Civil War, decades of corruption in Washington, and national greed. By eliminating the saloon and the liquor traffic, the source of the disease (or infection) would be removed, and the United States could look forward to an alcohol-free generation that would regard "drinking as a moral perversion and the purveyor as a felon."[18]

What is striking about these images is not so much their reliance on modern public health but their reliance on the medieval metaphors of the plague, casting national Prohibition as a kind of "plague-wall" against the depravity of a rich class of entrepreneurs and the weakness of the vicious lower orders. In this imagery, moral and physical pollution are deeply intertwined. As Antonin Artaud has written, "The plague . . . is the revelation, the bringing forth, the exteriorization of a depth of latent cruelty by means of which all the perverse possibilities of the mind are localized, either in an individual, or in a people."[19]

Prohibition at one time had its progressive side, and no doubt some features of a progressive public health's focus on changing the environment was behind the desire to rid the country of the saloon. But the Temperance and Prohibition movements lacked the singular features of the reform movements of the late nineteenth century: local and state bureaucracies staffed with clerks and inspectors. In other reform movements, fledgling bureaucrats checked on conditions, produced reports, and advocated change before elected bodies. As Oliver MacDonagh notes, these official agencies became the agents for the continual reform and change of society, but this process never happened for alcohol.[20]

In the second wave of Prohibition, which began after the Civil War, the Prohibition party, the Women's Christian Temperance Union, many Populists, and others saw Prohibition as a way to unite a society being industrialized and dividing along class lines. In this phase, Prohibitionists sought to ally themselves with other, more progressive, movements for reform.[21] But advocates of broad-gauged ideals about social justice could never shake Prohibition and the deeper and more entrenched view that eliminating alcohol from American society would move it closer to a virtuous and a just republic.

Actually, most reform movements of the nineteenth and early twentieth century mingled this kind of moralism with more progressive notions about changing the material conditions of the industrializing society. Thus, many Progressives embraced Prohibition to get at the evils of the city machine and the saloon, but many also agreed that Prohibition would remove from society a moral menace and purify society in all its limbs. Still, the moralizing of Progressivism ultimately took a back seat to the more liberal thought found in the writings of Herbert Croly, Walter Lippmann, Walter Weyl, and others.[22] These thinkers stressed not a politics of moral purity but the need to balance the individualism of the laissez-faire period with community controls over enterprise, thus building a national community and generally strengthening government to promote the common welfare.

Norman Clark has described the central feature of the Prohibition and earlier Temperance movements.[23] Because of the momentous changes occurring in America in the late eighteenth century and during the nineteenth century, the spheres of the public and the private became more sharply separated. Men and women departed the moral gaze of the small town into the impersonal anonymity of the cities, the factories, and the mines. America became a land of immigrants, factories, saloons, and slums as the moral homogeneity of family, church, and community began to diminish. A constant stream of immigrants further frightened some reformers. The tumult of the nineteenth century produced wave after wave of reform movements that sought not only to clean up the environment but to purge the environment of moral evils, seeking to protect the sphere of the private—the home, the family, women, and children—from contamination and pollution by the evils of a strange new world.

The problem with Prohibition was not that temperance cannot be legislated. National Prohibition proved that the law can encourage temperance. The adoption of national Prohibition, first with America's entry into World War I and later by constitutional amendment, *viewed only in public health terms*, was a striking success.[24] The consumption of alcohol fell by more than two-thirds, and cirrhosis rates fell to half the level that obtained in 1910. Although consumption gradually rose during Prohibition and the impact of Prohibition fell most clearly on the working class (beer consumption was hardest hit), nevertheless two years after repeal, total consumption of alcohol was only one-third of the 1910 level. And though Prohibition was unpopular with many segments of the population throughout the twenties, it was consumer capitalism and the shock of the Depression that doomed Prohibition, not public outrage. The organization that led the drive for repeal, the Association Against the Prohibition Amendment, was a right-wing group that reorganized the day after repeal as the Liberty Lobby, a group that opposed most of the Roosevelt economic program and advocated the repeal of the income tax.[25]

The Discovery of Alcoholism

After repeal a new set of ideas about alcohol problems arose. Determining to set aside moralistic and political approaches to society's alcohol problems and promising no more crusades to cure America's drinking habits, new groups — Alcoholics Anonymous (A.A.), the Yale Center for Alcohol Studies, and the National Council on Alcoholism — formed in the thirties and forties and adopted a "scientific" (i.e., nonmoralistic) approach to studying chronic addiction to alcohol, what they called alcoholism.[26]

It would be an oversimplification to claim that the collapse of Prohibition set the stage for the idea of alcoholism.

Actually, as the Prohibition experiment was occurring in America, some of the conditions for its unraveling were already well advanced. Obscenity standards were being relaxed, sexual standards were loosening, and the ethics of hard work and savings were shifting toward consumption and leisure. America was discovering a good time. The individual was moving even farther from the gaze of the law or the community, an emancipation celebrated in book, magazine, and film.

As part of this cultural emancipation, the advocates of the idea of alcoholism stressed two simple ideas. The first was to "de-moralize" alcohol, drinking, and drunkenness, and to remove the idea that alcohol was a central problem in American life. To many in the alcoholism movement, moralists like the Prohibitionist Carry Nation had the biggest alcohol problem of all; obsession with alcohol as an evil substance.[27]

The de-moralization project was to be accomplished through dissemination of the second major idea about alcoholism: The alcoholic suffered from a disease that could be treated. Making social problems into medical problems tends to privatize them; in the case of alcoholism this was especially true. The idea of alcoholism was based on the notion that most persons were immune to alcohol problems—that alcohol was a threat to only a small and vulnerable minority.[28]

Now the idea of addiction to alcohol was held by Benjamin Rush and even many Prohibitionists, as Harry Levine points out.[29] But contrary to the logic of Prohibitionism, alcoholism was a condition affecting only a minority of Americans, even though that minority numbered in the millions. It was a new fact of life that most individuals drank safely, drank as "social drinkers." The new conventional wisdom became that most Americans drank safely and had personal control over their drinking, a view Prohibitionists could not accept.

As social policy, the idea of alcoholism seems the very opposite from Prohibitionism—and in the early decades of the alcoholism movement it was very different. The concept of alcoholism, in the early going, shifted the focus of attention from "Why do we have such an alcohol problem?" to "Why do I have an alcohol problem?" The alcoholism experts continually stressed that a significant percentage of American drinkers—roughly 5 percent—were alcoholic, but they were not very interested in explaining the level of problems in society. They were more interested in what characterized alcoholics as a class of vulnerable individuals, seeking to explain why they, rather than others, suffered from the new disease.

The tradition of anonymity that eventually came to dominate A.A. expresses this private view of alcoholism perfectly. Despite the fact that A.A. had grown in size as a result of favorable publicity in a *Saturday Evening Post* story in the early forties, A.A. eventually decided to embrace the principle that its members could not identify themselves by name as members of A.A. and that A.A. would never associate with any cause, religion, sect, or controversy.[30] While the tradition of anonymity reflects the view that alcohol problems were individual ones, anonymity frustrated the mechanisms of publicity by which most problems in a democratic society are promoted; it also lent support to the view that alcohol, drunkenness, and drinking were in no way connected with larger alcohol problems in society.

Shielding the Industry

Thus, in order to *de-moralize* society's alcohol problems, the alcoholism movement sought to *depoliticize* alcohol problems, even shielding the industry from potential criticism. This way of viewing alcoholism would not create powerful enemies in the alcohol industry or among the vast majority of America's drinkers. As one leading writer in the movement noted, and many echoed, "Although alcoholism would be impossible without alcohol, alcohol can no more be considered its sole cause than marriage the sole cause of divorce, or the tubercle bacillus the sole cause of tuberculosis."[31] The idea of alcoholism, because it located the problem in the person rather than the bottle, was the perfect alibi for an industry desperately seeking to expand its sales after Prohibition.

Selden Bacon, a leading researcher in the alcoholism movement, wrote an influential article in 1958 arguing that "alcoholics don't drink."[32] His point was that the alcoholic drank for drastically different motives from the vast majority of drinkers, who drink for reasons of sociability and conviviality; the alcoholic was ingesting alcohol, not drinking at all in that sense.

Another leader of the alcoholism movement, Morris Chafetz, compared the progress made on alcoholism with that made with tuberculosis.

> For centuries, the focus was on the substance—alcohol. The belief that alcohol caused alcoholism was reinforced when specific organisms . . . were found to be related to the cause of some diseases. . . . Most people have the tubercle bacillus within them and have not developed active tuberculosis. Most people drink and do not become alcoholic.[33]

With the focus on the issue of "Why me," the alcoholism movement was at first not much interested in preventing alcohol problems; its focus was treatment. Indeed, it probably sensed that the idea of prevention might bring back the idea of inherent harm in alcohol itself, a development the alcoholism movement strongly wished to prevent.

Prevention as Domesticating Drinking

Eventually, however, the growing movement began to develop a theory of prevention that explained how alcohol problems occurred and what society must do about them. The new theory was in some ways the eerie negative of Prohibitionist logic. The Prohibitionist believed that society needed fundamental reform in order to protect the sanctity and the purity of the home. If the virus of the liquor traffic could be removed, all of society could rapidly move toward that stable familial order the Prohibitionist believed was captured in most small-town, Protestant, and abstemious life.

The alcoholism experts turned this idea inside out. The new idea was to prevent alcoholism by domesticating alcohol use in America, integrating it into everyday life. They saw society's moralizing as the problem; it was the American ambivalence toward alcohol that was the primary virus of alcoholism. Most Americans could drink safely; those who could not were impaired by a culture that created deep conflict about the use of alcohol.[34] Some even went so far as to argue that students should learn to drink at school, much as they learn to drive automobiles.[35] Because American society had an ambivalent tradition toward alcohol—largely attributed to American Puritanism—many in America grew up without much experience with the drug, believing on the one hand that it was an evil substance and on the other hand that it possessed powerful, even magical, properties. Other societies that had normalized alcohol use—the standard examples were Italy or orthodox Jewry—supposedly experienced few problems with alcohol.

Here we encounter one of the chief legacies of moralism. Moral crusades nearly always produce wild swings in the opposite direction; decades of treating all drug use as moral suicide led to the era of the sixties and early seventies, when many researchers regarded drug use as trivial in terms of health and social consequences. The alcoholism movement did force society to stop treating the alcoholic as a moral scapegoat. This victory of the movement is a primary safeguard against moralism's turning into neoprohibitionism. But the movement's unscientific and ideological opposition to prevention as regulating alcohol commerce only undermines another way in which alcohol could be approached in a more effective, stable, and nonmoralizing manner.

The Discovery of Prevention

Prevention—removed from the shadow of moralism—did not really get a start as an idea in the response to alcoholism until the National Institute on Alcohol Abuse and Alcoholism (NIAAA), primarily devoted to expanding treatment resources for the sick alcoholic and conducting research into the cause, cure, and prevention of alcoholism, was founded in 1971. The public health perspective for alcohol control began to gain ground during the seventies in the United States, building on international research of the preceding decade or so.[36] A major influence in making the federal government more receptive to preventing alcohol problems through legislation was the growth of consumer and public health legislation in the sixties and seventies.

The explosion of public health research into the risks of smoking, the automobile, alcohol, and the American high-fat diet undermined the logic of preventing alcohol problems by making alcohol more widely available. Researchers from around the world began to discover the links between high levels of societal drinking and high levels of alcohol problems.[37] That research demonstrated beyond any question that where alcohol is normative and widely used, and especially where wine is treated as a food and commonly served at meals, the result is a very high rate of per capita consumption of alcohol and high rates of disease and death related to heavy consumption of alcohol.[38] So much for the idea that, at least in modern industrial societies, where alcohol is domesticated, alcoholism and alcohol problems tend to vanish.

In countries where total consumption of alcohol is high, rates of cirrhosis tend to be correspondingly high.[39] This relationship appears causal: As alcohol consumption in the aggregate rises or falls sharply, cirrhosis rates—an excellent index of chronic consumption in a population—rise and fall. Researchers have also noted the strong relationship between alcohol availability—especially taxes and age restrictions—and the level of some alcohol problems in society.

Speaking very generally, the more alcohol is restricted in its availability, or the higher the effective price, the lower the rates of overall consumption and problems like cirrhosis and highway accidents due to alcohol. Studies also reveal that sharply curtailed alcohol availability (for example, during strikes by employees of state stores selling alcohol) reduces consumption and problems, and that the rapid liberalization of alcohol restrictions brings in its train sharply increased drinking and alcohol-related problems. Also, age restrictions and limits on the number of retail outlets reduce overall consumption and some problems. For example, James Blose and Harold Holder convincingly demonstrated that such marginal shifts in legal availability as permitting the sale of liquor by the drink resulted in significant increases in drinking levels and associated problems in North Carolina.[40]

Alcohol research began to attract official attention. A book on alcohol policy, *Alcohol Control Policies in Public Health Perspective*, by an international group of researchers and social scientists in the alcoholism field, appeared in 1974.[41] This book was instrumental in bringing the neglect of alcohol control policy to the attention of U.S. policy-makers. In 1978, the federal government asked the National Academy of Sciences to study the evidence supporting alcohol control measures and other preventive strategies. The result was *Alcohol and Public Policy: Beyond the Shadow of Prohibition*, a book that has had a major impact in creating a more favorable climate for alcohol policy.[42]

The new public health research created great tensions in the NIAAA. At least in its early years, the NIAAA's primary mission was to expand the nation's alcoholism treatment resources. Although it has no direct regulatory powers, it does have prevention responsibilities, primarily in providing public information and conducting research into effective prevention strategies. As the "public health perspective" for prevention began to build and gather support, pressures mounted for the agency to publicize these data and to abandon its earlier "responsible drinking campaigns" meant to placate the alcohol industry.

A principal focal point for this controversy was the *Special Reports to the U.S. Congress on Alcohol and Health*, modeled after the Surgeon General's reports on smoking and health.[43] Dr. Ernest Noble, an eminent alcoholism researcher and the second director of the NIAAA, took up the challenge and in a series of speeches argued that the nation should adopt the "per capita consumption" thesis, or the idea that limiting the growth of per capita consumption of alcohol was central to a successful alcohol strategy. This advocacy probably played a major role in his dismissal by superiors in the Department of Health, Education, and Welfare during the Carter administration.

The cuts in federal spending have reduced its role in treatment in the eighties, and there are indications that the NIAAA has in recent years sought the safer harbor of a new mission as a research institute; nonetheless, the new public health perspective has established a beachhead in the agency, and it cannot ignore the new temperance movement.

Moralism and the New Temperance

Actually, the label the "New Temperance" is potentially very misleading. The perspective that would treat alcohol like other public health risks and require more limits over the price, advertising, and physical availability of alcohol seeks only to expand the sphere of communal welfare to include alcohol controls. This approach, which is integral to a republican equality, differs in spirit from moral crusades based on a common and abstemious lifestyle that informs and purifies every other realm.

The difference between the two approaches is not easy to make or maintain. But it seems to me that there are two very different approaches to the common life in a democracy. In one, drug policy (and policy for sex and family life) is elevated to the status of a civil religion, which would underpin all other values in America, building its future by holding on to the virtues of an imagined past. This idea of the common life, based as it is on a mixture of religious and moralizing views, far from being open to more equality for all Americans, seeks to defend traditional values against egalitarian reforms. Proponents of the common life as a civil religion see a uniform and standard morality in matters of personal conduct and a stereotyped American family as the bedrock value for all the spheres of society and as the binding force for social cohesion. In this view, traditional and private virtues determine the public good in all spheres.

This was the central idea behind Prohibition, and of the purity crusades against prostitution, obscenity, birth control, sexual promiscuity, and so forth. In this view, because private conduct was the foundation of public virtue, public policy needed to protect the private realm vigorously. And because the problems that threatened the private realm were regarded as moral evils rather than problems, no compromises with evil—even a little evil—could be accepted.

In a more complex and republican equality, the common life of society rises from the interplay of a series of differentiated and interdependent spheres distributing different social goods. Immunizing the public against alcohol problems by radically safeguarding some idealized private conduct does not work. The public realm deserves protection in its own right through policy and regulation of the marketplace and of public practices. Private behavior is not off limits to public scrutiny; the notion that society has no interest whatsoever in whether people drink too much or whether they take drugs is not defensible, as I argued in Chapter Three, where I noted how a radical autonomy underlying all spheres of society undermines the integrity of the communal sphere.

Among new temperance advocates, there are disturbing signs that many who are interested in limiting alcohol are also interested in the dangerous idea that some specific set of traditional values, especially when inculcated in our young people, will preserve the republic. Thus, there are clear fault lines between the new temperance groups who are moralists and those who follow a more egalitarian emphasis on alcohol and other drugs as public health problems, not moral evils. The difference between the two groups is captured in the basic split over whether the ideal of a drug-free America is feasible given the ubiquity of alcohol and tobacco in our culture. For example, there are people seeking to label alcohol as a risk to pregnant mothers and as a danger to the fetus who also wish to make a larger moral statement about abortion and the fetus and who are often linked to the pro-life movement; another group wants to label alcohol for the same reason other consumer products are labeled: to enlarge the range of democratic controversy about alcohol and to overcome the influence of alcohol advertising as one means of protecting the public's health and safety.

Many who oppose teenage drinking and argue for abstinence for adolescents are also fighting a strong campaign against drug use in America that has moralistic overtones. The anti–drunk driving forces contain both those who want to raise the drinking age to protect the young as part of a broad strategy of shielding America's youth from a drug-oriented culture and others who want to raise the drinking age primarily on public health grounds, to demonstrate that legislation saves lives. Some want to ban advertising for beer and wine on television because advertising makes for bad public health generally, of which teenage drinking is only a part; others want to ban advertising principally because of its impact on teens and because of television's shaping of teen values.

The public health groups have the data and the momentum from the second Great Society; the new moralists have the "grass-roots horsepower" and can use the regulatory momentum and the data for their own ends. It is hard to predict where this will lead, and which of the several justifications for increasing the state's power over alcohol will prevail.

The Uses of Moralism

Prohibition today seems so alien, so restrictive and repressive—so illiberal and unmodern—as to be unthinkable to most Americans. The odds against another era of Prohibition, at least in the form it took during the earlier part of this century, are very great. The main reason the burden of proof falls to those who would argue for a new Prohibition is our own history of failure in cultural or moralizing politics and the genuine threat to personal liberty coming from moralism dominating public policy in a pluralistic, egalitarian society. Further, most of what we could accomplish in health and safety under Prohibition could be achieved through more stringent regulation of alcohol. Prohibition is something like ringing a doorbell with a cannon.

189

However, given the new, almost $2 billion "War on Drugs" now underway in the United States, it might be helpful to understand better the tremendous appeal of moralism in the field of drugs generally and why moralism is more likely to surface in our drug policy than in our alcohol policy.

The place to start looking for wisdom about Prohibition is the acknowledgement that our drinking practices have clearly changed as a result of the moral crusades of the past. Roughly one-third of the American populace does not drink, a rather astounding figure when one considers the international experience. This group of abstainers became smaller during the Great Society and the early seventies but seems to have returned to its historic size during most of the postrepeal era.

The other side of the coin is not that two-thirds of the American public does drink but that among those who do drink, the vast majority drinks very little. When we add it all up, roughly 60 to 66 percent of Americans are functional abstainers—abstainers or nominal drinkers. And that is not the whole story.

Dean Gerstein of the National Academy of Sciences constructed a table illustrating the distribution of drinking among the American public. Using a total of 2.65 gallons of alcohol consumed annually per capita (roughly today's level of consumption) he noted,

If we were to reduce the overall U.S. consumption curve to a representative sample of 10 drinking-age adults, their annual consumption of absolute ethanol would not be very different from the following rough approximation: 3 nondrinkers, 3 drinking a gallon among them, and the others drinking 1.5, 3, 6 and 15 gallons, respectively. . . . [O]ne drinker . . . consumes 57 percent of the total; two drinkers . . . consume 78 percent of the total.[44]

Put another way, 80 percent of all beer is drunk by 20 percent of all beer drinkers; alcohol consumption is concentrated in heavy consumers.

Thus, our overall consumption of alcohol is powerfully shaped by the moral crusades of the past, which have left many Americans nominal abstainers. A successful alcohol policy would not seek to eliminate the remnants of the past that encourage minimal or no use of alcohol, but would seek to prevent that past from breaking out in new crusades that divert attention from the steady task of building sensible limits to alcohol commerce, limits that hold the alcohol industry responsible for its practices rather than depict it as a pariah.

Thus, the beginning of wisdom in alcohol policy and policy for other drugs is to acknowledge our debts to the moralism of the past while avoiding the temptation to re-create its excesses, as with the moralistic rhetoric that surrounds the current "War on Drugs." Cries that America is being destroyed by drug use and that drug use in America is like the return of the plague in medieval Europe are common enough—and at a time when the use of all drugs, including alcohol, is declining in a decade-long trend.[45]

At the center of the new moralism is the exclusive focus on drug use among youth: Drugs threaten the very future of the republic by destroying our youth. This focus is an excellent example of what Nils Christie has termed the temptation of the state, in times of repression, to extend the duration and consequences of childhood.[46]

We see in this movement the difficulty posed for public health policy—we need more controls over alcohol without allowing those controls to turn into a new moral crusade. The answer seems to be not in abandoning democratic controls over alcohol—indeed, these need to be markedly expanded—but in making these controls conform to the larger sphere of collective protections any egalitarian society should seek. The middle road of limited but powerful public health protections like tax increases, curbs on advertising, the limits in general availability—measures aimed at the entire citizenry—is, along with treating alcoholics with respect, the safest path to avoid the "re-moralization" of alcohol.

Policy for Other Drugs

The difficulty of avoiding new moral crusades is even more acute in policy for other drugs. Here the issue is more complex because the task of prevention entails a much larger role by law enforcement. While treatment for the addict—including some form of drug maintenance—instead of jail has become the rule rather than the exception, this policy has had to overcome many decades of a strong, moralizing stance toward drug abuse that rejected most treatment programs for the addict, especially those that provided drug maintenance as treatment.

Many of the conflicts in establishing treatment for addicts can be traced to the federal Harrison Act of 1914 and subsequent Supreme Court decisions that, by 1919, had declared maintenance programs illegal. The history of conflict is too byzantine to relate in any detail; David Musto's *The American Disease* does this admirably, and I rely on Musto's history for the summary in the section that follows.[47]

In broad outline, the Harrison Act was a response to a growing campaign against drug addiction in the United States. It was aimed partly at drug use by Chinese and blacks but was also aware that the United States at the end of the nineteenth century had a very large addict population that was not black or Chinese. The number of addicts at that time has been estimated as perhaps as many as 250,000, and this number included many middle-class individuals.[48] Doctors and women were especially at risk for addiction.[49]

This unusual situation was the result of a fascinating set of circumstances in the nineteenth century, circumstances that echo those surrounding the abortion and contraception issues. Drug use in America, much like abortion, was relatively unregulated for most of the nineteenth century. Morphine and cocaine were widely used in proprietary drugs or were easily obtained from doctors for a wide range of maladies. Given the competition among doctors for patients, the parlous state of medical science, and the large number of doctors with very limited training, the widespread prescription of addictive drugs was common. In some periods these drugs were directly available from pharmacists. Cocaine was at one time added to shots of whiskey to increase the kick; in some regions it was peddled door to door.

The fear of drug addiction as a social problem nevertheless began to grow, partly because prominent physicians warned of the dangers of addiction and partly because drug use by those minorities was seen as symptomatic of a decaying moral order. At any rate, restriction of addictive drugs took its place alongside other campaigns for moral and environmental reform. As Paul Boyer argues, "At the heart of Progressive reform lay the dual convictions that human misery and social disorder were rooted in environmental maladjustments, and could be corrected by men of good will."[50] These men of good will, as we have seen with Prohibition, had differing ideas about how to alter the environment and eliminate human misery.

For those in the Progressive ranks who tended to see problems as moral evils (rather than as human problems), the temptation was to try and root out a problem altogether. Hence, Prohibition for alcohol, and prohibition for drugs, with the elimination of maintenance for those already addicted.

The problem of maintenance began to surface when the nation slowly began to tighten the availability of drugs, first with the Pure Food and Drugs Act of 1906, which required labels indicating the presence of addicting drugs in patent medicines. (States had already begun to take steps to limit the capacity of pharmacists and physicians to prescribe drugs, tough restrictions on the powerful proprietary industry were ignored). Labeling alone seemed to reduce consumption of narcotic-laced proprietary drugs to one-third its original level.[51]

The Harrison Act of 1914 went much further than labeling drugs sold in interstate commerce; it was intended to change the prescribing habits of American physicians, a proposition that at the time was probably not constitutional. The act was a revenues measure: A tax on certain drugs carried record-keeping functions for physicians and pharmacists with it. Addicts themselves were not permitted to register under the act. Persons who were found in possession of such drugs without a legal prescription could be prosecuted, as could the pharmacist and doctor who provided the drug.

Thus, long before the major expansion of the interstate commerce powers of the federal government after 1937, Congress used a revenue measure to regulate the practice of medicine directly and the behavior of every addict in the nation. At the heart of the legislation was the attempt to prevent doctors from prescribing a maintenance level of drugs for addicts and to close down pharmacies and clinics that did the same. For some physicians, prescribing for addicts was a minor part of their practice; for others it was their entire practice.

While American physicians generally were anxious to remove the moral cloud of "dope doctors" that hung over their profession, they were concerned when the federal government so suddenly and so directly interfered with their profession. Pharmacists were similarly alarmed. Yet physicians and pharmacists were anxious to strengthen the public reputation of their profession by excluding their poorly trained members. At the same time, many physicians and public health officials directly acquainted with the problem of addiction were concerned that the sudden drive

by the federal government (by way of the Treasury Department) to eliminate drug addiction would abruptly leave
tens of thousands of addicts stranded and drive them to
illegal sources, with their higher prices and the resultant
increase in crime.

In the first court test of the act, in *U.S. v. Jin Fuey Moy*,
the Court ruled that the Harrison Act as drafted did not
permit the federal government to prosecute physicians who
were maintaining addicts.[52] In 1919 the Court reversed
itself, holding that the act did not permit physicians to
prescribe maintaining dosages for addicts.[53] The majority
included Justice Holmes. It is likely that one factor in the
reversal of the Court was that only a few months earlier
national Prohibition had been ratified by the states. Public
opinion generally accepted the "hydraulic theory" of societal
drug use—the notion that the denial of alcohol would lead
to a surging demand for other drugs. With this Court ruling,
physicians fell under federal legislation that required them
to demonstrate that, in prescribing for addicts, they were
attempting to reduce their use and to "cure" them.

At the same time Internal Revenue agents moved against
a number of public clinics that had sprung up, mostly in the
second decade of this century, to provide a cheap, stable
source of supply for addicts. By 1925 these were largely
eliminated, although some local maintaining practices were
tolerated. Overall the policy that evolved was forced incarceration for addicts. Penalties for drug use continued to be
increased. A new special tax for marijuana was legislated in
1937.[54] Drug penalties were tightened again during the
early fifties, another period of domestic repression.

All of this began to change in the sixties as drug use
spread to the youth of the American middle class. It was one
thing to put poor blacks in prison for possession of marijuana, but quite another to put college students in jail for
such offenses. The Supreme Court in *Robinson v. California*
ruled that a person could not be incarcerated merely

for being an addict; it came close to the same decision in chronic drunkenness.[55] Increasingly, the emphasis in federal and state policy shifted toward treatment and civil commitment, not incarceration, for drug abuse.

Today, for the most part, simple possession of marijuana is rarely prosecuted except as a misdemeanor. Even simple possession of heroin is seldom prosecuted.[56] It is likely that the steep climb in marijuana use, at least on an experimental or occasional basis, has discouraged prosecution of this drug. As many as 50 million Americans admit to having tried marijuana at least once during their lives.[57] We are reaching the point at which more people try marijuana than smoke cigarettes regularly.

Heroin remains largely confined to an older, predominantly black population, one that now has very high levels of HIV infection. One of the most important issues in AIDS policy is to get heroin addicts to stop sharing needles, as this is a major source of HIV transmission. Many see an expansion of methadone maintenance programs as a way not only to reduce heroin use but also to stop the spread of AIDS.

While we still, at least in the media, treat drugs highly moralistically, as an unmitigated evil with which there can be no compromise, in practice we seem increasingly to accept the reality that drug abuse, like alcohol abuse, is a reality of modern society. The best we can hope for is to control this condition, a policy that combines legal suppression of supply, both here and abroad, with more humane and compassionate treatment of users and addicts, even offering some form of maintenance as an alternative to obtaining drugs in illegal settings. The difficulty is that we have yet to express that commitment to abandoning the moralism of the past by funding an adequate, extensive treatment and maintenance program for drug addicts, one that provides—for every addict who wants it—an alternative to the constant struggle of trying to maintain the habit.

Conclusion

Again, the purpose of examining the experience of Prohibition and its legacy is not simply to lay out a model policy for alcohol and drugs but rather to explore in some detail the structual features of a republican equality that seeks to limit the outbreak of moralism as much as it seeks to check the dominance of markets.

Moralism as a civil religion must be resisted in all of its forms; at the same time, paradoxically, the legacy of moralism in creating safer drinking practices should be preserved. The danger in modern-day moralism lies with movements that seek to exploit our preoccupation with drugs and their use among young people as a substitute for sensible policy. Refusing even to consider a careful test of the wisdom of providing clean needles to addicts, when the evidence clearly shows that sharing needles spreads HIV, is one striking example of moralizing in drug policy.

Focusing on drug prevention when the evidence suggests that drug use is epidemic among the unemployed poor of the nation's ghettos suggests that more equality in living conditions, jobs, and a promising future are the clearest ways to prevent drug use among America's youth. The government's campaign using simplistic slogans like "Just Say No" does not answer the claims of equality and is an obvious instance of moralism.

On the other hand, it is clear that moralism, in its milder forms, is playing a key role in discouraging smoking. People are quitting not only because smoking harms the smoker or others, but because smoking *offends* nonsmokers. We should welcome the reversal of attitudes of earlier decades that strongly approved of smoking; moralism as social disapproval of smoking (or of drinking and driving, to cite another example) is a welcome trend. But it can go too far:

One example is the placing of signs in drinking establishments warning women of the risks to the fetus. Why single out women? Why only the fetus? Why not put such notifications in the hands of physicians or clinics?

Moralism, like the market, is a permanent feature of American politics. The trick is not to make moralism disappear; that is impossible and probably undesirable. The goal can only be to prevent moralism from turning into a kind of civil religion, which when combined with the religion of the free market, subverts rather than promotes equality. Instead of the Pious Republic, the goal should be the Healthy Republic; a republic of equals that, in its policy for all drugs and in all other realms of health policy, always seeks to broaden the spheres of equality as ballast against the periodic reappearance of new crusades in the name of market efficiency or traditional morality.

AIDS AND THE
FAR SHORES OF
THE REPUBLIC

Let us suppose that a secret group—a kind of underground—with quite extensive membership has existed in
most countries of the world for centuries, perhaps since
civilization began. At its heart are certain rites or practices
that the larger society finds abominable and has declared
illegal; hence, members keep their participation in the group
secret, but at most times they live ordinary lives in the society at large. At some times in history, the group has been
tolerated, and indeed, one contemporary culture has gradually moved toward toleration. In some parts of that country,
the group's practices are no longer illegal, and in various
places, the group engages in these practices quite openly.
Nevertheless, prejudice against the society still runs deep.

Now suppose a deadly epidemic has broken out in the

group. It seems that the epidemic's spread is linked to the group's special practices and that it might decimate the group. Moreover, contact between members of the secret group and others creates a real, but lower risk that the epidemic will spread to society at large. Increasingly members of the larger society demand that the epidemic be combatted more vigorously, that carriers of the disease be identified with special tests. Some even want to quarantine members of the group. However, public health authorities recognize that identification is not possible because the members of the group are unwilling to step forward and risk prosecution. Health officials point out that the very measures society wants to impose—testing, isolation, or quarantine—are cut from the same cloth as laws that have been used to drive the group underground, making its members aliens and prisoners in their own land. Health authorities are concerned that not only are these vigorous techniques not feasible, but that they will simply drive the group farther underground and may make the epidemic spread more easily to the rest of society. What should the health authorities do?

The parable of the secret group and its epidemic alludes, of course, to the outbreak of AIDS that is decimating the gay community and is spreading rapidly among intravenous drug users in the United States. Fears that the disease will spread to heterosexuals who do not use drugs are responsible for a wealth of misinformation and public outcry for protection from infected individuals. My purpose in this chapter is not to separate fact from error, nor is it to address the specific moral issues that have become tangled in our debates about how to deal with AIDS. Rather, I want to challenge the idea that battling this epidemic is somehow a matter to be worked out between two great abstractions— the liberty of the individual and the welfare of the community. Drawing on the wisdom and vision of Walt Whitman, I suggest that the relation between the individual and the community is complex, and I argue that the principal task of public leadership in combatting the epidemic is to confront the civil war that lies beneath the great abstraction of the "welfare of the community." In my view, the task of leadership is to free the spheres of communal welfare, democratic discussion, and privacy from the tangles of moralism that surround drug addiction and homosexuality. I confine my analysis to the links between homosexuality, moralism, and AIDS, and do not address the tremendous problems of intravenous drug abusers because I think bringing to the surface the latent cruelties and hatreds—not to mention racism—behind this and other epidemics is as pertinent for drug addiction as it is for homosexuality.

AIDS has already killed over 35,000 men and women, most of them quite young—between the ages of twenty-five and forty; to date we have found roughly 65,000 cases. The Public Health Service (PHS) estimates that the cumulative case load of AIDS victims will increase from 19,000 at the start of 1986 to 270,000 at the end of 1991. The annual rate of deaths from AIDS will increase from 9,000 in 1986 to 54,000 in 1991. By the end of 1991, 179,000 persons will have died from AIDS.[1] Between one and two million people are believed to be infected with the AIDS virus, but the truth is that we do not really know how many people are infected. The PHS has initiated a national survey of seropositivity that should be concluded by the end of 1988.[2]

Over 90 percent of the victims of AIDS come from two at-risk groups: IV drug users and male homosexuals or bisexuals.[3] Women victims are nearly always intravenous drug addicts or married to addicts or bisexuals.[4] Heterosexual AIDS cases remain rare, but their incidence is steadily rising. By 1991, the level of heterosexual cases could rise from 7 to 9 percent of the total, but almost half of this total will comprise cases believed contracted outside the United States, where heterosexual transmission is more common.[5]

AIDS is actually not so much a disease as the collapse of the immune system induced by a virus—what we now call the HIV (human immunodeficiency virus)—and this collapse exposes the victims to a full range of what are called "opportunistic infections": cancers and pneumonias, attacks on the central nervous system that often result in dementia, and a host of other deadly complications. AIDS is a particularly painful, dreadful way to die.[6]

Many ethical and moral issues loom over this epidemic, but learning the central truth of the conflict—its basic nature—is more critical. If we don't understand what is going on, we can hardly be expected to develop adequate policies. The most common misreading is that the conflict is between the ethos of public health and that of civil liberty. As I noted in Chapter Three, Ronald Bayer has argued this view quite clearly:

> At the most fundamental level, the ethos of public health takes the well-being of the community as its highest good, and . . . would limit freedom or restrict . . . the realm of privacy in order to prevent morbidity from taking its toll. . . . From the point of view of civil liberties the situation is quite the reverse. . . . These two great abstractions, liberty and communal welfare, are always in a state of tension in the realm of public health policy.[7]

I think that the nature of the conflict over AIDS is different and that Mark Kleinman comes closest to the nature of the controversy when he defines this as a struggle between "moralists" and "libertarians."

> Moralists and libertarians alike perceive correctly that the epidemic gives at least apparent support to the moralists' claim that tolerating vice has disastrous consequences in the long run, making the public more likely to support moralist rather than libertarian positions on a wide range of issues. It is also possible that, comparing forms of social organization, those with less

respect for individual autonomy will tend to have greater success in controlling the epidemic.[8]

Kleinman describes the horrors of dying from AIDS and our present inability to do little more than ease the pain of that dying.[9] He concludes that while the

> more immediate interests of the infected involve being able to maintain their employment, their housing, their health insurance, their personal liberties, their lifestyles, and their anonymity, . . . I would assert that preventing new infections deserves almost complete precedence as an objective of policy.[10]

Kleinman argues that

> the rate of new infections can be reduced in three ways: by reducing the number of risky acts (penetrative sex and self-injection); by reducing the riskiness of each individual act (its "specific risk") (condom use, needle hygiene); and by decreasing the probability that any given act will involve a combination of infected and uninfected individuals.[11]

Kleinman lends support to the thesis that in an epidemic civil liberties and freedom from discrimination must take a back seat to preventing the spread of infection. Of course, it is very likely that, in specific instances in this epidemic, liberty and privacy may warrant secondary consideration, but as a generalization about epidemics, and particularly about the AIDS epidemic, this view is disastrously wrong.

I believe that the primary task of public health in this epidemic is not to isolate the afflicted group. It is just the opposite; to struggle to prevent society from joining forces with the epidemic, from attempting in various ways to imprison further the groups who are most at risk. This would not be the first time that public health has adopted this strategy. As Camus wrote in *The Plague*, "All I maintain is that on this earth there are pestilences and there are victims, and it's up to us, as far as possible, not to join forces with the pestilences."[12] Indeed, public health has often worked to liberate society from doctrines and practices that have held the larger society hostage to epidemics for centuries. This is especially the case when, as in the present epidemic, the conflict is clouded by centuries of persecution of a moral minority.

The history of public health has often been, as Bayer asserts, a struggle to expand communal provision. William Ryan made the same point in these words,

> Adherents of this approach tended to search for defects in the community and the environment rather than in the individual; to emphasize predictability and usualness rather than random deviance; they tried to think about predicting problems, rather than merely repairing or treating—to see social problems, in a word, as social.[13]

The emphasis on communal provision does sometimes come at the expense of individual liberty, in cases like antismoking campaigns, highway safety campaigns, alcohol policy, and some limited remnants of communicable disease controls. But typically, especially in the case of lifestyle risks, the restrictive measures are aimed as often at curtailing the freedom of producers as limiting the liberty of consumers.

Many of these modern public health reforms were loosely based on the analogy of controlling infectious diseases. For example, William Haddon, Jr., a physician, and the first head of the National Highway Traffic Safety Administration, developed a decade before the Great Society a general theory of injury prevention that separated human "hosts" from hazardous agents, which he termed dangerous energy exchanges, whether the agents of energy were biological, kinetic, ionizing, or chemical in nature.[14] But in Haddon's scheme restrictions on voluntary behavior were given very low priority—instead of seat belts, Haddon preferred air bags, primarily because these passive changes in the environment did not require the active cooperation of citizens and did not collide with their liberties.

As C.-E. A. Winslow recounted in his classic *The Evolution and Significance of the Modern Public Health Campaign*,[15] the principal foe of modern public health was centuries of religious and feudal thought that stressed a hatred of the body, glorified poverty and privation, ignored a robust diet, feared sexuality, and neglected municipal and personal hygiene. The chief contribution of the medieval period to public health was the quarantine, a method of fighting disease by separating those at risk from the community. Developed primarily to control leprosy, quarantine still symbolizes the archaic fears of epidemics as forms of divine retribution, and public health still is viewed by portions of the public as an instrument for protecting the community against moral and physical contamination.[16]

In fact, it was to reject these ideas that modern public health looked back past the Middle Ages to Rome and Greece, to their celebration of the body and emphasis on robust diet, a vigorous municipal and communal administration to provide fresh air, the control of filth, spaciousness, adequate waste disposal, and a safe food and water supply.

The modern public health movement began in the dawning modern world of nation–states, small republics, and mercantilism, when kings wanted to improve the health of their populace to increase the wealth and power of their realms.[17] But its more immediate impetus came in the late eighteenth and early nineteenth centuries with the rise of movements for prison, municipal, and factory reforms, measures that limited the liberties of slumlords, jailers, factory owners, and corrupt local officials more than individual citizens.[18]

Many of the most progressive public health reformers

were extremely critical of mass quarantine.[19] Advocates of quarantine believed that most diseases were spread by contagion; these people were usually mercantilist in economic philosophy, and their primary weapon in fighting yellow fever or small pox was isolation or quarantine (from the Italian *quarantiná*, "space of forty days," after the practice of making ships from foreign ports remain anchored offshore in isolation for at least forty days to make sure that they were not bringing in foreign infections).

The anticontagionists believed that diseases were caused by filth, and instead of the prison of quarantine advocated "domestic cleanliness" in the form of waste disposal, clean water, and the like.[20] They also lamented the destruction quarantine brought on the economies of cities as well as upon lives of communities. As Dr. Benjamin Rush, the Revolutionary physician and ardent anticontagionist argued:

> A belief in the contagious nature of yellow fever, which is so solemnly enforced by the execution of quarantine laws, has demoralized our citizens. It has, in many instances, extinguished friendship, annihilated religion, and violated the sacraments of nature, by resisting even the loud and vehement cries of filial and parental blood.[21]

Rush was wrong about yellow fever; it was contagious— not through association with other citizens, but through a virus carried by mosquitoes. But his mistaken science does not disguise the fact that progressive elements in public health have constantly battled the jail of mass quarantine and isolation, making them relics of a superstitious and distant past, using isolation only on a selected and highly limited basis.[22]

The accomplishments of the sanitary movement in breaking the hold of outdated doctrines on society became the platform for the modern welfare state in England and the

United States. In our time, domestic sanitation to improve the public's health, beyond decent housing, medical care, and safe working conditions, means the fresh air of more speech and privacy. Free speech would enlarge the right of the community to have at its disposal the frankest and fullest information about those aspects of sexuality and drug use that place individuals at heightened risk. More privacy would ensure the right of individuals to be free from discrimination because they are infected or at risk of being infected, and would guarantee individuals' right to make intimate decisions about their sexuality without fear of reprisal from employers, health insurers, schools, or the military. This battle for a new domestic sanitation, like earlier battles, is waged against centuries of religious moralizing, a tradition that imprisons all of us in a deep distrust of the body, of sexuality, of sexual variation.

The novelist Albert Camus, in *The Plague*, equated the calamity of Nazism with the return of the plague and the return of the town of Oran to the dark ages of isolation, fear, and suspicion. Camus used the metaphor of the quarantine as prison, creating the sense of society or a group under siege, imprisoned by fear, isolated, and made strangers in their own land. As Camus says in *The Plague*, "the first thing that plague brought to our town was exile. . . . We were much like those whom men's justice, or hatred, force to live behind prison bars . . . [even] if it was an exile . . . in one's home."[23] Camus quotes Daniel Defoe in his epigraph: "It is as reasonable to represent one kind of imprisonment by another, as it is to represent anything that really exists by that which exists not."[24]

Moralism, Deviance, and Public Health

The legal philosophy that makes the political isolation and exile of a moral minority possible is termed legal moralism.

Moralism is a theory of majority rule based on the use of the law to punish moral deviancy in order to protect the morality of the community, punishing behavior that is "offensive, degrading, vicious, sinful, corrupt, or otherwise immoral."[25] At its worst, moralism uses the law to perform what Harold Garfinkel calls "status degradation ceremonies," to publicly denounce a category of persons and to express the community's moral indignation.[26] In this view, moralism is more than a theory of government and majority rule, it is a form of symbolic politics aimed at strengthening the moral solidarity of the community, using shame to demoralize and control deviant minorities. As H. L. Mencken put it, "its aim is not to lift up saints, but to knock down sinners."[27]

Moralism may be religious in inspiration, but today it is better construed as a branch of politics, a ransacking of religion for the relics of ancient prejudice and superstition, fueling indignation against a constantly changing list of enemies of the republic: "Godless communists," "queers," "niggers," "secular humanists," or "Jews." And the moralist uses almost exactly the same tools as public health has used for fighting mass epidemics—isolation or exile of the contaminated group.

Thus it is no accident that the moralist constantly resorts to public health metaphors to describe his victims. In the nineteenth century, James F. Stephen said, "Vice is as infectious as disease, and happily virtue is infectious, though health is not. Both vice and virtue are transmittable, and, to a considerable extent, hereditary."[28] Justice William Rehnquist, in 1978, compared the workings of laws prohibiting the free association of homosexual students on college campuses to public health legislation preventing the spread of communicable disease, arguing that whether laws controlling homosexuals are constitutional is akin to "whether those suffering from measles have a constitutional right, in violation of quarantine regulations, to associate together and with others who do not presently have measles."[29]

The classic defense of moralism is found in Stephen's

Liberty, Equality, Fraternity, published in 1873 as a rebuttal to John Stuart Mill's "On Liberty." Stephen argued that the majority in any society is a moral majority.[30] In recent times, this view has been most forcefully stated by Lord Patrick Devlin in his critique of the Wolfenden Report, the English report that recommended removing criminal sanctions for private homosexual conduct between consenting adults.

> What makes a society of any sort is community of ideas, not only political ideas but also ideas about the way its members should behave and govern their lives; these latter ideas are its morals. . . . [W]ithout shared ideas on politics, morals and ethics no society can exist. . . . For society is not something that is kept together physically; it is held by the invisible bonds of common thought.[31]

Moralism and Homosexuality

What are the historical and religious roots of our moralizing attitudes toward homosexuality? It may not be true that, as Justice Burger argued in his concurring opinion in *Bowers v. Hardwick*, "proscriptions against sodomy have very 'ancient roots.'"[32] Burger went on to say that "decisions of individuals relating to homosexual conduct have been subject to state intervention throughout the history of Western Civilization. Condemnation of those practices is firmly rooted in Judeo-Christian moral and ethical standards. Homosexual sodomy was a capital crime under Roman law."[33]

This is only partially true. As John Boswell argues, Christianity has until very recent centuries evidenced only a fitful interest in suppressing homosexuality; moreover, for long periods of time homosexuals enjoyed a great deal of freedom and even influence in Europe.[34]

In both the Old and the New Testament, the fundamental biblical ethic was to attack religious formalism through identification with the outcast, the poor, the prisoner, or the stranger. Far from reinforcing "traditional values" with "ancient roots," the trajectory of biblical ethics, from the Prophets to Jesus, was to prevent those ancient roots from ossifying into ceremonies of moral indignation aimed at excluding the poor, the stranger, the prisoner, or the exile. In fact, homosexuality is explicitly forbidden in only one book in the Old Testament, Leviticus 18:22; 20:13 (RSV), and even there on the same plane as fornication or adultery or for reasons of ritual impurity (like the eating of pork), not as a fundamental sin.

In the New Testament, Jesus did not mention homosexuality at all, and his ministry to prostitutes, thieves, beggars, and the poor constituted a scandal to the moralists of his time.

And as Boswell argues in his *Christianity, Social Tolerance, and Homosexuality*, the most complete study of the issue of homosexuality, the Bible suggests that the famous destruction of Sodom occurred not because of the abomination of homosexuality but because the Sodomites refused hospitality to strangers (Matthew 10:14, 15).[35]

And if anyone will not receive you or listen to your words, shake off the dust of your feet as you leave that house or town. Truly I say to you, it shall be more tolerable on the day of judgment for the land of Sodom and Gomorrah than for that town.[36]

Jesus' attack on religious moralism and his elevation of a gospel of love and community were the principal reasons for his being put to death. As he said (Matthew 15:10, 17–20):

Not what goes into the mouth defiles a man but what comes out of the mouth, this defiles a man. . . .

Homosexual practices in republican Rome, as in classical Greece, were viewed with tolerance. Only in later imperial Rome was homosexuality made a capital crime, and then for reasons little related to sexual deviance.[37] And not until the thirteenth and fourteenth centuries was there a general shift toward intolerance for many different minorities. This period also marked the beginnings of absolute government, of a great increase in the codification of laws, and of actual persecution of religious deviance. It was a time when central authorities began to search for enemies against which to whip up popular passions and solidify moral cohesion. And the enemies were Jews, heretics, usurers, Muslims, and homosexuals.[38]

Until the late Middle Ages, the secular authorities had largely ignored homosexuality, leaving the regulation of this behavior to the Church. Then, as persecution of minorities began to increase (perhaps not coincidentally, at the same time that Europe was attacked by the bubonic plague), church authorities gave homosexuality more attention. Aquinas seems to have condemned homosexuality and other sexual deviations less on theological grounds than as a concession to changing political values.[39] But in the sixteenth century in England, to reduce the authority of the church, Henry VIII made sodomy or "buggery" a matter of the criminal law.

While the American colonists incorporated the English statutes wholesale, making homosexuality a capital offense, in the years before the American Revolution, apparently only one person was put to death under this law.[40] Such severe moralistic laws were relaxed or ignored in early nine-teenth-century America, but England was another story. According to one source, "Men were regularly hanged for homosexual relations in nineteenth-century England—sixty in the first three decades of the century and 'another score under naval regulations.' "[41]

In the United States today, roughly half of the states have

repealed antisodomy laws, and many localities have passed antidiscrimination statutes.[42] Yet half of the states retain these laws, and even if they are rarely enforced, the moral indignation and solidarity which these laws mean to conjure up are always there to keep in exile a large segment of the homosexual community.

Whitman and *Democratic Vistas*

To return to our secret group, we now grasp that the central task of public health is somehow to acknowledge that there are two epidemics, one a spreading, deadly disease, and a second shadow conflict, a civil persecution of a secret group whose practices society finds abominable. It is not too much to compare this hatred of the deviant as a kind of war. Alasdair MacIntyre sees our society as filled with such conflicts: "Modern politics cannot be a matter of genuine moral consensus. Modern politics is civil war carried on by other means, and *Bakke* [the Supreme Court decision on racial quotas for medical schools] was an engagement whose antecedents were at Gettysburg and Shiloh."[43]

MacIntyre's pessimism actually contains a clue for effective public health leadership: Realism demands that we confess that the basic issue of the epidemic is not communal welfare versus the rights of the victim; it is to prevent our fear of epidemics from encouraging us to join its ranks, turning on the victims, waging a civil war against them, a war that threatens the welfare of everyone alike.

Here we must see that a strong sense of individuality—an expanded private sphere—may be our best weapon against this epidemic. This thought brings me to Walt Whitman, often called America's greatest poet, and his theory of democracy forged in large part by his experiences during the American Civil War.[44] Because Whitman was forced to acknowledge the civil wars in the heart of America, his views about democracy could hold important ideas for fighting an epidemic that is also a civil conflict.

Whitman, in his poetry and especially in his great essay on democracy, *Democratic Vistas*, saw the republic as sustained by two opposed and paradoxical principles, the principle of individuality and the principle of the aggregate.[45] Of the two, "the noiseless operation of one's isolated Self" precedes community.[46] As Lewis Hyde comments in his brilliant essay on Whitman's politics, "The initial event in Whitman's democracy is not a political event at all."[47] Hyde goes on to say that, for Whitman, "our actions and character must spring from what is received in the ground of our being, else they will be merely derived behaviors, appliqué personalities."[48]

According to Hyde, Whitman believed that individual identity cannot thrive where some people count and others do not. "Democracy enfranchises every self—politically and spiritually. . . . [Whitman] places each citizen on . . . equal footing not only to protect the idiosyncratic self but to produce it as well."[49] Whitman begins with individual identity and adds community, but Hyde argues that for Whitman "in its action neither the One nor the Many is primary, each assists to produce the other so that the nation might be their union, [in Whitman's words] 'a common aggregate of living identities.' "[50]

But Whitman goes further and gives his democracy a sense of cohesion, which he calls "adhesiveness."[51] This adhesiveness has its erotic and artistic side. Whitman "assumes that the citizen, like the poet, will emerge from the centripetal isolation, in which character forms, with an appetite for sympathetic contact and an urge both to create and to bestow."[52]

Whitman penned a memorable line that celebrated his adhesiveness in imagery that is at once evocative of a deeper fraternity for all men and a cry for a freer sexuality within the life of the republic: "I confidently expect a time when there will be seen, running like a half-hid warp through all the myriad audible and visible worldly interests of America, threads of manly friendship, fond and loving, pure and sweet, strong and life-long, carried to degrees hitherto unknown."[53]

The source of Whitman's ideas about adhesiveness—phrenology, or the science that teaches that character can be determined through study of bumps on the head—despite its wide acceptance by many leading intellectuals of the period, was as incorrect as the science of the anticontagionists.[54] Yet such ideas opened our eyes to the bankruptcy of quarantine and isolation as a blanket technique for fighting epidemics. Whitman's idea of democracy as a comfortable marriage of deeply rooted individuality and community, in which the community is large enough to contain all measures of personhood, may help expose the foolishness of applying the discredited techniques of quarantine, isolation, or thoughtless mandatory mass screening to a twentieth-century epidemic.

My aim here is not to celebrate Whitman's homosexuality or the homoerotic elements of his notions of adhesiveness, although his sexuality clearly led him to this view of the meaning of democracy. Rather, my point is to note the paradox at the heart of his democratic vision, and to argue that it was the experience of the Civil War, and his encounter with the pain and suffering in the hospitals, that held for him the key to resolving this paradox. Whitman's experience bears directly on the current struggle against AIDS.

Whitman and the Hospitals

Whitman went to Washington, D.C., in 1862 to visit his wounded brother and to look for a government job, carrying a letter of recommendation from Emerson.[55] He didn't get the job. Secretary Chase did not approve of the *Leaves of Grass*; the notoriety of his poetry and his reputation had preceded him. As one friend wrote him, his difficulties in finding and holding employment were probably due to the fact that he was not sufficiently ashamed of his sexual organs.[56]

Whitman stayed in Washington because of his initial experiences in the hospitals of the Army of the Potomac, working part time as a copyist in the Army Paymaster's Office from 1863 to 1864. He immediately set about visiting the hospitals of the city and of the surrounding areas: There were forty to fifty army hospitals in Washington alone, and their population would swell at times to nearly seventy thousand, a number higher than the total population of the District only a few years earlier.[57]

He could stand and see most of the hospitals

> from any eminence . . . I use them as land marks. . . .
> That little town, as you might suppose it, off there on
> the brow of a hill, is indeed a town, but of wounds,
> sickness, and death. It is Finley hospital. . . . That other
> is Campbell. I have known these two alone to have
> from two thousand to twenty-five hundred inmates.
> Then there is Carver . . . , off east Lincoln hospital; and
> half a mile further Emory hospital.[58]

The hospitals were houses of horrible images—the "blue-face, glazy eye of the dying, the clotted rag, the odor of wounds and blood."[59] In one scene from *Specimen Days*, which contains his moving and rambling record of this part of his life, he writes:

> Out doors, at the foot of a tree, within ten yards of the
> front of the house, I notice a heap of amputated feet,
> legs, arms, hands, etc., a full load for a one-horse cart.
> Several dead bodies lie near, each cover'd with its
> brown woolen blanket.[60]

The hospitals transformed his life; he spent hours helping, bathing, holding, embracing, and loving the torn and dying young men, many barely more than boys. By his own estimate he made over six hundred visits during his stay, touching the lives of almost a hundred thousand.[61] His love for men obviously was a crucial part of this experience, but his love for America and its great, sad president was no less a part. The hospital experience seemed to revitalize him, to enlarge his spirit. As Lewis Hyde writes, "Death in particular focuses life."[62]

Whitman saw the hospitals as the great metaphor for the war—the "marrow" of the war concentrated in the nation's Capital, the place where the young of the North and South suffered alike. This was "America, brought to hospital in her fair youth," he wrote to Emerson.[63] The hospital experience shaped his great political essay, *Democratic Vistas*, begun a few years after the war. The book reflected the twin forces of the aggregate, as symbolized by the thousands of patients, and the spirit of the individual that he found in each bed he visited. For Whitman the Civil War was a symbol of the civil wars that raged constantly in all of our hearts, wars that could turn the nation into a vast hospital, ruining the hopes of union and of an enduring republic. Whitman's experience led him to appreciate the power of suffering and death as a source of transcendence, reconciliation, and community. And he conceived of a sense of community and fraternity arising out of the dying of thousands of young Americans, their sacrifice bringing a healing power to the nation. As it turned out, this did not occur; Lincoln was assassinated; after the North's victory those who wanted to prosecute the Civil War by other means prevailed.

Whitman insisted that democracy rests on the good of both the aggregate and the individual, that both can be strengthened by the sense of a shared community forged in the experience of a great calamity. The parallels with the AIDS epidemic are striking. The power and transcendence of death seems to be transforming the contemporary homosexual community; whether this transformation stretches to the entire nation, offering hope of reconciliation, remains to be seen.

The Rise of the Gay Subculture

America is still a land of deep divisions. The discrimination and prejudice against gays is widespread; recent surveys found that between 70 and 80 percent of the public thinks that homosexuality is either always or nearly always wrong, and that somewhere between 10 and 30 percent of the public favors imposition of a quarantine on AIDS victims. (In New York City as many as 40 percent of the populace favor such measures.)[64] The Supreme Court even vindicated this prejudice in 1986 in *Bowers v. Hardwick*.[65] On the other hand, homosexuals in some sections of the country over the past few decades have become one of the most influential and well-organized minorities or subcultures in the United States.[66] In the larger cities, the homosexual community has become a political force to be reckoned with. While homosexuals remain strangers in their own land, they are increasingly outspoken strangers, who have captured major strategic points in our nation's cities, in culture and the arts, and in segments of the business world; they are even carving out a place in the political agenda at all levels of government.

The emergence of a distinctive gay subculture and of gay power began in the sixties, a period of relaxed attitudes toward sexuality. As Altman, Gorman, White, and others have noted, three cities were the great forming grounds of a new homosexual identity: New York, Los Angeles, and especially San Francisco.[67] Sections of these cities became increasingly and almost exclusively populated by male homosexuals. The most famous of these gay districts was the Castro area in San Francisco. Gay businesses were opened, from gay travel agencies to real estate firms, clothing stores, restaurants, bath houses, and the like. The affluent gay ghettos became the neighborhoods for homosexuals who, out of the closet, worked as advertising executives, bankers, insurance brokers, or real estate speculators in the city's business district.

One of the demographic shifts helping the formation of the new gay identity and subculture was the gradual shift in American attitudes toward marriage and childbearing. As Kristen Luker documents in her *Abortion and the Politics of Motherhood*,[68] in the sixties women began to postpone having children, and men and women began to delay the age of marriage dramatically. Homosexuals, like the young professionals that followed them, carved out a new hedonistic, childless lifestyle, gentrifying the decaying neighborhoods of a retreating poor and largely minority population.

"I Sing the Body Electric"

At the center of much of the new gay lifestyle was sex—an astonishing sexual freedom, one that surpassed the wildest fantasies of young male heterosexuals. Gays in the large cities celebrated their new visibility by creating new institutions whose principal function was to facilitate sex among strangers. Indeed, this form of openly promiscuous sexuality, fostered by the emergence of new institutions like the gay bath house, was celebrated as the badge and emblem of a new gay identity.

While this new lifestyle was, to be sure, not widely recognized by the larger population, it was hardly hidden in New York, San Francisco, or Los Angeles. A central institution of the new gay subculture was the gay bathhouse. The baths were everywhere. There were even national chains of baths, one chain including bathhouses in forty-two cities in the United States and Canada.[69] In the baths and other gay establishments, gays could have frequent sex with complete strangers. Fellatio or anal sex several times every night was an ordinary experience for a substantial minority among the gay community. Indeed, frequent, anonymous sex was even canonized as a kind of fulfillment of Whitman's sexual prophecy of a time of "threads of Manly friendship, fond and loving, . . . carried to degrees hitherto unknown."[70]

Robert Martin, in analyzing sections of "Songs of Myself," one of Whitman's great poems, argues that it is, in part, a celebration of anonymous sex, sex in which there

> are no persons, but, rather a general feeling of the delight of sexual experiences regardless of the partner. They are totally tactile, since they could take place in the dream-world of closed eyes. Such experiences could well be repeated in almost any steam bath of a modern large city. But the important point is that not asking, not knowing, and not thinking are integral parts of Whitman's *democratic* vision, and anonymous sexuality is an important way-station on the path to the abolition of distinction of age, class, beauty, and gender. Whitman loves all being and will love and be loved by all being. It is perhaps at this juncture that the implications of his perspective become most revolutionary.[71]

Dennis Altman makes much the same point, arguing that

> the willingness to have sex immediately, promiscuously, with people about whom one knows nothing and from whom one demands only physical contact, can be seen as a sort of Whitmanesque democracy, a desire to know and trust other men in a type of brotherhood far removed from the male bonding of rank, hierarchy, and

competition that characterizes much of the outside world.[72]

Martin published his book, *The Homosexual Tradition in Poetry*, in 1979; Altman's book, *The Homosexualization of America*, was published in 1982. Altman also published an article in 1982 celebrating the gay sexual lifestyle as a search for community and communion, a new form of sexual politics.[73]

Today, these sentences sound tragic. What was going on in the gay ghettos in New York and San Francisco was not Whitman's dream of a "time when . . . manly friendship . . . [would be] carried to degrees hitherto unknown" but rather scenes that shocked even sympathetic gay writers recording the period. Edmund White, who in 1980 wrote *States of Desire*,[74] a book about his visits to the gay scenes in cities across America, was clearly disturbed by what he was seeing, especially in San Francisco and New York. In his view, New York's establishments, like the Flamingo, the Anvil, St. Mark's Baths, and the Mine Shaft, represented the turn from sexual liberation to sexual degradation.[75] These were modern houses of sexual exotica, including public sado-masochism, bookstores and public bathrooms featuring dreary "glory-holes" (holes in the wall for truly anonymous fellatio or anal intercourse),[76] and always the baths with endless rounds of sex with total strangers.[77] Moreover, such places provide another instance of, in Dennis Altman's words, the "commercialization of desire."[78] Ironically, the very visibility and presence of the baths and bars, and their protection from police harassment, resulted in risky sexual practices, like fisting (insertion of the fist into the anus of the partner) and repeated anal intercourse. Previously, gays engaged in furtive encounters in public rest rooms, parks, or alleyways, where the sexual encounter was more likely to include the less dangerous practices of fellatio or masturbation.[79]

"All This Diseasèd, Disproportionate *Adhesion*"[80]

An authoritative survey of gay sexual practices reveals that a minority engaged in this kind of strenuous sexual activity; nonetheless, the minority was significant. The survey found the baths the center of the new gay promiscuity.[81] Twenty-seven percent of all male homosexuals responding to a national survey reported that they had more than fifty to seventy sexual partners in the previous year.[82] If one definition of promiscuity is frequent sexual contact with persons unknown to each other—frequent, anonymous sex—some 50 percent reported that they have sex with some one they do not know very frequently or fairly frequently.[83]

Another index of the health risks of sexual practices of a minority of male homosexuals is the rate of infection from sexually transmitted diseases. Individuals who are exclusively homosexual for a major part of their lives constitute 5 to 10 percent of the adult white population, according to Kinsey.[84] If Kinsey's figures remain reliable, in the seventies and early eighties, gay men accounted for a third of all cases of infectious syphilis, a high rate of gonorrhea, and an increasing rate of hepatitis A and B.[85] Gay males were also at much greater risk for bacterial and enteric diseases like amebiasis and giardiasis. The risk of herpes and dermatologic disorders was much greater among gay males than in the straight population.[86]

In 1977, in New York City, 55 percent of all reported cases of syphilis occurred in homosexual males.[87] Despite the fact that syphilis among heterosexuals nationwide had, until recent years, been declining at a remarkable rate, the rate for homosexuals showed no decline and they were reported to be ten times more likely to contract syphilis than heterosexual males. The epidemic of sexually transmitted disease among homosexual males was in significant part a result of sexual liberation. The price many gays paid for this sexual democracy was a monthly shot of penicillin. But AIDS challenged this casual attitude toward sexually transmitted diseases, for there is no cure for AIDS, only protection through limiting partners or using condoms.

The New Gay Liberation

The story of gay liberation in the future will be focused less on the sexual liberation of the seventies than on the response to AIDS in the eighties, as AIDS transforms the gay community.

There are some hopeful signs that the growing media discussion of the AIDS epidemic and sexuality is changing sexual practices. Small-scale studies report sharp declines in sexually transmitted diseases among the gay population.[88] There have been three major studies of gay sexual practices, two focused on San Francisco and one on New York City. Although they have their limitations, they suggest that important changes are occurring in the sexual behavior of homosexuals. In San Francisco, the first studies suggest that the proportion of a sample of 655 gay men who reported five or more partners over a year declined between 1982 and 1983, as did the proportion who engaged in risky sexual acts (like anal intercourse).[89]

In New York City, sexual activity in the baths and other locations outside the place of residence has been reduced by one-third, and the number of partners in such locales over a year has declined from an average of twelve to four. Condom use rose from a negligible level to 20 percent. "The frequency of sexual episodes involving the exchange of body fluids and mucous membrane contact declined by 70 percent."[90] The report states that "measured in terms of the number of different sexual partners, sexual activity was reported to have declined by 78 percent since hearing about AIDS."[91]

We should not be complacent about such changes; there are enormous problems in developing representative samples of the homosexual population. The data suggest that very few gays have established monogamous relationships or have adopted celibacy as an alternative to promiscuity.[92] In cities where the prevalence of the virus may be well over 50 percent, the chance that even a few sexual contacts might expose an individual to infection is still great. We might well discover that changes far greater than those we now promulgate are needed to combat the spread of the epidemic.

Whitman recognized the hospital as the major institution through which soldiers returned to the community during the Civil War. The hospital became the setting in which civilians became aware that their losses as individuals occurred within the context of the community's unfolding tragedy.

> The hospital part of the [war] deserves . . . to be recorded. Of that many-threaded drama, with its sudden and strange surprises, its confounding of prophecies, its moments of despair, . . . —the immense money expenditure, like a heavy-pouring constant rain—with . . . an unending, universal mourning-wail of women, parents, orphans—the marrow of the tragedy concentrated in those Army hospitals—(it seem'd sometimes as if the whole interest of the land, North and South, was one vast central hospital, and all the rest of the affair but flanges). Think how much— . . . will be buried in the grave, in eternal darkness.[93]

Whitman was constantly struck by how death, even on a massive scale, renewed and revitalized life—how death and life were bride and bridegroom.[94] Whitman's perception applies to our own time as well. It speaks to the way AIDS has transformed the homosexual community. As Gorman states, never before has a community so marginal to the larger society become so unified and resolved in the face of death and tragedy.[95] The baths are still open, but the new centers of gay life are the hospital, the death bed, the hospice. Gays meet to organize AIDS relief activities, campaign for safe sex, and fuel the explosion of discourse on gay sexuality in the general media and in the specialized media for homosexuals.

As before, San Francisco leads the way.[96] The care and treatment for AIDS victims in San Francisco is universally acknowledged as the model for the rest of the country. The battle against the epidemic takes place in the community; its primary weapons include an emphasis on limited hospitalization, creation (after some opposition) of hospices for dying patients, generous funding for treatment costs at the public hospitals, and a very visible and public information campaign promoting safe sex. The costs for treatment in San Francisco, where the community and voluntary role is very great, is far less than in other parts of the United States.[97] By contrast, in New York City, where most AIDS patients now live, the emphasis has been more on bureaucratic solutions; a more central role is played by the city's municipal hospitals, and there is less volunteer involvement. Elsewhere, the local response has been paltry. The distressing side of this is that, as the epidemic spreads, in only a few short years 80 percent of the AIDS cases will come from places outside New York City or San Francisco.

But if it is a necessary truth that illness is the basis for allocating medical care,[98] and if the allocation of medical care is a touchstone of equality in society, we may expect that it will be the power of pain and suffering—the needs of AIDS victims for medical treatment and assistance—that will finally begin to dissolve the centuries of prejudice against an exiled minority. AIDS, our century's plague, may be the event that forces our society, for the first time, to *behold* the homosexual as a person, with rights like all other citizens, rights that include medical treatment. And this refusal to discriminate may be the beginning of a grudging acceptance by the larger society that gays should be entitled to fair equality of opportunity in places of residence, in the work place, and in public services.

Lydia Temoshok, Margaret Grade, and Jane Zich have recently completed a study of the role of the media in publicizing the risks of AIDS in San Francisco and London. They point out that the media are not only succeeding in informing the community of the dangers of AIDS and of the steps necessary to avoid infection; they are also helping to build both sympathy for victims, and a more realistic appraisal of the nature of the epidemic. By presenting the victims of AIDS in vivid stories and photographs, they prevent citizens from believing the epidemic is something happening to someone else.[99]

Further, there is at least the possibility that this publicity, with its poignant portrayal of lives cut short, will in the long run help defuse the stigma and prejudice against gays and drug addicts. Daniel Defoe, in his *Journal of the Plague Year*, had this to say about the effects of witnessing death first hand:

> Here we may observe . . . that a near view of death would soon reconcile men of good principles one to another, and that it is chiefly owing to our easy situation in life and our putting these things far from us that our breaches are fomented, ill blood continued, prejudices, breach of charity and of Christian union, so much kept and so far carried on among us as it is. . . . [A] close conversing with death, or with disease that threaten death, would scum off the gall from our tempers, remove the animosities among us, and bring us to see with differing eyes than those which we looked on things with before.[100]

For the immediate future, we will all have to come to a more realistic and honest appraisal of the role of sex in our common life, one that is neither repressive nor burdened

225

with false revolutionary hopes. I am struck by the insight of Edmund White on the meaning of the overwhelming importance placed on sex among gays during the seventies:

> If I were to venture my own generalizations, I would say that with the collapse of other social values (those of religion, patriotism, the family, and so on), sex has been forced to take up the slack, to become our sole mode of transcendence and our only touchstone of authenticity. . . . I feel that homosexuals, now identified as the element in our society most obsessed with sex, will in fact be the agent to cure the mania. Sex will be restored to its proper place as a pleasure, a communication, an appetite, an art; it will no longer pose as a religion.[101]

Edmund White could not know, when he predicted the shift in gay attitudes, that it would happen so fast, that AIDS was in the wings. While we must resist the temptation to, once again, institute repressive and moralizing attitudes toward sexuality in general, I think one lesson we will learn from this epidemic is that frequent, anonymous, impersonal sex is not a source of transcendence or community. The importance of the AIDS epidemic for the gay community is that the experience of solidarity in suffering offers a firmer, deeper source of community and transcendence, a suffering that is being met with courage and astonishing energy.

Rather than seeking to insulate ourselves further from the gay community, we need, as public health has done in the past, to expand the boundaries of community to include everyone. Our strongest hope lies in recognizing the "desirable life as one lived collectively,"[102] in a community that is spacious enough to contain many different types of people. Our best ideas about how to battle the epidemic will probably come from the extraordinary and extensive civic discourse going on now in the gay community; this discourse itself is the real education that is changing the lifestyles of gays everywhere. And this change will come because the experience of AIDS is forging a power and creative work among the gay community that is reaching out to all of us, rebuking all of us, provoking action and change.

Prevention of epidemics like AIDS begins with recognizing the injustice of a polarized society. Prevention means accepting others, and establishing union and community. Prevention begins with the slow, patient work of destroying centuries of moral bigotry, and with listening to the voices of suffering and alienation. Its first priority must be to minister to the suffering of an exiled and despised minority so that the epidemic will not spread further. Perhaps the most difficult task in curbing AIDS will be to acknowledge our own sexual fears, fears that we turn into nightmares for others. If we as a society can do this, the changes in the sodomy legislation and antidiscrimination statutes will come in their time.

In the end, Whitman's belief that democracy rested on the opposed but necessary elements of individuality and community finds an echo in Justice Blackmun's minority dissent in *Bowers v. Hardwick*.[103] Blackmun argues that

> we protect those rights not because they contribute, in some direct and material way, to the general public welfare, but because they form so central a part of an individual's life. . . . [T]he concept of privacy embodies the "moral fact that a person belongs to himself and not others nor to society as a whole." . . . [T]he ability independently to define one's identity that is central to any concept of liberty cannot truly be exercised in a vacuum; we all depend on the "emotional enrichment of close ties with others."[104]

And yet these rights do contribute to the safety and the unity of the republic.

It may well be that MacIntyre in his pessimistic view of

modern politics as a species of civil war from which there is little hope of escape is right, and Whitman is not justified in his optimism about the politics in the world's oldest republic.[105] But it is just possible that in the dying and suffering of AIDS we all, homosexual and otherwise, discover our common humanity and our common stake in being left alone to discover our own identity "amid real, independent, stormy life."[106] In truth, in the Civil War, we did not learn nearly enough about our common humanity.

We will never know whether, if Lincoln had lived, his sense of compassion and irony would have rebuilt the South and avoided the bitter years of the Reconstruction. For us, the question remains whether, in the midst of death, we can undertake the reconciliation and cessation of hostilities that will promote not only a healing of the body politic but its very safety.

AIDS and Citizenship

Myriad ethical and legal questions surround the AIDS epidemic. Who should be tested? Should the tests be mandatory? Should we use the technique of contact tracing, the notification of the sexual partners of an index case found to be viremic? If so, who should notify those sexual partners? Who should have access to the list of partners? If addicts have access to sterile needles, will this reduce the sharing of needles and the spread of the virus? Should health insurance companies be permitted to routinely screen applicants for AIDS, much as they now test for other diseases? Who will pay for the treatment of AIDS patients without insurance?[107]

In my view, there are political questions prior to and more important than these ethical dilemmas. Just as the Civil War did, the AIDS crisis calls into question the meaning of citizenship in our democratic republic.

AIDS is thus no different from the many other crises facing our health care system; resolving them depends less on ethics than on the answer to a single question: What is the connection between health policy and citizenship of the United States of America?

The single great failing of the Great Society period and after was our failure to adopt a national health program assuring health insurance to all as a matter of common citizenship. We are paying a grievous price for this neglect in the AIDS epidemic; the question now is whether the epidemic will destroy forever our hopes for equality in health care. If AIDS does not bring about a national health program, will this be our final answer to the challenge of equality in health care, a decision to adopt inequality as the guiding principle of health policy and to abandon the commitment to equality that is the very foundation of membership in a democratic community?

Weinberg and Murray estimate that by 1991 as many as 25 percent of all the medical-surgical beds in New York City's hospitals will be occupied by patients with AIDS or ARC (AIDS-related complex).[108] Currently an estimated 5 percent of New York City's hospital beds are taken by these patients. Such a dramatic increase, if these estimates prove accurate, though not typical for other parts of the United States, will profoundly alter the nature of medical care provided every patient in New York City.

At present there is no federal leadership to cope with this looming crisis. Will we leave the medical care system largely as it is, permitting state and local officials to struggle with meager, patchwork solutions and leaving thousands to fend for themselves with what they can squeeze out of Medicaid, private insurance, or uncompensated care? Will our response to the AIDS crisis signal for all time that being a citizen of the United States carries with it no protection against the risk that those suffering from a fearsome and fatal disease can spend the final months or years of their lives like modern-day lepers, desperately searching for decent medical treatment or a place to live while dying? If we are no more to each other than strangers, if we are permitted to turn away when some among us lose their jobs, their homes, or the right to attend school, leaving them to die without defense from the political community of their birth, what, as Rousseau asks, does citizenship mean for any one of us?[109]

The AIDS epidemic has not been the first to raise these questions, but its severe effects compel us to consider them again and to recognize that the failure to resolve them might mean the deaths of hundreds of thousands of young men and women as well as the death of a meaningful equal citizenship in our democracy. If our response to AIDS is to codify inequality permanently as the guiding principle of the health care system, eliminating for all time the ideal that equality in medical care is fundamental, then something far more ominous than the danger to those at risk for AIDS is closing in.

Perhaps even more shocking is the absence of federal leadership in prevention policy. The Great Society made an expanded national citizenship and an enlarged federal responsibility the center of protecting the public's health in the work place, the marketplace, and on the highways. It also witnessed the sharp expansion of a right to privacy and an invigorated democratic discussion as a formidable right of citizens and as a new means for promoting the public's health. To date, the federal response to the AIDS epidemic has ignored these precedents. Instead of federal standards for testing that would build confidence and trust among those at risk of being infected, instead of federal legislation protecting the infected against a breach of confidentiality and against discrimination, instead of federal legislation ensuring that the fullest and frankest discussion of sexuality and drug addiction ensues, we find hesitancy, confusion, and a thinly veiled moralism. Instead of a unified federal policy to combat a national and international epidemic, we are left to wait for fifty different approaches to emerge from the states.

The Chairman of the Presidential Commission on the Human Immunodeficiency Virus Epidemic, Admiral James D. Watkins, has recommended a several-billion-dollar program to establish a system of "treatment on demand" for all drug abusers, especially IV drug users. This group comprises 25 percent of all cases of AIDS and is the primary source of pediatric AIDS cases. In his recommendations, which also included major new health care funding programs for all AIDS victims, the chairman cited estimates that there are approximately 1.2 million IV drug abusers residing in the cities of the United States with only 150,000 in treatment. A key reason for the sparse figures is the lack of treatment facilities and dollars. The chairman estimates that perhaps three thousand new drug treatment facilities may be needed to provide an adequate treatment response to the AIDS epidemic.[110]

If we lived in a society held together by a greater trust, one in which homosexuals were free to live their lives in peace without fear of retribution from the majority; a society in which all had their medical or treatment needs met regardless of who they were; a society in which the basic information about one's person and state of health was held in the strictest confidentiality, to be overridden only by manifest evidence of a threat to the public safety; a society in which discrimination against moral minorities was not only forbidden by law but proscribed by our central practices; and where a fundamental privacy governed those intimate decisions that shape the course of our lives; perhaps then we could ask different questions about the relative merits and disadvantages of mandatory versus voluntary screening for AIDS, contact tracing, and even limited forms of coercion for people who wantonly disregard medical and public health guidelines for preventing the spread of infections. Perhaps then we could calmly and rationally discuss the question of testing more quietly and deliberately as well as devising an appropriate response to regulating high-risk sexual encounters in places like the baths in San Francisco or New York.[111] In such a society we could define the role of public health authorities in testing the efficacy and wisdom of providing safe and clean needles in ways that would not worsen our nation's drug problems.

Epidemics can derail a republic's journey, sidetracking its search for new regions of equality with civil and religious strife. The AIDS epidemic cast its shadow on the 1986 Supreme Court Decision, *Bower v. Hardwick*,[112] upholding state antisodomy laws. If the Court had overturned these laws, health experts would have found their hands strengthened in conducting frank AIDS education campaigns. We got instead a decision that could begin to unravel privacy as a right and a weapon in improving the health of the republic in abortion, birth control, or sex education.

If, at the close of the twentieth century, we succumb to our unconscious fears, permitting thousands to die because we cannot bear to hear or speak the brute facts of modern-day sexuality and intravenous drug use, we risk not only our citizens' lives, we also risk poisoning the free speech that is the life's blood of a democratic republic. On October 14, 1987, Jesse Helms (R-NC) in a Senate speech argued that "Every AIDS case can be traced back to a homosexual act,"[113] citing authorities like ex-Nixon aide and born-again Christian Chuck Colson and Monsignor Eugene Clark. Faced with such aggressive ignorance, the Senate voted 94 to 2 for legislation prohibiting the government from distributing educational materials that "promote, encourage, or condone" homosexual activities. Only Senators Lowell P. Weicker, Jr. (R-Conn) and Daniel Patrick Moynihan (D-NY) stood against this modern-day Comstockery. A belligerent moralism must not be permitted to return to limit what we ought to know, discuss, hear, or decide.

We may have, in the symbolic Brooklyn Bridge of Hart Crane's beautiful poem, *The Bridge*, a metaphor that suggests the stakes for our republic as the AIDS epidemic unfolds, "a symbol of hope for men who are beset by present peril."[114] Crane's bridge offers transport from a decaying cultural and moral order, across the bedlam of unchecked capitalism to a future where all citizens have their dignity affirmed. In Crane's words, "From gulfs unfolding, terrible of drums, Tall Vision-of-the-Voyage, . . . In myriad syllables,—Psalm of Cathay!"[115]

Neither republics nor bridges lead inexorably to democratic vistas. AIDS can lead us away to the dark days of a republic winding down, causing us to turn our backs on more than equality in health care. Or our response can become a shining moment—the Republic's rainbow spanning its far shores from the Brooklyn to the Golden Gate Bridge—carrying us into new territory, leaving centuries of religious bigotry behind on the receding shore. The travail of AIDS could deliver a long-overdue promise to give every American that deeper equality that is his or hers by right, as a token of mere citizenship: more speech, more privacy, and equal health care for all.

EQUALITY, TRUST, AND THE HEALTH OF THE REPUBLIC

Health policy and health care institutions should consider the needs of everyone equally to avoid serious injury and premature death and to be treated with dignity and respect. But health policy ought to mean more, deepening the loyalties and democratic trust that are the heart of a republican order.

But we have made distrust the reigning virtue of our democratic institutions. We have a long tradition of limited government, each branch jealously guarding its prerogatives against encroachment and suspicious of the powers of others, and our vision of citizenship enshrines the self as the only reliable guardian of interests. Many of our most pressing problems in health policy evade solution precisely because we lack the elemental trust that makes a democratic order possible, a trust flowing from a wellspring of shared loyalties, a basic respect for the rights of all groups, and a patriotism based not on nationalism or religious piety but a devotion to the best interests of the republic as a whole—a trust in the diversity of American spirits.

A democratic society's institutions depend more on its store of genuine patriotism and mutual trust than on its fund of intellectual capital. As our increasingly privatized and polarized society drifts further toward civic religion or commercialism, becoming a republic based on the "parochialisms of race or religion,"[1] we rob our republican political tradition of its deepest meaning: debt, obligation, and trust. Today it is likely that most citizens have long forgotten why we are a political community in the first place. As John Schaar notes, "Millions of Americans are simply without patriotism. . . . They do not think unpatriotic thoughts, but they do not think patriotic thoughts either. The republic for them is a vague and distant thing, absent from their hearts, lost to their eyes."[2]

The solidarity embodied in a common health care system in the face of our common death can be an enormous resource for renewing the trust of the citizenry in the decent purposes of government, helping reverse the drift toward mutual suspicion and radical self-interest in our society.

The absence of trust may be the greatest obstacle to fighting the AIDS epidemic. Questions about testing for the presence of the AIDS virus and issues of confidentiality, access to high-quality medical care, and freedom from discrimination must accompany an extensive health education to reduce the spread of the epidemic. But this education can occur only in an atmosphere of democratic trust. Trust can be nurtured only when all alike are assured of their right to adequate medical attention in the face of death and of the freedom to complete their lives without discrimination and hatred. This trust must be shown first in physicians' offices, in hospitals, and in health clinics; if the health community can shun the homosexual or the addict with AIDS, how can we possibly condemn the real estate industry, schools, employers, or the rest of society for its bigotry?

There could come a time in the course of the AIDS epidemic when its spread might require more extensive testing and surveillance than is now ethically justified.[3] Viruses and epidemics can suddenly change in their virulence and modes of transmission, taking the society into new and even more dangerous territory.

There is a growing debate over whether taking the AIDS test leads to safer sexual practices and whether those at risk should be more actively encouraged to determine their antibody status, if for no other reason than to protect their sexual partners.[4] But in the present atmosphere of mutual suspicion and distrust, a calm and intelligent discussion of all sides of the debate is not even possible. Meanwhile, we are in the eighth year of a worsening, terrible epidemic.

Our present policy of delay and abdication of national leadership on issues like confidentiality, testing, insurability, and discrimination against homosexuals and others at risk in employment, medical care, or housing, allows each state to shape its own policy. This default in national leadership only encourages local prejudices and narrow interests to spread distrust and disrespect for the rights of other citizens. Just as our need for trust and mutual respect increases, we are actively taking steps that add to the evidence that the majority is making a pact with the epidemic rather than defending its victims. The distrust and discord we sow not only jeopardize the rights of moral minorities, but gamble recklessly with the health and safety of the republic as a body.

The most important thing we can do to combat the present epidemic is to move rapidly to some form of national health insurance or national health program. Such a program would not only provide a common institution in which the civic virtues of trust and cooperation are encouraged, it would help us develop policies that could rapidly assure the most vulnerable in the epidemic that their basic rights are being respected.

The struggle for a national health program would certainly precipitate yet another civil war fought by the right-to-life movement and the Catholic Church to ensure that abortion and family planning were not covered services. Such a struggle would be a divisive, bloody battle, but it would at least reveal to all the dangerous mistrust that moralizing brings to the life of the republic. Such a conflict might in the long run be healthy, helping the majority see its clear interest in separating religion from politics, building trust among the citizens of a secular society where each determines his or her own ultimate ends.

Nowhere is the absence of republican trust more evident than in the discussions of rationing and controlling medical expenditures. Assuring adequate medical care to everyone while fairly rationing the benefits of medical technology is impossible without a common structure of provision that enables us to debate and evaluate the contradiction at the heart of a health care system: The needs of each of us as individuals do not add up to our needs as a republic. A system of common provision that stressed our common citizenship and common possession would help provide a framework of democratic trust that could ease the painful and difficult task of saying no to endless increases in marginal medical technology.

The alternative is wars and skirmishes fought over the spoils of the systems, with parents lobbying governors and state legislatures for liver transplants for their dying children, the working young increasingly resentful of a growing elderly population claiming a large and increasing share of hospital expenses, hospitals competing for the latest in expensive and redundant health technology, and millions of dollars spent on artificial hearts while millions of citizens lack basic medical care. These glaring inequities are not only wrong, they destroy the essence of trust and political obligation in a democratic society.

In 1987, in a series of articles in the *New England Journal of Medicine*, John Iglehart outlined the workings of the Canadian health care system and its celebrated success in controlling health expenditures.[5] In 1970, both the United States and Canada spent roughly 7 percent of their GNPs on health care. Today, Canada spends 8.5 percent of its GNP while we spend almost 11 percent. Moreover, our system is filled with glaring inequities; as many as 35 million Americans are without adequate health insurance, while Canadians have universal coverage.

The series brought an interesting rejoinder from Judith Feder, William Scanlon, and John Clark of Georgetown University's Center for Health Policy Studies, arguing that the fabled success of the Canadian system is just that—a fable.[6] Canada's health care costs, when computed per capita, actually grew *faster* than those in this country. During the period from 1970 to 1984, the per capita health expenditures (public and private) in the United States rose by an average annual rate of roughly 11 percent; Canada, during the same period, increased its per capita spending on health care at an annual rate of 12.2 percent.

Canada achieves considerable government control over spending through a system of annual budgetary ceilings established for hospitals and fee schedules for physicians; these data thus seem devastating to the thesis that a more centralized, top-down budgeting system for controlling costs is better than the American system for controlling costs. The authors argue that most analysts, when analyzing the rate of growth of health expenditures relative to GNP, pay far too little attention to the denominator—the rate of growth in GNP. Because Canada's GNP grew at a faster rate during the fourteen-year period studied, the rapid rise in prices and expenditures for health care were overshadowed by the far faster growing GNP and a more rapid rise in hourly output

239

of labor.[7] Iglehart, when faced with this response, complained that the Canadians he interviewed never mentioned this detail.

The comments of Feder, Scanlon, and Clark and the reaction by John Iglehart perfectly illustrate the damage done by the absence of a republican perspective on health policy. The issue is not, nor has it ever been, the rate of per capita growth of medical expenditures; the issue is whether the rate of growth in medical expenditures is wise, given the conditions of our economy, the resources of taxation, and the other needs of society, including housing, nutrition, and employment. In other words, what should we spend on medicine, given the health of our republic as a whole?

The Canadian system for allowing a rate of growth in health care costs consistent with their economic growth seems eminently successful and prudent. In contrast, our own incapacity to control the growth of medical expenditures during periods of rapid general inflation and slow gains in overall productivity seems disastrously imprudent.

Other American economists deny that there is a crisis in health care costs. Uwe Reinhardt, a frequent commentator on the economics of health care, asks us to imagine a favorite television newscaster beginning the evening news with the following item: "'There's good news and bad news on the national economic scene tonight. The good news: Consumer spending on automobiles continues to rise. The bad news: Health care expenditures are still going up, too.'"[8]

Reinhardt asks why an increase in spending on automobiles, with their social costs of pollution and highway injury and death, is always good news, while increases in health care expenditures are not. Reinhardt argues that our reliance on the personal automobile to fuel economic growth has been, in the long run, a disaster for the republic. Today, we have a national landscape shaped by the private convenience and aggregate calamity of too many automobiles. And we got to this point almost heedlessly, ignoring the

warnings of critics who noted the paradox of private afflu-
ence amid public squalor.[9]

This is precisely the danger we face in medical care. The
point is not that we should measure health expenditure
solely in terms of economic growth but rather that we
should decide collectively what level of growth we should
undertake, rather than accepting the rate of growth that our
present policy blindly levies on the republic. This policy
completely ignores millions of our fellow citizens who lack
the minimum assurances of almost every other democratic
society.

As Thomas Ferguson and Joel Rogers document, the turn
to the right in American politics is not reflected by a turn to
the right in public opinion polls.[10] They argue that the New
Deal coalition has not deserted the Democratic party; the
Democratic party has deserted the New Deal coalition and
its program of full employment, sustained economic growth,
defense of union rights, security in old age, unemployment
benefits, and health care for the people as a body. The New
Deal not only reached down to the poor and the powerless, it
also reached out to the middle class, whether Democrats,
independents, or Republicans.[11]

A signal contribution of universal health insurance in our
politics would be the revitalization of the political parties,
strengthening their role as the organizing force for a majority's sense of the needs of the republic. The party most likely
to take on that role is the Democratic party. The charge that
the Democratic party is a party of special interests sticks
because it is no longer trusted as the party standing for the
majority or the people as a body. Universal health insurance
would help change this, bringing the party a battle for a
stronger government role that people could understand, and
bringing the nation a clearer grasp that the purpose of a
party is to build trust in the wisdom of majority rule.

Despite the absence of political interest in universal
health insurance in Washington for almost ten years, there

is some reason to believe that this may be changing. New legislation has been introduced in the Senate by Senator Edward M. Kennedy mandating employer coverage of health insurance benefits. Washington may be responding to the end of the Reagan era as well as to the growing interest among the states in tackling the problem of the uninsured and the consequent burden of "uncompensated care" the uninsured levy on hospitals. Forty states have conducted studies of the problems of indigent care and of the uninsured. Because so many of the uninsured are employed, one favored approach is to require employers to carry health insurance. Hawaii enacted insurance of this kind in 1974, and the level of uninsured in Hawaii is estimated to be 5 percent, or less than half the national average. Massachusetts has attempted to pass a much more ambitious program, one combining mandated employer insurance and a public authority to examine and fix hospital budgets on an annual basis. This bill failed in the last days of the 1987 Massachusetts legislative session. A new and considerably weaker bill was signed into law in April 1988.[12]

A campaign for our own unique national health program will surely be met with charges of fiscal irresponsibility by members of both parties. But if the Democratic party in Congress could in 1981 capitulate to drastic cuts in taxes and domestic spending, and accept huge increases in defense spending, annual deficits, and a doubling of our national debt, surely it can now find the courage—not to speak of simple self-interest—to finance a project that might restore the trust of the nation in its role as the party of the majority.[13]

If universal health insurance is returned to the national agenda and is, miraculously, successfully developed and implemented, the Democratic party could raise its sights even farther, acknowledging the second-class status of far too many sections of our republic; our decaying infrastructure of bridges, sewers, and schools; our empty factories and eternal slums; our countryside filled with squalid trailer camps and vacant family farms overshadowed by giant agribusinesses; our water supply slowly souring from thousands of hazardous waste dumps; our urban environment befouled by smog and endless traffic jams; and our cities noted throughout the world for their violence and menace.

Perhaps the Democratic party can renew republican equality, replacing a belligerent nationalism and a resurgent religious bigotry with a calm devotion to our genuine needs as a people. Perhaps then we can trust in our courage and wisdom to sort through our many problems with the resources of renewed American spirits, traditions that leave to each individual what is properly his or her own and take up common challenges that require the resources of a community.

It is easy to despair in this cold season for the republic and for equality. But despair may turn to hope, as Robinson Jeffers suggests in his poem, "Shine, Perishing Republic":

> While this America settles in the mould of its vulgarity,
>   heavily thickening to empire,
> And protest, only a bubble in the molten mass, pops
>   and sighs out, and the mass hardens,
>
> I sadly smiling remember that the flower fades to make
>   fruit, the fruit rots to make earth.
> Out of the mother; and through the spring exultances,
>   ripeness and decadence; and home to the mother.
>
> You making haste haste on decay: not blameworthy; life
>   is good, be it stubbornly long or suddenly
> A mortal splendor: meteors are not needed less than
>   mountains: shine, perishing republic.[14]

NOTES

Chapter One

1. The idea of equality that informs this book is based on Michael Walzer's "complex equality." See his *Spheres of Justice: A Defense of Pluralism and Equality* (New·York: Basic, 1983). In contrast to "simple equality," Walzer's complex equality assumes that society is structurally complex, with different spheres allocating social goods by differing principles. Theories of equality must take into account this structural complexity.

There is a striking parallel between Walzer's ideas and Laurence Tribe's idea of "structural justice" in his *American Constitutional Law* (Mineola, N.Y.: The Foundation Press, 1978), chap. 17. Walzer's and Tribe's approaches to equality and justice differ from philosophical schemes of moral philosophy or jurisprudence based on a simple or small set of principles that underlie the entire enterprise; hence, Walzer's term, "simple equality." For a critique of Walzer, see Ronald Dworkin, "To Each His Own," a review of Walzer's *Spheres of Justice*, in *New York Review of Books*, April 14, 1983.

Thus, John Rawls's "justice as fairness" is a species of simple equality, based on breaking the tyranny of injustice by offering a "fair equality of opportunity" through a wider distribution of "primary goods" to all alike, as a way of remedying market and social inequalities. See John Rawls's *A Theory of Justice* (Cambridge: Harvard University Press, 1971). For a critique of this market-based idea of equality, see John Schaar, "Equality of Opportunity and Beyond," in *Equality, Nomos IX*, ed. J. Roland Pennock and John W. Chapman (New York: Atherton Press, 1967). For the best discussion of the varying liberal ideas of equality, see Amy Gutmann, *Liberal Equality* (New York: Cambridge University Press, 1980).

2. Bernard A. O. Williams, "The Idea of Equality," in Hugo A.

Bedau, *Justice and Equality* (Englewood Cliffs, N.J.: Prentice-Hall, 1971), 116–137.

3. My term, *republican equality*, is somewhat unusual. I chose the term, rejecting "democratic equality" (which I occasionally use) to emphasize the complexity of goods in a modern, differentiated republic, including community.

Most contemporary authors who embrace the "civic republican" tradition note its egalitarian side. See William M. Sullivan, *Reconstructing Public Philosophy* (Berkeley: University of California Press, 1986), for a discussion of equality in the civic republican tradition. While I clearly am in great sympathy with the critique of most versions of modern liberalism as having mislaid the republican roots of the American democracy, my project is not antiliberal. The basic idea of a liberal society as one that "presupposes a theory of the good, but within wide limits . . . does not prejudge the choice of the sort of persons that men want to be" belongs to John Rawls (see his *Theory of Justice*). Rawls makes this idea more explicit in works published after *A Theory of Justice*. See his "Justice as Fairness: Political not Metaphysical," *Philosophy and Public Affairs* 14 (1985): 223–251.

I believe that liberalism is large and complex enough to have within it a republican and strongly communitarian variant that seeks to marry the liberal emphasis on the autonomy of the individual with the necessity for community. See Robert N. Bellah, Richard Madsen, William M. Sullivan, Ann Swidler, and Steven Tipton, *Habits of the Heart* (Berkeley: University of California Press, 1985); see also Robert Paul Wolff, *The Poverty of Liberalism* (Boston: Beacon, 1968), for a useful communitarian critique of liberalism. See also R. H. Tawney and his theory of socialism as fellowship in *Equality* (New York: Capricorn, 1961). See Ross Terrill's *R. H. Tawney and His Times: Socialism as Fellowship* (Cambridge: Harvard University Press, 1973); George Sabine, "The Two Democratic Traditions," *Philosophical Review* 61 (1952): 451–474; Richard Titmuss, *The Gift Relationship* (New York: Vintage Books, 1971); and Dan Beauchamp, "Community: The Neglected Tradition of Public Health," *Hastings Center Report* 15 (December 1985): 28–36. One of the best communitarian justifications for public health is Jean Forster, "A Communitarian Ethical Model for Public Health Interventions: An Alternative to Individual Behavioral

Change Strategies," *Journal of Public Health Policy* 3 (1982): 150–163.

4. President's Commission for the Study of Ethical Problems in Medicine and Biomedical and Behavioral Research, *Securing Access to Health Care*, vol. 1 (Washington, D.C.: Government Printing Office, 1983).

5. See Robert Nozick, *Anarchy, State and Utopia* (New York: Basic, 1974), 234–235.

6. Centers for Disease Control, *Morbidity and Mortality Weekly Review* 37 (1988): 223–227.

7. For a good discussion of legal moralism, see Joel Feinberg, *Social Philosophy* (New York: Prentice-Hall, 1973). This dispute was articulated most clearly in the exchange between H. L. A. Hart and Lord Patrick Devlin. See H. L. A. Hart, *Law, Liberty, and Morality* (New York: Vintage, 1963), and Patrick Devlin, *The Enforcement of Morals* (London: Oxford University Press, 1965). The issue was the (London) *Report of the Committee on Homosexual Offences and Prostitution* (Cmnd. 247) 1957, otherwise known as the "Wolfenden Report."

8. President's Commission, *Securing Access to Health Care*.

9. Michael Pertschuk, *Revolt Against Regulation* (Berkeley: University of California Press, 1982).

10. Walzer, *Spheres of Justice*, 3–30.

11. Ibid., 10.

12. Ibid., 17.

13. Ibid., 10–13.

14. Ibid., 13–17.

15. The two best contemporary sources on the convergence of the biblical and civic republican traditions are Bellah et al., *Habits of the Heart*, and Sullivan, *Reconstructing Public Philosophy*. See also Michael J. Sandel, *Liberalism and Its Critics* (New York: New York University Press, 1984), especially part 2, 123–260. See Sandel's *Liberalism and the Limits of Justice* (Cambridge: Cambridge University Press, 1982). See also Chapter Four of the present work for a more detailed discussion of this tradition.

16. Ronald M. Peters, Jr., *The Massachusetts Constitution of 1780—A Social Compact* (Amherst: University of Massachusetts Press, 1978).

17. Amy Gutmann, "Communitarian Critics of Liberalism,"

Philosophy and Public Affairs 14 (Summer 1985): 308–322. For one of the best discussions of the theme of community in the American political tradition, see David Price, "Community and Control: Critical Democratic Theory in the Progressive Period," *American Political Science Review* 68 (1974): 1663–1678. See also Wolff, *The Poverty of Liberalism*.

18. Alasdair MacIntyre, *After Virtue*, 2d ed. (Notre Dame: Notre Dame University Press, 1981), 232–233. Quoted in Gutmann, "Communitarian Critics of Liberalism," 308.

19. Ibid.

20. Bellah et al., *Habits of the Heart*.

21. Ibid.

22. Alexis de Tocqueville, *Democracy in America* (Garden City, N.Y.: Anchor, 1969), 509–510.

23. Ibid.

24. Ibid. See Sullivan's *Reconstructing Public Philosophy*, 211–216, for a critique of Tocqueville. As Sullivan notes, it is not equality, but the absence of a sense of civic tradition in democratic capitalism that is the great danger. See esp. p. 214.

25. Raymond Williams, in *Keywords: A Vocabulary of Culture and Society* (New York: Oxford University Press, 1976), says that community has meant (a) the people of the common ranks (this is an archaic usage), (b) the people of a local area or district, (c) the quality of holding something in common, and (d) a sense of common identity and characteristics.

26. Ibid.

27. See Charles Forcey, *The Crossroads of Liberalism: Croly, Weyl, Lippmann, and the Progressive Era, 1900–1925* (New York: Oxford University Press, 1961), and Judith Walzer Leavitt, *The Healthiest City: Milwaukee and the Politics of Health Reform* (Princeton: Princeton University Press, 1982). See also Robert H. Wiebe, *The Search for Order: 1877–1920* (New York: Hill and Wang, 1967), 113–116; and C.-E. A. Winslow, *The Life of Herman Biggs, Physician and Statesman of the Public Health* (Philadelphia: Lea & Febiger, 1929). For a more restrictive interpretation of public health, see Paul Starr, *The Social Transformation of American Medicine* (New York: Basic, 1982), chap. 5, "The Boundaries of Public Health," 180–197.

28. John Dewey, *The Public and its Problems* (New York: Henry Holt, 1927), 149–150.

29. See Price, "Community and Control."
30. Rawls, *A Theory of Justice*, 97.
31. Ibid.
32. Ibid.
33. Ibid., 520–529 (social union) and 105–106 (fraternity).
34. I make this statement for two reasons. First, one of Rawls's leading interpreters, Norman Daniels, in his *Just Health Care* (New York: Cambridge University Press, 1985), basically ignores the idea of common provision. He does come close to arguing for a common framework for health care in his article, "Cost Containment, Justice, and Provider Autonomy," *New England Journal of Medicine* 314 (May 22, 1986): 1380–1383.

Second, the idea in "wide reflective equilibrium" or "ideal observer" approaches to ethics is to distance oneself so far from the world of shared meanings as to force into question those very notions of equality that exist in a democratic culture. See Norman Daniels, "Wide Reflective Equilibrium and Theory Acceptance in Ethics," *Journal of Philosophy* 76 (1979): 256–282. For a critique of the "ideal observer" approach in ethics see Larry R. Churchill, "The Place of the Ideal Observer in Medical Ethics," *Social Science and Medicine* 17 (1983): 897–901.

35. See Daniels, *Just Health Care*.
36. Ibid. Daniels is quoting Rawls.
37. Rawls, *A Theory of Justice*, 248–250.
38. Ibid., 250.
39. Daniels, *Just Health Care*, 153.
40. Oscar Wilde, *The Soul of Man Under Socialism* (London: Authur L. Humphreys, 1912). John Rawls's quote is from "Social Unity and Primary Goods," in *Utilitarianism and Beyond*, ed. Amartya Sen and Bernard Williams (Cambridge: Cambridge University Press, 1982). Rawls is talking here about stability in the life of a person, but the context and the many references in *A Theory of Justice* make it clear that stability is taken as a systemic need as well as a need for persons. However, as I argue, Rawls devotes little attention to how these systemic forces for stabilizing justice would be achieved.
41. Walzer, *Spheres of Justice*, 8.
42. The point about the modern hospital is taken from Judith Viorst, *Necessary Losses* (New York: Fawcett, 1986), 304. Viorst is quoting David Guttmann, "Psychoanalysis and Aging: A Develop-

mental View," *The Course of Life*, vol. 3. Department of Health and Human Services Pub. (ADM) 81-1000 (Washington, D.C.: Government Printing Office, 1981).

43. Walzer, *Spheres of Justice*, 64.

44. Ibid., 5–6.

45. Ibid., 8.

46. Joseph Tussman, *Obligation and the Body Politic* (New York: Oxford University Press, 1960), 27–28.

Chapter Two

1. That people should see themselves "as equal in some respects more fundamental than all the respects in which they are unequal" is taken from C. B. MacPherson, *The Political Theory of Possessive Individualism: Hobbes to Locke* (New York: Oxford University Press, 1962), 272.

2. Charles Lindblom, "The Market as Prison," *Journal of Politics* 44 (May 1982): 324–336.

3. President's Commission for the Study of Ethical Problems in Medicine and Biomedical and Behavioral Research, *Securing Access to Health Care*, vol. 1 (Washington, D.C.: Government Printing Office, 1983), 21. For a critical review of the commission's work, see John D. Arras, "Retreat from the Right to Health Care: The President's Commission and the Right to Health Care," *Cardozo Law Review* 6 (1984): 321–345.

4. John Rawls, *A Theory of Justice* (Cambridge: Harvard University Press, 1971), 270.

5. Michael Walzer, *Spheres of Justice: A Defense of Pluralism and Equality* (New York: Basic, 1983).

6. President's Commission, *Securing Access to Health Care*, 18.

7. Ibid.

8. Ibid., 22.

9. Ibid., 21.

10. Ibid., 17.

11. Amy Gutmann, "For and Against Equal Access to Health Care," *Milbank Memorial Fund Quarterly/Health and Society* 59 (1981): 542–560.

12. Rawls, *A Theory of Justice*, 454.

13. T. H. Marshall, *Citizenship and Social Class, and Other Essays* (Cambridge: Cambridge University Press, 1950), 56. One of the classic discussions of universalism as an organizing principle is found in Richard Titmuss, "Universal and Selective Social Services," in his *Commitment to Welfare* (London: George Allen & Unwin, 1968). For a good recent discussion of the distinction between universal and selective benefits see Neil Gilbert, *Capitalism and the Welfare State* (New Haven: Yale University Press, 1983). That universalism does not strive for equal incomes should not make us complacent about the distribution of income in the United States. This distribution is not only unequal—and growing more so—it is destabilizing to the prospects for a just society.

14. Norman Daniels, *Just Health Care* (New York: Cambridge University Press, 1985).

15. Ibid., 43. Daniels is quoting from John Rawls, "Social Unity and the Primary Goods," in *Utilitarianism and Beyond*, ed. A. K. Sen and Bernard Williams (New York: Cambridge University Press, 1982), 168.

16. John Schaar, "Equality of Opportunity and Beyond," *Equality, Nomos IX*, ed. J. Roland Pennock and John W. Chapman (New York: Atherton Press, 1967), 228–249. I mostly ignore the term "equal access" in my analysis, focusing on the norm of equity. I have done this because the term often means little more than providing the poor more access to some decent level of care, or equity, or that medicine ought to be reorganized in some optimal fashion to make it more accessible and affordable to all citizens, with little thought as to how that reorganization might be effected. For an excellent discussion of equal access in terms of the principle of equality, see Gutmann, "For and Against Equal Access to Health Care." Gutmann argues that "a principle of equal access to health care demands that every person who shares the same type and degree of health need must be given an equally effective chance of receiving appropriate treatment of equal quality so long as that treatment is available to anyone" (543). Gutmann argues that this principle leads to a one-class system and indeed a common system along the lines I have suggested, and that such a system would afford greater protection to the needs of the poor. I agree.

17. Olaf Palme, "In Praise of the Welfare State," *Harper's* (August 1984): 22–23.

18. Robert Wood Johnson Foundation, *Special Report: Updated Report on Access to Health Care for the American People* (Princeton, N.J.: Robert Wood Johnson Foundation, 1983).

19. Jack Hadley, *More Medical Care, Better Health?* (Washington, D.C.: The Urban Institute Press, 1983).

20. Judith Feder, Jack Hadley, and Ross Mullner, "Falling Through the Cracks: Poverty, Insurance Coverage, and Hospital Care for the Poor, 1980 and 1982," *Milbank Memorial Quarterly/ Health and Society* 62 (1984): 544–566.

21. Karen Davis and Diane Rowland, "Uninsured and Underserved: Inequities in Health Care in the United States," *Milbank Memorial Fund Quarterly/Health and Society* 61 (1983): 149–176. See also Gail Wilensky and Marc L. Berk, "Health Care, the Poor, and the Role of Medicaid," in *Health Affairs* 4 (Fall 1982): 93–100; Alan Monheit, Michael M. Hagan, Marc L. Berk, and Gail Wilensky, "Health Insurance for the Unemployed: Is Federal Legislation Needed?" *Health Affairs*: 101–111.

22. Davis and Rowland, "Uninsured and Underserved." For an analysis of Medicare's coverage, see Thomas Rice, "An Economic Assessment of Health Care Coverage for the Elderly," *Milbank Quarterly* 65 (1987): 488–502. Medicare covered 44 percent of the elderly's personal health care expenditures in 1986; coverage of nursing home expenditures by Medicare is virtually nonexistent.

23. Davis and Rowland, "Uninsured and Underserved."

24. Feder et al., "Falling Through the Cracks."

25. The data on the 1981 changes are based on Randall R. Bovbjerg and John Holahan, *Medicaid in the Reagan Era* (Washington, D.C.: The Urban Institute Press, 1982). See also Jerry Cromwell, Sylvia Hurdle, and Rachel Schurman, "Defederalizing Medicaid: Fair to the Poor, Fair to Taxpayers?" *Journal of Health Politics, Policy and Law* 12 (1987): 1–34. For a good discussion of the 1986 changes in the Medicaid legislation, see Intergovernmental Health Policy Project, *Major Changes in State Medicaid and Indigent Care Programs, January–December 1986* (Washington, D.C.: George Washington University Press, 1986). For a good overview of the limits of the Medicaid program written before the 1986 legislation, see Geraldine Dallek, "Six Myths of American Medical Care," *Health/PAC Bulletin* 16 (1985): 9–17. Dallek's article is the source for the estimate that 700,000 children lost Medicaid coverage because of the 1981 Budget Act as well as the point that Congress

repealed the provision that states provide comprehensive medical care for all the poor in 1972. See "Expanded Right to Medicaid Shatters Link to Welfare," *New York Times*, March 6, 1988, 1, 13.

26. Walzer, *Spheres of Justice*, 64.

27. The classic justification for pluralism is Robert Dahl's *A Preface to Democratic Theory* (Chicago: University of Chicago Press, 1956), 145.

28. Paul Starr, *The Social Transformation of American Medicine* (New York: Basic, 1982), 270–279. See also Theodore Marmor's *The Politics of Medicare* (Chicago: Aldine, 1973), and Richard Harris, *A Sacred Trust* (New York: New American Library, 1966).

29. Starr, *Social Transformation of American Medicine*, 286.

30. See Thomas Edsall, *The New Politics of Inequality* (New York: Norton, 1984), and Thomas Ferguson and Joel Rogers, *Right Turn: The Decline of the Democrats and the Future of American Politics* (New York: Hill and Wang, 1986).

31. Alan Wolfe, *America's Impasse: The Rise and Fall of the Politics of Growth* (Boston: South End Press, 1981), 81–88.

32. Starr, *Social Transformation of American Medicine*, 290–338.

33. See Dan Feschbach, "What's Inside the Black Box: A Case Study of Allocative Politics in the Hill-Burton Program," *International Journal of Health Services* 9 (1979): 313–339.

34. Gerald M. Oppenheimer and Robert A. Padgug, "AIDS: The Risks to Insurer, the Threat to Equity," *Hastings Center Report* 16 (1986): 18–22.

35. Judith Feder, *Medicare: The Politics of Federal Hospital Insurance* (Lexington, Mass.: Lexington Books, 1977).

36. John Kingdon, *Agendas, Alternatives, and Public Policies* (Boston: Little, Brown, 1984), 175. Emphasis in original.

37. Edsall, *New Politics of Inequality*. See also Morris Fiorina, *Congress: Keystone of the Washington Establishment* (New Haven: Yale University Press, 1977), for Congress's role in this pattern of politics.

38. Edsall, *New Politics of Inequality*, 23–66.

39. The seminal article in this area is Theodore J. Lowi's "American Business, Public Policy, Case Studies, and Political Theory," *World Politics* 16 (1964): 677–715. See also his "Distribution, Regulation, Redistribution: The Functions of Government," in *Readings in American Political Behavior*, ed. Raymond E. Wolfinger (Englewood Cliffs, N.J.: Prentice-Hall, 1970), 245–256.

40. Arthur Okun, *Equality and Efficiency: The Big Tradeoff* (Washington, D.C.: Brookings Institution, 1975), 119.

41. Charles L. Schultze, *The Public Use of Private Interest* (Washington, D.C.: Brookings Institution, 1977), 17–18.

42. Fred Hirsch, *Social Limits to Growth* (Cambridge: Harvard University Press, 1978).

43. Schultze, *Public Use of Private Interest*, 21.

44. Robert Heilbroner, *The Nature and Logic of Capitalism* (New York: Norton, 1985), 117–118. See also Hirsch, *Social Limits to Growth*, 84–114.

45. Ginzberg's article, "The Monetarization of Medical Care," is in *The New England Journal of Medicine* 310 (May 3, 1984): 1162–1165. Besides Ginzberg, the principal figures in the discussion of the commercialization of medicine have been Health Pac, *The American Health Empire* (New York: Random House, 1970); Starr, *Social Transformation of American Medicine*, 420–449; Arnold Relman, "The New Medical-Industrial Complex," *New England Journal of Medicine* 303 (October 23, 1980): 963–970; and Arnold Relman, "Investor-Owned Hospitals and Health-Care Costs," *New England Journal of Medicine* 309 (1983): 370–372.

46. Leonard Rosenfeld, "Costs of Health Care: Prospects and Contingencies," unpublished manuscript prepared for *Festschrift* in honor of Dr. Arthur M. Sackler, Department of Health Policy and Administration, School of Public Health, the University of North Carolina at Chapel Hill, January, 1986. Rosenfeld notes the marked increase in the number of residencies after World War II, with the number of residencies climbing from 5,000 in 1940 to more than 16,000 by 1948, to 32,000 by 1958. This dominance by specialists has likely been a major force in increasing costs of medical care in the United States (9–10).

47. Hirsch, *Social Limits to Growth*, 13–67.

48. Donald R. Cohodes, "Hospital Capital Formation in the 1980s: Is There a Crisis?" *Journal of Health Politics, Policy and Law* 8 (Spring 1983): 164–172.

49. Ibid.

50. This controversy was reported in Jeff Bendix, "Demarketing Speech Embroiled in Controversy," *Modern Healthcare* (January 1982).

51. Ibid. Berthold Brecht's line is from "Ballad on Approving the World," *Poems: 1919–1956* (New York: Methuen, 1976), 199.

52. Bradford H. Gray, *For-Profit Enterprise in Health Care*, The Institute of Medicine (Washington, D.C.: National Academy Press, 1986), 28–30.

53. Ibid.

54. Ibid. The quoted material is from the "Supplementary Statement on For-Profit Enterprise in Health Care" (205).

55. Ibid.

56. Ibid. See also Robert V. Pattison and Hallie M. Katz, "Investor-Owned and Not-for-Profit Hospitals," *New England Journal of Medicine* 309 (August 11, 1983): 347–353; and Lawrence Lewin, Robert Derzon, and Rhea Margulies, "Investor-owneds and Nonprofits Differ in Economic Performance," *Hospitals* 55 (July 1, 1981): 52–58. See Frank A. Sloan and R. A. Vraciu, "Investor-owned and Not-for-profit Hospitals," *Health Affairs* 2 (Spring 1983): 25–37, for a report of a Florida-based survey that reports that for-profit and nonprofit hospitals actually differ very little in terms of charges and treatment of the uninsured.

57. Gray, *For-Profit Enterprise in Health Care*.

58. David Starkweather, "Pros and Cons of Multi-hospital Systems," *Technical Assistance Memo* 57, Western Center for Health Planning, San Francisco, November 4, 1980.

59. Committee on the Costs of Medical Care, *Medical Care for the American People. The Final Report of the Committee on the Costs of Medical Care* (Chicago: University of Chicago Press, 1932).

60. Ibid., 108–118.

61. Ibid., 193. For the text of Hamilton's personal statement, see 189–200.

62. Ibid., 193.

63. Ibid., 195.

64. Ibid., 195–196.

65. James A. Morone and Andrew B. Dunham, "Slouching Toward National Health Insurance: The Unanticipated Politics of DRGs," *Bulletin of the New York Academy of Medicine* 62 (1986): 646–662.

66. Ibid., 648.

67. Ibid.

68. Ibid.
69. Ibid., 649.
70. Ibid., 646.
71. Ibid., 657–658.
72. Ibid., 658–659.

Chapter Three

1. Ronald Bayer, "AIDS, Power and Reason," *The Milbank Quarterly* 64, Supp. 1 (1986): 172–173.
2. Michael Pertschuk, *Revolt Against Regulation* (Berkeley: University of California Press, 1982).
3. Phyllis Tilson Piotrow, *World Population Crisis: The United States Response* (New York: Praeger, 1973).
4. The classic defense of freedom of speech is Alexander Meiklejohn, *Free Speech and Its Relation to Self-Government* (New York: Harper & Bros., 1948).
5. Daniel Patrick Moynihan, "Epidemic on the Highways," *The Reporter*, April 30, 1959, 16.
6. For a study of public interest lobbying see Jeffrey Berry, *Lobbying for the People* (Princeton: Princeton University Press, 1977). See also Pertschuk, *Revolt Against Regulation*.
7. Ralph Nader, *Unsafe at Any Speed* (New York: Grossman, 1965).
8. Rachel Carson, *Silent Spring* (Boston: Houghton Mifflin, 1962).
9. See James Q. Wilson, ed., *The Politics of Regulation* (New York: Basic, 1980), for a good review of this literature. The quotation from Wilson's book is taken from his chapter, "The Politics of Regulation," 366. For an excellent article summarizing other theories for the emergence of public interest lobbies, see Jeffrey Berry, "On the Origins of Public Interest Groups: A Test of Two Theories," *Polity* 10 (1978): 379–397.
10. Wilson, *The Politics of Regulation*, 366–372.
11. Ibid., 367.
12. Ibid., 370.
13. See Robert Dahl, *A Preface to Democratic Theory* (Chicago:

University of Chicago Press, 1957), 145, for a definition of "normal politics."

14. See Pertschuk, *Revolt Against Regulation*. See also Thomas Edsall, *The New Politics of Inequality* (New York: Norton, 1984), 107–140.

15. William M. Sullivan, *Reconstructing Public Philosophy* (Berkeley: University of California Press, 1986), 192–207.

16. Ibid., 196. Sullivan relies in this section on Richard Alan Ryerson, *The Revolution Is Now Begun* (Philadelphia: University of Pennsylvania Press, 1978), for the quotation.

17. Sullivan, *Reconstructing Public Philosophy*, 200–201.

18. Robert Reich, ed., *The Power of Public Ideas* (Cambridge: Ballinger, 1988), 4.

19. Government of Canada/Ministry of National Health and Welfare, *A New Perspective on the Health of Canadians* (Ottawa: Ministry of National Health and Welfare, 1974).

20. Aaron Wildavsky, "Can Health Be Planned?" The 1976 Michael M. Davis Lecture, the Center for Health Administration Studies, University of Chicago, April 23, 1976.

21. Alexis de Tocqueville, *Democracy in America*, ed. J. P. Mayer (Garden City, N.Y.: Anchor, 1969), 692.

22. U.S. Department of Health, Education and Welfare, *Forward Plan for Health* (Washington, D.C.: Government Printing Office, 1975).

23. Richard E. Palmer, M.D., "My Turn: The AMA's Health Plan," *Newsweek*, June 6, 1977, 11.

24. Leon Kass, "Regarding the End of Medicine and the Pursuit of Health," *Public Interest* 40 (1975): 11.

25. Chauncey Starr, "Social Benefit Versus Technological Risk," *Science* 165 (1969): 1232–1238.

26. Ibid.

27. National Safety Council, *Accident Facts* 1985 ed. (Chicago: National Safety Council, 1985), 40.

28. Geoffrey Rose, "Sick Individuals and Sick Populations," *International Journal of Epidemiology* 14 (1985): 32–38.

29. Mancur Olson, Jr., *The Logic of Collective Action* (Cambridge: Harvard University Press, 1965). For another excellent discussion of market failures, see Charles Lindblom's *Politics and Markets* (New York: Basic, 1977). See esp. chap. 6, "The Limited Compe-

tence of Markets." For a good discussion of collective consumption goods, see Norman Frohlich, Joe A. Oppenheimer, and Oran Young, *Political Leadership and Collective Goods* (Princeton: Princeton University Press, 1971). For a good discussion tying political obligation to the provision of collective goods, see Nannerl Henry, "Political Obligation and Collective Goods," *Political and Legal Obligation, Nomos XII*, ed. J. Roland Pennock and John W. Chapman (New York: Atherton, 1970), 263–289.

30. Adam Smith, *An Enquiry into the Nature and Causes of the Wealth of Nations*, ed. Edwin Cannan (New York: Modern Library, 1937), 681.

31. Brian Barry, *The Liberal Theory of Justice* (Oxford: Clarendon Press, 1973), 118–119.

32. Thomas Schelling, *Micromotives and Macrobehavior* (New York: Norton, 1978), 19.

33. The idea of scale is taken from Garrett Hardin, *Filters Against Folly* (New York: Penguin, 1985), 128–137.

34. Rose, "Sick Individuals and Sick Populations."

35. Mark Moore and Dean Gerstein, *Alcohol and Public Policy: Beyond the Shadow of Prohibition* (Washington, D.C.: National Academy Press, 1981); emphasis added.

36. Geoffrey Rose, "Strategy of Prevention: Lessons from Cardiovascular Disease," *British Medical Journal* 282 (1981): 1850.

37. Margaret E. Mattson, Earl S. Pollack, and Joseph W. Cullen, "What Are the Odds that Smoking Will Kill You?" *American Journal of Public Health* 77 (1987): 425–431.

38. Fred Hirsch, *Social Limits to Growth* (Cambridge: Harvard University Press, 1978).

39. The data on handgun availability are based on Philip J. Cook's "The Influence of Gun Availability on Violent Crime Patterns," in *Crime and Justice: An Annual Review of Research*, ed. Michael Tonry and Norval Morris (Chicago: University of Chicago Press, 1983).

40. The data on plastic guns are from Dan Bischoff, "I Just Want to Say One Word to You: Plastics," *Mother Jones Magazine* 11 (October 1986): 30–33, 54.

41. Gerald Dworkin, "Paternalism," *Monist* 56 (1972): 64–84. See also his "Paternalism," in *Morality and the Law*, ed. R. A. Wasserstrom (Belmont, Calif.: Wadsworth Press, 1971), 107–206.

42. Ronald Dworkin, "Liberty and Moralism," in *Taking Rights Seriously* (Cambridge: Harvard University Press, 1977), 263.

43. John Stuart Mill, *On Liberty*, ed. and with an introduction by Marshall Cohen (New York: Modern Library, 1961), 197.

44. Ibid., 276. Mill's reference to drunkenness is on p. 298.

45. Richard Bonnie, "Discouraging Unhealthy Personal Choices: Reflections on New Directions in Substance Abuse Policy," *Journal of Drug Issues* 8 (1978): 199–219. See also Bonnie, "The Efficacy of Law as a Paternalistic Instrument," *Nebraska Symposium on Motivation, 1985*, ed. G. Melton (Lincoln: University of Nebraska Press, 1986), 131–211.

46. Joel Feinberg, *Social Philosophy* (Englewood Cliffs, N.J.: Prentice-Hall, 1973), 50–52.

47. Dennis Thompson, "Paternalism in Medicine, Law, and Public Policy," in *Ethics Teaching in Higher Education*, ed. Daniel Callahan and Sissela Bok (New York: Plenum, 1980), 245–272.

48. Bonnie, "Discouraging Unhealthy Personal Choices."

49. Albert Weale, "Invisible Hand or Fatherly Hand? Problems of Paternalism in the New Perspective on Health," *Journal of Health Politics, Policy and Law* 7 (1983): 785–807.

50. Feinberg, *Social Philosophy*, 48.

51. D. D. Raphael, *Moral Judgment* (London: Allen & Unwin, 1955). For a communitarian alternative to paternalistic justifications for limiting lifestyle risks see Jean Forster, "A Communitarian Ethical Model of Public Health Interventions: An Alternative to Individual Behavior Change," *Journal of Public Health Policy* 3 (1982), 150–163.

52. Mill, *On Liberty*, 273.

53. Richard Flathman, *The Public Interest: An Essay Concerning the Normative Discourse of Politics* (New York: Wiley, 1966).

54. James Childress, *Who Should Decide? Paternalism in Health Care* (New York: Oxford University Press, 1982).

55. Ronald Dworkin, *Taking Rights Seriously*, 261.

56. Ibid., 263; emphasis added.

57. *Commonwealth v. Alger*, 7 Cushman 53 (1853).

58. See Pertschuk, *Revolt Against Regulation*, for a good discussion of the forces in favor of rolling back consumer protection legislation. For the market as prison idea, see Charles Lindblom, "The Market as Prison," *Journal of Politics* 44 (1982): 324–336.

59. These data are from Ronald Bayer and Jonathan Moreno, "The Limits of the Ledger in Public Health Promotion," *Hastings Center Report* 15 (December 1985): 37–41. Bayer and Moreno base the section of their article on helmet legislation on the unpublished paper by Stephen P. Teret, "Motorcycle Helmet Laws: Can the State Legislate Prudence?" Prepared for the Hastings Center Project, "Health Promotion: Ethical and Governmental Dilemmas," 1982. See Teret's "The Law and the Public's Health," *Biolaw—A Legal and Ethical Reporter on Medicine, Health Care, and Engineering* 1 (1986): 29–50.

60. Ralph Hingson, Suzette Levenson, Timothy Heeren, et al., "Repeal of the Massachusetts Seat Belt Law" (Washington, D.C.: Insurance Institute for Highway Safety, 1987).

61. Michael Pertschuk, *Revolt Against Regulation*, uses the phrase "National Nanny," which he found in a *Washington Post* editorial.

62. Leon Edel, *Stuff of Sleep and Dreams* (New York: Harper & Row, 1982), 47–65.

Chapter Four

1. Robert N. Bellah, Richard Madsen, William M. Sullivan, Ann Swidler, and Steven M. Tipton, *Habits of the Heart* (Berkeley: University of California Press, 1985).

2. Henry Steele Commager, *Majority Rule and Minority Rights* (New York: Peter Smith, 1950), 3.

3. John H. Schaar, "The Case for Patriotism," *American Review* 17 (New York: Bantam Books, 1973), 73.

4. For one of the best studies of English Puritanism, see Michael Walzer, *The Revolution of the Saints: A Study in the Origins of Radical Politics* (Cambridge: Harvard University Press, 1965). For a description of American Puritanism, see anything by Perry Miller, but especially his *Errand into the Wilderness* (Cambridge: Belknap Press of Harvard University Press, 1958).

5. Roland Berthoff, "Peasants and Artisans, Puritans and Republicans: Personal Liberty and Communal Equality in American History," *Journal of American History* 69 (December 1982): 579–598. The importance of the commonwealth tradition is discussed

in Leonard Levy, *The Law of the Commonwealth and Chief Justice Shaw* (Cambridge: Harvard University Press, 1957), 303–321. See also Oscar and Mary Handlin, *Commonwealth—A Study of the Role of Government in the American Economy: Massachusetts, 1774–1861* (Cambridge: Belknap, 1969).

6. The decision is *Jacobson v. Massachusetts*, 197 U.S. 11 (1905).

7. See Ronald M. Peters, Jr., *The Massachusetts Constitution of 1780—A Social Compact* (Amherst: University of Massachusetts Press, 1978).

8. See H. Richard Niebuhr, "The Idea of the Covenant and the American Political Tradition," in *Puritanism and the American Experience*, ed. Michael McGiffert (Reading, Mass.: Addison-Wesley, 1969), 219–226. See also Schaar, "The Case for Patriotism."

9. Lemuel Shattuck, *Report of the Sanitary Commission of Massachusetts, 1850* (Cambridge: Harvard University Press, 1948), 9–10.

10. Levy, *Chief Justice Shaw*. The present work is heavily indebted to Levy's study of the development of law and of the police power in Massachusetts under Justice Shaw. I also have been strongly influenced by Ernest Freund, *The Police Power—Public Policy and Constitutional Rights* (Chicago: Callaghan & Company, 1904). I have also relied on Scott M. Reznick's study of the police power, "Empiricism and the Principle of Conditions in the Evolution of the Police Power: A Model for Definitional Scrutiny," *Washington University Law Quarterly* (1978): 1–90, as well as Rodney L. Mott, *Due Process of Law* (Indianapolis: Bobbs-Merrill, 1926); and W. G. Hastings, "The Development of Law as Illustrated by the Decisions Relating to the Police Power of the State," *Proceedings of the American Philosophical Society* 39 (1900): 359–554. Among current scholars of this period, I have relied most heavily on Harry Scheiber, "Law and the Imperatives of Progress: Private Rights and Public Values in American Legal History," in *Ethics, Economics, and the Law, Nomos XXIV*, ed. J. R. Pennock and John W. Chapman (New York: New York University Press, 1982).

11. *Gibbons v. Ogden*, 9 Wheaton 1 (1824).

12. *Commonwealth v. Alger*, 7 Cushman 53 (1853).

13. Levy, *Chief Justice Shaw*, 246. Levy is actually referring here to *Commonwealth v. Tewksbury*, 11 Metcalf 55 (1846).

14. *Commonwealth v. Alger*, 82–83; my emphasis.

15. *Black's Law Dictionary*, 4th ed. (St. Paul, Minn.: West Publishing, 1968), 1551.
16. *Commonwealth v. Alger*, 96.
17. Levy, *Chief Justice Shaw*; emphasis added.
18. Freund, *The Police Power*, 25–26.
19. *Munn v. Illinois*, 94 U.S. 113 (1877).
20. Ibid.
21. Ibid.
22. The most influential nineteenth-century legal theorists holding this view were Thomas M. Cooley and Christopher G. Tiedeman. Cooley's most famous treatise is *A Treatise on the Constitutional Limitations Which Rest upon the Legislative Power of the States of the American Union* (Boston: Little, Brown, 1868). Tiedeman's best-known work on the police power is *A Treatise on the Limitations of Police Power in the United States*, 2 vols. (St. Louis: F. Thomas Law Book Co., 1900). A third voice belongs to Edwin Corwin, *Liberty Against Government* (Baton Rouge: Louisiana State University Press, 1948). But Levy, *Chief Justice Shaw*, and Freund, *The Police Power*, take the opposing view, as do W. W. Willoughby, *The Constitutional Law of the United States*, 2d ed. (New York: Baker, Voorhis & Co., 1929), and W. G. Hastings, "The Development of Law."
23. Freund, *The Police Power*, 6.
24. Hastings, "The Development of Law."
25. *Crowley v. Christensen*, 137 U.S. 86 (1890).
26. See Norman H. Clark, *Deliver Us from Evil* (New York: Norton, 1976); John Allen Krout, *The Origins of Prohibition* (New York: Knopf, 1925); and Paul Aaron and David Musto, "Temperance and Prohibition in America: An Overview," in *Alcohol and Public Policy: Beyond the Shadow of Prohibition*, ed. Mark H. Moore and Dean R. Gerstein (Washington, D.C.: National Academy Press, 1981), 140–142.
27. Quoted in Moore and Gerstein, *Alcohol and Public Policy*, 260, from *License Cases*, 5 Howard 504 (U.S.) (1847).
28. Quoted in Levy, *Chief Justice Shaw*, 261.
29. Ibid.
30. *Fisher v. McGirr*, 1 Gray 1 (Mass.) (1854). See Levy, *Chief Justice Shaw*, 261–262 for discussion of this case.
31. *Mugler v. Kansas*, 123 U.S. 623 (1887).
32. Ibid., 630.

33. Ibid., 662–663.

34. Leonard Glantz, "Constitutional Implications of Scientific and Technological Advances in Public Health" (Paper prepared for the Office of Technology Assessment, U.S. Congress, April 1987). My assessment of the role of the Court in the late-nineteenth and early-twentieth century is indebted to Benjamin F. Wright, *The Growth of American Constitutional Law* (New York: Houghton Mifflin, 1942). *Holden v. Hardy*, 169 U.S. 366 (1898).

35. Kenneth R. Wing, *The Law and the Public's Health*, 2d ed. (Ann Arbor, Mich.: Health Administration Press, 1985), 18.

36. For an excellent discussion of the tendency of courts to scrutinize public health restrictions in terms of their medical and procedural integrity, see Scott Burris, "Current Topics in Law and Policy: Fear Itself—AIDS, Herpes and Public Health Decisions," *Yale Law & Policy Review* 3 (1985): 479–518.

37. *Jacobson v. Massachusetts*, 197 U.S. 11 (1905).

38. Ibid.

39. Ibid. Glantz, "Constitutional Implications," 14–15, argues that the principal meaning of this passage is that Jacobson should understand that if he is to partake of the benefits of a community he must also accept its burdens, and that if he dissents from its policies he is free to move from Cambridge. I think this interpretation is too "localized" an interpretation of the police power. Generally, public health measures, especially reforms, were instituted to overcome the corruption and resistance of local municipalities to adequate health and safety measures.

40. See, for example, "Limiting the State's Police Power: Judicial Reaction to John Stuart Mill," *University of Chicago Law Review* 37 (1970): 605–627; Robert E. Clark and Michael M. Sophy, "Fluoridation: The Courts and the Opposition," *Wayne Law Review* 13 (1967): 338–375; George A. Strong, "Liberty, Religion and Fluoridation," *Santa Clara Lawyer* 8 (1967): 37–58; Kenneth M. Royalty, "Motorcycle Helmets and the Constitutionality of Self-Protective Legislation," *Ohio State Law Journal* 30 (1969): 355–381; *Notes*, Constitutional Law: "Police Power—Michigan Statute Requiring Motorcyclists to Wear Protective Helmets Held Unconstitutional," *Michigan Law Review* 67 (1968): 360–373.

41. See, for example, Clark and Sophy, "Fluoridation."

42. *Kaul v. City of Chehalis*, 45 Wash. 2d 616, 277 P. 2d 352 (1954): 356.

43. *Schuringa v. City of Chicago*, 30 Ill. 2d 504, 198 N.E. 2d 326 (1964).

44. See Earl Finbar Murphy, *Water Purity: A Study in Legal Control of Natural Resources* (Madison: University of Wisconsin Press, 1961).

45. See "Limiting the State's Police Power . . . "; The Illinois Supreme Court, in *The People v. Fries*, 42 Ill. 2d 446, 250 N.E. 2d 149 (1969), ruled that the helmet law was unconstitutional on the basis that the fundamental intent of the legislation was the regulation "of what is essentially a matter of personal safety" (151). The Illinois decision is atypical of the body of police regulations across the states.

46. *American Motorcycle Association v. Davids*, 11 Mich. App. 351, 158 N.W. 2d 72 (1968). A New York court, in rejecting the constitutionality of the helmet legislation, argued as follows: "As the police power is understood by this court it justifies the regulation of the conduct of one person because of the effect of the conduct upon other persons. Therefore the police power does not justify the statute on the basis of the direct effect alone. Is the indirect effect such that the police power authorizes the statute? In the opinion of this court it is not." *People v. Carmichael*, 53 Misc. 2d 584, 588, 279 N.Y.S. 2d 272, 277 (Genesee County Ct. Spec. Sess. 1967), rev'd, 56 Misc. 2d 388, 288 N.Y.S. 2d 931 (Genesee County Ct. 1968).

47. William F. Stone, "State's Power to Require an Individual to Protect Himself," *Washington and Lee Law Review* 26 (1969): 112–119.

48. *Griswold v. Connecticut*, 381 U.S. 479 (1965).

49. Wing, *The Law and the Public's Health*, chap. 4. Michael J. Perry, in "Abortion, the Public Morals, and the Police Power: The Ethical Function of Substantive Due Process," *U.C.L.A. Law Review* 23 (1976): 689–736, argues that, in the privacy cases the courts are returning to substantive due process, which they abandoned in the 1930s. In many ways this is true, but I believe that Perry's interpretation could easily be construed as a return of the Court to an earlier period, when it functioned as a "council of revision" over the work of Congress and state legislatures generally—a theory of judicial review advocated but rejected in the Constitutional Convention. On the role of the Court from 1890 to 1940, see Wright, *The*

Growth of American Constitutional Law, 16–17. I am more per-suaded by Laurence Tribe's thesis that the Court's modern role in protecting the rights of personhood is part of a larger, complex system of "structural justice." See his *American Constitutional Law* (Mineola, N.Y.: The Foundation Press, 1978), especially chap. 17.

50. Wing, *The Law and the Public's Health*.

51. *Griswold v. Connecticut*, 484.

52. Ibid., 485.

53. Ibid., 505.

54. Ibid., 506.

55. *Eisenstadt v. Baird*, 405 U.S. 438 (1972), 453.

56. Ibid., 448.

57. Ibid.

58. Ibid., 450.

59. *Carey v. Population Services International*, 431 U.S. 678 (1978).

60. Ibid.

61. *Roe v. Wade*, 410 U.S. 113 (1973). The companion case is *Doe v. Bolton*, 410 U.S. 179 (1973).

62. *Roe v. Wade*, 156–162.

63. Ibid., 162.

64. Roger Wertheimer, "Understanding the Abortion Argu-ment," *Philosophy and Public Affairs* 1 (1971): 67–95.

65. For a good discussion of legal moralism, see Joel Feinberg, *Social Philosophy* (Englewood Cliffs, N.J.: Prentice-Hall, 1973). See also Chapters Five, Six and Seven here.

66. *Bowers v. Hardwick*, 106 U.S. 2841 (1986). For a federal district court ruling that reached the opposite conclusion, see *Baker v. Wade*, 743 F. 2d 236 (1984).

67. *Posadas de Puerto Rico Associates, DBA Condado Holiday Inn v. Tourism Company of Puerto Rico*, 106 S. Ct. 2968 (1986).

68. *Central Hudson Gas and Electric Corp. v. Public Service Commission of New York*, 447 U.S. 557 (1980).

69. *Virginia State Board of Pharmacy v. Virginia Citizens Con-sumer Council, Inc.*, 425 U.S. 748 (1976).

70. Ibid.

71. *Central Hudson Gas and Electric Corp. v. Public Service Commission of New York*.

72. *Holiday Inn v. Tourism Company of Puerto Rico*.

73. Ibid.

74. Ibid. Rehnquist is here referring to *Carey v. Population Services*, 97 S. Ct. 2010 (1977).

75. Ibid.

76. Ibid.

77. Ibid.

78. Ibid.

79. Tribe, *American Constitutional Law*, 1137.

80. Ibid.

81. Ibid. Emphasis in original.

82. Ibid., 1139.

83. Bellah, et al., *Habits of the Heart*; Dan E. Beauchamp, "Community: The Neglected Tradition of Public Health," *Hastings Center Report* 15 (December 1985): 28–36.

Chapter Five

1. For an excellent discussion of the conflicts between the differing meanings of privacy in a public order, see Richard F. Hixson, *Privacy in a Public Society: Human Rights in Conflict* (New York: Oxford University Press, 1987). *The Power of Public Ideas*, ed. Robert Reich (Cambridge: Ballinger, 1988), was published as this book was in its final stages of production, but clearly its chapters on democracy as public deliberation and discussion parallel many of the ideas in this chapter.

2. Gary L. Bostwick, "Comment: A Taxonomy of Privacy: Repose, Sanctuary, and Intimate Decision," *California Law Review* 64 (1976): 1447–1483. The original article that stimulated the debate over a right to privacy concerned the invasion of privacy of well-known individuals by reporters and newspapers. See Samuel D. Warren and Louis D. Brandeis, "The Right to Privacy," *Harvard Law Review* 4 (1890): 193–220.

3. Nancy Milio, "Health Education = Health Instruction + Health News: Media Experiences in the United States, Finland, Australia, and England," in *The Media, Social Science, and Social Policy for Children*, ed. E. A. Rubenstein and Jane D. Brown (New Jersey: Ablex, 1985). For a good review of the difficulty of tracing changes in health practices due to specific mass media campaigns,

see Lawrence Wallack, "Mass Media Campaigns: The Odds Against Finding Behavior Change," *Health Education Quarterly* 8 (1981): 209–260. Wallack supports the larger point that publicity and controversy are potent forces in shaping the public health.

4. See Paul J. Quirk, "Food and Drug Administration," in *The Politics of Regulation*, ed. James Q. Wilson (New York: Basic, 1980), 191–235.

5. For a good account of the thalidomide scandal internationally, see Henning Sjoberg and Robert Nilsson, *Thalidomide and the Power of the Drug Companies* (Harmondsworth, England: Penguin, 1972).

6. See U.S. Department of Health, Education and Welfare, Public Health Service, National Institutes of Health, *Proceedings of the Conference on the Decline in Coronary Heart Disease Mortality* (Washington, D.C.: Government Printing Office, 1979).

7. Letitia Brewster and Michael F. Jacobson, *The Changing American Diet* (Washington, D.C.: Center for Science in the Public Interest, 1978), cited in Janet M. Levine, "The Politics of Diet and Heart Disease," in *Consuming Fears*, ed. Harvey M. Sapolsky (New York: Basic, 1986), 40–79.

8. Kenneth E. Warner, "The Effects of the Anti-Smoking Campaign on Cigarette Consumption," *American Journal of Public Health* 67 (1977): 645–650.

9. Kenneth E. Warner and Hillary Murt, "Premature Deaths Avoided by the Antismoking Campaign," *American Journal of Public Health* 73 (1983): 672–677.

10. Warner, "The Effects of the Anti-Smoking Campaign," 649.

11. Warner and Murt, "Premature Deaths Avoided by the Antismoking Campaign," 676.

12. See Lawrence Wallack, "Mass Media and Health Promotion: Ideological and Practical Foundations" (unpublished manuscript, School of Public Health, University of California, Berkeley, October 1987). Wallack provided much useful criticism for this chapter, and was especially helpful in getting me to see the need to draw the issues of privacy and democratic controversy closer together.

13. For results of surveys of changes in homosexual practices in San Francisco, see Leon McKusick, William Horstman, and Thomas J. Coates, "AIDS and Sexual Behavior Reported by Gay Men in San Francisco," *American Journal of Public Health* 75 (1985): 493–496. For a similar survey of gay sexual practices in New York,

see John L. Martin, "The Impact of AIDS on Gay Male Sexual Behavior Patterns in New York City," *American Journal of Public Health* 77 (1987): 578–581. For a case study of the role of the media in publicizing the risks for AIDS, even bringing up topics like anal sex, which a few years back would have been unthinkable to a newspaper editor, see Stephen Klaidman and Tom L. Beauchamp, *The Virtuous Journalist* (New York: Oxford University Press, 1987), 147–150.

14. See Lydia Temoshok, Margaret Grade, and Jane Zich, "Public Health, the Press, and AIDS: An Analysis of Newspaper Articles in London and San Francisco," in *AIDS: Principles, Practices, and Politics*, ed. Inge B. Corless, unabrg. (New York: Harper & Row, 1988).

15. Department of Health and Human Services, Assistant Secretary for Health, *Review of the Research Literature on the Effects of Health Warning Labels: A Report to the United States Congress* (Washington, D.C.: Government Printing Office, 1987). An earlier report by the Department of Health and Human Services and the Department of the Treasury recommended against warning labels on alcohol, mainly on grounds of efficacy; see U.S. Department of the Treasury and U.S. Department of Health and Human Services, *Report to the President and the Congress on Health Hazards Associated with Alcohol and Methods to Inform the General Public of these Hazards* (Washington, D.C.: Government Printing Office, November 1980). President Carter disagreed with these findings in his letter transmitting the report to Congress.

16. Alexander Meiklejohn, *Free Speech and Its Relation to Self-Government* (New York: Harper & Bros., 1948), 37.

17. R. C. Smith, "The Magazines' Smoking Habit," *Columbia Journalism Review* 16 (1978): 29–31. See also D. Owen, "The Cigarette Companies: How They Get Away with Murder, Part II," *Washington Monthly* (March 1985): 48–54, for a good discussion of the difficulties of a journalist in trying to place an article with a journal (*The New Republic*) that feared the loss of advertising revenues.

18. Kenneth E. Warner, *Selling Smoke: Cigarette Advertising and Public Health* (Washington, D.C.: American Public Health Association, 1986).

19. Kenneth E. Warner, "Cigarette Advertising and Media Cover-

age of Smoking and Health," *New England Journal of Medicine* 312 (1985): 384–388.

20. Kenneth E. Warner, Virginia L. Ernster, John L. Holbrook, et al., "Promotion of Tobacco Products," *Journal of Health Politics, Policy and Law* 11 (1986): 368.

21. J. L. Hamilton, "The Demand for Cigarettes: Advertising, the Health Scare, and the Cigarette Advertising Ban," *Review of Economics and Statistics* 54 (1972): 401–411.

22. George Seldes, *Witness to a Century* (New York: Ballantine Books, 1987), 459–462.

23. *Virginia State Board of Pharmacy v. Virginia Citizens Consumer Council, Inc.*, 425 U.S. 748 (1976), 770.

24. Kenneth E. Warner, *Selling Smoke*, 64.

25. *Bigelow v. Virginia*, 421 U.S. 809 (1975). The best account of the nineteenth-century connection between advertising and abortion is James C. Mohr, *Abortion in America: The Origins and Evolution of National Policy, 1800–1900* (New York: Oxford University Press, 1978).

26. *Bigelow v. Virginia*.

27. *Roe v. Wade*, 410 U.S. 113 (1973).

28. *Valentine v. Chrestensen*, 316 U.S. 52 (1942).

29. *Virginia State Board of Pharmacy v. Virginia Citizens Consumer Council, Inc.*

30. *Bigelow v. Virginia*, 759.

31. Ibid., 760.

32. *Virginia State Board of Pharmacy v. Virginia Citizens Consumer Council, Inc.*

33. Ibid., 765.

34. Meiklejohn, *Free Speech and Its Relation to Self-Government*.

35. Ibid., 91.

36. The central case for the commercial speech doctrine is *Central Hudson Gas & Electric Corp. v. Public Service Commission of New York*, 447 U.S. 557 (1980). In *Posadas de Puerto Rico Associates, DBA Condado Holiday Inn v. Tourism Company of Puerto Rico* (1986), Brennan in his dissent implied that the doctrine might not be applicable to public health hazards like alcohol or tobacco.

37. Justice William Rehnquist, dissenting, in *Virginia State Board of Pharmacy v. Virginia Citizens Consumer Council, Inc.*, 784.

38. Ibid., 787.

39. Ibid., 781.

40. *New York Times Co. v. Sullivan*, 376 U.S. 254 (1964).

41. *Virginia State Board of Pharmacy v. Virginia Citizens Consumer Council, Inc.*, 764.

42. *Abrams v. United States*, 250 U.S. 616 (1919), 630.

43. Meiklejohn, *Free Speech and Its Relation to Self-Government*, 87. Of course, Justice Holmes could have meant by "market" something closer to the Greek *agora*, a place of public assembly and deliberation, bringing his view closer to Meiklejohn's thesis.

44. My argument for more speech, and government's responsibility in assuring more speech, shifts the emphasis in the doctrine of free speech from limits on government to the affirmative duties of government to remove private limits. The classic case reviewing this issue for the broadcast media, or the Fairness Doctrine, is *Red Lion Broadcasting Co. v. FCC*, 395 U.S. 367 (1969), a case involving the duty of a Pennsylvania radio station to air opposing points of view. See also an earlier case, *Associated Press et al. v. U.S.*, 326 U.S. 1 (1945), where the Court argued that "freedom of the press from governmental interference under the First Amendment does not sanction repression of that freedom by private interests" (p. 20). For articles discussing the general notion of access to the media, see Lee C. Bollinger, Jr., "Freedom of the Press and Public Access: Toward a Theory of Partial Regulation of the Mass Media," *Michigan Law Review* 75 (1976), 1–42; and Kenneth L. Karst, "Equality as a Central Principle in the First Amendment," *The University of Chicago Law Review* 43 (1975): 20–68. Another possible reason the Courts took the path toward obliterating the distinction between free speech and commercial speech was the relatively minor role given free speech in the privacy (intimate decision) cases. For a study of the rise of the family planning and contraception issues that stress the key role that free discussion plays, see Phyllis Piotrow, *World Population Crisis: The United States Response* (New York: Praeger, 1973); James Reed, *From Private Vice to Public Virtue: The Birth Control Movement and American Society Since 1830* (New York: Basic, 1973); and Ernest Gruening, *Many Battles* (New York: Liveright, 1973). In *Griswold v. Connecticut*, 381 U.S. 479 (1965), Justice White uses something of a free speech argument in his concurring opinion, arguing that the Connecticut law did deprive couples of available knowledge about contraception (p. 503). Douglas, in the majority opinion, links the right to privacy to

the various guarantees of the First Amendment, including freedom of speech and assembly (see pp. 484–485).

45. Thomas Scanlon, "A Theory of Freedom of Expression," *Philosophy and Public Affairs* 1 (1972): 215, 212; emphasis in original.

46. Hannah Arendt, "Lying in Politics," in her *Crises of the Republic* (New York: Harcourt Brace Jovanovich, 1972), 1–47. See also Arendt's "Truth and Politics," in *Between Past and Future* (New York: Viking, 1961), 227–264. Fred Hirsch, in *Social Limits to Growth* (Cambridge: Harvard University Press, 1978), makes much the same point.

47. See note 44 for a discussion of the Fairness Doctrine. The quoted passage indicating the obligations of license holders is from *Red Lion Broadcasting Co. v. FCC*, 380.

48. Ben Bagdikian, *The Media Monopoly* (Boston: Beacon, 1983).

49. Christopher Lasch, *The Culture of Narcissism* (New York: Norton, 1978), 74. Quoted in Michael Schudson, *Advertising: The Uneasy Persuasion* (New York: Basic, 1984), 228.

50. Neil Postman, *Amusing Ourselves To Death: Public Discourse in the Age of Show Business* (New York: Viking/Penguin, 1985).

51. Harry Frankfurt, "On Bullshit," *Raritan* 6 (Fall 1986): 81–100.

52. Schudson, *Advertising: The Uneasy Persuasion*, 225–227.

53. Ibid., 209–223.

54. Ibid., 221–222.

55. Alan S. Levy and Raymond C. Stokes, "Effects of a Health Promotion Advertising Campaign on Sales of Ready-to-Eat Cereals," *Public Health Reports* 102 (1987): 398–403.

56. Daniel Callahan, "How Technology is Reframing the Abortion Debate," *Hastings Center Report* 16 (February 1986): 33–42.

57. William S. Nelson, *The Americanization of the Common Law* (Cambridge: Harvard University Press, 1975), 110–116.

58. Kristen Luker, *Abortion and the Politics of Motherhood* (Berkeley: University of California Press, 1984).

59. Mohr, *Abortion in America*.

60. Ibid., 6.

61. Ibid., 74.

62. Ibid.

63. See Aaron M. Powell, "The President's Opening Address," in *The National Purity Congress*, ed. Aaron M. Powell (New York: Arno

Press, 1976 [1896]), 1; quoted in C. Thomas Dienes, *Law, Politics, and Birth Control* (Urbana: University of Illinois Press, 1972), 37.

64. Mohr, *Abortion in America*, 18, 240.

65. This paragraph relies on Piotrow, *World Population Crisis: The United States Response*, and Reed, *From Private Vice to Public Virtue*.

66. See Piotrow, *World Population Crisis*.

67. Stanley K. Henshaw, Jacqueline D. Forrest, and Jennifer Van Vort, "Abortion Services in the United States, 1984 and 1985," *Family Planning Perspectives* 19 (March/April 1987): 63–70. About 40 million abortions are performed worldwide each year, and some experts see abortion as essential to a sound population control policy. See Stephen Mumford and Elton Kessel, "Is Wide Availability of Abortion Essential to National Population Growth Control Programs? Experiences of 116 Countries," *American Journal of Obstetrics and Gynecology* 149 (1984): 639–645.

68. Frederick J. Taussig, *Abortion, Spontaneous and Induced: Medical and Social Aspects* (St. Louis: C. V. Mosby, 1936). Cited in Mohr, *Abortion in America*, 254.

69. Christopher Tietze, "The Effects of Legalization of Abortion on Population Growth and Public Health," *Family Planning Perspectives* 7 (May/June 1975).

70. Roger Wertheimer, "Understanding the Abortion Argument," *Philosophy and Public Affairs* 1 (1971): 23–51.

71. Bostwick notes that in *Skinner v. Oklahoma ex rel. Williamson*, 316 U.S. 535 (1942), the Court overturned an Oklahoma law authorizing sterilization of persons convicted more than twice of certain felonies involving moral turpitude as violative of the equal protection of the law (p. 1468). The majority decisions in *Skinner* and in *Griswold* several decades later were written by Justice Douglas. In *Cleveland Board of Education v. LaFleur*, 414 U.S. 632 (1974), the Court invalidated a school board regulation that required pregnant teachers to take leave at least five months before delivery—a ruling patently designed to discourage pregnancy. Similarly, in *Loving v. Virginia*, 388 U.S. 1 (1967), the Court overturned a Virginia law prohibiting racially mixed marriages. In all of these cases the Court found these restrictions on the freedom of intimate decisions violative of the Constitution without mentioning privacy. See Bostwick, "A Taxonomy of Privacy," 1468–1469.

72. Hixson, *Privacy in a Public Society*, 85. Hixson is quoting Luker, *Abortion and the Politics of Motherhood*, and her point that to prolife groups the decision appears to move the question of when life begins to the private sphere, a move that to these groups seems roughly equivalent to making freedom of speech a mere matter of opinion. But Luker does not indicate that she accepts this view, and I do not find that the Court has made the entire abortion decision a matter of private opinion—only the question of when life begins. Hixson, in noting that the abortion decision is based on private criteria, is quoting Paul Bender, "The Privacies of Life," *Harper's* (April 1974): 41–44. Indeed, I find that abortion is declared a private right for public reasons: the unborn, particularly those in the earliest stages of pregnancy, are publicly declared not entitled to the legal protections of persons.

73. See *Roe v. Wade*, 410 U.S. 113 (1973), 158, where Justice Blackmun argues that "all this . . . persuades us that the word 'person,' so used in the 14th Amendment, does not include the unborn."

74. *Bowers v. Hardwick*, 106 S. Ct. 2841 (1986), 2854. Jackson's language is from *West Virginia Board of Education v. Barnette*, 319 U.S. 624 (1943), 641–642.

75. Cheryl D. Haynes, ed., *Risking the Future: Adolescent Sexuality, Pregnancy, and Childbearing* (Washington, D.C.: National Academy Press, 1987).

76. Bonnie Steinbock, "Baby Jane Doe in the Courts," *Hastings Center Report* 14 (February 1984): 13–19, and John Arras, "Toward an Ethic of Ambiguity," ibid. (April 1984): 25–33.

77. George Annas, "Women as Fetal Containers," *Hastings Center Report* 16 (December 1986): 13–14.

78. *Bowers v. Hardwick*, 2857–2858.

79. Ibid., 2851.

80. Ibid.

81. Ibid., 2855. In *Maher v. Roe*, 97 S. Ct. 2376 (1977), the Court overturned a federal district court opinion (408 F. Supp. 660 [1975]) that had declared unconstitutional federal bans on the use of Medicaid funding for abortion. The majority opinion, written by Justice Powell, reasoned that the right to an abortion did not mean that the government must supply the means for an abortion, even for poor women. This reveals one of the principal weaknesses of thinking about privacy as solely a right to withdraw from society.

Privacy is also the right of citizens to enjoy privileges, despite opposition from religious groups or even the majority. The right to an abortion is something like the right to a fair trial; it requires an implementing structure to give effect to that right, and the majority must not be permitted to take away what the courts have permitted.

Chapter Six

1. Alasdair MacIntyre, *After Virtue*, 2d ed. (Notre Dame, Ind.: Notre Dame University Press, 1984), 253–254.

2. John Stuart Mill, *On Liberty*, ed. and with an introduction by Marshall Cohen (New York: The Modern Library, 1961).

3. Richard Hofstadter, *The Age of Reform* (New York: Knopf, 1956), 287–288.

4. H. L. Mencken, *A Mencken Chrestomathy* (New York: Vintage, 1982), 624.

5. W. J. Rorabaugh, *The Alcoholic Republic* (New York: Oxford University Press, 1979). See also John Allen Krout, *The Origins of Prohibition* (New York: Knopf, 1925).

6. Rorabaugh, *The Alcoholic Republic*, 149–155.

7. Ibid.

8. See Paul Aaron and David F. Musto, "Temperance and Prohibition in America: A Historical Overview," in *Alcohol and Public Policy: Beyond the Shadow of Prohibition*, Report of the Panel on Alternative Policies for the Prevention of Alcohol Abuse and Alcoholism, National Academy of Sciences, ed. Mark Moore and Dean Gerstein (Washington, D.C.: National Academy Press, 1981), 127–181.

9. Alexander Hamilton, *The Federalist*, ed. Jacob E. Cooke (Middleton, Conn.: Wesleyan University Press, 1961), 78.

10. Aaron and Musto, "Temperance and Prohibition in America," 138.

11. Garry Wills, *Explaining America: The Federalist* (Garden City, N.Y.: Doubleday, 1981).

12. Aaron and Musto, "Temperance and Prohibition in America."

13. James H. Timberlake, *Prohibition and the Progressive Movement: 1900–1920* (Cambridge: Harvard University Press, 1966).

14. Daniel Bell, *The Cultural Contradictions of Capitalism* (New York: Basic, 1976).

15. Aaron and Musto, "Temperance and Prohibition in America."

16. David Musto, "Quarantine and the Problem of AIDS," *Milbank Quarterly* 64, supp. 1 (1986): 97–117.

17. Aaron and Musto, "Temperance and Prohibition in America," 151.

18. Ibid., 160. The authors are quoting R. C. Binkley, *Responsible Drinking: A Discreet Inquiry and a Modest Proposal* (New York: Vanguard, 1930), 25.

19. Antonin Artaud, *The Theatre and Its Double* (New York: Grove, 1958), 30.

20. Oliver MacDonagh, "The Nineteenth-Century Revolution in Government: A Reappraisal," *The Historical Journal* 1 (1958): 52–67. The point that alcohol and prohibition never were included in these beginnings of bureaucracy originated with Brian Harrison, *Drink and the Victorians—The Temperance Question in England, 1815–1872* (London: Faber and Faber, 1971).

21. Jack S. Blocker, Jr., *Retreat From Reform* (Westport, Conn.: Greenwood Press, 1976).

22. See Charles Forcey, *The Crossroads of Liberalism, 1900–1925* (New York: Oxford University Press, 1961), for a good discussion of the importance of these political intellectuals in the Progressive period. See also Robert Wiebe, *The Search for Order* (New York: Hill and Wang, 1967).

23. Norman H. Clark, *Deliver Us From Evil: An Interpretation of American Prohibition* (New York: Norton, 1976).

24. See Milton Terris, "Epidemiology of Cirrhosis of the Liver: National Mortality Data," *American Journal of Public Health* 57 (1967): 2076–2088. See also Aaron and Musto, "Temperance and Prohibition in America."

25. Alpheus T. Mason, *Security Through Freedom: American Political Thought and Practice* (Ithaca, N.Y.: Cornell University Press, 1955), 93–96.

26. See Dan E. Beauchamp, *Beyond Alcoholism: Alcohol and Public Health Policy* (Philadelphia: Temple University Press, 1980).

27. Morris Chafetz, "Carry Nation Had a Drinking Problem," *Johns Hopkins Magazine*, March 1976, 8–17.

28. See Beauchamp, *Beyond Alcoholism*.

29. Harry Gene Levine, "The Discovery of Addiction," *Journal of Studies on Alcohol* 39 (1978): 143–174.

30. See Beauchamp, *Beyond Alcoholism*, for a discussion of A.A.'s policy of anonymity.

31. National Center for Prevention and Control of Alcoholism, National Institute of Mental Health, *Alcohol and Alcoholism* (Washington, D.C.: Government Printing Office, 1969), 24.

32. Selden Bacon, "Alcoholics Do Not Drink," *Annals of the American Academy of Political and Social Science* 315 (January 1958): 63.

33. Morris Chafetz, *Why Drinking Could Be Good for You* (New York: Stein and Day, 1976), 109–110.

34. Abraham Myerson, "Alcohol: A Study of Social Ambivalence," *Quarterly Journal of Studies on Alcohol* 6 (1945/1946): 480–499. See also Albert D. Ullman, "Sociocultural Backgrounds Conducive to Alcoholism," *Annals of the American Academy of Political and Social Sciences* 315 (1958). See Beauchamp, *Beyond Alcoholism*, for a critical review of this literature.

35. Morris Chafetz, "Alcoholism Prevention and Reality," *Quarterly Journal of Studies on Alcohol* 28 (1967): 343.

36. The seminal work in this area in North America was by Jan deLint and Wolfgang Schmidt. Their early article was "The Distribution of Alcohol Consumption in Ontario," *Quarterly Journal of Studies on Alcohol* 29 (1968): 968–973.

37. This research was reviewed in the early seventies by Kettil Bruun, Griffith Edwards, M. Lumio, et al., *Alcohol Control Policies in Public Health Perspective* (Helsinki: Finnish Foundation for Alcohol Studies, 1975).

38. Ibid.

39. The distribution of consumption thesis was first proposed by the French demographer, Sully Ledermann. See his "Can One Reduce Alcoholism Without Changing Total Alcohol Consumption in a Population?" (Paper presented at the 27th International Congress on Alcohol and Alcoholism, Frankfurt-am-Main, 1964). For a relatively recent overview of this research, see Robin Room, *Annual Review of Public Health* 5 (1984): 293–317, for a review of studies

of availability, age limits, and the like, and public health consequences.

40. James Blose and Harold Holder, "Liquor-by-the-Drink and
Alcohol-Related Traffic Crashes: A Natural Experiment Using Time
Series Analysis," *Journal of Studies on Alcohol* 48 (1987): 52–60.

41. See Bruun, Edwards, Lumio, et al., *Alcohol Control Policies
in Public Health Perspective.*

42. Moore and Gerstein, *Alcohol and Public Policy.*

43. The most recent in this series is U.S. Department of Health
and Human Services, Public Health Service, Alcohol, Drug Abuse,
and Mental Health Administration, National Institute on Alcohol
Abuse and Alcoholism, *Sixth Special Report to the U.S. Congress on
Alcohol and Health* (Washington, D.C.: Government Printing Office,
1987).

44. Dean Gerstein, "Alcohol Use and Consequences," in Moore
and Gerstein, *Alcohol and Public Policy*, 193.

45. These data are based on National Institute on Drug Abuse,
"Highlights of the 1985 National Household Survey on Drug Abuse:
National Institute on Drug Abuse," *NIDA Capsules* (November
1986), and the University of Michigan Institute for Social Research,
Ann Arbor, Michigan, News and Information Service, February 20,
1987, reporting on the twelfth national survey of drug use in a sample of U.S. high schools. The "National Household Survey" found
that current users of marijuana (users during the past month)
declined from 20 million in 1982 to 18.2 million in 1985, while
current use of cocaine increased from 4.2 million in 1982 to 5.8
million, an increase from 2 percent of the household population to
3 percent. The Michigan survey reported that while well over half
of all high school seniors still report some experience with illicit
drugs, the gradual decline in most drug use observed over the past
decade is still continuing.

46. Nils Christie, "Foreword," in Klaus Mäkelä, Robin Room,
Eric Single, et al., *Alcohol, Society, and the State* (Toronto: Addiction Research Foundation, 1981), xiii–xvii.

47. David F. Musto, *The American Disease* (New Haven: Yale
University Press, 1973).

48. Ibid.

49. Ibid., 64.

50. See Paul S. Boyer, *Purity in Print: The Vice-Society Move-*

ment and Book Censorship in America (New York: Scribner's, 1968), 24. For other sources detailing the fascinating decades from 1880 to 1920, with their interesting admixture of moralism and environmental reforms, see David J. Pivar, *Purity Crusade: Sexual Morality and Social Control, 1868–1900* (Westport, Conn.: Greenwood Press, 1973). Pivar notes the many parallels between crusades against prostitution, immorality, obscenity, and alcohol. See also C. Thomas Dienes, *Law, Politics, and Birth Control* (Urbana: University of Illinois Press, 1972).

51. Musto, *The American Disease*, 22.

52. *U.S. v. Jin Fuey Moy*, 241 U.S. 394 (1916).

53. The Court reversed the *Jin Fuey Moy* decision in two 1919 decisions: *U.S. v. Doremus*, 249 U.S. 86 (1919), and *Webb et al. v. U.S.*, 249 U.S. 96 (1919).

54. John Kaplan, *Marijuana—The New Prohibition* (New York: World, 1969), 89–98.

55. In *Robinson v. California*, 370 U.S. 660 (1962), the Court ruled that the state cannot make narcotics addiction a crime. The public drunkenness case is *Powell v. Texas*, 392 U.S. 514 (1968).

56. See John Kaplan, *The Hardest Drug* (Chicago: University of Chicago Press, 1983).

57. See "Highlights of the 1985 Household Survey on Drug Abuse." Overall, 62 million Americans over twelve years of age (33 percent) have tried marijuana at least once in their lives. Current (during the past month) use of marijuana occurs among roughly 10 percent of the population aged twelve or older, or 18 million individuals.

Chapter Seven

1. These projections are taken from "PHS Plan for Prevention and Control of AIDS and the AIDS Virus," *Public Health Reports* 101 (July–August 1986): 341–348. The report is included as Appendix G in Institute of Medicine, National Academy of Sciences, *Confronting AIDS* (Washington, D.C.: National Academy Press, 1986), 326–333.

2. *New York Times*, June 5, 1987.

3. *Confronting AIDS*, 8.

4. Ibid.

5. Ibid.

6. Ibid., 42–50.

7. Ronald Bayer, "AIDS, Power and Reason," *Milbank Quarterly* 64, supp. 1 (1986): 172–173.

8. Mark Kleinman, "AIDS, Vice, and Public Policy" (paper presented at the Conference on Vice, Duke University, June 5–6, 1987), 2.

9. Ibid.

10. Ibid., 3.

11. Ibid., 4.

12. Albert Camus, *The Plague*, trans. Stuart Gilbert (New York: Modern Library, 1948), 229.

13. William Ryan, *Blaming the Victim* (New York: Vintage, 1971), 14–15.

14. William Haddon, Jr., "Energy Damage and the Ten Countermeasure Strategies," *The Journal of Trauma* 13 (1973): 321–331.

15. C.-E. A. Winslow, *The Evolution and Significance of the Modern Public Health Campaign* (New Haven: Yale University Press, 1923).

16. Ibid.

17. George Rosen, *A History of Public Health* (New York: MD Publications, 1958).

18. Ibid., 211 ff. for a discussion of Chadwick's report. See pp. 134–135 for a discussion of the influence of Jeremy Bentham. See also Winslow, *The Modern Public Health Campaign*.

19. For a good brief summary of the quarantine dispute, see David F. Musto, "Quarantine and the Problem of AIDS," *Milbank Quarterly* 64, supp. 1 (1986): 97–117. The classic article surveying this dispute is E. H. Ackerknecht, "Anti-contagionism Between 1821 and 1867," *Bulletin of the History of Medicine* 22 (1948): 562–593.

20. Musto, "Quarantine and the Problem of AIDS."

21. Rush is cited in Musto, "Quarantine and the Problem of AIDS." The quotation is taken from Benjamin Rush, *An Inquiry into the Various Sources of the Usual Forms of Summer and Autumnal Disease, in the United States and the Means of Preventing Them*, in his *Medical Inquiries and Observations*, 4th ed., vol. 4 (Philadelphia: Johnson and Warner, 1815), 107–139.

22. Musto, "Quarantine and the Problem of AIDS."

23. Camus, *The Plague.*

24. The quotation of Defoe appears as the epigraph of *The Plague* and is from *A Journal of the Plague Year*, ed. Anthony Burgess (Harmondsworth, England: Penguin, 1966). It was first published in 1722.

25. See Edwin M. Schur and Hugo A. Bedau, *Victimless Crimes* (Englewood Cliffs, N.J.: Prentice-Hall, 1974), 90. Bedau's section of this work is a good discussion of moralism. See also Joel Feinberg, *Social Philosophy* (Englewood Cliffs, N.J.: Prentice-Hall, 1973), 36–46, and Feinberg's *Rights, Justice, and the Bounds of Liberty* (Princeton, N.J.: Princeton University Press, 1980). See also Ronald Dworkin, *Taking Rights Seriously* (Cambridge: Harvard University Press, 1977), chap. 11; and A. D. Woozley, "Law and the Legislation of Morality," in *Ethics in Hard Times*, ed. Daniel Callahan and Arthur Caplan (New York: Plenum, 1981). See H. L. A. Hart, "Social Solidarity and the Enforcement of Morality," *The University of Chicago Law Review* 35 (1967): 1–13; and *Law, Liberty, and Morality* (New York: Vintage, 1963).

26. Harold Garfinkel, "Conditions of Successful Status Degradation Ceremonies," *American Journal of Sociology* 61 (March 1956): 420–424.

27. Quoted in C. Thomas Dienes, *Law, Politics and Birth Control* (Urbana: University of Illinois Press, 1972), 31.

28. James F. Stephen, *Liberty, Equality, and Fraternity*, ed. R. J. White (Cambridge: Cambridge University Press, 1967).

29. *Ratchford v. Gay Lib* 434 U.S. 1080, 1082 reh'g denied, 435 U.S. 981 (1978).

30. Stephen, *Liberty, Equality and Fraternity.*

31. Lord Patrick Devlin, *The Enforcement of Morals* (Oxford: Oxford University Press, 1959). Devlin's book is a reply to the "Wolfenden Report," the *Report of the Committee on Homosexual Offences and Prostitution* (London, Cmnd. 247), 1957. However, Ronald Dworkin argues that Devlin did not support the use of the criminal law to suppress private homosexual acts. See "The Bork Nomination," *The New York Review of Books* (August 13, 1987): 10. As Dworkin notes, "Devlin thinks the majority has a right to enforce its moral views only in unusual circumstances, when unorthodox behavior would actually threaten cultural continuity, and he does not think that his views would support making private homosexual acts between consenting adults criminal" (10).

32. Justice Burger, concurring opinion, *Bowers v. Hardwick*, 106 S. Ct. 2841 (1986), 2847. Burger is referring to the Justinian Code in sixth-century Rome. See note 37 below.

33. Ibid.

34. The source of this history of Roman and Christian attitudes toward homosexuality is John Boswell's *Christianity, Social Tolerance, and Homosexuality* (Chicago: The University of Chicago Press, 1980).

35. Ibid., 92–98.

36. Revised Standard Version.

37. Boswell, *Christianity, Social Intolerance, and Homosexuality*, 171. Justinian made homosexuality subject to the death penalty, at least potentially, but adultery was accorded the same treatment. Apparently, Justinian saw famine, pestilences, and earthquakes as signs of divine disfavor tied to sexual immorality.

38. Ibid., chaps. 10, 11.

39. Ibid.

40. See Robert Oaks, "Perceptions of Homosexuality by Justices of the Peace in Colonial Virginia," in *Homosexuality and the Law*, a special double issue of *The Journal of Homosexuality* 5 (1979/80): 35–42.

41. These data are found in Bernard Knox's book review, "Subversive Activities," *The New York Review of Books* (December 19, 1985): 3. Knox is reviewing Louis Crompton's *Byron and Greek Love: Homophobia in Nineteenth-Century England* (Berkeley: University of California Press, 1985), pp. 15–18.

42. Twenty-six states have repealed sodomy laws. Twenty-four states and the District of Columbia still retain them. See David A. J. Richards, "Homosexual Acts and the Constitutional Right to Privacy," and Joseph J. Bell, "Public Manifestations of Personal Morality: Limitations on the Use of Solicitation Statutes to Control Homosexual Cruising," in *Homosexuality and the Law*, a special double issue of *The Journal of Homosexuality* 5 (1979/80), for a good discussion of homosexuality and the law.

43. Alasdair MacIntyre, *After Virtue*, 2d ed. (Notre Dame, Ind.: Notre Dame University Press, 1984).

44. Walt Whitman, *Democratic Vistas*, in *The Portable Walt Whitman* (hereafter, *PWW*), ed. Mark Van Doren, rev. Malcolm Cowley (New York: Penguin, 1977), 317–382. Walt Whitman's ideas about democracy and his Civil War experiences visiting the

hospitals of the Union's Army of the Potomac in the Washington, D.C., area are beautifully described in Lewis Hyde's *The Gift* (New York: Random House, 1983), 160–215. This chapter would not have been conceived without my encounter with Hyde's essay on Whitman. For discussions of Whitman's homosexuality and the homoerotic side of his poetry, see Robert K. Martin, *The Homosexual Tradition in American Poetry* (Austin: University of Texas Press, 1979), 3–8; Martin Bauml Duberman, *About Time: Exploring the Gay Past* (New York City: Gay Presses of New York, 1986), 84–96; and Gay Wilson Allen, *The Solitary Singer* (New York: Macmillan, 1955), 421–425. The most recent and widely acclaimed biography passes over the subject obliquely, mentioning Whitman's "sexuality" in connection with his lifelong interest in phrenology and "adhesiveness." See Justin Kaplan, *Walt Whitman—A Life* (New York: Simon & Schuster, 1980), 148–156.

45. *PWW*.

46. Ibid., 353. Quoted in Hyde, *The Gift*, 195.

47. Hyde, *The Gift*, 196.

48. Ibid.

49. Ibid.

50. Ibid. Whitman's phrase is at *PWW*, 335.

51. See Hyde, *The Gift*, 196–202. Hyde treats adhesiveness as a species of fraternity and erotic love, a "gift" that binds up community, unlike market exchange. See also Allen, *The Solitary Singer*, 421–425.

52. Hyde, *The Gift*, 197.

53. Quoted in Martin, *The Homosexual Tradition in American Poetry*. See *Democratic Vistas*, *PWW*, p. 369.

54. See Kaplan, *Walt Whitman—A Life*, for a discussion of phrenology.

55. For this phase of Whitman's life I have relied on Whitman's *Specimen Days*, in *PWW* as well as Kaplan, *Walt Whitman—A Life*, Hyde, *The Gift*, and Allen, *Solitary Singer*.

56. See Kaplan, *Walt Whitman*, p. 276. The source of the comment was James Redpath. See also, Hyde, *The Gift*, p. 170.

57. The source of these estimates is Whitman, *Specimen Days*, in *PWW*, 438–439.

58. Ibid., 439.

59. Ibid.

60. Ibid. , 412.

61. Kaplan, *Walt Whitman*, 277.

62. Hyde, *The Gift*, 206.

63. See Kaplan, *Walt Whitman—A Life*, where Whitman uses the phrase in a letter to Emerson.

64. Poll data cited in Charles Turner, "Public Perceptions, Plural and Individual Behaviors in Response to AIDS Epidemic" (background paper submitted to the Committee on a National Strategy for AIDS, Institute of Medicine, National Academy of Sciences). See *Confronting AIDS*, 335.

65. *Bowers v. Hardwick*.

66. For the best discussion of the emergence of a gay subculture, see Dennis Altman, *The Homosexualization of America* (Boston: Beacon, 1982).

67. See E. Michael Gorman, "The AIDS Epidemic in San Francisco: Epidemiological and Anthropological Perspectives," in *Anthropology and Epidemiology*, ed. Craig R. Janes, Ron Stall, and Sandra M. Gifford (Boston: D. Reidel, 1986), 157–172; Edmund White, *States of Desire* (New York: E. P. Dutton, 1980); and Frances FitzGerald, *Cities on a Hill* (New York: Simon & Schuster, 1981). See also Randy Shilts, *And the Band Played On—Politics, People, and the AIDS Epidemic* (New York: St. Martin's, 1987).

68. Kristen Luker, *Abortion and the Politics of Motherhood* (Berkeley: University of California Press, 1984).

69. Altman, *AIDS in the Mind of America*, 14.

70. Walt Whitman, *Democratic Vistas*, *PWW*, 369. The section head is the title of one of Whitman's poems in *Leaves of Grass*, *PWW*, 126–133.

71. Martin, *The Homosexual Tradition in American Poetry*, 19–20.

72. Altman, *The Homosexualization of America*, 79–80.

73. Dennis Altman, "The New Frontline for Gay Politics," *Socialist Review*, September/October 1982.

74. White, *States of Desire*, 250–294.

75. Ibid., 282.

76. "Fisting" refers to inserting one's fist in the anus of the partner.

77. White, *States of Desire*.

78. Altman, *Homosexualization of America*, 80.

79. Altman, *AIDS in the Mind of America*.

80. This line is from a notebook kept by Whitman, quoted in Allen, *Solitary Singer*, 423.

81. Karla Jay and Allen Young, *The Gay Report* (New York: Summit Books, 1979), 500–501. Actually, this statement needs qualification. *The Gay Report* lists the bath as the site outside a residence where sex is "very" or "somewhat" frequently engaged in by a minority of gay men.

82. Ibid., 248.

83. Ibid., 251.

84. Terry A. Sandholzer, "Factors Affecting the Incidence and Management of Sexually Transmitted Diseases in Homosexual Men," in *Sexually Transmitted Diseases in Homosexual Men*, ed. D. G. Ostrow, T. A. Sandholzer, and Y. N. Felman (New York: Plenum, 1983), 3–12. Sandholzer is quoting *Sexual Behavior in the Human Male* by Alfred C. Kinsey, Wardell B. Pomeroy, and Clyde E. Martin (Philadelphia: W.B. Saunders, 1948).

85. Sandholzer, "Sexually Transmitted Diseases."

86. Ibid.

87. Ibid. See Centers for Disease Control, "Continuing Increase in Infectious Syphilis—United States," *Morbidity and Mortality Weekly Review* 37 (January 29, 1988): 35–38, for discussion of upsurge in syphilis among heterosexuals.

88. Leon McKusick, W. Horstman, T. J. Coates, "AIDS and Sexual Behavior Reported by Gay Men in San Francisco," *American Journal of Public Health* 75 (1985): 493–496; and Research and Decisions Corporation, "A Report on Designing an Effective AIDS Prevention Campaign Strategy for San Francisco: Results from the Second Probability Sample of an Urban Gay Male Community" (San Francisco: The San Francisco AIDS Foundation, 1985). Also, Centers for Disease Control, "Self-Reported Changes in Sexual Behaviors Among Homosexual and Bisexual Men from the San Francisco City Clinic Cohort," *Morbidity and Mortality Weekly Report* 36 (April 3, 1987): 187–189.

89. John L. Martin, "The Impact of AIDS on Gay Male Sexual Behavior Patterns in New York City," *American Journal of Public Health* 77 (1987): 578–581.

90. Ibid.

91. Ibid.

92. Ibid.

93. *PWW*, 484.

94. *PWW*.

95. Gorman, "The AIDS Epidemic in San Francisco," 167.

96. Ibid.; Altman, *AIDS in the Mind of America*.

97. Anne A. Scitovsky, Mary Lee Cline, Philip R. Lee, "Medical Care Costs of Patients with AIDS in San Francisco," *Journal of the American Medical Association* 256 (December 12, 1986): 3103–3106.

98. Bernard A. O. Williams, "The Idea of Equality," in Hugo A. Bedau, *Justice and Equality* (Englewood Cliffs, N.J.: Prentice-Hall, 1971), 116–137.

99. Lydia Temoshok, Margaret Grade, and Jane Zich, "Public Health, The Press, and AIDS: An Analysis of Newspaper Articles in London and San Francisco," in *AIDS: Principles, Practices, and Politics*, ed. Inge B. Corless, unabrg. (New York: Harper, 1988).

100. Defoe, *A Journal of the Plague Year*, 18.

101. White, *States of Desire*, 282.

102. The phrase is Anthony Burgess's, in his introduction to Defoe, *A Journal of the Plague Year*, 18.

103. *Bowers v. Hardwick*, 2848–2856.

104. Ibid., 2851.

105. MacIntyre, *After Virtue*.

106. *PWW*, 343–344.

107. For an excellent discussion of some of the leading ethical and legal issues in AIDS, see Larry Gostin and William J. Curran, "The Limits of Compulsion in Controlling AIDS," *Hastings Center Report* (December 1986), 24–29. See also Ron Bayer, Carol Levine, and Susan M. Wolf, "HIV Antibody Screening: An Ethical Framework for Evaluating Proposed Programs," *Journal of the American Medical Association* 254 (1985): 1342–1345. See also G. M. Oppenheimer and R. Padgug, "AIDS: The Risks to Insurers, the Threat to Equity," *Hastings Center Report* 16 (1986), 18–22, for a review of the limits of the private insurance market in protecting potential AIDS victims.

108. David S. Weinberg and Henry S. Murray, "Coping With AIDS: The Special Problems of New York City," *New England Journal of Medicine* 317 (1987): 1469–1472.

109. The actual line from Rousseau is "How shall men love their

country if it is nothing more for them than for strangers, and bestows on them only that which it can refuse to none?" See Jean-Jacques Rousseau, "A Discourse on Political Economy," in *The Social Contract and Discourses*, ed. G. D. H. Cole (New York: 1950), 302–303; quoted in Michael Walzer, *Spheres of Justice* (New York: Basic, 1983), 64.

110. James D. Watkins, "Chairman's Recommendations for the Full Presidential Commission on the Human Immunodeficiency Virus Epidemic," February 29, 1988, Washington, D.C.

111. See Michael J. Barry, Paul D. Cleary, and Harvey V. Fineberg, "Screening for HIV Infection: Risks, Benefits, and the Burden of Proof," *Law, Medicine and Health Care* 14 (December 1986): 259–267. For a good discussion of the issue of closing the bath houses, see Scott Burris, "Current Topics in Law and Policy: Fear Itself: AIDS, Herpes, and Public Health Decisions," *Yale Law and Policy Review* 3 (1985): 504–516.

112. 106 S. Ct. 2841 (1986). In *Watkins v. United States*, 837 F. 2d. 1428 (1988), the United States Court of Appeals for the Ninth Circuit held unconstitutional the Army's discharge of an enlisted man on the grounds of homosexuality, not on grounds of privacy, but because it denied homosexuals equal protection of the laws. In his dissent, although Judge Reinhardt felt compelled to adhere to *Hardwick*, he made plain that he believed that "the Supreme Court egregiously misinterpreted the Constitution in *Hardwick*. In my view, *Hardwick* improperly condones official bias and prejudice against homosexuals, and authorized the criminalization of conduct that is an essential part of the intimate sexual life of many of our homosexual citizens, a group that has historically been the victim of unfair and irrational treatment. I believe that history will view *Hardwick* much as it views *Plessy v. Ferguson*, 163 U.S. 537 (1896). And I am confident that, in the long run, *Hardwick*, like *Plessy*, will be overruled by a wiser and more enlightened Court."

113. *Congressional Record*, 100th Cong., 1st sess., 1987, vol. 133, Senate, S14204, October 14, 1987.

114. Hart Crane, *The Bridge* (New York: Liveright, 1970). The quotation is from Thomas A. Vogler's introduction. Crane's poem was originally published in 1930.

115. *The Bridge*, 74–75.

Chapter Eight

1. The inspiration for this last chapter, with its focus on re-membering the republic, is John H. Schaar's essay, "The Case for Patriotism," *American Review 17* (New York: Bantam Books, 1973), 59–99. The idea of a republic as "living together to accomplish things together" is from José Ortega y Gasset's *Invertebrate Spain*, trans. Mildred Adams (New York: Norton, 1937), 26.

2. Schaar, "The Case for Patriotism," 60.

3. For an excellent review of the issues in testing, see Ronald Bayer and Carol Levine, "HIV Antibody Screening: An Ethical Framework for Evaluating Proposed Programs," *Journal of the American Medical Association* 256 (1986): 1768–1774.

4. Several papers on this topic were presented at the Third International Conference on AIDS, Washington, D.C., June 1–5, 1987; most of them have not been published. An abstract of the paper by Charles Farthing, W. Jesson, A. G. Lawrence, and B. G. Gazzard, "The HIV Antibody Test: The Influence on Sexual Behavior of Homosexual Men," suggests that "the antibody test, administered with preliminary counselling, may be an important factor in preventing the spread of HIV infection." The authors go on to say that "except in exceptional circumstances, patients should only be tested with their consent and with time to consider the implications." Another paper presented on this issue was David W. Lyter, Ronald O. Valdiserri, Lawrence A. Kingsley, et al., "Factors Influencing the Decision to Learn HIV Antibody Results in Gay and Bisexual Men." For a study that suggests that learning antibody status did not result in safer sexual practices, see R. Fox, N. Odaka, and F. Polk, "Effect of Learning HTLV-III/LAV Antibody Status on Subsequent Sexual Activity" (Abstract, International Conference on AIDS, Paris, June 1986). For a published paper dealing with the issues this subject raises, see D. Miller, D. Jeffries, J. Greene, J. R. W. Harris, and A. Pinching, "HTLV: Should Testing Ever Be Routine?" *British Medical Journal* 292 (1986): 941–942.

Any consideration of increased testing should be accompanied by efforts to reform the nation's seriously outmoded laws on quarantine and sexually transmitted disease. For an excellent discussion of this topic, see Larry Gostin, "The Future of Communicable Disease Control: Toward a New Concept in Public Health Law," *Milbank Quarterly* 64, supp. 1 (1986): 79–96. See also Wendy Parmet, "AIDS and Quarantine: The Revival of an Archaic Doctrine," *Hofstra Law Review* 14 (Fall 1985): 53–90.

5. John Iglehart's series on the Canadian health system ran in *The New England Journal of Medicine* 316 (July 17, September 18, and December 18, 1986). Judith Feder, William Scanlon, and John Clark, "Canada's Health Care System," *New England Journal of Medicine* 317 (July 30, 1987): 320. Iglehart's reply to this letter is found on p. 321 of the same issue.

6. Feder, Scanlon, and Clark, "Canada's Health Care System."

7. Ibid. As Lester Thurow has argued in his *The Zero-Sum Solution* (New York: Simon & Schuster, 1985), if growth in the United States had continued at the pre-1965 rate of "slightly above 3 percent per year, today's health-care spending would absorb only 7 to 8 percent of the GNP and there would be much less pressure to control health care costs" (253).

8. Uwe Reinhardt, "We've Got a Health-Cost Crisis? Bunk," *Medical Economics*, July 23, 1984, 28.

9. John Kenneth Galbraith, *The Affluent Society* (Boston: Houghton Mifflin, 1958).

10. Thomas Ferguson and Joel Rogers, *Right Turn: The Decline of the Democrats and the Future of American Politics* (New York: Hill and Wang, 1986).

11. Samuel P. Huntington, "The Visions of the Democratic Party," *The Public Interest* 79 (Spring 1985): 63. Huntington argues that the Democrats ought to abandon policies that exclusively "reach down" in favor of policies that "reach out" to the middle class, many members of which are Independent or Republican.

12. The data for this section are taken from Patricia Butler, Molly Joel Coye, Edward P. Ehlinger, et al., "Report to the APHA Executive Board from the Task Force on State Health Insurance as Part of a National Health Program" (Washington, D.C.: American Public Health Association, January 1988). For information on the Massachusetts bill, see David A. Danielson and Susan Abrams, "The Massacre of MASSCARE: Dukakis' Health-Insurance Plan and Why It Was Defeated," *Health/PAC Bulletin* 17 (Winter 1987), 6–11.

13. One of the best accounts of this period is David Stockman's *The Triumph of Politics* (New York: Avon, 1987).

14. Robinson Jeffers, "Shine, Perishing Republic," in *The Selected Poems of Robinson Jeffers* (New York: Vintage, 1963), 9. Copyright © 1963 by Random House, Inc. and used here with permission of the publisher. I first found this poem in Garrett Epps's novel *The Floating Island* (Boston: Houghton Mifflin, 1985). William Sullivan also quotes Jeffers in his *Reconstructing Public Philosophy* (Berkeley: University of California Press, 1986).

INDEX

Aaron, Paul, 174–177

Abortion: advertising services for, 129, 144–146, 159; and autonomy, 162, 166; Court decision on, 126, 164; moralism and, 158–161, 163, 167, 238; in nineteenth century, 158–160; outlawing of, 160–161; right to privacy and, 71, 125–126, 157, 162, 166–167, 264n, 273n

Acquired Immunodeficiency Syndrome (AIDS), 6, 9, 28, 63, 199–233; absence of trust and, 236–237; citizenship and, 228–233; confidentiality and, 230–231, 237; defined, 201–202; drug addicts and, 196, 197, 201, 225, 228, 231; effects of publicity about, on sexual behavior, 139–140; extent of epidemic, 201, 224–233; heterosexual cases of, 201; homosexuals and, 201, 222–228, 231–232; moralism and, 201, 202–203, 207, 230–232

Adhesiveness, sense of, 213–214

Advertising, 12; as bullshit, 154–155; and commercial speech doctrine, 127–130, 144–146, 147–153; as limiting speech, 141–144, 152; role of, in promoting public health, 156

Aid to Families with Dependent Children (AFDC), 44, 54

Alcohol, 8, 12, 88, 91, 97, 98; addiction to, 180; advertising, 156, 189; and concept of alcoholism, 179–186; consumption, distribution of, 190–191, 276n; driving and, 84–85, 185, 189; in early America, 172–174; epidemics and, 176–177; industry, 181–182; moralism and, 169–170, 175, 189–192, 197; Prohibition and, 169–172, 174–179; taxes on, 28, 171, 173, 185; theory of prevention and, 183–186; U.S. Constitution and, 113–115; warning labels on, 140–141, 268n

Alcoholics Anonymous (A.A.), 179, 181

Altman, Dennis, 219, 220

American Hospital Association, 50, 58

American Medical Association, 50, 142

Amusing Ourselves to Death, 154

Annas, George, 166

Arendt, Hannah, on advertising and free speech, 152–153

Artaud, Antonin, 177

Autonomy: absolute, and paternalism, 89, 93–95, 99; Childress on, 94, 95; and communal sphere, 89, 93–96; (Ronald) Dworkin on, 94, 95; individual, 81, 162, 166; pluralism and, 89

Axelrod, David, 136

Baby Doe cases, 165

Bacon, Selden, 182

Baird, William, 124

Barry, Brian, 83

291

Index

292

Index

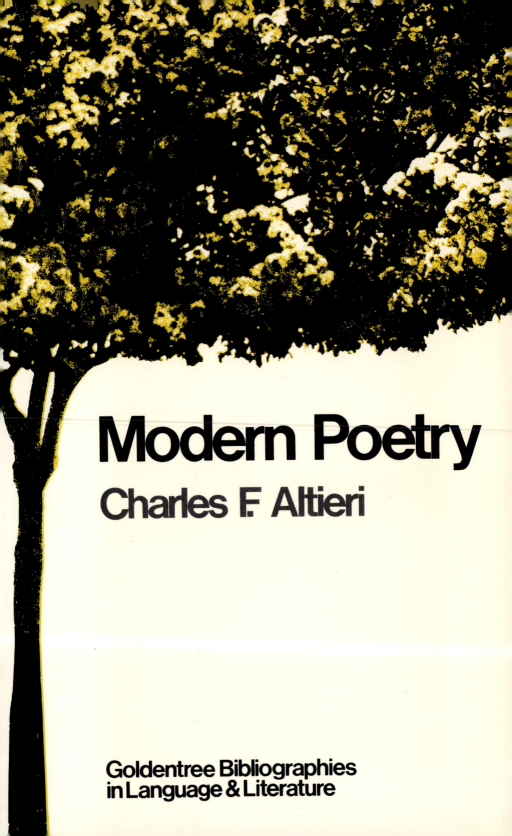

Modern Poetry

Charles F. Altieri

Goldentree Bibliographies in Language & Literature

MODERN POETRY

GOLDENTREE BIBLIOGRAPHIES

In Language and Literature
under the series editorship of
O. B. Hardison, Jr.

(MODERN POETRY)

compiled by

Charles F. Altieri

University of Washington

AHM Publishing Corporation
Arlington Heights, Illinois 60004

Copyright © 1979

AHM PUBLISHING CORPORATION

All rights reserved

ISBN: 0-88295-550-0, paper
ISBN: 0-88295-566-7, cloth

Library of Congress Card Number: 76-4656

PRINTED IN THE UNITED STATES OF AMERICA
769

Contents

Specific Works by and About the Poets
Specific works are arranged generally in the following
pattern: Works of Poetry
           Other Relevant Primary Materials
           Biography, Bibliography, and Other Reference Materials
           Collections of Critical Essays
           Critical Books and Essays

CONTENTS

Preface

I have tried here to guide the reader to what I consider the most significant criticism of modern and contemporary English and American poetry. This bibliography is intended primarily for teachers and for advanced students doing research projects, but I hope it will also enhance the pleasure of those seeking simply to deepen their knowledge of specific poets. Finally, this bibliography is intended to make easier the task of coming to terms with the challenge of contemporary poetry. I have listed several items that try to define what is new in contemporary poetry and I have tried to make available many of the different poets' statements on poetics, which are often difficult to locate.

What dealing with recent materials gives in an easy sense of relevance, it takes away in the anxieties of selection. With the modern poets the task of selection was not difficult since we have a kind of canon. But with the contemporaries I have felt constrained to include some poets whom I do not particularly like and to exclude some whom I like very much. My criteria here were the influence a poet has exerted on the writing scene in general and the amount of critical interest a poet has stirred. I also decided not to include poets who came to prominence only in the 1970s, in order to keep my work to manageable size.

I have used similar criteria in selecting critical materials. I have been guided by both my own sense of value and my sense of the material's influence on other critics. I have been more selective with respect to criticism of the modern poets than with criticism of the contemporaries because we have good studies which synthesize the former and render less useful and stimulating a variety of particular perspectives and insights. I have been strict about eliminating duplication. Thus when all of a poet's works are available in a collected edition, I list only that edition and expect that anyone interested in particular titles can consult the collected edition or a bibliography. I have also concentrated on recent criticism (up to the end of 1974) and have been very selective on bibliographic and reference guides, which tend to duplicate one another. I list only the most important older essays on a poet because most of the earlier work has been incorporated into later studies and

because the earlier work is often represented in anthologies. Finally, I have been highly selective in listing items from anthologies of
essays because I expect most readers to consult these works. This
bibliography was completed in 1975, and then delayed by a host of
problems. I have tried to bring it substantially up to date, but for
the period 1975-1978 I have listed only materials I considered really
necessary.

   This bibliography generally follows the standard format of the
Goldentree series. Items are numbered consecutively throughout
the book, and the index lists entry numbers, not pages. Journal entries are identified by the symbols used in the most recent Modern
Language Association bibliographies. (A guide to the most frequently used journals follows this preface.) When an essay is included in a collection or a previously mentioned book, I cross
reference the item simply with the entry number of its first mention. All cross references are given in boldface numbers. An
asterisk following an item indicates its special importance—either
as original criticism or as a very good general treatment of the
material for those who want only one or two representative
studies. Finally, I have indicated paperbound editions by placing in
brackets the abbreviations for publishers that are used in
Paperbound Books in Print.

   Bibliographies have a way of multiplying debts of gratitude owed
by the compiler, and this is one of their redeeming features. I am
especially grateful to Barbara Tomasi, Barbara Friedman, Jonas
Zdanys, Doreen Saar, Edna Cluff, Jerome Mazzaro and the staff of
the Poetry Room in the Lockwood Memorial Library at
SUNY/Buffalo. Without that room, its staff, and the aid given me
by my department, it would have taken much longer before I could
move on to the more pleasant task of writing materials for other
bibliographers to sift through.

C.F.A.

Journal Abbreviations

AION-SG	Annali dell'Istituto Universitario Oruntale, Napoli, Sezione Germanica
AL	American Literature
APR	American Poetry Review
ArQ	Arizona Quarterly
ASch	American Scholar
Ath	Athanor
BMR	Black Mountain Review
Bnd2	Boundary 2
BNYPL	Bulletin of the New York Public Library
BuR	Bucknell Review
CamQ	Cambridge Quarterly
CE	College English
CentR	Centennial Review
ChiR	Chicago Review
CLAJ	College Language Association Journal
CMLR	Canadian Modern Language Review
ConLit	Contemporary Literature (University of Wisconsin)
CP	Concerning Poetry
Crit	Critique: Studies in Modern Fiction (University of Minnesota)
CritQ	Critical Quarterly
DHLR	The D. H. Lawrence Review (University of Arkansas)
Diac	Diacritics: A Review of Contemporary Criticism
EDH	Essays by Divers Hands
EIC	Essays in Criticism (Oxford University)
ELH	Journal of English Literary History
ELN	English Language Notes (University of Colorado)
ES	English Studies
FP	The Far Point
GaR	Georgia Review
HC	The Hollins Critic (Hollins College, Virginia)
HudR	Hudson Review
IR	Iowa Review
JAAC	Journal of Aesthetics and Art Criticism
JML	Journal of Modern Literature
JPC	Journal of Popular Culture (Bowling Green University)
KanQ	Kansas Quarterly (formerly KM)
KenR	Kenyon Review
Lang&S	Language and Style
L&I	Literature and Ideology (Montreal)
LitR	Literary Review (Fairleigh Dickinson University)

ABBREVIATIONS

LM	London Magazine
MassR	Massachusetts Review
MHRev	Malahat Review
MissQ	Mississippi Quarterly
MLJ	Modern Language Journal
MLN	Modern Language Notes
MO	Modern Occasions
MP	Modern Philology
MPS	Modern Poetry Studies
MQ	Midwest Quarterly (Pittsburg, Kansas)
MQR	Michigan Quarterly Review
MSE	Massachusetts Studies in English
NEQ	New England Quarterly
NLH	New Literary History: A Journal of Theory and Interpretation (University of Virginia)
NMQ	New Mexico Quarterly
NR	The New Review
NYQ	New York Quarterly
NYRB	New York Review of Books
NYTB	New York Times Book Review
OhR	Ohio Review: A Journal of the Humanities
Parn	Parnassus
ParR	Paris Review
PBA	Proceedings of the British Academy
PC	Poet and Critic
PLL	Papers on Language and Literature
PMLA	Publications of the Modern Language Association of America
PoetryR	Poetry Review (London)
PR	Partisan Review
PrS	Prairie Schooner
QQ	Queen's Quarterly
RALS	Resources for American Literary Study
REN	Renascence
Rev	The Review
Sal	Salamagundi
SAQ	South Atlantic Quarterly
SEL	Studies in English Literature, 1500 – 1900 (Rice University)
Sev	The Seventies
SewR	Sewanee Review
Shen	Shenandoah
SM	Speech Monographs
SoR	Southern Review (Louisiana State University)
TC	Twentieth Century
TCL	Twentieth Century Literature
TPJ	Tennessee Poetry Journal
TriQ	Tri-Quarterly
TSE	Tulane Studies in English
TSLL	Texas Studies in Literature and Language
UKCR	University of Kansas City Review
UWR	University of Windsor Review (Windsor, Ontario)
VQR	Virginia Quarterly Review
WAL	Western American Literature

ABBREVIATIONS

WCR	West Coast Review
WR	Western Review
WSCL	Wisconsin Studies in Contemporary Literature (later *ConLit*)
XR	X, A Quarterly Review
YR	Yale Review

Note: *The publisher and compiler invite suggestions for additions to future editions of the bibliography.*

General Bibliographies and Literary Histories

1 *Academy of American Poets Newsletter.* 1078 Madison Ave. N.Y., N.Y. [Semi-annual checklist of newly published volumes of poetry.]

1a AKEROYD, Joanne, and George BUTTERICK, comps. *Where Are Their Papers? A Union List Locating the Papers of Forty-two Contemporary American Poets.* Storrs: Univ. of Connecticut Library, 1976.

1b "Annual Retrospect of the Year's Poetry." *MassR.* From 1967 to the present.

2 "Annual Review Number." *JML.* [A thorough bibliography with review of books published. First issued in 1971 with review of 1970 materials.]*

3 BRYER, Jackson R., ed. *Sixteen Modern American Authors.* New York: Norton, 1973. [Annotated bibliographies up to 1972 for Crane, Frost, Eliot, Pound, E. A. Robinson, Stevens, and Williams.] [Norton]

3a CHICOREL, Marietta. *Chicorel Index to Poetry in Collections in Print, on Discs, and on Tapes.* New York: Chicorel Library, 1972. [Index both by poet and by record.]

4 "Current Bibliography of Twentieth Century Literature, 1954—." Appears annually in *TCL*, 1955—present. [Highly selective, but with brief summaries.]

5 DAICHES, David. *The Present Age in British Literature.* Bloomington: Indiana Univ. Press, 1969.

5a DAVIS, Lloyd, and Robert IRWIN. *Contemporary American Poetry: A Checklist.* Metuchen, N.J.: Scarecrow, 1975.

6 *MLA International Bibliography*, every May in *PMLA*. [Abstracts were published between 1970 and 1976.]

7 MELLOWN, Elgin W. *A Descriptive Catalogue of the Bibliographies of Twentieth Century British Writers.* Troy, N.Y.: Whitston, 1972.

8 MURPHY, Rosalie, ed. *Contemporary Poets.* New York: St. Martin's, 1971. [Biography, bibliography, critical studies the poets consider important, comments by poets on their work, etc.]

8a PERKINS, David. *A History of Modern Poetry: From the 1890's to the High Modernist Mode.* Cambridge: Harvard Univ. Press, 1976.

8b *National Union Catalog: Music and Phonorecords*, 5 vols. Ann Arbor: J. W. Edwards, 1973. [A continuing catalog of records, including poetry records, collected by the Library of Congress.]

9 ROBSON, W. W. *Modern English Literature.* New York: Oxford Univ. Press, 1970.

10 WALCUTT, Charles G., and J. E. WHITSELL, eds. *The Explicator Cyclopedia*, vol. 1. Chicago: Quadrangle Books, 1965. [This volume devoted to modern poetry.]

11 WILLISON, I. R., comp. *Cambridge Bibliography of English Literature*, vol. 4. Cambridge: Cambridge Univ. Press. [Covers critical materials through 1969 on English literature from 1900 to 1950.]

11a WOODRESS, James, ed. *American Literary Scholarship*. Durham, N.C.: Duke Univ. Press, 1963—75. [An annual review of scholarship, complete through 1977, with review essays on "American Poetry 1900—1930" and "American Poetry, 1930—Present.]*

12 "The Writers Forum: Poets on Video-Tape." [A continuing project. Consult Ms. B. H. Poulin, 92 Park Avenue, Brockport, N.Y. 14420.]

Social, Intellectual, and Artistic Contexts

13 ALLSOP, Kenneth. *The Angry Decade: A Survey of the Cultural Revolt of the Nineteen-Fifties*. London: P. Owen, 1958. [The Movement.]

14 ALVAREZ, A. *The Savage God: A Study of Suicide*. New York: Random House, 1972. [Especially Plath and Berryman.] [Bantam]

14a ATLAS, James. *Delmore Schwartz: The Life of An American Poet*. New York: Harcourt, Farrar, Straus and Giroux, 1977.

14b BERGONZI, Bernard. *Reading the Thirties: Texts and Contexts*. London: Macmillan, 1978.

15 BRADBURY, Malcolm. *The Social Context of Modern English Literature*. New York: Schocken, 1971. [The best sociological study of modern literature.]*

16 BRUNS, Gerald. *Modern Poetry and the Idea of Language*. New Haven: Yale Univ. Press, 1974.

17 BULLOCK, Alan, ed. *The Twentieth Century: A Promethean Age*. New York: McGraw-Hill, 1971. [14 essays on social, political, philosophical, and other aspects of the age.]

17a BURKE, Kenneth. *Counter-Statement*. Berkeley: Univ. of California Press, 1968. [U Cal Pr]

18 COX, C. B., and A. E. DYSON, eds. *The Twentieth Century Mind: History, Ideas, and Literature in Britain*, 3 vols. New York: Oxford Univ. Press, 1972. [Summary essays and bibliography on British social and intellectual history; volume 1—from 1900 to 1918; vol. 2—from 1918 to 1945; vol. 3—from 1945 to 1965.] [Oxford U Pr]

18a DICKSTEIN, Morris. *American Culture in the Sixties*. New York: Basic Books, 1977.

19 EDWARDS, Thomas. *Imagination and Power: A Study of Poetry on Public Themes*. New York: Oxford Univ. Press, 1971.

20 ELLMANN, Richard, and Charles FEIDELSON, eds. *The Modern Tradition*. New York: Oxford Univ. Press, 1965. [A masterful anthology of cultural documents for the study of modernism.]*

20a FRANK, Joseph. *The Widening Gyre*. New Brunswick, N.J.: Rutgers Univ. Press, 1963. [Especially important on spatial form in modern literature.]

21 FRIEDRICH, Hugo. *The Structure of Modern Poetry: From the Mid-Nineteenth to the Mid-Twentieth Century.* Princeton: Princeton Univ. Press, 1974. [On Continental Poetry.]

21a FUSSELL, Paul. *The Great War and Modern Memory.* New York: Oxford Univ. Press, 1975. [Oxford]*

22 GRUEN, John. *The Party's Over Now: Reminiscences of the Fifties—New York's Artists, Writers, Musicians, and their Friends.* New York: Viking, 1972.

23 HOFFMAN, Frederic J. *Freudianism and the Literary Mind,* rev. ed. Baton Rouge: Louisiana State Univ. Press, 1957. [La State U Pr]

24 HOFFMAN, Frederic J. *The Mortal No: Death and the Modern Imagination.* Princeton: Princeton Univ. Press, 1964.*

24a HOFFMAN, Frederic J. *The Twenties,* 2nd ed. New York: Collier Books, 1962.

25 HYNES, Samuel. *The Edwardian Turn of Mind.* Princeton: Princeton Univ. Press, 1968.

26 JACKSON, Blyden, and Louis RUBIN. *Black Poetry in America: Two Essays in Historical Interpretation.* Baton Rouge: Louisiana State Univ. Press, 1974.

27 JOHNSTON, John H. *English Poetry of the First World War.* Princeton: Princeton Univ. Press, 1964.

28 KRIEGER, Murray. *The New Apologists for Poetry.* Bloomington: Indiana Univ. Press, 1963. [Best book on the New Criticism.]

29 MOORE, Stephen. "Contemporary Criticism and the End of a Revolution." *CentR,* 15 (1971), 144—61.

29a MORGAN, Robert B. "On the Analysis of Recent Music." *Critical Inquiry,* 4 (1977), 33—53.

30 MYERS, Rollo H., ed. *Twentieth Century Music.* New York: Orion, 1968.

31 POGGIOLI, Renato. *The Theory of the Avant-Garde,* trans. Gerald Fitzgerald. Cambridge, Mass.: Belknap, 1968.

32 POIRIER, Richard. *The Performing Self: Compositions and Decompositions in the Languages of Contemporary Life.* New York: Oxford Univ. Press, 1971.

33 PONDROM, Cyrena. *The Road From Paris: The French Influence on English Poetry 1900—1920.* Cambridge, Mass.: Cambridge Univ. Press, 1974. [Anthology of essays and letters on the subject, with a long introduction.]

33a PREMINGER, Alex, ed. *Princeton Encyclopedia of Poetry and Poetics.* Princeton: Princeton Univ. Press, 1965. [Excellent reference work, international in scope.]

34 ROSENBERG, Harold. *Artworks and Packages.* New York: Horizon, 1969. [Dell]

35 ROSENBERG, Harold. *The Tradition of the New.* New York: Horizon, 1959. [Modern painting since 1945.] [McGraw]

35a ROSS, Robert H. *The Georgian Revolt 1910—1922: Rise and Fall of a Poetic Ideal.* Carbondale: Southern Illinois Univ. Press, 1965.

36 SEARS, Sallie, and Georgianna LORD, eds. *The Discontinuous Universe.* New York: Basic Books, 1972. [Anthology updating *The Modern Tradition.*] [Basic]

3

36a SONTAG, Susan. "The Aesthetics of Silence." *Styles of Radical Will.* New York: Dell, 1969.

36b STANSKY, Peter, and William ABRAHAMS. *Journey to the Frontier: Two Roads to the Spanish Civil War.* Boston: Little, Brown, 1966.

36c VICKERY, John. *The Literary Impact of the Golden Bough.* Princeton: Princeton Univ. Press, 1973.

36d VICKERY, John, ed. *Myth and Literature: Contemporary Theory and Practice.* Lincoln: Nebraska Univ. Press, 1966.

37 WILLIAMS, Raymond. *Culture and Society 1780–1950.* London: Chatto and Windus, 1958.

General Studies of Modern Poetry

38 AIKEN, Conrad. *Collected Criticism.* New York: Oxford Univ. Press, 1968.

38a ALTIERI, Charles. "Objective Image and Act of Mind in Modern Poetry." *PMLA,* 91 (1976), 101–14.*

38b ALVAREZ, A. *Stewards of Excellence.* New York: Scribner's, 1958.

39 BAYLEY, John. *The Romantic Survival: A Study in Poetic Evolution.* Fairlawn, N.J.: Essential Books, 1957.

39a BLACKMUR, R. P. *Form and Value in Modern Poetry.* Garden City: Doubleday, 1952.

39b BORNSTEIN, George. *Transformations of Romanticism in Yeats, Eliot, and Stevens.* Chicago: Univ. of Chicago Press, 1976.*

40 BROOKS, Cleanth. *Modern Poetry and the Tradition.* Chapel Hill: Univ. of North Carolina Press, 1939. [U of NC Pr]

40a COOK, Albert. *Prisms: Studies in Modern Literature.* Bloomington: Indiana Univ. Press, 1967.

41 DAICHES, David. *Poetry and the Modern World: A Study of Poetry in England Between 1900 and 1939.* Chicago: Univ. of Chicago Press, 1940.

42 DAVIE, Donald. *Articulate Energy: An Inquiry into the Syntax of English Poetry.* New York: Harcourt, Brace, 1958.

43 DAVIE, Donald. *Thomas Hardy and British Poetry.* New York: Oxford Univ. Press, 1972.*

44 DE MAN, Paul. "Literary History and Literary Modernity" and "Lyric and Modernity." *Blindness and Insight.* New York: Oxford Univ. Press, 1971.*

45 DEMBO, L. S. *Conceptions of Reality in Modern American Poetry.* Berkeley: Univ. of California Press, 1966.

46 DONOGHUE, Denis. *Connoisseurs of Chaos, Ideas of Order in Modern American Poetry.* New York: Macmillan, 1965. [Essays on Frost, Roethke, Stevens, Robinson, Cunningham, and Robert Lowell.]

47 DONOGHUE, Denis. "The Holy Language of Modernism." In *Literary English Since Shakespeare,* ed. George Watson. London: Oxford Univ. Press, 1970, 386–407.

48 DONOGHUE, Denis. *The Ordinary Universe.* New York: Macmillan, 1968.*

49 DURRELL, Lawrence. *A Key to Modern British Poetry.* Norman: Univ. of Oklahoma Press, 1952.

50 EAGLETON, Terence. *Exiles and Emigrés: Studies in Modern Literature.* New York: Schocken, 1970. [Eliot, Auden, and Lawrence.]

51 FEDER, Lillian. *Ancient Myth in Modern Poetry.* Princeton: Princeton Univ. Press, 1971.

52 FRASER, G. S. *The Modern Writer and His World.* New York: British Book Centre, 1953. Revised edition: Harmondsworth: Penguin, 1964.

53 FRIAR, Kimon, and John Malcom BRINNIN. "Myth and Metaphysics: An Introduction to Modern Poetry." *Modern Poetry: British and American,* ed. Friar and Brinnin. New York: Appleton-Century-Crofts, 1951, 421–43. [Good example of basic critical themes of the fifties.]

54 FUSSELL, Edwin. *Lucifer in Harness: American Meter, Metaphor and Diction.* Princeton: Princeton Univ. Press, 1973.

55 GROSS, Harvey. *Sound and Form in Modern Poetry.* Ann Arbor: Univ. of Michigan Press, 1964.

56 GROSS, Harvey. *The Contrived Corridor: History and Fatality in Modern Literature.* Ann Arbor: Univ. of Michigan Press, 1971.

57 HAMBURGER, Michael. *The Truth of Poetry: Tensions in Modern Poetry from Baudelaire to the 1960's.* London: Weidenfeld & Nicolson, 1969. [Har Brace J]*

58 HARRISON, John. *The Reactionaries: Yeats, Lewis, Pound, Eliot, Lawrence: A Study of the Anti-Democratic Intelligentsia.* New York: Schocken, 1967. [Schocken]

59 HARTMAN, Geoffrey. "The Maze of Modernism: Reflections on MacNiece, Graves, Hope, Lowell and Others." *Beyond Formalism.* New Haven: Yale Univ. Press, 1970. [Yale U Pr]

60 HOUGH, Graham. *The Last Romantics.* New York: Barnes and Noble, 1962. [B&N]

61 HOUGH, Graham. *Reflections on a Literary Revolution.* New York: Catholic Univ. Press, 1949. *Image and Experience: Studies in a Literary Revolution.* London: Duckworth, 1960.

62 JARRELL, Randall. *Poetry and the Age.* New York: Farrar, Straus and Giroux, 1953. [Essays on Frost, Ransom, Stevens, Moore, and Williams.] [FS&G]*

63 JARRELL, Randall. *The Third Book of Criticism.* New York: Farrar, Strauss and Giroux, 1969. [Essays on Auden, Stevens, Frost, Graves, and "Fifty Years of American Poetry."] [FS&G]*

64 JOHNSEN, William A. "Toward a Redefinition of Modernism." *Bnd2,* 2 (1974), 539–56.

65 JUHASZ, Suzanne. *Metaphor and the Poetry of Williams, Pound, and Stevens.* Lewisburg, Pa.: Bucknell Univ. Press, 1974.

66 KALSTONE, David. "Conjuring with Nature: Some Twentieth Century Readings of Pastoral." See **161.**

67 KARTIGANER, Donald. "Process and Product: A Study of Modern Literary Form." *MassR,* 12 (1971), pts. I–IV, 297–328.

67a KENNER, Hugh. *A Homemade World: American Modernist Writers.* New York: Morrow, 1975. [Especially Williams, Stevens and Zukofsky.]

68 KENNER, Hugh. *The Pound Era.* Berkeley: Univ. of California Press, 1971. [U of Cal Pr]*

69 KERMODE, Frank. *Romantic Image.* New York: Macmillan, 1957.*

69a LANGBAUM, Robert. *The Mysteries of Identity: A Theme in Modern Literature.* New York: Oxford Univ. Press, 1977.*

70 LANGBAUM, Robert. "The New Nature Poetry" and "Mysteries of Identity: A Theme in Modern Literature." *The Modern Spirit.* New York: Oxford Univ. Press, 1970. [Oxford U Pr]

71 LANGBAUM, Robert. *The Poetry of Experience: The Dramatic Monologue in Modern Literary Tradition.* New York: Random House, 1957. [Norton]*

72 LEAVIS, F. R. *New Bearings in English Poetry: A Study of the Contemporary Situation.* London: Chatto & Windus, 1932; rev. ed., 1950.

72a LODGE, David. *The Modes of Modern Writing.* London: Edward Arnold, 1977.*

73 MARTZ, Louis L. *The Poem of the Mind.* New York: Oxford Univ. Press, 1966. [On Eliot, Stevens, Williams, and Roethke.] [Oxford U Pr]*

74 MAXWELL, D. E. S. *Poets of the Thirties.* London: Routledge & Kegan Paul, 1969.

75 MILES, Josephine. *Poetry and Change: Donne, Milton, Wordsworth, and the Equilibrium of the Present.* Berkeley: Univ. of California Press, 1974.

76 MILES, Josephine. *The Primary Language of Poetry in the 1940's.* Berkeley: Univ. of California Press, 1951.

77 MILLER, Joseph Hillis. *Poets of Reality: Six Twentieth-Century Writers.* Cambridge: Harvard Univ. Press, 1965. [Ground-breaking essays on Yeats, Eliot, Thomas, Stevens, and Williams.] [Atheneum]*

78 MOORE, Marianne. *Predilections.* New York: Viking, 1955.

79 OBERG, Arthur. "The Modern British and American Lyric: What will Suffice." *PLL*, 8 (1972), 70 – 88.

79a PAZ, Ottavio. *Children of the Mire: Modern Poetry from Romanticism to the Avant Garde.* Cambridge: Harvard Univ. Press, 1974. [Harvard]*

80 PEARCE, Roy H. *The Continuity of American Poetry.* Princeton: Princeton Univ. Press, 1961. [Princeton U Pr]*

81 QUINN, Sr. M. Bernetta. *The Metamorphic Tradition in Modern Poetry: Essays on the Work of Ezra Pound, Wallace Stevens, William Carlos Williams, T. S. Eliot, Hart Crane, Randall Jarrell and William Butler Yeats.* New Brunswick, N.J.: Rutgers Univ. Press, 1955.

82 ROSENTHAL, M. L. *The Modern Poets: A Critical Introduction.* New York: Oxford Univ. Press, 1965. [Oxford U Pr]

83 RUBIN, Louis D. "The Concept of Nature in Modern Southern Poetry." *AQ*, 9 (1957), 63 – 71.

83a SCHNEIDAU, Herbert. "Style and Sacrament in Modernist Writing." *Ga R*, 31 (1977), 427 – 53.*

84 SCHWARTZ, Delmore. *Selected Essays*, ed. Donald A. Dike and David H. Zucker. Chicago: Univ. of Chicago Press, 1970. [Essays on general themes and on Pound, Eliot, Auden, Tate, Ransom, and Stevens.]

84a SCOTT, Nathan. *The Poetry of Civic Virtue: Eliot, Malraux, and Auden.* Philadelphia: Fortress, 1976.

84b SHAPIRO, Karl. *In Defense of Ignorance.* New York: Random House, 1960.

85 SPEARS, Monroe. *Dionysus and the City: Modernism in Twentieth Century Poetry.* New York: Oxford Univ. Press, 1970. [Oxford U Pr]

86 SPENDER, Stephen. *The Destructive Element.* Philadelphia: Landsdowne, 1971. [First published in 1935.]

86a STAUFFER, Donald. *A Short History of American Poetry.* New York: Dutton, 1974.

87 STEAD, C. K. *The New Poetic.* London: Hutchinson Univ. Library, 1964.

88 THURLEY, Geoffrey. *The Ironic Harvest: English Poetry in the Twentieth Century.* New York: St. Martin's, 1974.

88a TOLLEY, A. T. *The Poetry of the Thirties.* London: Victor Gollancz, 1975.

89 VERNON, John. *The Garden and the Map: Schizophrenia in Twentieth-Century Literature and Culture.* Urbana: Univ. of Illinois Press, 1973.

90 WAGGONER, Hyatt H. *American Poetry: From the Puritans to the Present.* Boston: Houghton-Mifflin, 1968. [Dell]

90a WAGGONER, Hyatt H. *The Heel of Elohim: Science and Values in Modern Poetry.* Norman: Univ. of Oklahoma Press, 1950.

91 WESLING, Donald. *Wordsworth and the Adequacy of Landscape.* New York: Barnes and Noble, 1971. [Good on the limits of imagism.]

92 WHITAKER, Thomas R. "Voices in the Open: Wordsworth, Eliot, and Stevens." *IR*, 11 (Summer 1970), 322–32.

93 WHITE, Gina. "Modes of Being in Yeats and Eliot." *MO*, 1 (1971), 227–37.

94 WILSON, Edmund. *Axel's Castle.* New York: Scribner's, 1959. [First published in 1931.] [Scribner]

95 WINTERS, Yvor. *In Defense of Reason.* Denver: Univ. of Denver Press, 1947. [Includes "Primitivism and Decadence" and other important essays.]*

96 WINTERS, Yvor. *On Modern Poets.* New York: Meridian, 1959. [Stevens, Eliot, Ransom, Crane, Hopkins, and Frost.]

97 WRIGHT, George T. *The Poet in the Poem: The Personae of Eliot, Yeats and Pound.* Berkeley and Los Angeles: Univ. of California Press, 1960.

General Studies of Post-Modern Poetry, 1950–1970

98 ALTIERI, Charles. *Enlarging the Temple: New Directions in American Poetry of the Sixties.* Lewisburg, Pa.: Bucknell Univ. Press, 1979.

98a ALTIERI, Charles. "From Symbolist Thought to Immanence: The Logic of Post-Modern American Poetics." *Bnd2*, (1973), 605–41.*

99 ANTIN, David. "Modernism and Post-Modernism: Approaching the Present in American Poetry." *Bnd2*, 1 (1972), 98–113.

100 BEDIENT, Calvin. *Eight Contemporary Poets.* New York: Oxford Univ. Press, 1974. [Bibliography of primary materials and chapters on Tomlinson, Davie, Stevie Smith, R. S. Thomas, Ted Hughes, Kinsella, Larkin, and W. S. Graham.]*

101   BERRY, Wendell. "A Secular Pilgrimage." *HudR*, 23 (1970), 401 – 24.*

102   CARROLL, Paul. *The Poem in its Skin.* Chicago: Follet, 1968. [Follet]

103   CHARTERS, Samuel. *Some Poems/Poets: Studies in American Underground Poetry Since 1945.* Berkeley: Oyez, 1971. [Duncan, Snyder, Creeley, Olson, and Ginsberg.]

103a GILBERT, Sandra. " 'My Name is Darkness': The Poetry of Self-Definition." *ConLit,* 18 (1977), 443 – 57. [Women's Confessional Poetry.]

104   HALL, Donald. "Introduction." *Contemporary American Poetry*, ed. Hall. Baltimore: Penguin, 1962.

105   HALL, David. "The New Poetry: Notes on the Past Fifteen Years in America." *New World Writing, Seventh Mentor Selection.* New York: New American Library, 1955.

106   HAMILTON, Ian. *A Poetry Chronicle: Essays and Reviews.* New York: Barnes and Noble, 1973. [On Berryman, *Waste Land*, MacNeice, the forties, Fuller, Lowell, the Movement, Larkin, Davie, and short reviews.]

107   HASSAN, Ihab. "POSTmodernISM." *NLH*, 3 (1971), 5 – 31.

108   HOWARD, Richard. *Alone with America.* New York: Atheneum, 1969. [Essays on 41 poets first published after 1950.] [Atheneum]*

108a KALSTONE, David. *Five Temperaments: Elizabeth Bishop, Robert Lowell, James Merrill, Adrienne Rich, John Ashbery.* New York: Oxford Univ. Press, 1977.*

109   KERMODE, Frank. *Continuities.* New York: Random House, 1968. [Part I, pp. 1 – 32, is on the relationship of modernism to post-modernism.]

109a KERN, Robert. "Gary Snyder and the Modernist Imperative." *Crit,* 19 (1977), 158 – 77.

110   KINNELL, Galway. "The Poetics of the Physical World." *IR*, 11 (Summer 1971), 113 – 26.

111   LACEY, Paul. *The Inner War: Forms and Themes in Recent American Poetry.* Philadelphia: Fortress, 1972.

112   LEVERTOV, Denise. *The Poet in the World.* New York: New Directions, 1973. [New Directions]

112a MILLS, Ralph. *Cry of the Human: Essays on Contemporary American Poetry.* Urbana: Univ. of Illinois Press, 1974.

112b MOLESWORTH, Charles. "We Have Come This Far: Audience and Form in Contemporary American Poetry." *Soundings,* 29 (1977), 204 – 25.*

113   MORAN, Ronald, and George LENSING. "The Emotive Imagination: A New Departure in American Poetry." *SoR,* 3 (1967), 52 – 67.*

113a OBERG, Arthur. *Modern American Lyric: Lowell, Berryman, Creeley, and Plath.* New Brunswick: Rutgers, 1977.

114   PEARCE, Roy Harvey. "The Burden of Romanticism: Toward the New Poetry." *IR*, 11 (Spring 1970), 109 – 28.

115   PERLOFF, Marjorie. "The Corn-Porn Lyric: Poetry 1972 – 73." *ConLit,* 16 (1975), 84 – 125.

116   PHILLIPS, Robert. *The Confessional Poets.* Carbondale: Southern Illinois Univ. Press, 1973.

116a PINSKY, Robert. *The Situation of Poetry: Contemporary Poetry and Its Traditions.* Princeton: Princeton Univ. Press, 1976.*

116b PLUMLY, Stanley. "Chapter and Verse." *APR*, 7,1 (1978), 19—31. [A concise statement of the poetic values of many younger poets.]

117 POULIN, A., Jr. "Contemporary American Poetry: The Radical Tradition." *CP*, 3 (Fall 1970), 5—21.*

117a QUASHA, George. "DiaLogos: Between the Written and the Oral in Contemporary Poetry." *NLH*, 8 (1977), 485—506.

117b REXROTH, Kenneth. *The Alternate Society*. New York: Herder and Herder, 1970. [This book best represents a position developed in Rexroth's various writings.]

118 ROSENTHAL, M. L. "Dynamics of Form and Motive in Some Representative Twentieth-Century Lyric Poems." *ELH*, 37 (1970), 136—51.

118a ROSENTHAL, M. L. *The New Poets: American and British Poetry Since World War II*. New York: Oxford Univ. Press, 1967. [Oxford U Pr]

119 ROSENTHAL, M. L. "Some Thoughts on American Poetry Today." *Sal*, nos. 22—23 (1973), 57—70.

120 RYAN, Michael. "A Symposium of Young Poets." *IR*, 4, 4 (1973), 52—112.

120a SCOTT, Nathan. *Wild Prayer of Longing*. New Haven: Yale Univ. Press, 1971.

120b ZWEIG, Paul. "The New Surrealism." *Sal*, nos. 22—23 (1973), 269—84.

121 ZWEIG, Paul. "The Raw and the Cooked." *PR*, 41 (1974), 604—12. [Discusses Stafford and Ammons in particular.]

Special Topics and Movements in Modern and Post-Modern Poetry

122 BALAKIAN, Anna. *The Symbolist Movement*. New York: Random House, 1967.

123 CAWS, Mary Ann. *The Poetry of Dada and Surrealism: Aragon, Breton, Tzara, Eluard, Desnos*. Princeton: Princeton Univ. Press, 1970.

124 COFFMAN, Stanley K., Jr. *Imagism: A Chapter in the History of Modern Poetry*. Norman: Oklahoma Univ. Press, 1951.

125 COOK, Bruce. *The Beat Generation*. New York: Scribner's, 1971. [Scribner]

126 COWAN, Louise. *The Fugitive Group: A Literary History*. Baton Rouge: Louisiana State Univ. Press, 1959.

127 DIJKSTRA, Bram. "Wallace Stevens and William Carlos Williams: Poetry Painting, and the Function of Reality." *Encounters: Essays on Literature and the Visual Arts*, ed. John Dixon Hunt. New York: Norton, 1971.

128 DOUGLAS, Wallace. "Deliberate Exiles: The Social Sources of Agrarian Poetics." See **173**.

129 DUBERMAN, Martin. *Black Mountain: An Exploration in Community*. New York: Doubleday, 1971. [Doubleday]

130 ENGELBERG, Edward. "Introduction." *The Symbolist Poem*, ed. Engelberg. New York: Dutton, 1967, 17 – 46. [Dutton]

131 GAYLE, Addison, Jr., ed. *The Black Aesthetic*. Garden City: Doubleday, 1971. [A wide spectrum of essays on blacks and the arts.] [Doubleday]

132 HUGGINS, Nathan. *Harlem Renaissance*. New York: Oxford Univ. Press, 1971.

133 JONES, Peter, ed. *Imagist Poetry*. London: Penguin, 1972.

134 LAWLER, James. *The Language of French Symbolism*. Princeton: Princeton Univ. Press, 1969.

135 MARTIN, Wallace. "The Sources of the Imagist Aesthetic." *PMLA*, 85 (1970), 196 – 204.

136 NAREMORE, James. "The Imagists and the French Generation of 1900." *ConLit*, 11 (1970), 354 – 74.

137 PARKINSON, Thomas, ed. *A Casebook on the Beat*. New York: Crowell, 1961.

138 RAY, Paul. *The Surrealist Movement in England*. Ithaca: Cornell Univ. Press, 1971.

139 RAYMOND, Marcel. *From Baudelaire to Surrealism*, translated from the French. New York: Barnes and Noble, 1970. [First published in 1950; on French poetry but very suggestive.] [B&N]

139a SCHNEIDAU, Herbert. *Ezra Pound: The Image and the Real*. Baton Rouge: Louisiana State Univ. Press, 1969. [Contains the best recent treatment of imagism.]*

140 SENIOR, John. *The Way Down and Out: The Occult in Symbolist Literature*. Ithaca: Cornell Univ. Press, 1959.

140a SIMON, Myron. *The Georgian Poetic*. Berkeley: Univ. of California Press, 1975.

141 SOLT, Mary Ellen, ed. *Concrete Poetry: A World View*. Bloomington: Indiana Univ. Press, 1968. [Anthology with critical introduction.]

142 STEWART, John L. *The Burden of Time: The Fugitives and Agrarians*. Princeton: Princeton Univ. Press, 1965.

143 SYMONS, Arthur. *The Symbolist Movement in Literature*. New York: Dutton, 1958. [First published in 1899, 1914.] [Dutton]

143a TASHJIAN, Dickran. *Skyscraper Primitives: Dada and the American Avant Garde*. Middletown, Conn.: Wesleyan Univ. Press, 1975. [Williams, Crane, Cummings.]

144 Twelve Southerners. *I'll Take my Stand: The South and the Agrarian Tradition*. New York: Harper, 1962. [First published in 1929.] [Har-Row]

145 WEES, William C. *Vorticism and the English Avant-Garde*. Toronto: Univ. of Toronto Press, 1972.

146 WESLING, Donald. "The Prosodies of Free Verse." See **161**.

Anthologies of Modern and Post-Modern Poetry and Poetics

147 ALLEN, Donald M. *The New American Poetry, 1945– 1960.* New York: Grove, 1960. [The first self-consciously post-modernist anthology.] [Grove]

147a ALLEN, Donald M., and Warren TALLMAN, eds. *The Poetics of the New American Poetry.* New York: Grove, 1973. [Grove]*

148 CONQUEST, Robert, ed. *New Lines.* London: Macmillan, 1955.

149 ELLMANN, Richard, and Robert O'CLAIR, eds. *The Norton Anthology of Modern Poetry.* New York: Norton, 1973. [Excellent bibliography.] [Norton]*

149a HALPERN, Daniel, ed. *The American Poetry Anthology.* New York: Avon, 1975. [Represents poets born after 1934.] [Avon]

150 HEWITT, Geof, ed. *Quickly Aging Here: Some Poets of the 1970's.* Garden City: Doubleday, 1969. [Doubleday]

150a HEYEN, William, ed. *American Poets in 1976.* Indianapolis: Bobbs Merrill, 1976. [Anthology, plus 29 poets writing on their own work. With selected bibliography of primary and secondary works.]* [Bobbs]

150b HUGGINS, Nathan, ed. *Voices from the Harlem Renaissance.* New York: Oxford Univ. Press, 1976.

151 JONES, Leroi, and Larry NEAL. *Black Fire: An Anthology of Afro-American Writing.* New York: Morrow, 1968. [Morrow]

152 MATTHIAS, John, ed. *23 Modern British Poets.* Chicago: Swallow, 1971.

153 POULIN, Al, Jr., ed. *Contemporary American Poetry,* 2nd ed. Boston: Houghton-Mifflin, 1975. [H-M]*

154 POULIN, Al, Jr., ed. *Making in All Its Forms: Contemporary American Poetics and Criticism.* New York: Dutton, 1974. [Dutton]*

155 RANDALL, Dudley, ed. *The Black Poets.* New York: Bantam, 1971. [Bantam]

155a REXROTH, Kenneth, ed. *The New British Poets.* Norfolk, Conn.: New Directions, n.d. [Early 1940s; it announced the end of ideological poetry and called for a new Romanticism.]

156 ROBSON, Jeremy, ed. *The Young British Poets.* New York: St. Martin's, 1971.

157 SANDERS, G. D., J. H. NELSON, and M. L. ROSENTHAL, eds. *Chief Modern Poets of England and America,* 2 vols., 5th ed. New York: Macmillan, 1970. [Macmillan]

158 SCULLY, James, ed. *Modern Poetics.* New York: McGraw-Hill, 1965. [McGraw]

159 SERGEANT, Howard, and Dannie ABSE, eds. *The Mavericks.* London: Editions Poetry and Poverty, 1957.

160 SHAPIRO, Karl, ed. *Prose Keys to Modern Poetry.* New York: Harper & Row, 1962. [Har-Row]

Anthologies of Interviews and Critical Essays

160a BAKER, Houston, ed. *A Dark and Sudden Beauty: Two Essays in Contemporary Black American Poetry: 1962–1977.* Philadelphia: Univ. of Pennsylvania Press, 1977.

160b BORNSTEIN, George, ed. *Romantic and Modern: Revaluations of Literary Tradition.* Pittsburgh: Univ. of Pittsburgh Press, 1977.

160c BOYERS, Robert, ed. *Contemporary Poetry in America: Essays and Interviews.* New York: Schocken, 1974.* [Schocken]

161 BROWER, Reuben, ed. *Twentieth Century Literature in Retrospect.* Cambridge: Harvard Univ. Press, 1971. [Harvard U Pr]

162 COWLEY, M., VanWyck BROOKS, and George PLIMPTON, eds. *Writers at Work: The Paris Review Interviews,* 3 vols. New York: Viking, 1959, 1963, 1967. [R. P. Warren, Eliot, Moore, Frost, Pound, Lowell, and Williams.] [Viking]

163 DEMBO, L. S., and Cyrena PONDROM, eds. *The Contemporary Writer: Interviews With Sixteen Novelists and Poets.* Madison: Univ. of Wisconsin Press, 1972. [U of Wis Pr]

164 DODSWORTH, Martin, ed. *The Survival of Poetry: A Contemporary Survey.* London: Faber, 1970.

165 EHRENPREIS, Irvin, ed. *American Poetry.* London: Edward Arnold, 1965.

165a FASS, Ekbert, ed. *Towards a New American Poetics.* Santa Barbara: Black Sparrow Press, 1978. [Includes interviews with Duncan, Snyder, Creeley, Bly, and Ginsberg.]

166 FORD, Boris, ed. *The Modern Age,* 3rd ed. Baltimore: Penguin, 1973. [Penguin]

167 FRENCH, Warren, ed. *The Fifties: Fiction, Poetry, Drama.* DeLand, Fla: Everett/Edwards, 1970.

168 GIBSON, Donald, ed. *Modern Black Poets: A Collection of Critical Essays.* Englewood Cliffs, N.J.: Prentice-Hall, 1973. [P-H]

169 HAMILTON, Ian, ed. *The Modern Poet: Essays from the Review.* London: McDonald, 1968.

170 HOLLANDER, John, ed. *Modern American Poetry: Essays in Criticism.* New York: Oxford Univ. Press, 1968. [Oxford U Pr]*

171 HOWE, Irving, ed. *Literary Modernism.* New York: Fawcett, 1967. [Fawcett]

172 HUNGERFORD, Edward, ed. *Poets in Progress.* Evanston: Northwestern Univ. Press, 1962. [Essays on Lowell, Roethke, Levertov, and others.] [Northwestern U Pr]

173 LUDWIG, Richard M., ed. *Aspects of Modern Poetry.* Columbus: Ohio State Univ. Press, 1962.

173a MARTIN, Graham, and P. N. FURBANK, eds. *Twentieth Century Poetry: Critical Essays and Documents.* Atlantic Highlands, N.J.: Open Univ. Press, 1975.

174 MAZZARO, Jerome, ed. *Modern American Poetry: Essays in Criticism.* New York: David McKay, 1970. [McKay]

175 MILLER, James, Jr., Karl SHAPIRO, and Bernice SLOTE, eds. *Start with the Sun: Studies in Cosmic Poetry.* Lincoln: Univ. of Nebraska Press, 1960. [Anti-Eliot perspectives on Lawrence, Crane, and Thomas.]

176 NEMEROV, Howard, ed. *Poets on Poetry.* New York: Basic Books, 1966.

177 NORMAN, Charles, ed. *Poets on Poetry.* New York: Collier Books, 1962.

178 OSSMAN, David. *The Sullen Art: Interviews with Modern American Poets.* New York: Corinth, 1963. [Bly, Logan, Creeley, Merwin, Levertov, Ginsberg, and others.][Corinth]

179 OSTROFF, Anthony, ed. *The Contemporary Poet as Artist and Critic.* Boston: Little, Brown, 1964. [Wilbur, Roethke, Lowell, Ransom, Auden, and others.][Little]

180 OWEN, Guy, ed. *Modern American Poetry: Essays in Criticism.* Deland, Fla.: Everett/Edwards, 1972.

180a PACKARD, William, ed. *The Craft of Poetry: Interviews from the New York Quarterly.* Garden City: Doubleday, 1974. [Anchor]

181 PERRY, John Oliver, ed. *Backgrounds to Modern Literature.* San Francisco: Chandler, 1968. [Chandler]

181a Rogers, Timothy, ed. *Georgian Poetry, 1911—1922: The Critical Heritage.* London: Routledge, 1977.

Important Literary Magazines of the Period and Bibliographic Guides

Bibliographic Material for the Study of Literary Periodicals

182 BRADBURY, Malcolm. "The Climate of Literary Culture and the Literary Periodical." See **15.**

183 FULTON, Len, ed. *International Directory of Little Magazines and Small Presses.* Paradise, Cal.: Dustbooks. [Published annually since 1965.]

184 HOFFMAN, Frederick J. *The Little Magazine: A History and a Bibliography.* Princeton: Princeton Univ. Press, 1947. [Description of a wide variety of little magazines.]*

185 *Index to Little Magazines.* Several editors. Denver: Swallow. [Annual indexes from 1943 to 1967 of poetry and essays in American small literary magazines.]

186 ZULAUF, Sander, and Irwin H. WEISER, eds. *Index of American Periodical Verse*. Metuchen, N.J.: Scarecrow. [First volume published in 1973 for year 1971; to be an annual review. Indexes periodical verse by poet.]

Important Literary Periodicals

187 *Accent*, ed. Kerker Quinn and others, 1940 – 60.

187a *American Poetry Review*, ed. Stephen Berg and Stephen Parker, 1972 – present.

188 *Black Mountain Review*, ed. Robert Creeley, 1954 – 57.

189 *Blast*, ed. Wyndham Lewis, 1914 – 15.

189a *Boundary 2*, ed. William Spanos, 1972 – present.

190 *Choice*, ed. John Logan and others, 1961 – present.

191 *Contact*, ed. William Carlos Williams and others, 1920 – 23.

192 *The Criterion*, ed. T. S. Eliot, 1922 – 39.

193 *The Dial*, ed. Scofield Thayer, Marianne Moore, and others, 1920 – 29. [The basic modernist journal in America.]

194 *The Egoist*, ed. Harriet Weaver, 1914 – 19. [Published experimental work by the major modern writers.]

195 *Field*, ed. Stuart Friebert and David Young, 1969 – present. [Important interviews on poetics.]

196 *The Fifties*, *The Sixties*, and *The Seventies*, ed. Robert Bly, 1958 – present.

197 *The Fugitive*, ed. John Crowe Ransom and others, 1922 – 25.

198 *Furioso*, ed. Reed Whittemore and others, 1939 – 53.

199 *Hudson Review*, ed. Frederick Morgan and others, 1948 – present.

200 *Iowa Review*, ed. Merle Brown, Thomas Whitaker, and David Hamilton, 1970 – present. [Probably the best critical journal on contemporary poetry.]

201 *Kayak*, ed. George Hitchcock, 1964 – present.

202 *The Kenyon Review*, ed. John Crowe Ransom and others, 1939 – 70.

203 *The Little Review*, ed. Margaret Anderson, 1914 – 29.

204 *The New Age*, ed. A. R. Orage and others, 1884 – 1938.

205 *New Directions in Prose and Poetry*, ed. James Laughlin, 1936 – present. [An annual devoted to experimental writing.]

206 *New Masses*, ed. Michael Gold and others, 1926 – 48. [The basic left-wing literary journal.]

207 *New Verse*, ed. Geoffrey Grigson, 1933 – 39. [The most important British literary journal of the 1930s.]

208 *Others*, ed. Alfred Kreymborg, 1915 – 19.

209 *Parnassus: Poetry in Review*, ed. Herbert Leibowitz, 1972 – present.

210 *Partisan Review*, ed. Delmore Schwartz, Dwight MacDonald, and others, 1943 – present. [Basic journal of the non-Stalinist left.]

211   *Poetry*, ed. Harriet Monroe and others, 1912 – present.

212   *Prairie Schooner*, ed. Karl Shapiro and others, 1944 – present.

213   *The Review*, ed. Ian Hamilton, 1962 – 72.

214   *Sewanee Review*, ed. Allen Tate and others, 1892 – present.

215   *The Transatlantic Review*, ed. Ford Madox Ford, 1924 – 25. [Much discussion of exile and America by major American writers.]

216   *Transition*, ed. Eugene Jolas and Eliot Paul, 1927 – 38.

Specific Works By and About The Poets

A. R. Ammons

Works of Poetry

217   *Collected Poems: 1951 – 1971*. New York: Norton, 1972.

217a *Diversifications*. New York: Norton, 1975.

217b *The Selected Poems 1951 – 1977*. New York: Norton, 1977. [Norton]

217c *The Snow Poems*. New York: Norton, 1977.

218   *Sphere: The Form of a Motion*. New York: Norton, 1974. [Norton]

218a *Tape for the Turn of the Year*. New York: Norton, 1965.

Other Relevant Primary Materials

219   "Essays on Poetics: A Long Poem." *HudR*, 22, 3 (1970), 425 – 48. [Also in **215**, but his basic theoretical statement.]

220   "Interview." *Diac*, 3, 4 (1973), 47 – 53.

221   "A Poem is a Walk." *Epoch*, 18, 1 (Fall 1968), 114 – 19.

222   "Pray Without Ceasing." *HudR*, 26 (1973), 471 – 85. [Another statement of his poetics.]

Collections of Critical Essays

223   *Diac*, 3, 4 (1973). [Ammons issue.]

Critical Books and Essays

223a BLOOM, Harold. "A. R. Ammons: The Breaking of the Vessels." *Sal*, 31 – 32 (1975), 185 – 203.

224 BLOOM, Harold. "A. R. Ammons and Mark Strand: Dark and Radiant Peripheries." *SoR*, 8 (1972), 133 – 49.

225 BLOOM, Harold. "The New Transcendentalism: The Visionary Strain in Merwin, Ashbery and Ammons." *ChiR*, 24, 3 (Winter 1973), 25 – 43. Reprinted in Bloom, *The Ringers in the Tower*. Chicago: Univ. of Chicago Press, 1971.*

226 HOWARD, Richard. "A. R. Ammons: The Spent Seer Consigns Order to the Vehicle of Change." See **108**.

227 KALSTONE, David. "Ammons' Radiant Toys." *Diac*, 3, 4 (1973), 13 – 20.

228 MATTHEWS, William. "Some Notes on the Self in A. R. Ammons' *Uplands and Briefings*." *Apple*, no. 5 (Summer 1971), 16 – 22.

229 MAZZARO, Jerome. "Reconstruction in Art." *Diac*, 3, 4 (1973), 39 – 44.

230 MORGAN, Robert. "The Compound Vision of A. R. Ammons' Early Poems." *Epoch*, 22, 3 (Spring 1973), 343 – 63.

231 ORR, Linda. "The Cosmic Backyard of A. R. Ammons." *Diac*, 3, 4 (1973), 3 – 12.

232 TATE, James. "Ammons' Canon." *Lillabulero*, nos. 10 and 11, ser. 2 (1971), 63 – 70.

233 WAGGONER, Hyatt H. "The Poetry of A. R. Ammons: Some Notes and Reflections." *Sal*, nos. 22 – 23 (Spring – Summer 1973), 285 – 93.

John Ashbery

Works of Poetry

234 *The Double Dream of Spring*. New York: Dutton, 1970. [Dutton]

234a *Houseboat Days*. New York: Viking Press, 1977. [Penguin]

235 *Rivers and Mountains*. New York: Holt, Rinehart and Winston, 1966. [HR &W]

236 *Self-Portrait in a Convex Mirror*. New York: Viking, 1975. [Penguin]

237 *Some Trees*. New Haven: Yale Univ. Press, 1956. [Corinth]

238 *The Tennis-Court Oath*. Middletown, Conn.: Wesleyan Univ. Press, 1962. [Wesleyan U Pr]

239 *Three Poems*. New York: Viking, 1972. [Viking]

240 *Turnadot and Other Poems*. New York: Tibor de Nagy Gallery, 1953.

240a *The Vermont Notebooks*. Santa Barbara: Black Sparrow, 1977. [Black Sparrow]

Other Relevant Primary Materials

241 ''Absence and Illusion.'' *ARTnews*, 71, 3 (May 1972), 33; 60 – 62. [Review of abstract-expressionist Esteban Vicente.]

242 *The Compromise.* In *Hasty Papers*. New York: Alfred Leslie, 1960. [Play]

243 *A Conversation between John Ashbery and Kenneth Koch.* Tucson, Ariz.: Interview, 1966.

244 ''Craft Interview with John Ashbery.'' *NYQ*, no. 9 (Winter 1972), 11 – 33.

245 ''G.M.P.'' *ARTnews*, 69, 10 (February 1971), 44 – 47; 73 – 74. [Review of Gertrude, Michael, and Sarah Stein collection exhibition at the Museum of Modern Art.]

246 ''The Heroes.'' *Artist's Theatre*, ed. Herbert Machiz. New York: Grove, 1960. [Play]

247 ''Introduction'' to *Collected Poems of Frank O'Hara*, ed. Donald Allen. New York: Alfred Knopf, 1971.

248 ''Jacquet.'' *Catalogue for Jacquet Exhibition*. New York: Alexander Jolas Gallery, 1964.

249 ''The Joys and Enigmas of a Strange Hour.'' *The Grand Eccentrics*, ed. Thomas B. Hess and John Ashbery. New York: Collier Books, 1966. [Essay.]

250 *A Nest of Ninnies* [by Ashbery and James Schuyler]. New York: Dutton, 1969. [Novel]

251 ''The New Realism.'' *Catalogue of Sidney Janis Gallery*. New York: Sidney Janis Gallery, 1962.

251a *Three Plays.* Calais, Vt.: Z Press, 1978.

Biography, Bibliography, and Other Reference Materials

251b KERMANI, David K. *John Ashbery: A Comprehensive Bibliography Including His Art Criticism and with Selected Notes from Unpublished Materials.* New York: Garland, 1976.

Critical Essays

251c Altieri, Charles. ''Metaphor as Motive: John Ashbery and the Modernist Long Poem.'' *Genre*, 11 (1978) , 653 – 87.

252 BLOOM, Harold. ''John Ashbery: The Charity of the Hard Moments.'' *Sal*, no. 22 – 23 (Spring – Summer 1973), 103 – 33.

253 BLOOM, Harold. ''The New Transcendentalism: The Visionary Strain in Merwin, Ashbery and Ammons.'' *ChiR*, 24, 3 (Winter 1973), 25 – 43. See **225.**

254 CARROL, Paul. "John Ashbery—'Leaving the Atocha Station': If only He Had Left from the Finland Station." See **102.**

255 DiPIERO, W. S. "John Ashbery: The Romantic as Problem Solver." *APR*, 2, 4 (July—August 1973), 39—42.

256 HOWARD, Richard. "John Ashbery: 'You May Never Know How Much is Pushed Back into the Night, Nor What May Return'." See **108.***

256a KALSTONE. *Five Temperaments.* See **108a.***

257 KOETHE, John. "Ashbery's Meditations." *Parn*, 1, 1 (1972), 89—93.

257a LEHMANN, David, ed. Forthcoming (1980) collection of critical essays. Probably Cornell Univ. Press.

257b MOLESWORTH, Charles. "This Leaving Out Business: The Poetry of John Ashbery." *Sal*, 38—39 (1977), 20—41.

257c MORAMARCO, Fred. "John Ashbery and Frank O'Hara: The Painterly Poets." *JML*, 5 (1976), 436—62.

258 SHAPIRO, David. "Urgent Masks: an Introduction to John Ashbery's Poetry." *Field*, no. 5 (Fall 1971), 32—45.

W. H. Auden

Works of Poetry

259 *About the House.* New York: Random House, 1965.

260 *Academic Graffiti.* New York: Random House, 1972.

261 *City Without Walls and Other Poems.* New York: Random House, 1969.

262 *Collected Poems.* New York: Random House, 1945. [Earlier versions of many of his poems.]

263 *Collected Longer Poems.* New York: Random House, 1968.

264 *Collected Shorter Poems, 1927— 1957.* New York: Random House, 1970.

265 *Epistle of a Godson.* New York: Random House, 1972.

266 *Homage to Clio.* New York: Random House, 1960.

267 *Thank You Fog: Last Poems by W. H. Auden.* New York: Random House, 1974.

Other Relevant Primary Materials

268 *A Certain World: A Commonplace Book.* New York: Random House, 1970.

269 *The Dyers Hand.* New York: Random House, 1962. [Important essays.] [Random]

270 *The Enchafed Flood.* New York: Random House, 1950. [On Romanticism.] [Random]

271 *Forewords and Afterwords*, selected by Edward Mendelson. New York: Random House, 1973.

272 *Secondary Worlds*. New York: Random House, 1968. [Essentially on literature and Christianity.]

Biography, Bibliography, and Other Reference Materials

273 BLOOMFIELD, Barry Cambray, and Edward MENDELSON. *W. H. Auden: A Bibliography 1924– 1969*. Charlottesville: Univ. Press of Virginia, 1972.

273a SPENDER, Stephen, ed. *W. H. Auden: A Tribute*. New York: Macmillan, 1975.

Collections of Critical Essays

274 SPEARS, Monroe. *Auden, A Collection of Critical Essays*. Englewood Cliffs, N.J.: Prentice-Hall, 1964. [P-I]

275 *Shen*, 18 (1968), no. 1. [An Auden issue.]

Critical Books and Essays

276 BAHLKE, George W. *The Later Auden: From "New Year Letter" to "About the House."* New Brunswick, N.J.: Rutgers Univ. Press, 1970.

277 BAYLEY, John. "W. H. Auden." See **39.**

278 BEACH, Joseph Warren. *The Making of the Auden Canon*. Minneapolis: Univ. of Minnesota Press, 1957.

279 BLAIR, John G. *The Poetic Art of W. H. Auden*. Princeton: Princeton Univ. Press, 1965.

280 BLOOM, Robert. "W. H. Auden's Bestiary of the Human." *VQR*, 42 (1966), 207 – 33.

281 BLOOM, Robert. "Auden's Essays at Man: Some Long Views in the Early Poetry." *Shen*, 18 (1967), 23 – 43.

282 BLOOM, Robert. "The Humanization of Auden's Early Style." *PMLA*, 83 (1968), 443 – 54.

283 BLUESTONE, Max. "The Iconographic Sources of Auden's 'Musee des Beaux Arts'." *MLN*, 76 (1961), 331 – 36.

284 BROOKS, Cleanth. "W. H. Auden as a Critic." *KenR*, 26 (1964), 173 – 89.

285 BUELL, Frederick. *W. H. Auden as a Social Poet*. Ithaca: Cornell Univ. Press, 1973.

286 CALLAN, Edward. "W. H. Auden: The Farming of a Verse." *SoR*, 3 (1967), 341 – 56.

287 DAVISON, Dennis. *W. H. Auden.* London: Evans Bros., 1970.

288 DUCHÊNE, François. *The Case of the Wounded Airman: A Study of W. H. Auden's Poetry.* London: Chatto and Windus, 1972.

289 FRASER, G. S. *Vision and Rhetoric: Studies in Modern Poetry.* London: Faber and Faber, 1959. Reprinted in **274.**

290 FULLER, John. *A Reader's Guide to W. H. Auden.* New York: Farrar, Straus and Giroux, 1970. [FS&G]*

291 GREENBERG, Herbert. *Quest for the Necessary: W. H. Auden and the Dilemma of Divided Consciousness.* Cambridge: Harvard Univ. Press, 1968.*

292 HARDY, Barbara. "W. H. Auden: Thirties to Sixties: A Face and a Map." *SoR,* 5 (1969), 655—72.

293 HARDY, Barbara. "The Reticence of W. H. Auden." *Review,* 11—12 (1964), 54—64.

294 ISHERWOOD, Christopher. *Exhumations.* London: Methuen, 1966.

295 JARRELL, Randall. "Changes of Attitude and Rhetoric in Auden's Poetry" and "Freud to Paul: The Stages of Auden's Ideology." See **63.***

296 JOHNSON, Richard. *Man's Place, An Essay on Auden.* Ithaca: Cornell Univ. Press, 1973.

297 McDOWELL, Frederick P. "The Situation of Our Time: Auden in His American Phase." See **173.**

298 MAXWELL, D. E. S. "W. H. Auden: The Island and the City." See **74.**

299 NELSON, Gerald. *Changes of Heart: a Study of the Poetry of W. H. Auden.* Berkeley: Univ. of California Press, 1969.

300 PARKIN, Rebecca Price. "The Facsimile of Immediacy in W. H. Auden's 'In Praise of Limestone'." *TSLL,* 7 (1965), 295—304.

301 REPLOGLE, Justin Maynard. *Auden's Poetry.* Seattle: Univ. of Washington Press, 1969. [U of Wash Pr]*

302 SPEARS, Monroe K. *The Poetry of W. H. Auden: The Disenchanted Island.* New York: Oxford Univ. Press, 1963. [Oxford U Pr]

303 STEAD, C. K. "Auden's 'Spain'." *LM,* 7 (March 1968), 41—54.

Imamu Amiri Baraka
[Leroi Jones]

Works of Poetry

304 *The Dead Lecturer: Poems.* New York: Grove, 1964. [Grove]

305 *Preface to a Twenty Volume Suicide Note.* New York: Totem/Corinth, 1961.

306 *Spirit Reach.* Newark: Jihad Productions, 1972.

Other Relevant Primary Materials

307   *Afrikan Revolution.* Newark: Jihad Productions, 1973.

308   *The Baptism and the Toilet.* New York: Grove, 1967. [Grove]

309   *Black Magic: Sabotage, Target Study, Black Art: Collected Poetry, 1961 – 1967.* Indianapolis: Bobbs-Merrill, 1969. [Bobbs]

310   *A Black Value System.* Newark: Jihad Productions, 1970.

311   *Dutchman and the Slave, Two Plays.* New York: Morrow, 1964. [Morrow.]

312   *Four Black Revolutionary Plays, All Praises to The Black Man.* Indianapolis: Bobbs-Merrill, 1969. [Bobbs]

313   *Home: Social Essays.* New York: Morrow, 1966. [Morrow]

314   *In Our Terribleness (some elements and meaning in Black style),* ed. Leroi Jones/Baraka and Fundy/Billy Abernathy. Indianapolis: Bobbs-Merrill, 1970.

315   "Introduction" to *The Moderns: An Anthology of New Writing in America.* New York: Corinth, 1963.

316   *It's Nation Time.* Chicago: Third World, 1970. [Third World]

317   *Jello.* Chicago: Third World, 1970.

318   *Kawaida Studies: The New Nationalism.* Chicago: Third World, 1972. [Third World]

318a   *The Motion of History and Other Plays.* New York: Morrow, 1978. [Morrow]

319   *Raise Race Rays Raze: Essays since 1965.* New York: Random House, 1971. [Random]

320   *Slave Ship.* Newark: Jihad Productions, 1966.

321   *The System of Dante's Hell.* New York: Grove, 1965. [A novel.] [Grove]

322   *Tales.* New York: Grove, 1967. [Grove]

322a   "Why I Changed My Ideology: Black Nationalism and Socialist Revolution." *Black World,* 24, 9 (1975), 30 – 42.

Biography, Bibliography, and Other Reference Materials

323   DACE, Letitia. *Leroi Jones (Imamu Amiri Baraka): A Checklist of Works by and About Him.* London: Nether, 1971.

Collections of Critical Essays

323a   "Supplement on Amiri Baraka." *Bnd. 2,* 6 (1978), 303 – 442. [Includes poems and an interview.]

21

Critical Books and Essays

323b BENSTON, Kimberly. *Baraka: The Renegade and the Mask.* New Haven: Yale Univ. Press, 1976.

324 BROWN, Lloyd W. "Comic-Strip Heroes: Leroi Jones and the Myth of American Innocence." *JPC*, 3, 2 (Fall 1969), 191 – 204.

325 GALLAGHER, Kathleen. "The Art(s) of Poetry: Jones and MacLeish." *MQ*, 12 (1971), 383 – 92.

326 HENDERSON, Stephen. *Understanding the New Black Poetry: Black Speech and Black Music as Poetic References.* New York: Morrow, 1973.

327 HUDSON, Theodore R. *From Leroi Jones to Amiri Baraka: The Literary Works.* Durham, N.C.: Duke Univ. Press, 1973. [With bibliography.]

327a JACKSON, Esther. "Leroi Jones: Form and the Progression of Consciousness." *CLAJ*, 17 (1973), 33 – 56.

328 JACOBUS, Lee. "Imamu Amiri Baraka: The Quest for Moral Order." See **168.**

329 OTTEN, Charlotte F. "Leroi Jones: Napalm Poet." *CP*, 3, 1 (Spring 1970), 5 – 11.

329a SOLLARS, Werner. *Amiri Baraka / Leroi Jones: The Quest for a Populist Modernism.* New York: Columbia Univ. Press, 1978.

330 TAYLOR, Clyde. "Baraka as Poet." See **168.**

George Barker

Works of Poetry

331 BARKER, George Granvill. *Collected Poems 1930– 1965.* New York: October House, 1965.

Other Relevant Primary Materials

332 *Essays.* London: MacGibbon and Kee, 1970.

333 "An Interview with George Barker," with Cyrena Pondrom. *ConLit*, 12 (1971), 375 – 401.

Critical Books and Essays

334 DAICHES, David. "The Lyricism of Barker." *The Modern World: A Study of Poetry in England Between 1900 and 1939.* Chicago: Univ. of Chicago Press, 1940.

335   FODASKI, Martha. *George Barker*. New York: Twayne, 1969.
336   SWIFT, P. "Prolegomenon to Barker." *XR*, I (1960), 215 – 27.

John Berryman

Works of Poetry

337   *Berryman's Sonnets*. New York: Farrar, Straus and Giroux, 1967. [FS&G]
338   *Delusions, Etc*. New York: Farrar, Straus and Giroux, 1972. [FS&G]
339   *The Dream Songs*. New York: Farrar, Straus and Giroux, 1969. [FS&G]
339a *Henry's Fate and Other Poems*. New York: Farrar, Straus and Giroux, 1977. [Noonday]
340   *Homage to Mistress Bradstreet*. New York: Farrar, Straus and Giroux, 1969.
341   *Homage to Mistress Bradstreet and other Poems*. New York: Noonday, 1968. [Good paperback selection of shorter poems.] [FS&G]
342   *Recovery/Delusions, Etc*. New York: Delta, 1973. [Dell]
343   *Short Poems*. New York: Farrar, Straus and Giroux, 1967.

Other Relevant Primary Materials

344   Numerous uncollected critical essays by Berryman listed in **352**.
345   "Conversation with Berryman," by Richard Kostelanetz. *MassR*, 11 (1970), 340 – 47.
345a *The Freedom of the Poet*. New York: Farrar, Straus and Giroux, 1976. [Noonday]
346   "Interview: The Art of Poetry," with Peter Stitt. *ParR*, 14 (1972), 177 – 207.
347   *Stephen Crane*. New York: William Sloane Associates, 1950.
348   *Recovery*. New York: Farrar, Straus and Giroux, 1973. [Novel]

Biography, Bibliography, and Other Reference Materials

348a ARPIN, Gary. *John Berryman: A Reference Guide*. Boston: Hall, 1976.
349   HEYEN, William. "John Berryman: A Memoir and an Interview." *OhR*, 15, 2 (1974), 46 – 65.
350   KELLY, Richard J., comp. *John Berryman: A Checklist*. Metuchen, N.J.: Scarecrow, 1972.

351 STEFANIK, Ernest. "Bibliography of John Berryman Criticism." *WCR*, 8, 2 (1973), 45 – 52.

352 STEFANIK, Ernest. *John Berryman: A Descriptive Bibliography.* Pittsburgh: Univ. of Pittsburgh Press, 1974.

Critical Books and Essays

353 ALVAREZ, A. *Beyond All This Fiddle.* London: Penguin, 1968.

353a BAYLEY, John. "John Berryman: A Question of Imperial Sway." *Sal*, nos. 22 – 23 (1973), 84 – 102.

354 BROWNE, Michael Dennis. "Henry Fermenting: Debts to the Dream Songs." *OhR*, 15, 2 (Winter 1974), 46 – 75.

354a CONNAROE, Joel. *John Berryman: An Introduction to the Poetry.* New York: Columbia Univ. Press, 1977.

355 DODSWORTH, Martin. "John Berryman: An Introduction." See **164**.

356 HOLDER, Alan. "Anne Bradstreet Resurrected." *CP*, 2 (1969), 11 – 18.

357 LINEBARGER, J. M. *John Berryman.* New York: Twayne, 1974. [Good bibliography.]*

358 MARTZ, William J. *John Berryman.* Minneapolis: Univ. of Minnesota Pamphlets, 1969.

359 MAZZARO, Jerome. "John Berryman and the Yeatsian Mask." *Review of Existential Psychology and Psychiatry*, 12 (1973), 141 – 62.

360 OBERG, Arthur. "John Berryman: The Dream Songs and the Horror of Unlove." *UWR*, 6 (1970), 1 – 11.

361 PEARSON, Gabriel. "John Berryman." See **169**.*

362 STITT, Peter. "Berryman's Last Poems." *CP*, 6 (1973), 5 – 12.

363 STITT, Peter. "John Berryman: The Dispossessed Poet." *OhR*, 15, 2 (1974), 66 – 74.

364 VONALT, Larry. "Berryman's Most Bright Candle." *Parn*, I (1972), 180 – 87.

365 WASSERSTROM, William. "Cagey John: Berryman as Medicine Man." *CentR*, 12 (1968), 334 – 54.

John Betjeman

Works of Poetry

366 BETJEMAN, John. *John Betjeman's Collected Poems, Compiled and with*

an Introduction by the Earl of Birkenhead, ed. and introduction by Philip Larkin. Boston: Houghton-Mifflin, 1971.

366a   *A Nip in the Air*. New York: Norton, 1976. [Norton]

Critical Books and Essays

366b   BROOKE, Jocelyn. *Ronald Firbank and John Betjeman*. London: Longmans, Green, 1962.

366c   HARVEY, G. M. "Poetry of Commitment: John Betjeman's Later Writings." *Dalhousie Review*, 56 (1976), 112 – 24.

367   KERMODE, Frank. "Henry Miller and Betjeman." *Encounter*, 16, 3 (1961), 69 – 75.

367a   SCHRÖDER, Rheinhard. *Die Lyrik John Betjemans*. Hamburg: Verlag, 1972. [With good bibliography.]

368   STANFORD, Derek. *John Betjeman: A Study*. London: Neville Spearman, 1961.

369   WIEHE, R. E. "Summoned by Nostalgia: Betjeman's Poetry." *ArQ*, 19, 1 (Spring 1963), 37 – 49.

Elizabeth Bishop

Works of Poetry

370   *The Ballad of the Burglar of Babylon*. New York: Farrar, Straus and Giroux, 1968.

371   *Complete Poems*. New York: Farrar, Straus and Giroux, 1969. [FS&G]

371a   *Geography III*. New York: Farrar, Straus and Giroux, 1976. [Noonday]

Other Relevant Primary Materials

372   "Introduction" to *An Anthology of Twentieth Century Brazilian Poetry*, ed. Elizabeth Bishop and Emanuel Brazil. Middletown, Conn.: Wesleyan Univ. Press, 1972. [Wesleyan U Pr]

373   *The Diary of "Helena Morley,"* trans. and ed. Elizabeth Bishop. New York: Farrar, Straus and Cudahy, 1977.

373a   " 'The Work': A Conversation with Elizabeth Bishop." *Ploughshares*, 3 (1977), 11 – 29.

Critical Books and Essays

374 ASHBERY, John. "Review of Elizabeth Bishop, *Complete Poems*." *NYTB*, 8 (June 1, 1969), 25.

375 GORDON, Jan B. "Days and Distances: The Cartographic Imagination of Elizabeth Bishop." *Sal*, nos. 22 – 23 (1973), 294 – 305.*

375a "Homage to Elizabeth Bishop, Our 1978 Laureate." *World Literature Today*, 5, 1 (1977), 1 – 52.

375b KALSTONE, David. See **108a**.

376 MAZZARO, Jerome. "Elizabeth Bishop and the Poetics of Impediment." *Sal*, no. 27 (1974), 118 – 44.

377 SHEEHAN, Donald. "The Silver Sensibility: Five Recent Books of American Poetry." *ConLit*, 12 (1971), 98 – 121.

378 STEVENSON, Anne. *Elizabeth Bishop*. New York: Twayne, 1966.

Robert Bly

Works of Poetry

378a *The Body Is Made of Camphor and Gopherwood*. New York: Harper and Row, 1977.

379 *The Light Around the Body*. New York: Harper & Row, 1967. [Har-Row]

379a *The Morning Glory*. Harper and Row, 1975.

380 *Silence in the Snowy Fields*. Middletown, Conn.: Wesleyan Univ. Press, 1962. [Wesleyan U Pr]

381 *Sleepers Joining Hands*. New York: Harper & Row, 1973. [Har-Row]

382 *The Teeth Mother Naked at Last*. San Francisco: City Lights, 1970. [City Lights]

Other Relevant Primary Materials

383 Many essays—in *The Fifties, The Sixties*, and *The Seventies*, all edited by Bly, often signed "Crunk."

384 "The Dead World and the Live World." *The Sixties*, 8 (1966), 2 – 7.*

385 "Interview with Robert Bly." *TPJ*, 2 (Winter 1969), 29 – 48.

385a Interviews with Robert Bly. See **150a, 165a**.

385b *Leaping Poetry: An Idea with Poems and Translations*. Boston: Beacon, 1975.

386 *Lorca and Jimenez*. Boston: Beacon, 1973. [Translations.]

387   "Prose vs. Poetry." *Choice*, 2 (1962), 65 – 80.*

388   "Reflections of the Origins of Poetic Form." *Field*, 10 (Spring 1974), 31 – 35.

389   A series of essays. *Sev*, no. 1 (Spring 1972), 3 – 8; 16 – 21; 30 – 32; 48 – 49; 50 – 51; 54 – 56; 61 – 69; 74 – 76.

390   *Twenty Poems by Tomas Transtromer*. Boston: Beacon, 1970. [Translations.]

391   "A Wrong Turning in American Poetry." *Choice*, 3 (1963), 33 – 47.

392   *Neruda and Vallejo*. Boston: Beacon, 1971. [Bly also did some of the translations.]

Biography, Bibliography, and Other Reference Materials

393   BLY, Robert. "Robert Bly Checklist." *Schist*, no. 1 (Fall 1973), 48 – 51.

394   McMILLAN, Samuel. "On Robert Bly and His Poems: A Selected Bibliography." *TPJ*, 2, 2 (Winter 1969), 48 – 50. [A Bly issue.]

Critical Books and Essays

394a   ATKINSON, Michael. "Robert Bly's Sleepers Joining Hands." *IR*, 7, 4 (1976), 135 – 53.

395   HEYEN, William. "Inward to the World: The Poetry of Robert Bly." *FP*, no. 3 (Fall – Winter 1969), 42 – 50.

396   HOWARD, Richard. "Robert Bly: 'Like Those Before, We Move to the Death We Love'." See **108.**

397   LACEY, Paul. "The Live World." See **111.**

398   LIBBY, Anthony. "Robert Bly Alive in Darkness." *IR*, 3, 3 (Summer 1972), 78 – 89.

399   LIBBY, Anthony. "Fire and Light, Four Poets to the End and Beyond." *IR*, 4, 2 (Spring 1973), 111 – 26.

400   MATTHEWS, William. "Thinking about Robert Bly." *TPJ*, 2 (Winter 1969), 49 – 57.

Hart Crane

Works of Poetry

401   *The Complete Poems and Selected Letters and Prose of Hart Crane*, ed. Brom Weber. Garden City: Doubleday, 1966. [Doubleday]

Other Relevant Primary Materials

402 *The Letters of Hart Crane, 1916— 1932*, ed. Brom Weber. Berkeley: Univ. of California Press, 1965. [Reprint, with silent corrections.]

403 *Letters of Hart Crane and His Family*, ed. Thomas S. W. Lewis. New York: Columbia Univ. Press, 1974.

404 *Robber Rocks: Letters and Memoirs of Hart Crane, 1923— 1932*, ed. Susan Jenkins Brown. Middletown, Conn.: Wesleyan Univ. Press, 1969.

Biography, Bibliography, and Other Reference Materials

405 HORTON, Philip. *Hart Crane: The Life of an American Poet*. New York: Norton, 1937.

406 SCHWARTZ, Joseph. *Hart Crane: An Annotated Critical Bibliography*. New York: David Lewis, 1970.

407 SCHWARTZ, Joseph, and Robert C. SCWEIK. *Hart Crane: A Descriptive Bibliography*. Pittsburgh: Univ. of Pittsburgh Press, 1972.

408 UNTERECKER, John. *Voyager: A Life of Hart Crane*. New York: Farrar, Straus and Giroux, 1969.*

408a WEBER, Brom. *Hart Crane: A Biographical and Critical Study*. New York: Bodley, 1948.

Critical Books and Essays

409 ANDREACH, Robert J. "Crane." *Studies in Structure: The Stages of Spiritual Life in Four Modern Authors*. New York: Fordham Univ. Press, 1964.

410 ARPAD, Joseph. "Hart Crane's Platonic Myth: The Brooklyn Bridge." *AL*, 39 (1967), 75— 86.

411 BUTTERFIELD, R. W. *The Broken Arc: A Study of Hart Crane's Poetry*. Edinburgh: Oliver and Boyd, 1969.

412 COFFMAN, Stanley K., Jr. "Symbolism in the Bridge." *PMLA*, 66 (March 1951), 65— 77.

413 DEMBO, L. S. "Hart Crane: The 'Nuclear Self' and the Fatal Object." See **45.**

414 DEMBO, L. S. *Hart Crane's Sanskrit Charge: A Study of the Bridge*. Ithaca: Cornell Univ. Press, 1960.

415 HAZO, Samuel. *Hart Crane: An Introduction and Interpretation*. New York: Barnes and Noble, 1963.

416 HERMAN, Barbara. "The Language of Hart Crane." *SewR*, 58 (January— March 1950), 52— 67.

417 HOFFMAN, Fredrick J. "The Technological Fallacy in Contemporary Poetry: Hart Crane and MacKnight Black." *AL*, 21 (1949), 94—107.

418 HOPKINS, Konrad. "Make the Dark Poems Light." *Writers and Their Critics*. Tallahassee: Florida State Univ. Studies (#19), (1955), 125—42.

419 HUTSON, Richard. "Exile Guise: Irony and Hart Crane." *Mosaic*, 2, iv (1969), 71—86.

420 LEIBOWITZ, Herbert A. *Hart Crane: An Introduction to the Poetry*. New York: Columbia Univ. Press, 1968. [Columbia Univ Pr]*

421 LEWIS, R. W. B. *The Poetry of Hart Crane: A Critical Study*. Princeton: Princeton Univ. Press, 1967.

422 LOGAN, John. "Introduction." *White Buildings: Poems by Hart Crane*. New York: Liveright, 1972.

423 MCMICHAEL, James. "Hart Crane." *SoR*, 8 (1972), 290—309.

424 MORRIS, H. C. "Crane's 'Voyages' as a Single Poem." *Accent*, 14 (1954), 291—99.

425 NASSAR, Eugene Paul. "Hart Crane's *The Bridge* and its Critics." *The Rape of Cinderella: Essays in Literary Continuity*. Bloomington: Indiana Univ. Press, 1970.

426 PAUL, Sherman. *Hart's Bridge*. Urbana: Univ. of Illinois Press, 1972.*

426a PAUL, Sherman. "Lyricism and Modernism: The Example of Hart Crane." *English Symposium Papers III*, ed. Douglas Shepard. Fredonia: SUNY College at Fredonia, 1972.

427 RIDDLE, Joseph. "Hart Crane's Poetics of Failure." *ELH*, 33 (1966), 473—96.*

428 TATE, Allen. "Hart Crane." *Reactionary Essays on Poetry and Ideas*. New York: Scribner's, 1936. Reprinted in **1457**.*

429 TATE, Allen. "Crane: The Poet as Hero." See **1457**.

430 TRACHTENBERG, Allen. *Brooklyn Bridge: Fact and Symbol*. New York: Oxford Univ. Press, 1965.

431 UROFF, M. D. *Hart Crane: The Patterns of His Poetry*. Urbana: Univ. of Illinois Press, 1974.

432 VOGLER, Thomas. "Crane: A Myth to God." *Preludes to Vision: The Epic Venture in Blake, Wordsworth, Keats, and Hart Crane*. Berkeley: Univ. of California Press, 1971.

433 WINTERS, Yvor. "Hart Crane's Poems." *Poetry*, 30 (April 1927), 47—51.*

434 WINTERS, Yvor. "The Significance of *The Bridge* by Hart Crane." See **95**. Reprinted in **170**.*

435 YANELLA, Phillip. "Toward Apotheosis: Hart Crane's Visionary Lyrics." *Crit*, 10 (1968), 313—33.

Robert Creeley

Works of Poetry

435a *Away*. Santa Barbara: Black Sparrow, 1976.

436 *The Charm: Early and Uncollected Poems.* New York: Scribner's, 1969. [Four Seasons Foun]

437 *A Day Book.* New York: Scribner's, 1972. [Scribner]

438 *For Love: Poems 1950— 1960.* New York: Scribner's, 1962. [Scribner]

438a *Hello: A Journal, Feb. 29— May 3, 1976.* New Directions, 1976. [New Directions]

438b *Listen.* Los Angeles: Black Sparrow, 1972.

439 *Pieces.* New York: Scribner's, 1969. [Scribner]

439a *St. Martin's.* Los Angeles: Black Sparrow, 1974.

439b *Selected Poems.* New York: Scribner's, 1976.

439c *Thirty Things.* Los Angeles: Black Sparrow, 1974.

440 *Words.* New York: Scribner's, 1967. [Scribner]

Other Relevant Primary Materials

441 *Contexts of Poetry: Interviews 1961— 71,* ed. Donald Allen. Bolinas, Cal.: Four Seasons Foundation, 1973.

442 *The Gold Diggers and Other Stories.* New York: Scribner's, 1965. [Scribner]

443 *The Island.* New York: Scribner's, 1963. [Novel.] [Scribner]

443a "Life at All Its Points: An Interview with Robert Creeley." By Philip Milner. *Antigonish Review,* 26 (1976), 37 — 47.

443b Interviews. See **150a** and **165a**.

443c *Mabel: A Story.* London: Marion Boyars, 1976.

443d *Presences: A Text for Marisol.* New York: Scribner's, 1976.

444 *A Quick Graph.* San Francisco: Four Seasons Foundation, 1970. [Collected essays.] [Four Seasons Foun]

445 "Craft Interview with Robert Creeley." *NYQ,* no. 13 (Winter 1973), 18 — 47.

Biography, Bibliography, and Other Reference Materials

446 NOVIK, Mary. *Robert Creeley: An Inventory, 1945— 70.* Kent, Ohio: Kent State Univ. Press, 1973.

Collections of Critical Essays

447 "Robert Creeley Issue." *Ath,* no. 4 (Spring 1973).

447a SPANOS, William, ed. "Robert Creeley: A Gathering." *Bnd 2*, 6 – 7 (1978), 1 – 570. [A collection of critical essays with poems and an interview.]*

Critical Books and Essays

448 ALTIERI, Charles. "The Unsure Egoist: Robert Creeley and the Theme of Nothingness." *ConLit*, 13 (1972), 162 – 85.

449 CAMERON, Allen Barry. "Love Comes Quietly: The Poetry of Robert Creeley." *ChiR*, 19, 2 (1967), 92 – 103.

450 CARROLL, Paul. "Robert Creeley—'A Wicker Basket': The Scene in the Wicker Basket." See **102**.

451 COX, Kenneth. "Address and Posture in the Poetry of Robert Creeley." *CamQ*, 4 (1969), 237 – 43.

452 DORN, Ed. "Review of *Pieces.*" *Caterpillar*, 10 (January 1970), 248 – 50.

453 HOWARD, Richard. "Robert Creeley: 'I Begin Where I Can, and End When I See the Whole Thing Returning'." See **108**.

454 LEWIS, Peter Elfred. "Robert Creeley and Gary Snyder, A British Assessment." *Stand*, 13, 4 (1972), 42 – 47.

455 MANDEL, Ann. *Measures: Robert Creeley's Poetry*. Toronto: Coach House, 1974.

456 MARTZ, Louis L. "Review of *Pieces*," *YR*, 59 (1969), 256 – 61.

457 MAZZARO, Jerome. "Robert Creeley, The Domestic Muse, and Post-Modernism." *Ath*, no. 4 (Spring 1973), 16 – 33.

458 TALLMAN, Warren. *Three Essays on Creeley*. Toronto: Coach House, 1973.*

E. E. Cummings

Works of Poetry

459 *The Complete Poems*. New York: Harcourt, Brace, 1973.

460 *100 Selected Poems*. New York: Grove, 1959.

Other Relevant Primary Materials

461 *The Enormous Room*. New York: Modern Library, 1934. [First published in 1922.] [Liveright]

462 *E. E. Cummings: A Miscellany*, ed. George J. Firmage. New York: October House, 1965.

463 *Eimi*. New York: Grove, 1958. [Novel first published in 1933.]

464 *Fairy Tales*. New York: Harcourt, Brace, 1965.

465 . . . *Him*. . . . New York: Liveright, 1927. [Drama.] [Liveright]

466 *i: Six Nonlectures*. Cambridge: Harvard Univ. Press, 1953. [Harvard U Pr]

467 *Selected Letters of E. E. Cummings*, eds. F. W. Dupee and George Stade. New York: Harcourt, Brace and World, 1969.

Biography, Bibliography, and Other Reference Materials

468 ECKLEY, Wilton. *Checklist of E. E. Cummings*. Columbus, Ohio: C. E. Merrill, 1970.

469 FIRMAGE, George J. *E. E. Cummings: A Bibliography*. Middletown, Conn.: Wesleyan Univ. Press, 1960.

470 LAUTER, Paul. *Index to 1st Lines and Bibliography of Works by and about the Poet*. Denver: Swallow, 1955.

471 NORMAN, Charles. *E. E. Cummings: The Magic Maker*. Indianapolis: Bobbs-Merrill, 1972. [Biography.]

Collections of Critical Essays

472 FRIEDMAN, Norman, ed. *E. E. Cummings: A Collection of Critical Essays*. Englewood Cliffs, N.J.: Prentice-Hall, 1972. [With annotated selected bibliography.] [P-H]

Critical Books and Essays

473 BAUM, Stanley Vergil. *'Eoxi:e.e.c.: E. E. Cummings and the Critics*. East Lansing: Michigan State Univ. Press, 1962.

474 BLACKMUR, R. P. "Notes on E. E. Cummings' Language." *Hound and Horn*, 4 (Winter 1931), 163–92. Reprinted in **39a**.

475 CLARK, David R. *Lyric Resonance: Glosses on Some Poems of Yeats, Frost, Crane, Cummings*. Amherst: Univ. of Massachusetts Press, 1972. [Includes Cummings letters, ed. Robert G. Tucker and David R. Clark.]

476 CLINE, Patricia Buchanan Tal-Maun. "The Whole E. E. Cummings." *TCL*, 14 (1968), 90–97. Reprinted in **472**.

476a COWLEY, Malcolm. "Cummings: One Man Alone." *YR*, 62 (1973), 332–54.

477 DEMBO, L. S. "E. E. Cummings: The Now Man." See **45.**

478 ECKLEY, Wilton. *Guide to E. E. Cummings.* Columbus, Ohio: C. E. Merrill, 1970.

479 FRIEDMAN, Norman. *E. E. Cummings, The Art of His Poetry.* Baltimore: Johns Hopkins Univ. Press, 1960. [Johns Hopkins]

480 FRIEDMAN, Norman. *E. E. Cummings: The Growth of a Writer.* Carbondale: Southern Illinois Univ. Press, 1964.

481 LOGAN, John. "The Organ-Grinder and the Cockatoo: an Introduction to E. E. Cummings." See **174.**

482 MARKS, Barry Alan. *E. E. Cummings.* New York: Twayne, 1964.

483 MAURER, Robert. "Latter-Day Notes on E. E. Cumming's Language." *BuR,* 5 (1955), 1 – 23. Reprinted in **472.**

484 POUND, Ezra. "E. E. Cummings," "e.e. cummings/examined." *"If this be treason . . ."* Siena, Italy: Printed for Olga Rudge by Tip. Nueva, 1948.

485 RIDING, Laura, and Robert GRAVES. "William Shakespeare and E. E. Cummings." *A Survey of Modernist Poetry.* London: Heinemann, 1927, 59 – 82.

486 SHAPIRO, Karl. "Prosody as Meaning," *Poetry,* 73, 3 (1949), 336 – 51.

487 TRIEM, Eve. *E. E. Cummings.* Minneapolis: Univ. of Minnesota Press, 1969.

488 WEGNER, Robert E. *The Poetry and Prose of E. E. Cummings.* New York: Harcourt, Brace and World, 1965.

James Dickey

Works of Poetry

489 *The Eye-Beaters, Blood, Victory, Madness, Bulkhead and Mercy.* Garden City: Doubleday, 1970. [Doubleday]

490 *Poems, 1957– 1967.* Middletown, Conn.: Wesleyan Univ. Press, 1967. [Macmillan]

490a *The Strength of Fields.* Bloomfield Hills, Mich. Bruccoli Clark, 1977. [Poem written for Carter's inauguration.]

490b *The Zodiac.* Garden City: Doubleday, 1976. [A "rewriting" of Horsman's poem.]

Other Relevant Primary Materials

491 *Babel to Byzantium: Poets and Poetry Now.* New York: Farrar, Straus and Giroux, 1968. [G & D]

492 "Conversation with James Dickey," by William Heyen. *SoR*, 9 (1973), 883 – 94.

493 "A Conversation with James Dickey," with Carolyn Kizer and James Boatwright. *Shen*, 17 (Autumn 1966), 3 – 28. Reprinted in **503**.

494 *Deliverance*. Boston: Houghton-Mifflin, 1970. [Novel.][Dell]

494a "Interview with James Dickey." By David Arnett. *Con Lit*, 16 (1975), 286 – 300.

494b "Interview." In Matthew Bruccoli, et al., *Conversations with Writers*, I. Detroit: Gale, 1977.

495 "Introduction" to *The Wreck of the Deutschland*, by G. M. Hopkins. Boston: David Godine, 1971.

496 *Metaphor as Pure Adventure*. Lecture at Library of Congress, December 1967.

497 *Self-Interviews*. Garden City: Doubleday, 1970. [Dell]

498 *Spinning the Crystal Ball*. Garden City: Doubleday, 1971.

499 *Sorties: Journals and New Essays*. Garden City: Doubleday, 1971.

500 *The Suspect in Poetry*. Madison: Sixties, 1964.

Biography, Bibliography, and Other Reference Materials

501 ASHLEY, Franklin. *James Dickey: A Checklist*. Detroit: Gale, 1972.

502 GLANCY, Eileen. *James Dickey: The Critic as Poet: an Annotated Bibliography with an Introductory Essay*. Troy, N.Y.: Whitson, 1971.

Collections of Critical Essays

503 CALHOUN, Richard S., ed. *James Dickey: The Expansive Imagination*. Deland, Fla.: Everett/Edwards, 1973. [With checklist.]

Critical Books and Essays

504 BLY, Robert. "The Work of James Dickey." *The Sixties*, 7 (Winter 1964), 41 – 57.*

505 BLY, Robert. "The Collapse of James Dickey." *The Sixties*, 9 (Spring 1967), 70 – 79.*

506 CARROLL, Paul. "James Dickey—'The Heaven of Animals'; The Smell of Blood in Paradise." See **102**.

507 GUILLORY, Daniel L. "Water Magic in the Poetry of James Dickey." *ELN*, 8 (1970), 131 – 37.

508 HOWARD, Richard. "James Dickey: 'We Never Can Really Tell Whether Nature Condemns Us Or Loves Us'." See **108**.

509 LENSING, George. "James Dickey and the Movements of Imagination." See **503**.

510 LIEBERMAN, Laurence. "Notes on James Dickey's Style." *FP*, I (Spring – Summer 1969), 57 – 63. Reprinted in **503**.

511 LIEBERMAN, Laurence. "The Worldly Mystic." *HudR*, 20 (1967). Reprinted in **503**.

512 NIFLIE, N. Michael. "A Special Kind of Fantasy: James Dickey on the Razor's Edge." *SWR*, 57 (1972), 311 – 17.

513 RAMSEY, Paul. "James Dickey: Meter and Structure." See **503**.

514 SILVERSTEIN, Norman. "James Dickey's Muscular Eschatology." *Sal*, no. 22 – 23 (1973), 258 – 68.

515 SMITH, Raymond. "The Poetic Faith of James Dickey." *MPS*, 2, 6 (1972), 259 – 71.

516 WEATHERBY, H. L. "Way of Exchange in James Dickey's Poetry." *SewR*, 74 (Summer 1966), 669 – 80. Reprinted in **503**.

Hilda Doolittle (H.D.)

Works of Poetry

517 *Collected Poems of H.D.* New York: Liveright, 1925.

518 *Selected Poems.* New York: Grove, 1957. [Grove]

519 *Helen in Egypt.* New York: Grove, 1961.

520 *Hermetic Definition.* New York: New Directions, 1972.

521 Trilogy. New York: New Directions, 1973. [Contains Tribute to the Angels (1945), *The Walls Do Not Fall* (1944), *The Flowering of the Rod* (1946).] [New Directions]

Other Relevant Primary Materials

522 *Bid Me to Live* (A Madrigal). New York: Grove, 1960.

523 *Palimpset.* Carbondale: Southern Illinois Univ. Press, 1968. [Three stories, first published in 1926.]

524 *Tribute to Freud.* Boston: David Godine, 1974. [A much fuller text than the 1956 edition.]

Biography, Bibliography, and Other Reference Materials

525 BRYER, Jackson, and Pamela ROBLYER. "H.D.: A Preliminary Checklist." *ConLit*, 10 (1969), 632 – 75.

Critical Books and Essays

526 DUNCAN, Robert. "Two Chapters from H.D." *TriQ*, no. 12 (Spring 1968), 67 – 98.*

527 ENGEL, Bernard F. "H.D.: Poems that Matter and Dilutations." *ConLit*, 10 (1969), 507 – 23.

528 GREENWOOD, E. B. "H.D. and the Problem of Escapism." *EIC*, 21 (1971), 365 – 76.

529 HOLLAND, Norman. "H.D. and the Blameless Physician." *ConLit*, 10 (1969), 474 – 506.

529a PECK, John. "Passio Perpetuae H.D." *Parn*, 3, no. 2 (1975), 42 – 74.

530 QUINN, Vincent. *Hilda Doolittle*. New York: Twayne, 1967.*

531 RIDDEL, Joseph W. "H.D. and the Poetics of 'Spiritual Realism'." *ConLit*, 10 (1969), 447 – 73.*

532 SWANN, Thomas B. *The Classical World of H.D.* Lincoln: Univ. of Nebraska Press, 1962.

533 WAGNER, Linda Welshimer. " 'Helen in Egypt': A Culmination." *ConLit*, 10 (1969), 523 – 37.

Robert Duncan

Works of Poetry

534 *Bending the Bow.* New York: New Directions, 1968. [New Directions]

534a "Circulations of the Song after Jalāl Al-Dīn Rūmī." *Par R*, 44, 1 (1977), 87 – 97.

535 *Derivations: Selected Poems, 1950– 56.* London: Fulcrum, 1968.

535a *First Decade.* Belfast, Maine: Bern Porter, 1978.

536 *The Opening of the Field.* New York: Grove, 1960. [New Directions]

537 *Roots and Branches.* New York: New Directions, 1964. [New Directions]

538 *The Years as Catches: First Poems (1939– 46).* Berkeley: Oyez, 1966. [Oyez]

Other Relevant Primary Materials

539 *As Testimony.* San Francisco: White Rabbit, 1968.

540 "Beginnings." *Coyote's Journal*, nos. 5 – 6 (1966), 8 – 31. [Chap. I of H.D.]

541 *Robert Duncan: An Interview*, by George Bowering and Robert Hogg. Toronto: Coach House, 1971.

542 "The H.D. Book, Part II, Chapter 5." *Stonybrook*, 1 – 2 (Fall 1968), 4 – 19; 3 – 4 (1969), 27 – 60.

543 "The H.D. Book, Part II, Nights and Days, Chapter 4." *Caterpillar*, 7 (April 1969), 27 – 60.

543a *The Male Muse: Gay Poetry Anthology.* Ed. Duncan, et al. Trumansburg, N.Y.: Crossings, 1977.

544 *The Sweetness and Greatness of Dante's Divine Comedy.* San Francisco: Open Spaces, 1965.

545 "Towards an Open Universe." See **176.**

546 *The Truth and Life of Myth.* New York: House of Books, 1968.

547 "Two Chapters From H.D." *TriQ*, no. 12 (Spring 1968), 67 – 99.

Critical Books and Essays

547a ALTIERI, Charles. "The Book of the World: Robert Duncan's Poetics of Presence." *Sun and Moon*, 1 (1976), 66 – 94.

548 LACEY, Paul. "A Poetry of Exploration." See **111.**

548a REID, Ian. " 'Towards Possible Music': The Poetry of Robert Duncan." *New Poetry*, 21, 2 (April 1973), 17 – 27.

549 ROSENTHAL, M. L. "Robert Duncan." See **119.**

T. S. Eliot

Works of Poetry

550 *Collected Poems, 1909 – 1962.* New York: Harcourt, Brace and World, 1963.

551 *Complete Poems and Plays.* London: Faber and Faber, 1969.

552 *Poems Written in Early Youth.* London: Faber and Faber, 1967. [FS&G]

553 *Selected Poems.* London: Faber and Faber, 1954. [Har Brace J]

554 *The Wasteland: A Facsimile and Transcript of the Original Drafts Including the Annotations of Ezra Pound*, ed. Valerie Eliot. New York: Harcourt, Brace, Jovanovich, 1971. [Har Brace J]

Other Relevant Primary Materials

555 "The Art of Poetry I: T. S. Eliot, an Interview." *ParR*, 21 (Spring – Summer 1959), 47 – 70. Reprinted in **162**, vol. 2.

556 *Christianity and Culture.* New York: Harvest Book, 1949. [Combines in one volume *The Idea of a Christian Society* and *Notes Towards a Definition of Culture.*] [Har Brace J]

557 *Collected Plays.* London: Faber and Faber, 1962.

558 *Knowledge and Experience in the Philosophy of F. H. Bradley.* London: Faber and Faber, 1964. [Doctoral dissertation.]

559 *On Poetry and Poets.* London: Faber and Faber, 1957. [Collection of later essays.] [FS & G]

560 *Selected Essays.* New York: Harcourt, Brace, 1950. [Virtually all the important essays up to 1935.]

561 *To Criticize the Critic.* New York: Farrar, Strauss and Giroux, 1965. [FS & G]

Biography, Bibliography, and Other Reference Materials

562 BERGONZI, Bernard. *T. S. Eliot.* New York: Collier Books, 1972. [Macmillan]

563 DYSON, Anthony E., ed. "Thomas Sterns Eliot." *English Poetry; Select Bibliographical Guides.* London: Oxford Univ. Press, 1971.

564 GALLUP, Donald. *T. S. Eliot: A Bibliography.* New York: Harcourt, Brace and World, 1969.

564a GORDON, Lyndall. *Eliot's Early Years.* New York: Oxford Univ. Press, 1977.* [Oxford]

565 MARTIN, Mildred. *A Half-Century of Eliot Criticism 1916 – 1965.* Lewisburg, Pa.: Bucknell Univ. Press, 1972.

Collections of Critical Essays

566 BERGONZI, Bernard, ed. *T. S. Eliot: "Four Quartets": A Casebook.* London: Macmillan, 1969.

567 KENNER, Hugh, ed. *T. S. Eliot, A Collection of Critical Essays.* Englewood Cliffs, N.J.: Prentice-Hall, 1962. [P-H]

568 LITZ, A. Walton, ed. *Eliot and His Time; Essays on the Occasion of the Fiftieth Anniversary of "The Waste Land."* Princeton: Princeton Univ. Press, 1973.

569 MARTIN, Graham, ed. *Eliot in Perspective, A Symposium.* New York: Humanities, 1970.*

570 MARTIN, Jay, ed. *Twentieth Century Interpretations of the Waste Land.* Englewood Cliffs, N.J.: Prentice-Hall, 1968.

570a MOODY, A. D., ed. *The Waste Land in Different Voices.* London: Edward Arnold, 1974. [Originally 12 lectures presented in 1972.]

571 RAJAN, B., ed. *T. S. Eliot: A Study of His Writings by Several Hands.* London: Dennis Dobson, 1947.

572 SAN JUAN, Epifanio, Jr., ed. *A Casebook on Gerontion.* Columbus, Ohio: C. E. Merrill, 1970. [Merrill]

573 TATE, Allen, ed. "T. S. Eliot (1888–1965)." *SewR,* 74, 1 (January–March 1966), [Important collection for Eliot's effect on modernism.]

Critical Books and Essays

573a ABEL, Richard. "The Influence of St. John Perse on T. S. Eliot." *ConLit,* 14 (1973), 213–39.

574 ADAMS, Robert M. "Precipitating Eliot." See **568.** [Eliot's modernism.]

575 ALVAREZ, A. "Eliot and Yeats: Orthodoxy and Tradition." See **38a.**

576 ANTRIM, Harry T. *T. S. Eliot's Concept of Language: A Study of its Development.* Gainesville: Univ. of Florida Press, 1971.

577 AUSTIN, Allen. *T. S. Eliot; The Literary and Social Criticism.* Bloomington: Indiana Univ. Press, 1971.

578 BLAMIRES, Harry. *Word Unheard: A Guide through Eliot's 'Four Quartets.'* London: Methuen, 1969.

579 BODELSEN, C. A. *T. S. Eliot's Four Quartets: A Commentary.* Copenhagen: Rosenkilde and Bagger, 1958.

580 BOLGAN, Anne C. *What the Thunder Really Said: A Retrospective Essay on the Making of The Waste Land.* Montreal: McGill-Queen's Univ. Press, 1973.

581 BRADBROOK, Muriel Clara. *T. S. Eliot: The Making of 'The Waste Land.'* Harlow, England: Longman Group, 1972.

582 BROOKS, Cleanth. "The Wasteland: An Analysis." See **40.** Reprinted in **570** and **571.**

583 BROOKS, Harold. "Four Quartets: The Structure in Relation to the Themes." See **569.***

584 CHACE, William M. *The Political Identities of Ezra Pound and T. S. Eliot.* Stanford: Stanford Univ. Press, 1973.

585 DAVIE, Donald. "Pound and Eliot: A Distinction." See **569.***

586 DAVIE, Donald. "T. S. Eliot: The End of an Era." *TC,* 159 (1956), 350–62. Reprinted in **566** and **567.** [Mostly on "Dry Salvages."]

587 DONOGHUE, Denis. "A Reading of *Four Quartets.*" See **48.**

588 DUNCAN JONES, E. E. "Ash Wednesday." See **571.**

589 EAGLETON, Terry. "Eliot and a Common Culture." See **569.***

590 ELLMANN, Richard. "The First *Waste Land.*" See **568.**

591 EMPSON, William. "My God Man There's Bears on it." *EIC,* 22 (1972), 417–29. [Review article on Wasteland facsimile.]

592 FRYE, Northrop. *T. S. Eliot.* London: Oliver and Boyd, 1963. [Putnam]*

593 GARDNER, Helen. *The Art of T. S. Eliot.* London: Cresset, 1949.*

594 GARDNER, Helen. "T. S. Eliot." See **161.**

595 GARDNER, Helen. "The Landscapes of Eliot's Poetry." *CritQ*, 10 (1968), 313 – 31.

596 GERSTENBERGER, D. "The Saint and the Circle: The Dramatic Potential of an Image." *Crit*, 2 (1960), 336 – 41.

597 HAMILTON, Ian. *"The Waste Land."* See **579.**

598 HARDING, D. W. " 'Little Gidding'." *Scrutiny*, 11 (1943), 216 – 19. Reprinted in **567.**

598a HARMON, William. "T. S. Eliot's Raids on the Inarticulate." *PMLA*, 9 (1976), 450 – 59.

598b HOUGH, Graham. "Vision and Doctrine in *Four Quartets.*" *CritQ*, 15 (1973), 107 – 27.

599 HOWARTH, Herbert. *Notes on Some Figures Behind T. S. Eliot.* Boston: Houghton-Mifflin, 1964.

600 KENNER, Hugh. *The Invisible Poet: T. S. Eliot.* New York: McDowell, McDowell, Obolensky, 1959. [Har Brace J]*

601 KENNER, Hugh. "The Urban Apocalypse." See **568.**

602 KIRK, Russell. *Eliot and His Age: T. S. Eliot's Moral Imagination in the Twentieth Century.* New York: Random House, 1971.

603 KOJECKY, Roger. *T. S. Eliot's Social Criticism.* New York: Farrar, Straus and Giroux, 1972.

604 KUMAR, Jitendra. "Consciousness and its Correlates: Eliot and Husserl." *PPR*, 28 (1968), 332 – 52.

605 LANGBAUM, Robert. "New Modes of Characterization in *The Waste Land.*" See **568.***

605a LEAVIS, F. R. *The Living Principle: English As a Discipline of Thought.* New York: Oxford Univ. Press, 1975. [Contains a long reading of *Four Quartets.*]

606 LITZ, A. Walton. "The Waste Land Fifty Years After." See **568.**

607 LU, Fei-Pai. *T. S. Eliot: The Dialectical Structure of His Theory of Poetry.* Chicago: Univ. of Chicago Press, 1966.

608 MACCALLUM, Reid. "Time Lost and Regained: The Theme of Eliot's *Four Quartet's.*" *Imitation and Design.* Toronto: Univ. of Toronto Press, 1953.

609 MARGOLIS, John D. *T. S. Eliot's Intellectual Development: 1922 – 1939.* Chicago: Univ. of Chicago Press, 1972.

610 MATTHIESSEN, F. O. *The Achievement of T. S. Eliot, an Essay on the Nature of Poetry.* New York: Oxford Univ. Press, 1947.

611 MILLER, J. Hillis. "T. S. Eliot." See **77.***

612 MILLER, Milton. "What the Thunder Meant." *ELH*, 36 (1969), 440 – 54.

613 MOYNIHAN, William T. "Character and Action in the *Four Quartets.*" *Mosaic* 6 (1972), 203 – 28. [This issue of *Mosaic* is an Eliot number.]

614 PATTERSON, Gertrude. *T. S. Eliot: Poems in the Making.* New York: Barnes and Noble, 1971.

615 PUCKETT, Harry. "T. S. Eliot on Knowing: The Word Unheard." *NEQ*, 44 (1971), 179—96.

616 PRAZ, Mario. "T. S. Eliot and Dante." *SoR*, 2 (1973), 525—48. Reprinted in *The Flaming Heart*. Glouchester, Mass.: P. Smith, 1966.

617 RODGERS, Audrey. "T. S. Eliot's Purgatorio: The Structure of *Ash Wednesday*." *CLS*, 7 (1970), 97—112.

618 SCHNEIDER, Elisabeth. *T. S. Eliot: The Pattern in the Carpet*. Berkeley: Univ. of California Press, 1974.

619 SCHWARTZ, Delmore. "The Literary Dictatorship of T. S. Eliot." *PR*, 16 (February 1949), 119—37.

620 SCHWARZ, Daniel R. "The Unity of Eliot's 'Gerontion': The Failure of Meditation." *BuR*, 19 (1971), 55—76.

621 SHAPIRO, Karl. "The Death of Literary Judgement." *In Defense of Ignorance*. New York: Random House, 1960.

622 SMITH, Grover. *T. S. Eliot's Poetry and Plays: A Study in Sources and Meaning*. Chicago: Univ. of Chicago Press, 1956. [Good on background information and allusions.] [Univ of Chicago Pr]*

623 STEAD, C. K. "Eliot's 'Dark Embryo' The Merger of Morals and Aesthetics" and "The Poetry of T. S. Eliot: Affirmation and the Image." See **87.**

624 TATE, Allen. "Ash Wednesday." See **567.**

624a TRAVERSI, Derek. *T. S. Eliot: The Longer Poems*. New York: Harcourt, 1976.

625 UNGER, Leonard. *T. S. Eliot: Movements and Patterns*. Minneapolis: Univ. of Minnesota Press, 1966. [Univ of Minn Pr]

625a WARD, David. *T. S. Eliot Between Two Worlds: A Reading of T. S. Eliot's Poetry and Plays*. London: Routledge and Kegan Paul, 1973.

626 WARREN, Austin. "Continuity and Coherence in the Criticism of T. S. Eliot. *Connections*. Ann Arbor: Univ. of Michigan Press, 1970.

627 WEITZ, Morris. "T. S. Eliot: Time as a Mode of Salvation." *SewR*, 60 (1952), 48—64. Reprinted in **583.**

628 WHEELWRIGHT, Philip. "Eliot's Philosophical Themes." See **571.**

629 WHITESIDE, George. "T. S. Eliot's Dissertation." *ELH*, 34 (1967), 400—425.*

630 WILSON, Edmund. "T. S. Eliot." See **94.**

631 WOLLHEIM, Richard. "Eliot and F. H. Bradley." See **569.***

Robert Frost

Works of Poetry

632 *Robert Frost: Poetry and Prose*, ed. Edward C. Lathem and Lawrance Thompson. New York: Holt, Rinehart and Winston, 1972.

633 *Selected Poems of Robert Frost.* New York: Holt, Rinehart and Winston, 1963. [HR & W]

Other Relevant Primary Materials

634 *Family Letters of Robert and Elinor Frost*, ed. Arnold Grade. Albany: State Univ. of New York Press, 1972.

635 *Interviews With Robert Frost*, ed. Edward Lathem. New York: Holt, Rinehart and Winston, 1966.

636 *Robert Frost on Writing*, ed. Elaine Barry. Brunswick, N.J.: Rutgers Univ. Press, 1973.

637 MERTINS, Louis. *Robert Frost: Life and Talks Walking.* Norman: Univ. of Oklahoma Press, 1965.

638 SMYTHE, Daniel. *Robert Frost Speaks.* New York: Twayne, 1964.

639 *Selected Letters of Robert Frost*, ed. Lawrance Thompson. New York: Holt, Rinehart and Winston, 1964.

640 *Selected Prose*, ed. Hyde Cox and Edward Connery Lathem. New York: Holt, Rinehart and Winston, 1966.

Biography, Bibliography, and Other Reference Materials

641 GREINER, Donald. *The Merrill Guide to Robert Frost.* Columbus, Ohio: C. E. Merrill, 1969.

642 LATHEM, Edward Connery. *A Concordance to the Poetry of Robert Frost.* New York: Holt Information Systems, 1971.

642a LENTRICCHIA, Frank and Melissa Christensen LENTRICCHIA. *Robert Frost: A Bibliography, 1913— 1974.* Metuchen, N.J.: Scarecrow, 1976.

643 THOMPSON, Lawrance. *Robert Frost: The Early Years, 1874— 1915.* New York: Holt, Rinehart and Winston, 1966. [Univ of Minn Pr]

644 THOMPSON, Lawrance. *Robert Frost: The Years of Triumph, 1915— 1938.* New York: Holt, Rinehart and Winston, 1970. [Univ of Minn Pr]

645a THOMPSON, Laurance, and R. H. WINNICK. *Robert Frost: The Later Years: 1938— 1963.* New York: Holt, Rinehart and Winston, 1976.

Collections of Critical Essays

645 *Frost Centennial Essays*, compiled by the Committee on the Frost Centennial. Jackson: Univ. of Mississippi Press, 1974.

646 COX, James M., ed. *Robert Frost: A Collection of Critical Essays.* Englewood Cliffs, N.J.: Prentice-Hall, 1962. [P-H]

647 GREENBERG, Robert A., and James G. HEPBURN, eds. *Robert Frost: An Introduction.* New York: Holt, Rinehart and Winston, 1961. [Has a section with several reprinted commentaries on specific poems.]

657a WAGNER, Linda, ed. *Robert Frost: The Critical Reception.* New York: Franklin, 1977.

Critical Books and Essays

648 BORROFF, Marie. "Robert Frost's New Testament: Language and the Poem." *MP*, 69 (1971), 36 – 56.

649 BROWER, Reuben. *The Poetry of Robert Frost: Constellations of Intention.* New York: Oxford Univ. Press, 1963. [Oxford U Pr]*

650 COOK, Reginald L. *Robert Frost: A Living Voice.* Amherst: Univ. of Massachusetts Press, 1974.

651 DONOGHUE, Denis. "Robert Frost." See **46.***

652 GORDON, Jan B. "Robert Frost's Circle of Enchantment." See **174.***

653 HAYNES, Donald T. "The Narrative Unity of *A Boy's Will.*" *PMLA* 87 (1972), 452 – 64.

654 IRWIN, W. R. "The Unity of Frost's Masques." *AL*, 32 (1960), 302 – 12.

655 JARRELL, Randall. "To the Laodiceans." See **62.** Reprinted in **646.***

655a JAYNE, Edward. "Up Against the 'Mending Wall': The Psychoanalysis of a Poem by Frost." *CE*, 34 (1973), 934 – 51.

656 JENNINGS, Elizabeth. *Frost.* Edinburgh and London: Oliver and Boyd, 1964.

657 JONES, Howard Mumford. "The Cosmic Loneliness of Robert Frost." *Belief and Disbelief in American Literature.* Chicago: Univ. of Chicago Press, 1967.

658 LANGBAUM, Robert. "The New Nature Poetry." *AmSch*, 28 (1959), 323 – 40.

659 LATHEM, Edward Connery. *The Poetry of Robert Frost.* New York: Holt, Rinehart and Winston, 1969.

660 LENTRICCHIA, Frank. *Robert Frost: Modern Poetics and the Landscapes of the Self.* Durham: Duke Univ. Press, 1975.

661 LYNEN, John F. *The Pastoral Art of Robert Frost.* New Haven: Yale Univ. Press, 1960.*

662 MONTGOMERY, Marion. "Robert Frost and His Use of Barriers: Man vs. Nature Toward God." *SAQ*, 57 (1958), 339 – 53. Reprinted in **646.**

663 MORRIS, John. "The Poet as Philosopher: Robert Frost." *MQR*, 11 (1972), 127 – 34.

664 MORRISON, Theodore. "Frost: Country Poet and Cosmopolitan Poet." *YR*, 59 (1970), 179 – 96.

665 NITCHIE, George W. *Human Values in the Poetry of Robert Frost.* Durham, N.C.: Duke Univ. Press, 1961.

665a POIRIER, Richard. *Robert Frost: The Work of Knowing.* New York: Oxford Univ. Press, 1977.*

666 SQUIRES, Radcliffe. *The Major Themes of Robert Frost.* Ann Arbor: Univ. of Michigan Press, 1963. [Univ of Mich Pr]

667 THOMPSON, Lawrance. *Fire and Ice: The Art and Thought of Robert Frost.* New York: H. Holt, 1942.

668 TRILLING, Lionel. "A Speech on Robert Frost: A Cultural Episode." *PR,* 26 (Summer 1959), 445—52. Reprinted in **646.***

669 WINTERS, Yvor. "Robert Frost: or, the Spiritual Drifter as Poet." *The Function of Criticism: Problems and Exercises.* Denver: Swallow, 1957. Reprinted in **646.**

Allen Ginsberg

Works of Poetry

670 *Empty Mirror: Early Poems.* New York: Corinth, 1961. [Corinth]

671 *The Fall of America: Poems of These States 1965—71.* San Francisco: City Lights, 1972. [City Lights]

672 *The Gates of Wrath: Rhymed Poems: 1948—52.* Bolinas, Cal.: Grey Fox, 1972. [Grey Fox]

673 *Howl and Other Poems.* San Francisco: City Lights, 1956. [City Lights]

674 *Kaddish and Other Poems.* San Francisco: City Lights, 1968. [City Lights]

674a *Mind Breaths: Poems 1972—1977.* San Francisco: City Lights, 1978.

675 *Planet News 1961—67.* San Francisco: City Lights, 1968. [City Lights]

676 *Reality Sandwiches.* San Francisco: City Lights, 1963. [City Lights]

Other Relevant Primary Materials

677 *Allen Verbatim: Lectures on Poetry, Politics, Consciousness,* ed. Gordon Ball. New York: McGraw-Hill, 1974.

678 "Art of Poetry, VIII." *ParR,* 37 (Spring 1966), 13—61. Reprinted in **162,** vol. 3.

679 "A Conversation Between Ezra Pound and Allen Ginsberg," by Michael Reck. *Evergreen,* 55 (June 1968), 27—29.

680 "A Conversation With Allen Ginsberg," by John Tytell, *PR,* 41 (1974), 253—62.

680a "A Conversation with Allen Ginsberg." By Paul Geneson. *Chi R,* 27 (1975), 27—35.

681 "Craft Interview With Allen Ginsberg." *NYQ*, 6 (1971), 11–40.

682 *Gay Sunshine Interview With Allen Young*. Bolinas, Cal.: Grey Fox, 1974.

683 *Improvised Poetics*, ed. Mark Robison. San Francisco: Anonym, 1972.

684 *Indian Journals*. San Francisco: City Lights, 1970.

684a "Interview." See **165a**.

684b "Interview." With Paul Portugés. *Boston Univ. Journal*, 25, 1 (1977), 47–59.

684c *Journals: Early Fifties, Early Sixties*, ed. Gordon Ball. New York: Grove, 1977.

685 "Playboy Interview." *Playboy*, 16, 4 (1969), 81–92; 236–44.

686 "A Talk With Allen Ginsberg," by Alison Colbert. *PR*, 38 (1971), 289–309.

686a *To Eberhart from Ginsberg*. Lincoln, MA: Penmaen, 1976. [Mostly on "Howl" and an essay of Eberhart's.]

Biography, Bibliography, and Other Reference Materials

687 DOWDEN, George. *A Bibliography of Works by Allen Ginsberg, October 1943 to July 1, 1967*. San Francisco: City Lights, 1971.

688 KRAMER, Jane. *Allen Ginsberg in America*. New York: Random House, 1969. [Essentially on Ginsberg's social world.]

Critical Books and Essays

689 BOWERING, George. *How I Hear Howl*. Toronto: Beaver Kosmos Folio One, 1969.

689a BRESLIN, James. "Allen Ginsberg: The Origins of 'Howl' and 'Kaddish.' " *IR*, 8, 2 (1977), 82–108.*

690 DAVIE, Donald. "On Sincerity: From Wordsworth to Ginsberg." *Encounter*, 31, 4 (1968), 61–66.

691 HOWARD, Richard. "Allen Ginsberg: 'O Brothers of the Laurel, Is the World Real? Is the Laurel a Joke or a Crown of Thorns?" See **108**. [The opening paragraph is the funniest story in modern criticism.]

692 MERRILL, Thomas F. *Allen Ginsberg*. New York: Twayne, 1969. [With bibliography.]

693 MOTTRAM, Eric. *Allen Ginsberg in the Sixties*. Brighton, U.K.: Unicorn Bookshop, 1972.

694 ROSZAK, Theodore. "Journey to the East . . . and Points Beyond; Allen Ginsberg and Alan Watts." *The Making of a Counter Culture*. Garden City: Doubleday, 1969. [Doubleday]

695 RUMAKER, Michael. "Allen Ginsberg's Howl." *BMR*, 3 (Autumn 1957), 228–37.

696 SISK, John. "Beatniks and Tradition." *Commonweal*, 70 (April 17, 1959), 74–77.

Robert Graves

Works of Poetry

697   *Collected Poems*. Garden City: Doubleday, 1966. [Doubleday]

697a   *New Collected Poems*. Garden City: Doubleday, 1977.

698   *Poems 1965– 1968*. Garden City: Doubleday, 1969.

699   *Poems 1968– 1970*. Garden City: Doubleday, 1972.

700   *Poems 1970– 1972*. Garden City: Doubleday, 1973.

701   *Poems About Love*. Garden City: Doubleday, 1969. [Collects his love poems.]

Other Relevant Primary Materials

702   *The Crowning Privilege: Collected Essays on Poetry*. London: Penguin, 1959.

703   *Difficult Questions Easy Answers*. Garden City: Doubleday, 1973.

704   *Goodbye to all That: an Autobiography*. Garden City: Doubleday, 1957. [Doubleday]

704a   *On Poetry: Collected Talks and Essays*. Garden City: Doubleday, 1969.

705   *The White Goddess: A Historical Grammar of Poetic Myth*. New York: Vintage, 1959. [New and enlarged.] [FS & G]

Biography, Bibliography, and Other Reference Materials

706   HIGGINSON, Fred H. *A Bibliography of the Works of Robert Graves*. Hamden, Conn.: Archon Books, 1966. [Selected list of criticism.]

706a   POWNALL, David. "An Annotated Bibliography on Robert Graves." *Focus*, 2 (1973), 17 – 23. [More bibliography, pp. 27 – 32.]

Critical Books and Essays

707   DAY, Douglas. *Swifter than Reason: The Poetry and Criticism of Robert Graves*. Chapel Hill: Univ. of North Carolina Press, 1963. [U of NC Press]*

708   ENRIGHT, D. J. "Robert Graves and the Decline of Modernism." *EIC*, 11 (1961), 319 – 66.

709 GASKELL, Ronald. "The Poetry of Robert Graves." *CritQ*, 3 (1961), 213–22.

709a "Graves Issue." *Malakat Review*, 35 (1975).

710 HIJMANS, B. L. "Graves, The White Goddess and Vergil." *Mosaic*, 2 (1969), 58–73.

711 HOFFMAN, Daniel. *Barbarous Knowledge in the Poetry of Yeats, Graves, and Muir.* New York: Oxford Univ. Press, 1967. [Oxford U Pr]

712 JARRELL, Randall, "Graves and the White Goddess." *YR*, 65 (1956), 302–14; 467–78. Reprinted in **63**.*

713 KIRKHAM, Michael. *The Poetry of Graves.* New York: Oxford Univ. Press, 1969.

714 READ, Herbert, and Edward DAHLBERG. "Robert Graves and T. S. Eliot." *TC*, 166 (1959), 54–62.

715 SINCLAIR, J. McH. "A Technique of Stylistic Description." *Lang&S*, 1 (1968), 215–42. [On "The Legs."]

716 STADE, George. *Robert Graves.* New York: Columbia Univ. Press, 1967.

717 STEINER, George. "The Genius of Robert Graves." *KenR*, 22 (1960), 340–65. [Reply by George Stade, 22, 675–77, and rejoinder by Steiner, 22, 677–79.]

718 TRILLING, Lionel. *A Gathering of Fugitives.* Boston: Beacon, 1956.

719 VICKERY, John B. *Robert Graves and the White Goddess.* Lincoln: Univ. of Nebraska Press, 1972.

Ted Hughes

Works of Poetry

720 *Crow: From the Life and Songs of the Crow.* London: Faber and Faber, 1970. Revised printing, 1972. [Har-Row]

721 *The Hawk in the Rain.* London: Faber and Faber, 1957.

722 *Lupercal.* London: Faber and Faber, 1960.

723 *Prometheus on His Crag.* London: Rainbow, 1973.

724 *Selected Poems, 1957–1967.* London: Faber and Faber, 1973. [Har-Row]

725 *Wodwo.* London: Faber and Faber, 1967.

Other Relevant Primary Materials

726 Numerous children's books. See bibliography in **100**.

726a *Cave Bride: An Alchemical Drama.* New York: Viking, 1978.

727 *Eat Crow.* London: Rainbow, 1971. [Play]

728   *Seneca's Oedipus*, adapted by Ted Hughes. Garden City: Doubleday, 1972. [Doubleday]

729   "Ted Hughes and Crow," interview with Egbert Hass. *LM*, 10, 10 (January 1971), 5 – 20.

Biography, Bibliography, and Other Reference Materials

730   SMITH, A. C. H. *Orghast at Persepolis: An Account of the Experiment in Theatre Directed by Peter Brook and Written by Ted Hughes.* London: Methuen, 1972.

Critical Books and Essays

731   BEDIENT, Calvin. "Ted Hughes." See **100.**

731a   BOLD, Allan N. *Gunn and Hughes: Thom Gunn and Ted Hughes.* New York: Barnes and Noble, 1976.

732   HOFFMAN, Daniel. "Talking Beasts: The 'Single Adventure' in the Poems of Ted Hughes." *Shen*, 19, 4 (Summer 1968), 49 – 68.

733   LIBBY, Anthony. "God's Lioness and the Priest of Sycorax: Plath and Hughes." *ConLit*, 15 (1974), 386 – 405.

734   LODGE, David. " 'Crow' and the Cartoons." *CritQ*, 13 (1971), 37 – 42; 68.

735   RIFE, David. "Rectifying Illusion in the Poetry of Ted Hughes." *MinnR*, 10, 3 – 4 (1970), 95 – 99.

736   ROBINSON, Ian, and David SIMS. "Ted Hughes's Crow." *The Human World*, 9 (November 1972), 31 – 40.

737   SAGAR, Keith. *The Art of Ted Hughes.* Cambridge Univ. Press, 2nd ed., 1977.

Randall Jarrell

Works of Poetry

738   *Randall Jarrell: The Complete Poems.* New York: Farrar, Straus and Giroux, 1969. [FS & G]

Other Relevant Primary Materials

739 "Answers and Questions." *Mid-Century American Poets*, ed. John Ciardi. New York: Twayne, 1950.

740 *Jerome: The Biography of a Poem.* New York: Grossman, 1971.

741 *The Juniper Tree and Other Tales from Grimm*, 2 vols, trans. Lore Segal. New York: Farrar, Straus and Giroux, 1973. [Four tales trans. by Jarrell.]

742 *Pictures From an Institution.* New York: Alfred Knopf, 1954. [Novel.]

743 *Poetry and the Age.* New York: Farrar, Straus and Giroux, 1953. [FS & G]

744 *A Sad Heart at the Supermarket.* New York: Farrar, Straus and Giroux, 1962.

745 *The Third Book of Criticism.* New York: Farrar, Straus and Giroux, 1969. [FS & G]

Biography, Bibliography, and Other Reference Materials

746 *Alumni News.* Univ. of North Carolina, Greensboro, 54 (Spring 1966). [Memorial issue for Jarrell—mostly memoirs.]

747 ADAMS, Charles M. *Randall Jarrell: A Bibliography.* Chapel Hill: Univ. of North Carolina Press, 1958. [Supplement by Adams in *Analects*, 1 (Spring 1961), 49−56.]

748 GILLIKIN, Dure Jo. "A Check List of Criticism on Randall Jarrell, 1941−1970: With an Introduction and a List of His Major Works." *BNYPL*, 75 (1971), 176−94.

Collections of Critical Essays

749 LOWELL, Robert, Peter TAYLOR, and R. P. WARREN, eds. *Randall Jarrell, 1914−1965.* New York: Farrar, Straus and Giroux, 1967. [Mostly short pieces by poets and friends.] [FS & G]

Critical Books and Essays

750 DICKEY, James. "Randall Jarrell." See **500.** Reprinted in **766.**

751 FERGUSON, Frances. "Randall Jarrell and the Flotations of Voice." *GaR*, 28 (1974), 423−39.

752 FERGUSON, Suzanne. *The Poetry of Randall Jarrell.* Baton Rouge: Louisiana State Univ. Press, 1971. [With selected bibliography.]*

753 FOWLER, Russell. "Randall Jarrell's 'Eland': A Key to Motive and Technique in His Poetry." *IR*, 5, 2 (1974), 113—26.

754 FULLER, John. "Randall Jarrell." See **169**.*

755 HOFFMAN, Frederick. "Randall Jarrell—A Profound Record," introduction to *The Achievement of Randall Jarrell.* Glenview, Ill.: Scott, Foresman, 1970.

756 MAZZARO, Jerome. "Between Two Worlds: The Post-Modernism of Randall Jarrell." *Sal*, 22—23 (1973), 164—86.*

757 NITCHIE, George. "Randall Jarrell: A Stand-In's View." *SoR*, 9 (1973), 883—94.

758 QUINN, Sister M. Bernetta. "Landscapes of Life and *Life*." *Shen*, 20, 2 (Winter 1969), 49—78.

759 RANSOM, John Crowe. "The Rugged Way of Genius." *SoR*, 3 (1967), 263—81. Reprinted in **749**.

760 ROSENTHAL, M. L. *Randall Jarrell.* Minneapolis: Univ. of Minnesota Press, 1972.

761 SHAPIRO, Karl. *Randall Jarrell.* Washington, D.C.: Library of Congress, 1967. [With bibliography of Jarrell materials in Library of Congress.] Reprinted in **749**.

762 WEISBERG, Robert. "Randall Jarrell: The Integrity of His Poetry." *CentR*, 17 (1973), 237—55.

Robinson Jeffers

Works of Poetry

763 *Be Angry at the Sun.* New York: Random House, 1941.

764 *The Beginning and the End and Other Poems.* New York: Random House, 1963.

765 *Californians.* New York: Macmillan, 1916.

766 *Cawdor and Other Poems.* New York: Liveright, 1928.

767 *Dear Judas and Other Poems.* New York: Liveright, 1929.

768 *The Double Axe and Other Poems.* New York: Random House, 1948.

769 *Give your Heart to the Hawks and Other Poems.* New York: Random House, 1933.

770 *Hungerfield and Other Poems.* New York: Random House, 1954.

771 *Roan Stallion, Tamar, and Other Poems.* New York: Boni and Liveright, 1925.

772 *Robinson Jeffers, Selected Poems.* New York: Random House, 1938. [Jeffers' own selections.] [Random]

773 *Solstice and Other Poems.* New York: Random House, 1935.

774 *Such Counsels You Gave to Me and Other Poems.* New York: Random House, 1937.

775 *Thurso's Landing and Other Poems.* New York: Liveright, 1932.

776 *The Women at Point Sur.* New York: Boni and Liveright, 1927.

Other Relevant Primary Materials

777 *Cawdor and Medea.* New York: New Directions, 1970. [Contains Jeffers' adaptation of Euripedes.][New Directions]

778 *Poetry, Gongorism and a Thousand Years.* Los Angeles: Ward Ritchie, 1949.

779 *The Selected Letters of Robinson Jeffers,* ed. Ann Ridgeway. Baltimore: Johns Hopkins Univ. Press, 1968.

780 *Themes in My Poems.* San Francisco: Book Club of California, 1956.

Biography, Bibliography, and Other Reference Materials

781 BENNETT, Melba Berry. *The Stone Mason of Tor House.* Los Angeles: Ward Ritchie, 1966.

782 NOLTE, William. *The Merrill Guide to Robinson Jeffers.* Columbus, Ohio: C. E. Merrill, 1970.

783 POWELL, Lawrence Clark. *Robinson Jeffers, The Man and His Work.* Pasadena: San Pasqual, 1940. [The most reliable biography.]

784 VARDAMIS, Alex. *The Critical Reputation of Robinson Jeffers: A Bibliographical Study.* Hamden, Conn.: Archon Books, 1972.

Critical Books and Essays

785 ALEXANDER, John. "Conflict in the Narrative Poetry of Robinson Jeffers." *SewR,* 80 (1972), 85 – 99.

786 ANTONINUS, Brother [William Everson]. *Robinson Jeffers: Fragments of an Older Fury.* Berkeley: Oyez, 1968.

787 BOYERS, Robert. "A Sovereign Voice: The Poetry of Robinson Jeffers." *SewR,* 77 (1969), 487 – 507. Reprinted in **174.**

788 BROPHY, Robert. *Robinson Jeffers: Myth, Ritual, and Symbol in His Narrative Poems.* Cleveland: Case Western Reserve Univ. Press, 1973. [Has good bibliographical notes.]*

789 CARPENTER, Frederic I. *Robinson Jeffers.* New York: Twayne, 1962.

790 COFFIN, Arthur. *Robinson Jeffers: Poet of Inhumanism*. Madison: Univ. of Wisconsin Press, 1971.*

791 GREGORY, Horace. "Poet Without Critics: A Note on Robinson Jeffers." *The Dying Gladiator and Other Essays*. New York: Grove, 1961.

792 NOLTE, William. "Robinson Jeffers as Didactic Poet." *VQR*, 42 (1966), 257—71.

792a SHEBL, James. *In This Wild Water: The Suppressed Poems of Robinson Jeffers*. Pasadena, Calif.: Ward, Ritchie, 1976. [Describes and prints poems suppressed from *Double Axe*.]

793 SQUIRES, James Radcliffe. *The Loyalties of Robinson Jeffers*. Ann Arbor: Univ. of Michigan Press, 1956. [U of Mich Pr]

794 WINTERS, Yvor. "Robinson Jeffers." *Poetry*, 35 (1930), 279—86.

David Jones

Works of Poetry

795 *The Anathemata*. London: Faber and Faber, 1952. [Viking]

796 *In Parentheses*. London: Faber and Faber, 1973. [Viking]

796a *The Sleeping Lord*. London: Faber and Faber, 1974. [Collects work after *Anathemata*.]

796b *David Jones, Letters to Vernon Watkins*. Ed. Ruth Pryor. Cardiff: Univ. of Wales Press, 1976.

796c *The Dying Gaul and Other Writings*. London: Faber and Faber, 1978.

Other Relevant Primary Materials

797 *Epoch and Artists*, ed. Harmon Grisewood. London: Faber and Faber, 1959. [Selection of essays and prefaces.][Faber]

798 "Interview." *The Poet Speaks*, ed. Peter Orr. London: Routledge and Kegan Paul, 1966.

799 *An Introduction to the Rhyme of the Ancient Mariner*. London: Clover Hill Editions, 1972.

800 "Looking Back at the Thirties." *LM*, 5 (1965), 47—54.

Collections of Critical Essays

801 *Agenda*. 5 (1967). [Special David Jones issue on the writing and the painting.]

802 *Agenda.* 11, 4, and 12, 1 (1973 — 74). [Mostly a special Jones issue on his recent writings.]

802a MATHIAS, Roland, ed. *David Jones: Eight Essays on His Work as Writer and Artist.* Llandyssol, Wales: Gomer, 1976.

803 *Poetry Wales.* 8, 3 (1972).

Critical Books and Essays

804 AUDEN, W. H. "A Contemporary Epic." *Encounter*, 12, 2 (1954), 67 — 71. [On *Anathemata*.]

805 BLAMIRES, David. *David Jones: Artist and Writer.* Manchester: Manchester Univ. Press, 1971. [With selected bibliography.]

806 BLISSET, William. "David Jones: Himself at the Cave Mouth." *UTQ*, 36 (1966 — 67), 259 — 73.

807 GEMMILL, Janet Powers. "*In Parenthesis*: A Study of Narrative Technique." *JML*, 1 (1971), 311 — 28.

807a HAGUE, René. *A Commentary on The Anathemata of David Jones.* Toronto: Univ. of Toronto Press, 1977.

807b HAGUE, René. "Myth and Mystery in the Poetry of David Jones." *Agenda*, 15, 2 — 3 (1977), 37 — 79.

808 HILLS, Paul. "The Romantic Tradition in David Jones." *MHRev*, no. 27 (July 1973), 39 — 64.

808a HOOKER, Jeremy. "On the *Anathemata*." *Anglo-Welsh Review*, 22 (Autumn 1973), 31 — 43.

809 JOHNSTON, John H. See **27.**

809a RAINE, Kathleen. *David Jones: Solitary Perfectionist.* Ipswich, U.K.: Golgonooza, 1974. [First published in *SewR*, 75 (1967), 740 — 46.]

810 REES, Samuel. "The Poetry of David Jones." *MPS*, 3 (1972), 161 — 69.

810a SPEARS, Monroe K. "Shapes and Surfaces: David Jones, with a Glance at Charles Tomlinson." *ConLit*, 12 (1971), 402 — 19.

811 STONEBURNER, Tony. "Notes on Prophecy and Apocalypse in a Time of Anarchy and Revolution: A Trying Out." *TriQ*, no. 23 — 24 (1972), 246 — 82.

Philip Larkin

Works of Poetry

812 *High Windows.* New York: Farrar, Straus and Giroux, 1974.

813 *The Less Deceived.* Hessle, East Yorkshire: Marvell, 1955.

814 *The North Ship.* London: Fortune, 1945.

815 *20 Poems*. Privately printed, 1951.

816 *The Whitsun Weddings*. London: Faber and Faber, 1964.

Other Relevant Primary Materials

817 "A Conversation with Philip Larkin." *Tracks*, 1 (Summer 1967), 5—10.

818 *All What Jazz: A Record Diary, 1961—68*. London: Faber and Faber, 1970.

819 "Four Conversations with Philip Larkin," with Ian Hamilton. *LM*, 4 (November 1964), 71—77.

820 *A Girl in Winter*. New York: St. Martin's, 1962. [Novel, first published in 1957.]

821 "Introduction" to Jenny Stratford (Lewis). *The Arts Council Collection of Modern Literary Manuscripts*. London: Turret Books, 1974.

822 *Jik*. London: Fortune, 1946. [Novel.]

823 "Preface" to *The Oxford Book of Twentieth Century English Verse*. Oxford: Clarendon, 1973.

Critical Books and Essays

824 BAYLEY, John. "Too Good for This World." *TLS*, 772, no. 3 (June 21, 1974), 653.

825 BEDIENT, Calvin. "Philip Larkin." See **100.***

826 FALCK, Colin. "Philip Larkin." See **169.**

827 JACOBSON, Dan. "Philip Larkin: A Profile." *NR*, 1, no. 4 (June 1974), 25—29.

828 NAREMORE, James. "Philip Larkin's 'Lost World'." *ConLit*, 15 (Summer 1974), 331—44.*

829 TIMMS, David. *Philip Larkin*. Edinburgh: Oliver Boyd, 1973. [With bibliography.]

829a WEATHERHEAD, A. "Philip Larkin of England." *ELH*, 38 (1971), 616—30.

830 WELZ, Dieter. "A Winter Landscape in Neutral Colors: Some Notes on Philip Larkin's Vision of Reality." *Theoria*, 39 (1973), 61—73.

D. H. Lawrence

Works of Poetry

831   *Collected Poems*, ed. Vivian deSola-Pinto and Warren Roberts, rev. ed., 2 vols. New York: Viking, 1971. [Lawrence's prose introductions to his volumes are important and are included here.] [Viking]

Other Relevant Primary Materials

832   *Collected Letters*, ed. Harry Moore, 2 vols. New York: Viking, 1962.

833   *Psychoanalysis and the Unconscious (1921) and Fantasia of the Unconscious (1922).* New York: Viking, 1960. [Viking]

834   *Selected Literary Criticism*, ed. Anthony Beal. New York: Viking, 1956. [Viking]

835   *Selected Poems*, ed. Keith Sagar. Harmondsworth: Penguin, 1972.

836   *Studies in Classic American Literature.* New York: Viking, 1961. [First published in 1923.] [Viking]

Biography, Bibliography, and Other Reference Materials

837   *Bibliography.* Annual Checklist in the *D. H. Lawrence Review*, 1968 – present.

837a   FERRIER, Carole. "D. H. Lawrence's Pre-1920 Poetry: A Descriptive Bibliography of Manuscripts, Typescripts and Proofs." *DHLR*, 6 (1973), 333 – 59.

838   GARCIA, Reloy, and James KARABATSOS. *A Concordance to the Poetry of D. H. Lawrence.* Lincoln: Univ. of Nebraska Press, 1970.

839   MOORE, Harry T. *The Priest of Love: A Life of D. H. Lawrence*, rev. ed. New York: Farrar, Straus and Giroux, 1974.

840   NEHLS, Edward, ed. *D. H. Lawrence: A Composite Biography*, 3 vols. Madison: Univ. of Wisconsin Press, 1957 – 59.

Collections of Critical Essays

841 COOMBES, H., ed. *D. H. Lawrence: A Critical Anthology*. Harmondsworth: Penguin, 1973. [Many early letters and reviews.]

842 DRAPER, R. P., ed. *D. H. Lawrence: The Critical Heritage*. New York: Barnes and Noble, 1970. [St. Martin's]

843 MOORE, Harry, and Frederick HOFFMAN, eds. *The Achievement of D. H. Lawrence*. Norman: Univ. of Oklahoma Press, 1953.

844 MOORE, Harry, ed. *A D. H. Lawrence Miscellany*. Carbondale: Southern Illinois Univ. Press, 1959.

845 SPENDER, Stephen, ed. *D. H. Lawrence: Novelist, Poet, Prophet*. London: Weidenfeld and Nicolson, 1973.

Critical Books and Essays

846 ALVAREZ, A. "D. H. Lawrence: The Single State of Mind." See **38**. Reprinted in **844** and **845**.*

847 BLACKMUR, R. P. "D. H. Lawrence and Expressive Form: See **39a**.*

848 BLOOM, Harold. "Lawrence, Blackmur, Eliot and the Tortoise." See **844**.

849 CIPOLA, Elizabeth. "The Last Poems of Lawrence." *DHLR*, 2 (1969), 103−19.

850 CLARKE, Colin. *River of Dissolution: D. H. Lawrence and English Romanticism*. London: Routledge and Kegan Paul, 1969.*

851 ELLMANN, Richard. "Lawrence and His Demon." *NMQ*, 22 (1952), 385−93. Reprinted in Moore and Hoffman, eds., **843**.

852 ENRIGHT, D. J. "A Haste for Wisdom: The Poetry of D. H. Lawrence." *Conspirators and Poets*. London: Chatto and Windus, 1966.

853 GILBERT, Sandra M. *Acts of Attention: The Poems of D. H. Lawrence*. Ithaca: Cornell Univ. Press, 1972.*

854 GREGORY, Horace. "D. H. Lawrence." *Pilgrim of the Apocalypse*. New York: Viking, 1933. Reprinted in **843**.

855 GUTIERREZ, Donald. "Circles and Arcs: The Rhythm of Circularity and Centrifugality in D. H. Lawrence's *Last Poems*." *DHLR*, 4 (1971), 319−33.

856 LUCIE-SMITH, Edward. "The Poetry of D. H. Lawrence—With a Glance at Shelley." See **845**.

857 MARSHALL, Tom. *The Psychic Mariner: A Reading of the Poems of D. H. Lawrence*. New York: Viking, 1970.

858 OATES, Joyce Carol. *The Hostile Sun: The Poetry of D. H. Lawrence*. Los Angeles: Black Sparrow, 1973. [Black Sparrow]

859 SHAPIRO, Karl. "The Unemployed Magician." *In Defence of Ignorance*. New York: Random House, 1960. Reprinted in **844**.

860 SPENDER, Stephen. "Notes on D. H. Lawrence." See **1355**.

861 WOOD, Frank. "Rilke and D. H. Lawrence." *GR*, 15 (1940), 212−23.

862 YOUNGBLOOD, Sarah. "Substance and Shadow: The Self in the Poetry of D. H. Lawrence." *DHLR*, 1 (1968), 114−28.

Denise Levertov

Works of Poetry

863   *The Double Image.* London: Cresset, 1946.

864   *Footprints.* New York: New Directions, 1972. [New Directions]

864a *The Freeing of the Dust.* New York: New Directions, 1975.

865   *Here and Now.* San Francisco: City Lights, 1957.

866   *The Jacob's Ladder.* New York: New Directions, 1961. [New Directions]

866a *Life in the Forest.* New York: New Directions, 1978.

867   *O Taste and See.* New York: New Directions, 1964. [New Directions]

868   *Overland to the Islands.* Highlands, N.C.: Jargon, 1958.

869   *Relearning the Alphabet.* New York: New Directions, 1970. [New Directions]

870   *The Sorrow Dance.* New York: New Directions, 1967. [New Directions]

871   *To Stay Alive.* New York: New Directions, 1971. [New Directions]

872   *With Eyes at the Back of our Heads.* New York: New Directions, 1959. [New Directions]

Other Relevant Primary Materials

873   *Guillevic: Selected Poems.* New York: New Directions, 1969. [Translation.] [New Directions]

874   *Jules Superveille: Selected Writings.* New York: New Directions, 1967. [New Directions]

875   *The Poet in the World.* New York: New Directions, 1973. [Essays and interviews.] [New Directions]

Biography, Bibliography, and Other Reference Materials

876   WILSON, Robert. *A Bibliography of Denise Levertov.* New York: Phoenix Book Shop, 1972. [Only primary materials.]

Critical Books and Essays

877   BOWERING, George. "Denise Levertov." *The Antigonish Review*, no. 7 (Autumn 1971), 76–87.

878   DUDDY, Thomas A. "To Celebrate: A Reading of Denise Levertov." *Crit*, 10 (1968), 138 – 52.

878a   DU PLESSIS, Rachel Blau. "The Critique of Consciousness and Myth in Levertov, Rich and Rukeyser." *Feminist Studies*, 3, 1 – 2 (1975), 199 – 221.

879   HOWARD, Richard. "Denise Levertov: 'I Don't Want to Escape, Only to See the Enactment of Rites'." See *Alone with America*.

879a   KYLE, Carol. "Every Step An Arrival: *Six Variations* and the Musical Structure of Denise Levertov's Poetry." *CentR*, 17 (1973), 281 – 96.

880   MILLS, Ralph. "Denise Levertov: The Poetry of the Immediate." See **172**.

881   WAGNER, Linda. *Denise Levertov*. New York: Twayne, 1967. [Coll & U Pr]

John Logan

Works of Poetry

882   *The Anonymous Lover: New Poems*. New York: Liveright, 1973. [Liveright]

883   *Cycle for Mother Cabrini*. New York: Grove, 1955.

884   *Ghosts of the Heart*. Chicago: Univ. of Chicago Press, 1960. [U of Chicago Pr]

884a   *Poem in Progress*. Washington, D.C.: Dryad Press, 1976.

885   *Spring of the Thief*. New York: Alfred Knopf, 1963.

886   *The Zigzag Walk: Poems 1965– 68*. New York: Dutton, 1969. [Dutton]

Other Relevant Primary Materials

887   *The House that Jack Built*. Omaha: Univ. of Nebraska Press, 1974. [Memoir.]

888   "Interview." See **178**.

889   "John Logan: An Interview." *Salted Feathers*, 3 (July 1966), n.p.

890   "John Logan on Poets and Poetry Today." *Voyages*, 4, 3 and 4 (1971 – 72), 17 – 24.

891   "A Note on the Inarticulate as Hero." *NMQ*, 38 – 39 (1969), 148 – 53.

Critical Books and Essays

892 ALTIERI, Charles. "Poetry as Resurrection: John Logan's Structures of Metaphysical Solace." *MPS*, 3 (1973), 193—224.

893 BLY, Robert. "John Logan's Force Field." *Voyages*, 4, 3 and 4 (1971—72), 29—36.*

894 CARROLL, Paul. "John Logan—'A Century Piece for Poor Heine': Was Frau Heine a Monster? or Yung and Easily Freudened in Dusseldorf, Hamburg, Berlin, Paris and New York City." See **102.**

895 CHAPLIN, William. "Identity and Spirit in the Recent Poetry of John Logan." *APR*, 2, 3 (May—June 1973), 19—24.*

896 HOWARD, Richard. "John Logan, 'I am Interested in the Unicorn Underneath the Wound'." See **108.**

897 ISBELL, Harold. "Growth and Change: John Logan's Poems." *MPS*, 2 (1971), 213—23.

898 MAZZARO, Jerome. "Venture Into Evening: Self-Parody in the Poetry of John Logan." *Sal*, 2, 4 (Fall 1968), 78—95.

899 RUST, Michael. "Singing for the Shadow: Elaborations on John Logan's 'Lines for Michael in the Picture'." *Voyages*, 4, 3 and 4 (1971—72), 40—47.

Robert Lowell

Works of Poetry

900   *Day by Day.* New York: Farrar, Straus and Giroux, 1977. [F, S and G]

900a *The Dolphin.* New York: Farrar, Straus and Giroux, 1973. [FS & G]

901   *For Lizzie and Harriet.* New York: Farrar, Straus and Giroux, 1973.

902   *For the Union Dead.* New York: Farrar, Straus and Giroux, 1964. [With **905**—FS & G]

903   *History.* New York: Farrar, Straus and Giroux, 1973. [Revision of and addition to Notebook.]

904   *Imitations.* New York: Farrar, Straus and Giroux, 1961.

905   *Life Studies.* New York: Farrar, Straus and Giroux, 1959. [FS & G]

906   *Land of Unlikeness.* Cummington, Mass.: Cummington, 1944.

907   *Lord Weary's Castle.* New York: Harcourt, Brace, 1946. [Har Brace]

908   *The Mills of the Kavanaughs.* New York: Harcourt, Brace, 1951. [With **907**—Har Brace]

909   *Near the Ocean.* New York: Farrar, Straus and Giroux, 1967. [FS & G]

910 *Notebook: Revised and Expanded Edition.* New York: Farrar, Straus and Giroux, 1970. [FS & G]

910a *Selected Poems.* New York: Farrar, Straus and Giroux, 1976. [F, S and G]

Other Relevant Primary Materials

911 "Conversation with Robert Lowell," with D. S. Carne-Ross. *Delos*, 1 (1968), 165 – 75. [Interview on translation.] Reprinted in **923**.

912 "Et in America Ego," with V. S. Naipaul. *The Listener*, 82 (September 4, 1969), 302 – 304. [Interview.] Reprinted in **923**.

913 "Lowell in England: 14 Poems and an Interview." *Rev*, 26 (Summer 1971), 3 – 29.

914 *The Old Glory.* New York: Farrar, Straus and Giroux, 1965. [Three plays.] [FS & G]

915 "On 'Skunk Hour'." *New World Writing*, 21. Reprinted in **179**.

916 *Phaedra.* New York: Farrar, Straus and Giroux, 1961. [Translation.]

917 *Prometheus Bound.* New York: Farrar, Straus and Giroux, 1969. [Translation.] [FS & G]

918 "Robert Lowell." See **162**, vol. 2. Reprinted in **922**. [Interview.]

919 "Robert Lowell in Conversation," with Anthony Alvarez. See **923**.

920 "A Talk with Robert Lowell," with A. Alvarez. *Encounter*, 24 (February 1965), 39 – 43. Reprinted in **923**.

Biography, Bibliography, and Other Reference Materials

921 MAZZARO, Jerome. "Checklist: 1939 – 1968." See **922**.

Collections of Critical Essays

921a BOYERS, Robert, ed. "Special Issue for Lowell's 60th Birthday." *Sal*, 37 (1977).

922 BOYERS, Robert, and Michael LONDON, eds. *Robert Lowell: A Portrait of the Artist in His Time.* New York: David Lewis, 1970. [Collects mostly intelligent reviews.]

923 MAZZARO, Jerome, ed. *Profile of Robert Lowell.* Columbus, Ohio: C. E. Merrill, 1971. [Merrill]

924 PARKINSON, Thomas, ed. *Robert Lowell: A Collection of Critical Essays.* Englewood Cliffs, N.J.: Prentice-Hall, 1968. [Collects mostly important reviews and parts of books.] [P-H]

925 PRICE, Jonathan, ed. *Critics on Robert Lowell.* Coral Gables: Univ. of Miami Press, 1971.

Critical Books and Essays

926 ALTIERI, Charles. "Poetry in a Prose World: Robert Lowell's *Life Studies.*" *MPS*, 1 (1970), 182 – 99. Reprinted in **923.**

927 AXELROD, Stephen. "Baudelaire and the Poetry of Robert Lowell." *TCL*, 17 (October 1971), 257 – 74.

928 BAYLEY, John. "The Poetry of Cancellation." *LM*, 6 (June 1966), 76 – 85. Reprinted in **922.**

928a BERRYMAN, John. "Lowell, Thomas, & c." *PR*, 14 (1947), 73 – 85.

929 BERRYMAN, John. "On Skunk Hour." See **179.**

929a BERRYMAN, John. "The Poetry of Robert Lowell." *NYRB*, 2 (May 28, 1964), 3 – 4.

930 BLY, Robert. "Prose vs. Poetry." *Choice*, 2 (1962), 65 – 80.*

931 BLY, Robert. "A Wrong Turning in American Poetry." *Choice*, 3 (1962), 33 – 47.

932 BOWEN, Roger. "Confession and Equilibrium: Robert Lowell's Poetic Development." *Crit*, 11 (1969), 78 – 93.

933 BOYERS, Robert. "On Robert Lowell." *Sal*, 13 (Summer 1970), 36 – 44. Reprinted in **923.**

934 CARNE-ROSS, D. S. "The Two Voices of Translation." See **924.**

935 CARRUTH, Hayden. "A Meaning of Robert Lowell." *HudR*, 20 (1967), 429 – 47. Reprinted in **922.**

936 COOPER, Philip. *The Autobiographical Myth of Robert Lowell.* Chapel Hill: Univ. of North Carolina Press, 1970.

937 COSGRAVE, Patrick. *The Public Poetry of Robert Lowell.* London: V. Golancz, 1970.

938 EDWARDS, Thomas. "The Liberal Imagination and Robert Lowell." See **18.**

939 EHRENPREIS, Irvin. "The Age of Lowell." *American Poetry*, ed. I. Ehrenpreis. London: Stratford-Upon-Avon Studies No. 7 (1965). Reprinted in **922** and **924.***

940 FEIN, Richard. "Mary and Bellona: The War Poetry of Robert Lowell." *SoR*, n.s., 1 (1965), 820 – 34.

941 FEIN, Richard. *Robert Lowell.* New York: Twayne, 1970.

942 HAMILTON, Ian. "Robert Lowell." See **169.**

943 HARDISON, O. B., Jr. "Robert Lowell: The Poet and the World's Body." *Shen*, 14 (Winter 1963), 24 – 32.

944 HOLDER, A. "The Flintlocks of the Fathers: Robert Lowell's Treatment of the American Past." *NEQ*, 44 (March 1971), 40 – 65.

945 HOLLOWAY, John. "Robert Lowell and the Public Dimension." *Encounter*, 30 (April 1968), 73 – 79.

946 JARRELL, Randall. "From the Kingdom of Necessity." See **62**. Reprinted in **922**.

947 JONES, A. R. "Necessity and Freedom: The Poetry of Robert Lowell, Sylvia Plath and Anne Sexton." *CritQ*, 7 (Spring 1965), 11 – 30.

948 LEIBOWITZ, Herbert. "Robert Lowell: Ancestral Voices." *Sal*, 1, 4 (1966 – 67), 25 – 43. Reprinted in **922**.*

949 MARTIN, Jay. *Robert Lowell*. Minneapolis: Univ. of Minnesota Press, 1970.

950 MAZZARO, Jerome. "Lowell after *For the Union Dead*." *Sal*, 1, 4 (1966 – 67), 57 – 68.

951 MAZZARO, Jerome. *The Poetic Themes of Robert Lowell*. Ann Arbor: Univ. of Michigan Press, 1965.

952 MAZZARO, Jerome. "Robert Lowell and the Kavanaugh Collapse." *UWR*, 5 (Autumn 1969), 1 – 24.*

953 MAZZARO, Jerome. "Robert Lowell's Early Politics of Apocalypse." *Modern American Poetry: Essays in Criticism*, ed. Jerome Mazzaro. New York: David McKay, 1970.

954 MCFADDEN, George. " 'Life Studies': Robert Lowell's Comic Breakthrough." *PMLA*, 90 (1975), 96 – 106.

955 MEINERS, R. K. *Everything to be Endured: An Essay on Robert Lowell and Modern Poetry*. Columbia: Univ. of Missouri Press, 1970.*

956 MILLER, Terry. "The Prosodies of Robert Lowell." *SM*, 35 (1968), 425 – 34.

957 NITCHIE, George. "The Importance of Robert Lowell." *SoR*, 8 (1972), 118 – 32.

958 OBERG, Arthur. " 'Lowell' Had Been Misspelled 'Lovel'." *IR*, 5, 3 (Summer 1974), 89 – 121.

959 PARKINSON, Thomas. "For the Union Dead." *Sal*, 1, 4 (1966 – 67), 87 – 95.*

960 PEARSON, Gabriel. "Robert Lowell." *Rev*, no. 20 (March 1969), 3 – 36.*

961 PERLOFF, Marjorie. *The Poetic Art of Robert Lowell*. Ithaca: Cornell Univ. Press, 1973.

962 REED, John. "Going Back: The Ironic Progress of Robert Lowell's Poetry." *MPS*, 1 (1970), 162 – 81. Reprinted in **923**.

963 RICKS, Christopher. "Authority in Poems." *SoR*, 5 (1969), 203 – 208.

964 ROSENTHAL, M. L. See **119**.

965 SPACKS, Patricia M. "From Satire to Description." *YR*, 58 (1969), 232 – 48.

966 STAPLES, Hugh B. *Robert Lowell: The First Twenty Years*. New York: Farrar, Straus and Cudahy, 1962.

967 VOGLER, Thomas. "Robert Lowell: Payment Gat He Nane." *IR*, 2, 3 (1971), 64 – 95.

968 WILLIAMSON, Alan. *Pity the Monsters: The Political Vision of Robert Lowell*. New Haven: Yale Univ. Press, 1974.

968a YENSER, Stephen. *Circle to Circle: The Poetry of Robert Lowell*. Berkeley: Univ. of California Press, 1975.*

Hugh MacDiarmid

Works of Poetry

969 *Collected Poems.* New York: MacMillan, 1967.

Other Relevant Primary Materials

970 *The Company I've Kept.* Berkeley: Univ. of California Press, 1971.

971 *Lucky Poet: A Self-Study in Literature and Political Ideas, Being the Autobiography of Hugh MacDiarmid (Christopher Murray Grieve.)* London: Methuen, 1943.

972 "Preface." *A Bibliography of Scottish Poets From Stevenson to 1974*, comp. Duncan Glen. Preston, England: Akros Publications, 1974.

973 *The Uncanny Scot: A Selection of Prose by MacDiarmid*, ed. K. Buthlay. London: MacGibbon and Kee, 1968.

Biography, Bibliography, and Other Reference Materials

973a AITKEN, W. R. "A Hugh MacDiarmid Bibliography." See **975a**.

Collections of Critical Essays

974 DUVAL, K. D., and S. G. SMITH, eds. *Hugh MacDiarmid: A Festschrift.* Edinburgh: K. D. Duval, 1962.

975 DUVAL, K. D. "Hugh MacDiarmid and Scottish Poetry." *Agenda*, 5–6, 4, 1 (Autumn–Winter 1967–68). [Issue devoted to the topic.]

975a GLEN, Duncan. *Hugh MacDiarmid: A Critical Survey.* Edinburgh: Scottish Academic Press, 1972. [Reprinted essays.]

Critical Books and Essays

976 ARUNDEL, Honor. "MacDiarmid and the Scottish Tradition." *Essays in Honour of William Gallacher*, ed. E. Lingner. Berlin: Humboldt Univ. Press, 1966.

977 BOUTELLE, Ann E. "Language and Vision in the Early Poetry of Hugh MacDiarmid." *ConLit*, 12 (1971), 495 – 509.

978 CRAIG, David. "MacDiarmid the Marxist Poet." See **974.**

979 DAICHES, David. "Hugh MacDiarmid: The Early Poems." See **974.***

980 GLEN, Duncan. *Hugh MacDiarmid (Christopher Murray Grieve) and the Scottish Renaissance.* Edinburgh: W. and R. Chambers, 1964.

981 MORGAN, Edwin. "Poetry and Knowledge in MacDiarmid's Later Work." See **974.**

982 SMITH, I. C. *The Golden Lyric: An Essay on the Poetry of MacDiarmid.* Preston, England: Akros Publications, 1967.

Louis MacNeice

Works of Poetry

983 *The Collected Poems*, ed. E. R. Dodds. London: Faber and Faber, 1966.

Other Relevant Primary Materials

984 *Modern Poetry: A Personal Essay*, 2nd ed. Oxford: Clarendon, 1968.

985 *The Strings are False: An Unfinished Autobiography.* New York: Oxford Univ. Press, 1966.

Biography, Bibliography, and Other Reference Materials

986 ARMITAGE, C. M., and Neil CLARK. *A Bibliography of the Works of Louis MacNeice.* London: Kaye and Ward, 1973.

Critical Books and Essays

987 ALLEN, W. "Louis MacNeice." *EDH*, 35 (1969), 1 – 17.

988 BROWN, Terence. *Sceptical Vines: The Poetry of Louis MacNeice.* New York: Barnes and Noble, 1974.

989 FRASER, G. S. "Evasive Honesty: The Poetry of MacNeice." *Vision and Rhetoric.* New York: Barnes and Noble, 1959.

990 GITZEN, Julian. "Louis MacNeice: The Last Decade." *TCL*, 19, 3 (October 1968), 133–41.

991 HOUGH, Graham. "MacNeice and Auden." *CQ*, 9, 1 (Spring 1967), 9–18.

992 IRWIN, John T. "MacNeice, Auden and the Art Ballad." *ConLit*, 11 (1970), 58–79.

993 MATTHIESSEN, F. O. "Louis MacNeice." *The Responsibilities of the Critic.* New York: Oxford Univ. Press, 1952.

994 MCKINNON, William T. *Apollo's Blended Dream: A Study of the Poetry of Louis MacNeice.* London: Oxford, 1971.*

994a MCKINNON, William T. "MacNeice's Pale Panther: An Exercise in Dream Logic." *EIC*, 23 (1973), 388–98.

995 MOORE, Donald B. *The Poetry of Louis MacNeice.* New York: Humanities, 1972.

996 SMITH, Elton E. *Louis MacNeice.* New York: Twayne, 1970.

997 WAIN, John. "MacNeice as Critic." *Encounter*, 27, 5 (1966), 49–55.

998 WALL, S. "Louis MacNeice and the Line of Least Resistance." *Rev*, 11–12 (1964), 91–94.

W. S. Merwin

Works of Poetry

999 *The Carrier of Ladders.* New York: Atheneum, 1970. [Atheneum]

999a *Compass Flower.* New York: Atheneum, 1976. [Atheneum]

1000 *The Dancing Bears.* New Haven: Yale Univ. Press, 1954.

1001 *The Drunk in the Furnace.* New York: Macmillan, 1960. [Macmillan]

1001a *The First Four Books of Poems.* New York: Atheneum, 1975. [Collects 1000, 1001, 1002, 1004.] [Atheneum]

1002 *Green With Beasts.* New York: Alfred Knopf, 1956.

1003 *The Lice.* New York: Atheneum, 1967. [Atheneum]

1004 *A Mask for Janus.* New Haven: Yale Univ. Press, 1952.

1005 *The Moving Target.* New York: Atheneum, 1963. [Atheneum]

1006 *Writings to an Unfinished Accompaniment.* New York: Atheneum, 1973. [Atheneum]

Other Relevant Primary Materials

1007   *Asian Figures.* New York: Atheneum, 1973. [Translations.] [Atheneum]

1008   "Favor Island." *New World Writing.* New York: New American Library, 1957. [Play.]

1008a *Houses and Travelers.* New York: Atheneum, 1977. [Prose pieces.] [Atheneum]

1009   "Interview." *Road Apple Review*, 1 (1969), 35 – 36.

1010   *The Miner's Pale Children.* New York: Atheneum, 1970. [Short prose pieces.]

1011   *Osip Mandelstam: Selected Poems*, trans. Clarence Brown and Merwin. New York: Atheneum, 1973.

1012   *The Poem of the Cid.* New York: New American Library, 1959. [Translation.]

1013   "A Portrait of W. S. Merwin," by Frank McShane. *Shen*, 21 (Winter 1970), 3 – 17. [An essay and interview.]

1014   *Selected Translations, 1948 – 68.* New York: Atheneum, 1968. [Atheneum]

1014a *Selected Translations, 1968 – 78.* New York: Atheneum, 1978.

1015   *The Song of Roland.* New York: Random House, 1963. [Translation.] [Random]

1016   *Spanish Ballads.* New York: Anchor, 1960.

1017   "Statement." *The Distinctive Voice*, ed. William Martz. Glencoe, Ill.: Macmillan Free, 1966.

1018   "The Story of Everyman." *The Nation*, 195, 22 (December 29, 1962), 463 – 80.

1019   *Transparence of the World: Poems by Jean Follain.* New York: Atheneum, 1969. [Translation.]

1020   *Voices: Poems by Antonio Porchia.* Chicago: Big Table Books, 1969. [Translation.]

Critical Books and Essays

1021   BENSTON, Alice. "Myth in the Poetry of W. S. Merwin." See **172.**

1022   BLOOM, Harold. "The New Transcendentalism: The Visionary Strain in Merwin, Ashbery and Ammons." See **225.**

1023   CARROLL, Paul. " 'Lemuels Blessing': The Spirit With Long Ears and Paws." See **102.**

1024   GORDON, Jan B. "The Dwelling of Disappearance: W. S. Merwin's *The Lice.*" *MPS*, 3 (1972), 119 – 38.

1025   GROSS, Harvey. "The Writing on the Void: The Poetry of W. S. Merwin." *IR*, 1, 3 (Summer 1970), 92 – 106.

1026 GUSTAFSON, Richard. "What is Merwin Trying To Do?" *PC*, 7, 1 (1972), 29—35.

1027 HOWARD, Richard. "W. S. Merwin: 'We Survived the Selves that we Remembered'." See **108**.*

1028 KYLE, Carol. "A Riddle for the New Year: Affirmation in W. S. Merwin." *MPS*, 4 (1973), 288—303.

1029 LIBBY, Anthony. "W. S. Merwin and the Nothing that is." *ConLit*, 16 (1975), 19—40.

1029a NELSON, Cary. "The Resources of Failure: W. S. Merwin's Deconstructive Career." *Bnd 2*, 5 (1977), 573—98.

1030 RAMSEY, Jarold. "The Continuities of W. S. Merwin: 'What has Escaped us we Bring with us'." *MassR*, 14 (1973), 569—90.

1031 VOGELSANG, John. "Toward the Great Language: W. S. Merwin." *MPS*, 3 (1972), 97—118.

1031a WATKINS, Evan. "W. S. Merwin: A Critical Accompaniment." *Bnd 2*, 4 (1975), 187—99.

Marianne Moore

Works of Poetry

1032 *The Complete Poems of Marianne Moore.* New York: Macmillan, 1967.

1033 *A Marianne Moore Reader.* New York: Viking, 1961. [Viking]

Other Relevant Primary Materials

1034 *The Fables of La Fontaine: A Complete New Translation.* New York: Viking, 1954.

1035 "Marianne Moore." See **162**, vol. 2. Reprinted in **1037**. [Interview.]

1036 *Predilections.* New York: Viking, 1955.

Biography, Bibliography, and Other Reference Materials

1036a ABBOT, Craig. *Marianne Moore: A Descriptive Bibliography.* Pittsburgh: Univ. of Pittsburgh Press, 1977.

Collections of Critical Essays

1037 TOMLINSON, Charles, ed. *Marianne Moore: A Collection of Critical Essays*. Englewood Cliffs, N.J.: Prentice-Hall, 1969. [With selected bibliography.][P-H]

Critical Books and Essays

1038 BELOOF, Robert. "Prosody and Tone: The 'Mathematics' of Marianne Moore." *KenR*, 20 (1958), 116−23. Reprinted in **1037**.

1039 BLACKMUR, R. P. "The Method of Marianne Moore." See **39a**. Reprinted in **1037**.

1040 BURKE, Kenneth. "Motives and Motifs in the Poetry of Marianne Moore." *A Grammar of Motives*. Berkeley: Univ. of California Press, 1969. Reprinted in **1037**.

1041 DEMBO, L. S. "Marianne Moore: Unparticularities." See **45**.

1042 DODSWORTH, Martin. "Marianne Moore." See **169**.

1043 DONOGHUE, Denis. "The Proper Plenitude of Fact." See **48**. Reprinted in **1037**.*

1043a HADAS, Pamela White. *Marianne Moore, Poet of Affection*. Syracuse: Syracuse Univ. Press, 1977.

1044 HALL, Donald. *Marianne Moore: The Cage and the Animal*. New York: Pegasus, 1969.*

1045 JARRELL, Randall. "The Humble Animal" and "Her Shield." See **62**.

1046 KENNER, Hugh. "Meditation and Enactment." *Poetry*, 52 (1963), 109−15. Reprinted in **1037**.

1046a KENNER, Hugh. "Supreme in her Abnormality." *Gnomon*. New York: McDowell, Obolensky, 1958.

1047 NITCHIE, George W. *Marianne Moore: An Introduction to Her Poetry*. New York: Columbia Univ. Press, 1969. [Columbia U Pr]

1048 REPLOGLE, Justin M. "Marianne Moore and the Art of Intonation." *ConLit*, 12 (1971), 1−17.

1049 SPRAGUE, Rosemary. *Imaginary Gardens: A Study of Five American Poets*. Philadelphia: Chilton, 1969.

1050 TOMLINSON, Charles. "Marianne Moore: Her Poetry and Her Critics." *Agenda*, 6 (1968), 137−42.

1051 VONALT, Larry P. "Marianne Moore's Medicines." *SewR*, 78 (1970), 669−78.

1052 WEATHERHEAD, A. Kingsley. *The Edge of the Image: Marianne Moore, William Carlos Williams and Some Other Poets*. Seattle: Univ. of Washington Press, 1967.

1053 WILLIAMS, William Carlos. "Marianne Moore" (1931) and "Marianne Moore" (1948). See **1592.**

Frank O'Hara

Works of Poetry

1054 *The Collected Poems of Frank O'Hara*, ed. Donald Allen. New York: Alfred Knopf, 1971. [Also contains O'Hara's essays on poetry.]

1054a *Early Writings, 1946– 1951*, ed. Donald Allen. Bolinas: Grey Fox, 1977.

1055 *The Selected Poems of Frank O'Hara*, ed. Donald Allen. New York: Alfred Knopf, 1974. [Random]

Other Relevant Primary Materials

1056 *Art Chronicles 1954– 1966.* New York: Braziller, 1975. [Braziller]

1056a *Jackson Pollock.* New York: George Braziller, 1959.

1057 *Nakian.* Garden City: Doubleday, 1966.

1058 "Nature and New Painting." *Folder II*, no. 1 (1954– 55), n.p.

1059 *Robert Mothewell.* New York: Museum of Modern Art, 1965.

1060 "Try, Try." *Artists Theatre: Four Plays*, ed. Herbert Machiz. New York: Grove, 1960.

Critical Books and Essays

1061 ALTIERI, Charles. "The Significance of Frank O'Hara." *IR*, 4, 1 (1973), 90– 104.*

1062 BERKSON, B. V. "Frank O'Hara and His Poems." *Art and Literature*, no. 12 (Spring 1967), 53– 63.

1063 CARROLL, Paul. "Frank O'Hara: 'The Day Lady Died': An Impure Poem About July 17, 1959." See **102.**

1064 HOWARD, Richard. "Frank O'Hara: 'Since We are We Always Will Be in This Life Come What May." See **108.***

1064a MOLESWORTH, Charles. " 'The Clear Architecture of Nerves': The Poetry of Frank O'Hara." *IR*, 6, 3– 4 (1975), 61– 74.*

1064b PERLOFF, Marjorie. *Frank O'Hara: Poet Among Painters*. New York: Braziller, 1977.*

1065 VENDLER, Helen. "The Virtues of the Alterable." *Parn*, 1 (1972), 5—20.

Charles Olson

Works of Poetry

1066 *Archaeologist of Morning*. London: Cape Goliard, 1970, in association with Grossman, New York. [Collects his shorter poems.] [Grossman]

1067 *The Distances*. New York: Grove, 1960. [Grove]

1068 *The Maximus Poems*. New York: Corinth, 1960. [Corinth]

1069 *Maximus Poems, IV, V, VI*. London: Cape Goliard, 1968, in association with Grossman, New York. [Grossman]

1069a *The Maximus Poems: Volume Three*. New York: Grossman, 1975. [Grossman]

1069b *Some Early Poems*. Ed. Sherman Paul. Iowa City: Windhover Press, 1978.

Other Relevant Primary Materials

1070 *Additional Prose: A Bibliography on America, Proprioception and Other Notes and Essays*, ed. George Butterick. San Francisco: Four Seasons Foundation, 1974. [Four Seasons Foun]

1071 "The Art of Poetry: Charles Olson," with Gerald Melanga. *ParR*, 49 (Summer 1970), 177—204.

1072 *Call Me Ishmael: A Study of Melville*. New York: City Lights, 1947. [City Lights]

1073 *Causal Mythology*, ed. Donald Allen. San Francisco: Four Seasons Foundation, 1969. [Four Seasons Foun]

1073a *Charles Olson and Ezra Pound: An Encounter at St. Elizabeths*, ed. Catherine Seelye. New York: Grossman, 1975. [Olson's reflections on Pound.]

1073b *The Fiery Hunt and Other Plays*, ed. George Butterick. Bolinas: Four Seasons Foundation, 1977.

1074 *Human Universe and Other Essays*, ed. Donald Allen. New York: Grove, 1967. [Grove]

1075 *Letters For Origin: 1950—55*, ed. Albert Glover. London: Cape Goliard, 1969, in association with Grossman, New York. [Grossman]

1075a *Muthologos: The Collected Lectures and Interviews*, vol. I., ed. George Butterick. Bolinas: Four Seasons Foundation, 1978.

1076   *Poetry and Truth: The Beloit Lectures and Poems*, transcribed and ed. George Butterick. San Francisco: Four Seasons Foundation, 1971. [Four Seasons Foun]

1076a *The Post Office: A Memoir of His Father.* Bolinas: Grey Fox, 1975.

1077   *Reading at Berkeley*, transcribed Zoe Brown. San Francisco: Coyote, 1966.

1078   *Selected Writings of Charles Olson*, ed. Robert Creeley. New York: New Directions, 1966. [Contains *Apollonius of Tyana* and selections from *Mayan Letters*.] [New Directions]

1079   *The Special View of History*, ed. Ann Charters. Berkeley: Oyez, 1970. [Oyez]

1080   "A Syllabary For A Dancer." *Maps*, no. 4 (1971), 9–15.

Biography, Bibliography, and Other Reference Materials

1081   BUTTERICK, George, and Albert GLOVER. *A Bibliography of Works by Charles Olson.* New York: Phoenix Book Shop, 1967.

1081a BUTTERICK, George. "A Bibliography of Writings by Charles Olson: Posthumous Publications." *Olson*, 7 (1977), 43–60.

1081b BUTTERICK, George. *A Guide to the Maximus Poems of Charles Olson.* Berkeley: Univ. of California Press, 1978.

Collections of Critical Essays

1082   BUTTERICK, George, ed. *Olson: The Journal of the Charles Olson Archives.* [Vol. i—Spring 1974.]

1083   CORRIGAN, Matthew, ed. *Charles Olson: Essays, Reminiscences, Reviews. Bnd2* (Fall 73/Winter 74). [Special Olson issue.]

1084   *Olson Issue. Ath*, 2 (Fall–Winter 1971).

Critical Books and Essays

1085   AIKEN, William. "Charles Olson: A Preface." *MassR*, 12 (1971), 57–58.*

1086   ALTIERI, Charles. "Olson's Poetics and the Tradition." See **1083.**

1087   CHARTERS, Ann. *Olson/Melville: A Study in Affinity.* Berkeley: Oyez, 1968. [Oyez]

1088   CORRIGAN, Matthew. "Materials for A Nexus." See **1083.**

1089   DAVENPORT, Guy. "Scholia and Conjectures for Olson's 'The Kingfishers'." See **1083.**

1090   DAVEY, Frank. "Six Readings of Olson's *Maximus*." See **1083**.

1091   DEMBO, L. S. "Postscript: Charles Olson and Robert Duncan: The Mystique of Speech and Rhythm." See **45**.

1092   DORIA, Charles. "Pound, Olson, and the Classical Tradition." See **1083**.

1092a   DORN, Edward. *What I see in the Maximus Poems.* Ventura, Cal.: Migrant Pamphlet, 1960. [Reprinted in *Kulchur*, 4 (1961), 31 – 44.]

1093   DUNCAN, Robert. "Notes on Poetics: Regarding Olson's Maximus." *Rev*, no. 10 (January 1964), 36 – 42.

1093a   LIEBERMAN, Marcia R., and Philip LIEBERMAN. "Olson's Projective Verse and the Use of Breath Control as a Structural Element." *Lang&S*, 5 (1972), 287 – 92.

1094   MOTTRAM, Eric. "Charles Olson's Apollonius of Tyana." *Sixpack*, nos. 3 – 4 (March 1973), n.p. (12 pp.)

1094a   PAUL, Sherman. *Olson's Push: Origin, Black Mountain, and Recent American Poetry.* Baton Rouge: Louisiana State Univ. Press, 1978. [Contains Paul's important essays on the *Maximus Poems*.]*

1095   PERLOFF, Marjorie. "Charles Olson and the 'Inferior Predecessors': 'Projective Verse' Revisited." *ELH*, 40 (1973), 285 – 306.

1096   POPS, Martin L. "Melville; To Him, Olson." *MPS*, 2 (1971), 61 – 96. Reprinted in **1083**.

1097   PRYNNE, J. H. "Charles Olson, Maximus Poems IV, V, VI." *Io*, no. 16 (Winter 1972 – 73), 89 – 92.

1098   ROSENBERG, Jim. *Notes for the Foundations of a Theory of Meter: An Essay Towards an Understanding of Charles Olson's "Projective Verse."* San Francisco: Grabhorn-Hoyem, 1970.

1099   ROSENTHAL, M. L. "Olson/His Poetry." *MassR*, 12 (1971), 45 – 57.

1100   SCOGGAN, John. "The Larger Setting." *Maps*, 4 (1971), 83 – 96.*

1100a   VON HALLBERG, Robert. *Charles Olson: The Scholar's Art.* Cambridge: Harvard Univ. Press, 1978.

1101   VON HALLBERG, Robert. "Olson's Relation to Pound and Williams." *ConLit*, 15 (1974), 15 – 48.

1102   VON HALLBERG, Robert. "Olson, Whitehead and the Objectivists." See **1083**.

Wilfred Owen

Works of Poetry

1103   *The Collected Poems of Wilfred Owen*, ed. C. Day Lewis. London: Chatto and Windus, 1963. [New Directions]

Other Relevant Primary Materials

1104   *Collected Letters of Wilfred Owen*, ed. John Bell and Harold Owen. London: Oxford Univ. Press, 1967.

Biography, Bibliography, and Other Reference Materials

1105   OWEN, William. *Journey from Obscurity: Wilfred Owen 1893– 1918*, 3 vols. New York: Oxford Univ. Press, 1963. [Memoirs of the family.]

1105a   WHITE, William. *Wilfred Owen (1893– 1918): A Bibliography*. Kent, Ohio: Kent State Univ. Press, 1967.

Critical Books and Essays

1106   BERGONZI, Bernard. "Rosenberg and Owen." *Heroes Twilight: A Study of the Literature of the Great War*. London: Constable, 1965.

1107   GRUBB, Frederic. "The Embattled Truth: Wilfred Owen and Isaac Rosenberg." *A Vision of Reality: A Study of Liberalism in Twentieth Century Verse*. London: Chatto and Windus, 1965.

1108   JOHNSTON, John H. See **27**.

1109   LANE, Arthur E. *An Adequate Response: The War Poetry of Wilfred Owen and Siegfried Sassoon*. Detroit: Wayne State Univ. Press, 1972.

1110   PARSONS, I. "The Poems of Wilfred Owen (1893– 1918)." *New Criterion*, 10 (1931), 658– 69.

1111   STALLWORTHY, Jon. "Wilfred Owen." *PBA*, 56 (1970), 241– 62.*

1112   THOMAS, Dylan. "Wilfred Owen." *Quite Early One Morning*. New York: New Directions, 1954.

1113   WELLAND, Dennis S. *Wilfred Owen, A Critical Study*. London: Chatto and Windus, 1960.

1114   WHITE, Gertrude M. *Wilfred Owen*. New York: Twayne, 1969. [With useful bibliography.]

Sylvia Plath

Works of Poetry

1115   *Ariel.* New York: Harper & Row, 1966. [Har-Row]

1116   *The Colossus and Other Poems.* New York: Alfred Knopf, 1962. [Random]

1117   *Crossing the Water.* London: Faber and Faber, 1971. [Poems from 1960 – 61.]

1118   *Fiesta Meloni.* Exeter, U.K.: Rougemont, 1971. [Early poems and drawings.]

1119   *Pursuit.* London: Rainbow, 1973.

1120   *Winter Trees.* New York: Harper & Row, 1972.

Other Relevant Primary Materials

1121   *The Bell Jar.* New York: Harper & Row, 1971. [Novel.] [Bantam]

1121a   *Johnny Panic and the Bible of Dreams: Short Stories, Prose, and Diary Excerpts.* New York: Harper and Row, 1979.

1121b   *Letters Home by Sylvia Plath: Correspondence 1950– 1963.* Ed. Aurelia Schober Plath. New York: Harper and Row, 1975.

Biography, Bibliography, and Other Reference Materials

1122   AIRD, Eileen. *Sylvia Plath: Her Life and Work.* New York: Barnes and Noble, 1973.

1123   KINZIE, Mary, and others. "Critical Bibliography" and "Bibliography." See **1126**. [Critical bibliography is annotated.]

1124   KINZIE, Mary, and others. "Part III." See **1126**. [Biographical essays by Lois Ames, Anne Sexton, Wendy Campbell, and Ted Hughes—on the chronological order of her poems.]

1125   STEINER, Nancy Hunter. *A Closer Look at Ariel: A Memory of Sylvia Plath.* New York: Harper's Magazine Press, 1973.

Collections of Critical Essays

1126 NEWMAN, Charles, ed. *The Art of Sylvia Plath*. Bloomington: Indiana Univ. Press, 1970. [Ind U Pr]

Critical Books and Essays

1127 ALVAREZ, A. *The Savage God: A Study of Suicide*. New York: Random House, 1972. [Bantam]

1128 ALVAREZ, A. "Sylvia Plath." See **1126**.*

1129 BAGG, Robert. "The Rise of Lady Lazarus." *Mosaic*, 2, 4 (1969), 9 – 36.

1130 BLODGETT, E. D. "Sylvia Plath: Another View." *MPS*, 2 (1971), 97 – 106.

1131 BOYERS, Robert. "Sylvia Plath: The Trepanned Veteran." *CR*, 13 (Spring 1968), 138 – 53.

1131a BUTSCHER, Edward. *Sylvia Plath: Method and Madness*. New York: Seabury, 1976.

1132 DAVIS, William V. "Sylvia Plath's 'Ariel'." *MPS*, 3 (1972), 176 – 84.

1133 GORDON, Jan B. "Who Is Sylvia? The Art of Sylvia Plath." *MPS*, 1 (1970), 6 – 34.

1134 HARDWICK, Elizabeth. "Sylvia Plath." *Seduction and Betrayal: Women and Literature*. New York: Random House, 1974.

1135 HARDY, Barbara. "Sylvia Plath." See **169**.

1136 HOLBROOK, David. "R. D. Laing and the Death Circuit." *Encounter*, 31, 2 (1968), 35 – 45.*

1137 HOLBROOK, David. *Sylvia Plath: Poetry and Existence*. London: Athlone, 1976.*

1138 HOWARD, Richard. "Sylvia Plath: 'And I Have No Face, I Have Wanted To Efface Myself . . .'." See **108**. Reprinted in **1126**.

1139 HUGHES, Ted. "Sylvia Plath's *Crossing the Water*: Some Reflections." *CritQ*, 13 (1971), 165 – 72.

1140 KAMEL, Rose. " 'A Self to Recover': Sylvia Plath's Bee Cycle Poems." *MPS*, 4 (1973), 304 – 18.

1140a KROLL, Judith. *Chapters in a Mythology: The Poetry of Sylvia Plath*. New York: Harper and Row, 1976.

1141 LAVERS, Annette. "The World As Icon: On Sylvia Plath's Themes." See **1126**.

1142 LIBBY, Anthony. "God's Lioness and the Priest of Sycorax: Plath and Hughes." *ConLit*, 15 (1974), 386 – 405.

1143 MEISSNER, William. "The Rise of the Angel: Life Through Death in the Poetry of Sylvia Plath." *MSE*, 3 (1970), 34 – 39.

1144 NEWMAN, Charles. "Candor is the Only Wile: The Art of Sylvia Plath." See **1126.***

1145 NIMS, John Frederick. "The Poetry of Sylvia Plath: A Technical Analysis." See **1126.**

1146 OATES, Joyce Carol. "The Death Throes of Romanticism: The Poems of Sylvia Plath." *SoR*, 9 (October 1973), 501 – 22.*

1147 OBERG, Arthur K. "Sylvia Plath and the New Decadence." *ChiR*, 20, 1 (1968), 66 – 73.

1148 OSTRIKER, Alicia. " 'Fact' as Style: The Americanization of Sylvia." *Lang&S*, 1 (1968), 201 – 12.*

1149 PERLOFF, Majorie. " 'Angst' and Animism in the Poetry of Sylvia Plath." *JML*, 1 (1969), 57 – 74.

1149a PERLOFF, Majorie. "On the Road to *Ariel*: The 'Transitional' Poetry of Sylvia Plath." *IR*, 4, 2 (1973), 94 – 110.

1149b SCHWARTZ, Murray, and Christopher BOLLAS. "The Absence at the Center: Sylvia Plath and Suicide." *Crit*, 18 (1976), 147 – 72.

1150 STEINER, George. "In Extremis." *CamR*, 90 (February 7, 1969), 247 – 49.

Ezra Pound

Works of Poetry

1151 *The Cantos of Ezra Pound (I– CXVIII)*. New York: New Directions, 1970.

1151a *Collected Early Poems of Ezra Pound*. Ed. Michael King. New York: New Directions, 1976.

1152 *Personae*. New York: New Directions, 1949.

1153 *Selected Poems of Ezra Pound*. New York: New Directions, 1957. [New Directions]

Other Relevant Primary Materials

1154 *ABC of Reading*. New York: New Directions, 1960. [First published in 1934.] [New Directions]

1155 "The Art of Poetry: Ezra Pound." See **162**, vol. 3. [Interview.]

1156 *The Confucian Odes: The Classic Anthology Defined by Confucius*. New York: New Directions, 1959. [New Directions]

1157 *Gaudier-Brzeska*. New York: New Directions, 1970. [First published in 1916.][New Directions]

1158 *Guide to Kulchur*. Norfolk, Conn.: New Directions, 1938. [New Directions]

1159 *Indiscretions; or, Une Revue de Deux Mondes*. Paris: Three Mountains, 1923.

1160 *The Letters of Ezra Pound 1907—1941*, ed. D. D. Paige. New York: Harcourt, Brace, 1950.

1161 *The Literary Essays of Ezra Pound*, ed. T. S. Eliot. Norfolk, Conn.: New Directions, 1954. [New Directions]

1162 *Pound/Joyce: Letters & Essays*, ed. Forrest Read. New York: New Directions, 1967. [New Directions]

1162a *Selected Prose, 1909—1965*, ed. William Cookson. New York: New Directions, 1973.

1163 *The Spirit of Romance*. New York: New Directions, 1968. [First published in 1910.] [New Directions]

1164 *Translations*. New York: New Directions, 1963. [New Directions]

Biography, Bibliography, and Other Reference Materials

1165 CORRIGAN, Robert. "The First Quarter Century of Ezra Pound Criticism: An Annotated Checklist." *RALS*, 2 (1972), 157—207.

1166 DE RASCHEWILTZ, Mary. *Discretions*. Boston: Little, Brown, 1971. [Memoir by Pound's daughter.]

1167 EDWARDS, John H., and William W. VASSE. *The Annotated Index to the Cantos of Ezra Pound*. Berkeley: Univ. of California Press, 1957.

1168 GALLUP, Donald. *A Bibliography of Ezra Pound*. London: Hart-Davis, 1963.

1169 HUTCHINS, Patricia. *Ezra Pound's Kensington*. London: Faber and Faber, 1965.

1169a LANE, Gary. *A Concordance to Personae*. New York: Haskell House, 1972.

1170 MEACHAM, Harry M. *The Caged Panther: Ezra Pound at Saint Elizabeth's*. New York: Twayne, 1968.

1170a SLATIN, Myles. "A History of Pound's Cantos I—XVI, 1915—1925." *AL*, 35 (1963), 183—95.

1171 STOCK, Noel. *The Life of Ezra Pound*. New York: Pantheon Books, 1970.

Collections of Critical Essays

1172 HOMBERGER, Eric, ed. *Ezra Pound: The Critical Heritage*. London: Routledge and Kegan Paul, 1972. [Wide variety of reviews and a bibliography.]

1173 LEARY, Lewis, ed. *Motive and Method in the Cantos of Ezra Pound*. New York: Columbia Univ. Press, 1954. [Columbia U Pr]

1174　*Paideuma: A Journal Devoted to Ezra Pound Scholarship*, 1 (Spring—Summer 1972).

1175　SAN JUAN, Epifanio, Jr., ed. *Critics on Ezra Pound*. Coral Gables: University of Miami Press, 1972. [With selected bibliography.]

1176　SUTTON, Walter, ed. *Ezra Pound*. Englewood Cliffs, N.J.: Prentice-Hall, 1963. [P-H]

Critical Books and Essays

1177　ALVAREZ, A. "Ezra Pound: Craft and Morals." See **38a.**

1178　BAAR, Ron. "Ezra Pound: Poet as Historian." *AL*, 42 (January 1971), 531—43.

1178a　BAUMANN, Walter. *The Rose in the Steel Dust: An Examination of the Cantos of Ezra Pound*. Bern: Francke Verlag, 1967.

1179　BROOKE-ROSE, Christine. *ABZ of Ezra Pound*. Berkeley: Univ. of California Press, 1971.* [U Cal Pr]

1179a　BROOKE-ROSE, Christine. *A Structural Analysis of Pound's Usura Canto: Jakobson's Method Extended and Applied to Free Verse*. The Hague: Mouton, 1976.*

1179b　BUSH, Ronald. *The Genesis of Ezra Pound's Cantos*. Princeton: Princeton Univ. Press, 1976.

1179c　CARNE-ROSS, D. S. " 'The Music of a Lost Dynasty': Pound in the Classroom." *Boston University Journal*, 21, 1 (1972), 25—41.

1180　CHACE, William M. *The Political Identities of Ezra Pound and T. S. Eliot*. Stanford: Stanford Univ. Press, 1973.

1181　DAVIE, Donald. "The Cantos: Towards a Pedestrian Reading." *Paideuma*, 1 (1972), 55—62.

1182　DAVIE, Donald. *Ezra Pound: Poet as Sculptor*. New York: Oxford Univ. Press, 1964.*

1183　DEKKER, George. *The Cantos of Ezra Pound: A Critical Study*. New York: Barnes and Noble, 1963.

1184　DEMBO, L. S. *The Confucian Odes of Ezra Pound: A Critical Appraisal*. Berkeley: Univ. of California Press, 1963.

1185　DEMBO, L. S. "Ezra Pound: Fac Deum." See **45.**

1185a　EHRENPREIS, Irvin. "Love, Hate and Ezra Pound." *NYRB*, 27 (May, 1976), 6—12.

1186　ELIOT, T. S. *Ezra Pound: His Metric and Poetry*. New York: Alfred Knopf, 1917.

1187　ESPEY, John. *Ezra Pound's 'Mauberley': A Study in Composition*. Berkeley: Univ. of California Press, 1955.

1188　FUSSELL, Edwin. "Dante and Pound's *Cantos*." *JML*, 1 (1974), 75—87.

1188a　HARMON, William. *Time in Ezra Pound's Work*. Chapel Hill: Univ. of North Carolina Pr., 1977.

1189 JACKSON, Thomas H. *The Early Poetry of Ezra Pound.* Cambridge: Harvard Univ. Press, 1968.

1190 KENNER, Hugh. *The Poetry of Ezra Pound.* London: Faber and Faber, 1951.*

1191 KENNER, Hugh. *The Pound Era.* Berkeley: Univ. of California Press, 1971. [Univ of Cal Pr]*

1192 KORG, Jacob. "The Music of Lost Dynasties: Browning, Pound and History." *ELH*, 39 (1972), 420 – 40.

1193 MC DOUGAL, Stuart. *Ezra Pound and the Troubador Tradition.* Princeton: Princeton Univ. Press, 1972.

1194 MINER, Earl. "Ezra Pound." *The Japanese Tradition in British and American Literature.* Princeton: Princeton Univ. Press, 1958.

1195 OLSON, Paul A. "Pound and the Poetry of Perception." *Thought*, 35 (1960), 331 – 48. Reprinted in **1175**.

1196 PEARCE, Roy Harvey. "Pound, Whitman and the American Epic." See **80**.

1197 PEARLMAN, Daniel D. *The Barb of Time: On the Unity of Ezra Pound's "Cantos."* New York: Oxford Univ. Press, 1969.

1198 PECK, John. "Pound's Lexical Mythography." *Paideuma*, 1 (1972), 3 – 36.

1199 PEVEAR, Richard. "Notes on the Cantos of Ezra Pound." *HudR*, 25 (1972), 51 – 70.

1200 READ, Forrest. "A Man of No Fortune." See **1172**. Reprinted in **1176**.

1200a RIDDEL, Joseph. "Pound and the Decentered Image." *Ga R*, 29 (1975), 565 – 91.

1201 RUTHVEN, K. K. *A Guide to Ezra Pound's "Personae."* Berkeley: Univ. of California Press, 1969.

1202 SAN JUAN, Epifanio, Jr. "Ezra Pound's Craftmanship: An Interpretation of *Hugh Selwyn Mauberly.*" See **1175**.

1203 SCHNEIDAU, Herbert N. *Ezra Pound: The Image and the Real.* Baton Rouge: Louisiana State Univ. Press, 1969.*

1203a SCHNEIDAU, Herbert. "Style and Sacrament in Modernist Writing." See **83a**.*

1203b SCHNEIDAU, Herbert. "Wisdom Past Metaphor: Another View of Pound, Fenollosa and Objective Verse." *Paideuma*, 5 (1976), 15 – 29.

1204 SPANOS, William V. "The Modulating Voice of Hugh Selwyn Mauberley." *WSCL*, 6 (1965), 73 – 96.

1204a SULLIVAN, John. *Ezra Pound and Sextus Propertius: A Study in Creative Translation.* Austin: Univ. of Texas Press, 1964.

1205 SULLIVAN, John. "Pound's *Homage to Propertius*: The Structure of a Mask." *EIC*, 10 (1960), 239 – 49. Reprinted in **1176**.

1206 WILHELM, James. "Guido Cavalcanti as a Mask for Ezra Pound." *PMLA*, 89 (1974), 332 – 40.

1207 WITEMEYER, Hugh. *The Poetry of Ezra Pound: Forms and Renewals 1908 – 1920.* Berkeley: Univ. of California Press, 1969.

John Crowe Ransom

Works of Poetry

1208   *Chills and Fever*. New York: Alfred Knopf, 1924.

1209   *Grace After Meat*. London: Hogarth, 1924.

1210   *Poems About God*. New York: H. Holt, 1919.

1211   *Poems and Essays*. New York: Vintage, 1955. [Random]

1212   *Selected Poems*, rev. and enlarged ed. New York: Alfred Knopf, 1969.

1212a   *Selected Poems*, 3rd rev. ed. New York: Ecco, 1978.

1213   *Two Gentlemen in Bonds*. New York: Alfred Knopf, 1927.

Other Relevant Primary Materials

1214   *God Without Thunder: An Unorthodox Defense of Orthodoxy*. New York: Harcourt, Brace, 1930.

1215   *The New Criticism*. Norfolk, Conn.: New Directions, 1941.

1216   *The World's Body*. New York: Scribner's, 1938. [Essays.] [La State U Pr]

Biography, Bibliography, and Other Reference Materials

1217   PETERS, Mildred Brooks. "Bibliography." See **1219**. [Very important because of the number of Ransom's uncollected essays and poems.]

1218   YOUNG, Thomas Daniel. *Gentleman in a Dustcoat: A Biography of John Crowe Ransom*. New York: Random House, 1976.

Collections of Critical Essays

1218a   "Random Issue." *Miss Q*, 30 (1977).

1219   YOUNG, Thomas Daniel. *John Crowe Ransom: Critical Essays and a Bibliography*. Baton Rouge: Louisiana State Univ. Press, 1968.

Critical Books and Essays

1220 AMES, Van Meter. "Expression and Aesthetic Experience." *JAAC*, 6 (December 1947), 172—79.

1221 BRADBURY, John M. "Ransom as Poet." *Accent*, 11 (Winter 1951), 45—57.

1222 BUFFINGTON, Robert. *The Equilibrist: A Study of John Crowe Ransom's Poems, 1916— 1963.* Nashville: Vanderbilt Univ. Press, 1967.*

1223 BUFFINGTON, Robert. "The Poetry of the Master's Old Age." *GaR*, 25 (1971), 5—16.

1224 BUFFINGTON, Robert. "Ransom's Poetics: 'Only God, My Dear'." *MQR*, 12, 4 (Fall 1973), 353—60.

1225 CORE, George. "Mr. Ransom and The House of Poetry." *SewR*, 82, 4 (1974), 619—38.

1226 HOUGH, Graham. "John Crowe Ransom: The Poet and the Critic." *SoR*, 1 (January 1965), 1—21. Reprinted in **1219.**

1227 JARRELL, Randall. "John Ransom's Poetry." See **62.** Reprinted in **1219.**

1228 MACCAFFREY, Isabel Gamble. "Ceremonies of Bravery: John Crowe Ransom." *South: Modern Southern Literature in its Cultural Setting*, ed. Louis D. Rubin, Jr. and Robert D. Jacobs. Garden City: Doubleday, 1961.

1229 MANN, David, and Samuel H. WOODS, Jr. "John Crowe Ransom's Poetic Revisions." *PMLA*, 83 (1968), 15—21.

1230 NEMEROV, Howard. "Summer's Flare and Winter's Flaw." *SewR*, 56 (Summer 1948), 416—25.

1231 OWEN, Guy. "John Crowe Ransom: The Evolution of His Style." *The Twenties: Poetry and Prose*, ed. Richard E. Langford and William E. Taylor. Deland, Fla.: Everett/Edwards, 1966.

1232 PARSONS, Thornton H. *John Crowe Ransom.* New York: Twayne, Inc., 1969.

1233 PRATT, William. "In Pursuit of the Fugitives." *The Fugitive Poets: Modern Southern Poetry in Perspective.* New York: Dutton, 1965, 13—46. [Dutton]

1234 RUBIN, Louis D., Jr. "The Wary Fugitive, John Crowe Ransom." *SewR*, 82 (1974), 583—618.

1235 STEWART, John L. *John Crowe Ransom.* Minneapolis: Univ. of Minnesota Press, 1962.

1236 TATE, Allen. "Reflections on the Death of John Crowe Ransom." *SewR*, 82 (1974), 545—51.

1237 WARREN, Robert Penn. "John Crowe Ransom: A Study in Irony." *VQR*, 11 (1935), 93—112. Reprinted in **1219.***

1238 WARREN, Robert Penn. "Notes on the Poetry of John Crowe Ransom at His Eightieth Birthday." *KenR*, 30 (1968), 319—49.

1239 WASSERMAN, G. R. "The Irony of John Crowe Ransom." *UKCR*, 23 (Winter 1956), 151—60. Reprinted in **1219.**

1240 WILLIAMS, Miller. *The Poetry of John Crowe Ransom.* New Brunswick, N.J.: Rutgers Univ. Press, 1972.

1241 WINTERS, Yvor. "John Crowe Ransom; or, Thunder Without God." See **96.**

1242 YOUNG, Thomas Daniel. "A Kind of Centering." *GaR*, 28 (Spring 1974), 58 – 82.

1243 YOUNG, Thomas Daniel. "Mostly Nurtured from England." *SewR*, 82 (1974), 552 – 82.

Adrienne Rich

Works of Poetry

1243a *Adrienne Rich's Poetry.* Ed. Barbara Charlesworth Gelpi and Albert Gelpi. New York: Norton, 1975. [Norton Critical Edition with bibliography.]

1244 *A Change of World.* New Haven: Yale Univ. Press, 1951.

1245 *The Diamond Cutters.* New York: Harper & Row, 1955.

1246 *Diving Into the Wreck: Poems 1971 – 1972.* New York: Norton, 1973. [Norton]

1246a *The Dream of a Common Language: Poems, 1974 – 1977.* New York: Norton, 1978.

1247 *Leaflets: Poems, 1965 – 68.* New York: Norton, 1969. [Norton]

1248 *Necessities of Life.* New York: Norton, 1966. [Norton]

1249 *Poems: Selected and New, 1951 – 74.* New York: Norton, 1975.

1250 *Snapshots of a Daughter-in-Law.* New York: Harper & Row, 1963. [Norton]

1251 *The Will To Change.* New York: Norton, 1971. [Norton]

1251a *Of Woman Born: Motherhood as Experience and Institution.* New York: Norton, 1976. [Bantam]

Other Relevant Primary Materials

1252 "Poetry, Personality and Wholeness: A Response to Galway Kinnell." *Field*, 7 (Fall 1972), 11 – 18.

1253 "Talking With Adrienne Rich," with Stanley Plumly, Wayne Dodd, and Walter Trevis. *OhR*, 13, 1 (1971), 28 – 46. [Followed by her "Trying to Talk with a Man," 47 – 48.]

1254 "When We Dead Awaken: Writing as Re-Vision." *CE*, 34 (1972), 18 – 30.

Critical Books and Essays

1255 BOYERS, Robert. "On Adrienne Rich: Intelligence and Will." *Sal*, 22–23 (1973), 132–48.

1255a DU PLESSIS, Rachel Blau. "The Critique of Consciousness . . ." See **878a**.

1255b FLYNN, Gale. "The Radicalization of Adrienne Rich." *HC*, no. 4 (1974), 1–15.

1255c GELPI, Albert. "Adrienne Rich: The Poetics of Change." See **1243a**.

1255d HOWARD, Richard. "Adrienne Rich: 'What Lends Us Anchor But the Mutable'." See **108**.

1255e KALSTONE, David. *Five Temperaments*. See **108a**.*

1255f VAN DYNE, Susan. "The Mirrored Vision of Adrienne Rich." *MPS*, 8 (1977), 140–77.

1256 VENDLER, Helen. "Ghostlier Demarcations, Keener Sounds." *Parn* 2, 1 (1973), 5–10; 15–16; 18–24.*

Theodore Roethke

Works of Poetry

1257 *The Collected Poems of Theodore Roethke*. Garden City: Doubleday, 1966. [Doubleday]

Other Relevant Primary Materials

1258 *On the Poet and His Craft: The Selected Prose of Theodore Roethke*, ed. Ralph Mills. Seattle: Univ. of Washington Press, 1965. [U of Wash Pr]

1259 *Selected Letters of Theodore Roethke*, ed. Ralph Mills. Seattle: Univ. of Washington Press, 1968.

1260 *Straw for the Fire: From the Notebooks of Theodore Roethke*, selected by David Wagoner. Garden City: Doubleday, 1972.

Biography, Bibliography, and Other Reference Materials

1261 LANE, Gary, ed. *A Concordance to the Poems of Theodore Roethke.* Metuchen, N.J.: Scarecrow, 1972.

1262 MCLEOD, James Richard. *Theodore Roethke: A Bibliography.* Kent, Ohio: Kent State Univ. Press, 1971.

1263 MCLEOD, James Richard. *Theodore Roethke: A Manuscript Checklist.* Kent, Ohio: Kent State Univ. Press, 1971.

1263a MOUL, Keith R. *Theodore Roethke's Career: An Annotated Bibliography.* Boston: Hall, 1977.

1264 SEAGER, Allen. *The Glass House: The Life of Theodore Roethke.* New York: McGraw-Hill, 1968.

Collections of Critical Essays

1265 HEYEN, William, ed. *Profile of Theodore Roethke.* Columbus, Ohio: C. E. Merrill, 1971.

1266 STEIN, Arnold, ed. *Theodore Roethke: Essays on the Poetry.* Seattle: Univ. of Washington Press, 1965.*

Critical Books and Essays

1267 BLESSING, Richard. *Theodore Roethke's Dynamic Vision.* Bloomington: Univ. of Indiana Press, 1974.*

1268 BOYD, J. D. "Texture and Form in Theodore Roethke's Greenhouse Poems." *MLQ*, 32 (1971), 409 – 24.

1269 BURKE, Kenneth. "The Vegetal Radicalism of Theodore Roethke." *SewR*, 58 (1950), 68 – 108.*

1270 DONOGHUE, Denis. 'Theodore Roethke." See **46.** Reprinted in **1266.***

1271 HEYEN, William. "The Divine Abyss: Theodore Roethke's Mysticism." *TSLL*, 11 (1969), 1051 – 68. Reprinted in **1265.**

1272 HEYEN, William. "Theodore Roethke's Minimals." *MinnR*, 8 (1968), 359 – 75.

1273 HOFFMAN, Fred. "Theodore Roethke: The Poetic Shape of Death." See **1266.**

1273a LA BELLE, Jenijoy. *The Echoing Wood of Theodore Roethke.* Princeton: Princeton Univ. Press, 1976.

1274 LUCAS, John. "The Poetry of Theodore Roethke." *The Oxford Review,* 7 (1968), 39 – 64.

1275 MCMICHAEL, James. "The Poetry of Theodore Roethke." *SoR*, 5 (1969), 4—25. Reprinted in **1265.**

1276 MALKOFF, Karl. *Theodore Roethke: An Introduction to the Poetry.* New York: Columbia Univ. Press, 1968.

1277 MAZZARO, Jerome. "Theodore Roethke and the Failures of Language." *MPS*, 1 (1970), 73—96. Reprinted in **1265.**

1278 SCOTT, Nathan A. "The Example of Roethke." See **121.**

1279 SNODGRASS, W. D. "That Anguish of Concreteness—Theodore Roethke's Career." See **1266.**

1280 STAPLES, Hugh B. "Rose in the Sea-Wind: A Reading of Theodore Roethke's 'North American Sequence'." *AL*, 36 (1964), 189—203.

1280a SULLIVAN, Rosemary. *Theodore Roethke: The Garden Master.* Seattle: Univ. of Washington Press, 1975.

1281 VERNON, John. "Theodore Roethke's Praise to the End! Poems." *IR*, 2 (Fall 1971), 60—74. Reprinted and expanded in **89.***

Anne Sexton

Works of Poetry

1282 *All My Pretty Ones.* Boston: Houghton-Mifflin, 1962 [HM]

1282a *The Awful Rowing Toward God.* Boston: Houghton-Mifflin, 1975. [HM]

1283 *The Book of Folly.* Boston: Houghton-Mifflin, 1972. [HM]

1284 *The Death Notebooks.* Boston: Houghton-Mifflin, 1974, [HM]

1284a *45 Mercy Street.* Ed. Linda Sexton. Boston: Houghton-Mifflin, 1976.

1285 *Live or Die.* Boston: Houghton-Mifflin, 1966. [HM]

1286 *Love Poems.* Boston: Houghton-Mifflin, 1969. [HM]

1287 *To Bedlam and Part Way Back.* Boston: Houghton-Mifflin, 1960. [HM]

1288 *Transformations.* Boston: Houghton-Mifflin, 1971. [HM]

Other Relevant Primary Materials

1289 "Anne Sexton: The Art of Poetry XV." *ParR*, no. 52 (Summer 1971), 158—91. [Interview.]

1289a *Anne Sexton: A Self Portrait in Letters.* Ed. Linda Sexton and Lois Ames. Boston: Houghton-Mifflin, 1977.

1290 "Craft Interview with Anne Sexton." *NYQ*, no. 3 (Summer 1970), 8—12.

1290a "From 1928 to Whenever: A Conversation with Anne Sexton." See **150a.**

1291   *Joey and the Birthday Present* [by Sexton and Maxine Kumin]. New York: McGraw-Hill, 1971. [Child's book.]

1292   *More Eggs of Things* [by Sexton and Maxine Kumin]. New York: Putnam, 1964. [Child's book.]

1292a   "A Nurturing Relationship: A Conversation with Anne Sexton and Maxine Kumin." By Elaine Showalter and Carol Smith. *Women's Studies,* 4 (1976), 115 – 36.

1293   "Suicide Note" and "Worksheets." *NYQ,* no. 4 (Fall 1970), 81 – 94.

1294   "Anne Sexton: Worksheets." *MHRev,* 6 (1968), 105 – 14.

Collections of Critical Essays

1294a   McCLATCHY, J.D., ed. *Anne Sexton: The Author and Her Critics.* Bloomington: Indiana Univ. Press, 1978. [With bibliography.]

Critical Books and Essays

1295   AXELROD, Rise B. "The Transforming Art of Anne Sexton." *CP,* 7 (Spring 1974), 6 – 13.

1296   FIELDS, Beverly. "The Poetry of Anne Sexton." See **172.**

1297   HOFFMAN, Nancy J. "Reading Women's Poetry: The Meaning and Our Lives." *CE,* 34 (1972), 48 – 62.

1298   HOWARD, Richard. "Anne Sexton: 'Some Tribal Female who is Known but Forbidden'." See **108.**

1299   JONG, Erica. "Remembering Anne Sexton." *NYTB* (October 27, 1974), 63.

1300   LACEY, Paul. "The Sacrament of Confession." See **111.**

1300a   McCLATCHY, J. D. "Anne Sexton: Somehow to Endure." *Cent R,* 19, 2 (1975), 1 – 36.

1301   MOOD, John J. " 'A Bird Full of Bones': Anne Sexton—A Visit and a Reading." *ChiR,* 23, 4 and 24, 1 (1972), 107 – 23.

1302   ZOLLMAN, Sol. "Criticism, Self-Criticism, No Transformation: The Poetry of Robert Lowell and Anne Sexton." *L&I,* no. 9 (1971), 29 – 36.

Louis Simpson

Work of Poetry

1303   *Adventures of the Letter I.* London: Oxford Univ. Press, 1971. [Har-Row]

1304   *The Arrivistes: Poems 1940– 1949.* New York: Fine Editions, n.d.

1305   *At the End of the Open Road.* Middletown, Conn.: Wesleyan Univ. Press, 1963. [Wesleyan U Pr]

1306   *A Dream of Governors.* Middletown, Conn.: Wesleyan Univ. Press, 1959. [Wesleyan U Pr]

1307   *Good News of Death and other Poems.* In *Poets of Today, II,* ed. John Hall Whelock, New York: Scribner's, 1955.

1308   *Riverside Drive.* New York: Atheneum, 1962. [Manor]

1308a   *Searching for the Ox.* New York: Morrow, 1976.

1309   *Selected Poems.* New York: Harcourt, Brace and World, 1965. [Harbrace J]

Other Relevant Primary Materials

1309a   ''A Conversation with Louis Simpson.'' By Lawrence Smith. *Chi R,* 27 (1975), 99– 109.

1310   *An Introduction to Poetry.* New York: St. Martin's, 1967. [Anthology.] [St. Martin's]

1311   *James Hogg: A Critical Study.* Edinburgh: Oliver and Boyd, 1962.

1312   *North of Jamaica.* New York: Harper & Row, 1972. [Autobiography.]

1313   ''Opinion.'' *Rev,* no. 25 (Spring 1971), 29– 38.

1313a   *A Revolution in Taste: Studies of Dylan Thomas, Allen Ginsberg, Sylvia Plath and Robert Lowell.* New York: Macmillan, 1978.

1313b   ''Rolling Up.'' See **150a.** [Statement on his poetry.]

1313c   *Three on the Tower: The Lives and Works of Ezra Pound, T. S. Eliot, and William Carlos Williams.* New York: Morrow, 1975.

Critical Books and Essays

1314   GRAY, Yohma. ''The Poetry of Louis Simpson.'' See **172.**

1315   HOWARD, Richard. ''Louis Simpson: 'The Hunger in My Vitals is for Some Credible Extravaganza'.'' See **108.**

1315a HYMES, Dell. "Louis Simpson's 'The Deserted Boy.' " *Poetics,* 5 (1976), 119–55.

1316 MORAN, Ronald. *Louis Simpson.* New York: Twayne, 1972.*

1317 MORAN, Ronald. "Louis Simpson: The Absence of Criticism and the Presence of Poetry." *FP*, 1, 1 (Fall/Winter 1968), 60–66.

Edith Sitwell

Works of Poetry

1318 *Collected Poems.* New York: Vanguard, 1954.

Other Relevant Primary Materials

1319 *Aspects of Modern Poetry.* London: Duckworth, 1934.

1320 *Poetry and Criticism.* New York: H. Holt, 1926.

1321 *A Poet's Notebook.* Boston: Little, Brown, 1950.

1322 *The Queens and the Hive.* Boston: Little, Brown, 1962.

1323 *Selected Letters of Edith Sitwell, 1919–1966,* ed. John Lehmann and Derek Parker. New York: Vanguard, 1970.

1324 *Taken Care Of: The Autobiography of Edith Sitwell.* New York: Atheneum, 1965.

Biography, Bibliography, and Other Reference Materials

1325 FIFOOT, Richard. *A Bibliography of Edith, Osbert and Sachaverell Sitwell.* London: Rupert Hart-Davis, 1963. [Up to 1958.]

Critical Books and Essays

1326 BROPHY, James D. *Edith Sitwell: The Symbolist Order.* Carbondale: Southern Illinois Univ. Press, 1968.

1327 HARRINGTON, David. "The 'Metamorphosis' of Edith Sitwell." *Crit*, 9 (Winter 1968), 80 – 91.

1328 MILLS, Ralph. *Edith Sitwell: A Critical Essay*. Grand Rapids: Eerdmans, 1968.

1329 OWER, John. "Cosmic Aristocracy and Cosmic Democracy in Edith Sitwell." *ConLit*, 12 (1970), 527 – 53.

1330 OWER, John. "Edith Sitwell's Metaphysical Medium and Metaphysical Message." *TCL*, 16 (1970), 253 – 67.

1331 OWER, John. "A Golden Labyrinth: Edith Sitwell and the Theme of Time." *REN*, 26 (1974), 207 – 17.

1332 SINGLETON, Geoffrey. *Edith Sitwell: The Hymn to Life*. London: Fortune, 1968.

Gary Snyder

Works of Poetry

1333 *The Back Country*. New York: New Directions, 1968. [New Directions]

1334 *Myths and Texts*. New York: Totem, 1960.

1335 *A Range of Poems*, ed. Stuart Montgomery. London: Fulcrum, 1966. [Contains *Riprap* and other early materials not otherwise in print.]

1336 *The Regarding Wave*. New York: New Directions, 1970. [New Directions]

1337 *Riprap*. New York: Origin, 1959.

1338 *Six Sections from Mountains and Rivers Without End Plus One*. San Francisco: Four Seasons Foundation, 1970. [Four Seasons Foun]

1339 *Turtle Island*. New York: New Directions, 1974. [New Directions]

Other Relevant Primary Materials

1340 "Changes: A Discussion." *Reprinted in Notes from the New Underground*, ed. Jesse Kornbluth. New York: Viking, 1968.

1341 *Earth House Hold*. New York: New Directions, 1970. [New Directions]

1341a "The Incredible Survival of Coyote." *Western American Literature*, 9 (1975), 255 – 72.

1342 "Interview." *Road Apple Review*, 1, 4 (1969), 59 – 68.

1342a "Interview." See **165a.**

1342b "An Interview with Gary Snyder." By Paul Geneson. *Oh R*, 18, 3 (1977), 67-105.

1343   "Letters From Gary Snyder," ed. Robert Bertholf. *Io*, no. 14 (1972), 76 – 113.

1343a   *The Old Ways: Six Essays*. San Francisco: City Lights, 1977.

1344   "On Earth Geography," with Richard Grossinger. *Io*, no. 12 (1972), 5 – 18. [Interview.]

1344a   "The Politics of Ethnopoetics." *Alcheringa*, 2, 2 (1976), 6 – 12.

Biography, Bibliography, and Other Reference Materials

1345   MCCORD, Howard. *Some Notes to Gary Snyder's "Myths and Texts."* Berkeley: Sand Dollar, 1971. [Many of the notes are given by Snyder.]

1346   NORTON, David. "Gary Snyder Checklist." *Schist*, no. 2 (Summer 1974), 58 – 66.

Critical Books and Essays

1347   ALTIERI, Charles. "Gary Snyder's Lyric Poetry: Dialectic as Ecology." *FP*, no. 4 (1970), 55 – 65.

1348   GITZEN, Julian. "Gary Snyder and the Poetry of Compassion." *CritQ*, 15 (1973), 341 – 57.

1349   HOWARD, Richard. "Gary Snyder: 'To Hold Both History and Wilderness in the Mind'." See **108.**

1349a   KERN, Robert. "Gary Snyder and the Modernist Imperative." See **109a.**

1349b   KERN, Robert. "Recipes, Catalogues, Open Form Poetics: Gary Snyder's Archetypal Voice." *Con Lit*, 18 (1977), 173 – 97.

1350   PARKINSON, Thomas. "The Poetry of Gary Snyder." *SoR*, 4 (1968), 616 – 32.

1351   PAUL, Sherman. "From Lookout to Ashram: The Way of Gary Snyder." *IR*, 1, 3 and 4 (1970), 76 – 89; 70 – 85.*

Stephen Spender

Works of Poetry

1352   *Collected Poems, 1928 – 1953*. New York: Random House, 1955.

1353   *The Generous Days*. New York: Random House, 1972. [Random]

Other Relevant Primary Materials

1354   *The Creative Element: A Study of Vision, Despair and Orthodoxy Among Some Modern Writers.* London: Hamish Hamilton, 1953.

1355   *The Destructive Element: A Study of Modern Writers and Beliefs.* London: Jonathan cape, 1935.

1356   *Love-Hate Relations: English and American Sensibilities.* New York: Random House, 1974.

1357   *The Struggle of the Modern.* Berkeley: Univ. of California Press, 1963. [U of Cal Pr]

1357a *T. S. Eliot.* New York: Viking, 1976. [Viking]

1358   *World Within World.* London: Hamish Hamilton, 1951. [Autobiography.] [U of Cal Pr]

Critical Books and Essays

1359   FRASER, G. S. "A Poetry of Search: Spender." *Vision and Rhetoric.* New York: Barnes and Noble, 1959.

1360   HEATH-STUBBS, John. *Stephen Spender.* Harmondsworth: Penguin, 1971.*

1361   KULKARNI, H. B. *Stephen Spender: Poet in Crisis.* Glasgow: Blackie and Son, 1970.

1362   REPLOGLE, Justin. "The Auden Group." *WSCL*, 5 (1964), 133–50.

1363   SEIF, M. "The Impact of T. S. Eliot on Auden and Spender." *SAQ*, 53 (1954), 61–69.

1364   SELLERS, W. H. "Wordsworth and Spender: Some Speculations on the Use of Rhyme." *SEL 1500– 1900*, 5 (1965), 641–50.

1365   STANFORD, Derek. *Stephen Spender, Louis MacNeice, Cecil Day Lewis: A Critical Essay.* Grand Rapids: Eerdmans, 1969.

1366   WEATHERHEAD, A. K. "Stephen Spender: Lyric Impulse and Will." *ConLit*, 12 (1971), 451–65.

William Stafford

Works of Poetry

1367   *Allegiances.* New York: Harper & Row, 1970. [Har-Row]

1368   *Eleven Untitled Poems.* Mt. Horeb, Wisc.: Perishable, 1968.

1369   *In the Clock of Reason.* Victoria, B.C.: Soft, 1973.

1370   *The Rescued Year.* New York: Harper & Row, 1966. [Har-Row]

1371   *Someday, Maybe.* New York: Harper & Row, 1973.

1371a *Stories That Could Be True: New and Collected Poems.* New York: Harper and Row, 1977.

1372   *Temporary Facts.* Athens, Ohio: D. Schneider, 1970.

1373   *That Other Alone.* Mt. Horeb, Wisc.: Perishable, 1973.

1374   *Travelling Through the Dark.* New York: Harper & Row, 1962.

1375   *Weather.* Mt. Horeb, Wisc.: Perishable, 1969.

1376   *West of Your City.* Los Gatos, Cal.: Talisman, 1960.

Other Relevant Primary Materials

1377   ''An Interview with William Stafford,'' with Cynthia Lofsness. *IR*, 3, 3 (Summer 1972), 92 – 107.

1378   ''An Interview with William Stafford,'' with Beth Bentley. *Madrona*, 2, 5 (1972), 5 – 18.

1379   ''Introduction.'' *The Achievement of Brother Antonius.* Glenview, Ill.: Scott, Foresman, 1967. [Scott F]

1380   ''Keeping the Lines Wet: A Conversation with William Stafford,'' with Philip Gerba and Robert Gemmett. *PrS*, 44, 2 (Summer 1970), 123 – 36.

1380a ''Making A Poem / Starting a Car on Ice.'' See **150a.**

1381   ''Reciprocity vs. Suicide: An Interview with William Stafford,'' with Sam Bradley. *Trace*, 46 (Summer 1962), 223 – 26.

1382   ''The Sar Interview: William Stafford,'' with Sam Ragan and Ronald Bayes. *St. Andrews Review*, 2, 1 (Fall – Winter 1972), 29 – 30.

1383   ''A Way Of Writing.'' *Field*, no. 2 (Spring 1970), 10 – 12.

Biography, Bibliography, and Other Reference Materials

1384   MACMILLAN, Samuel H. ''Selected Bibliography.'' *TPJ*, 2, 3 (Spring 1969), 21 – 22.

Critical Books and Essays

1385   CARRUTH, Hayden. ''In Spite of Artifice.'' *HudR*, 19 (Winter 1966 – 67), 689 – 700. [Review of *The Rescued Year.*]

1386 CREELEY, Robert. "Think What's Got Away . . . ." *Poetry*, 102 (April 1963), 42 – 48. [Review of *Travelling Through the Dark*.]

1386a HOLDEN, Jonathan. *The Mark to Turn: A Reading of William Stafford's Poetry*. Lawrence: Univ. Press of Kansas, 1976.

1387 HOWARD, Richard. "William Stafford: 'Tell Us What You Deserve, The Whole World Said'." See **108.**

1388 HUGO, Richard. "Problems with Landscape in Early Stafford Poems." *KanQ*, 2, 2 (1970), 33 – 38.

1389 KYLE, Carol. "Point of View in 'Returned to Say' and the Wilderness of William Stafford." *WAL*, 7 (1972), 191 – 201.

1390 LAUBER, John. "The World's Guest—William Stafford." *IR*, 5, 2 (Spring 1974), 88 – 100.

1391 LIEBERMAN, Laurence. "The Expansional Poet: A Return to Personality." *YR*, 57 (Winter 1968), 258 – 71. [Review of *The Rescued Year*.]

Wallace Stevens   *

Works of Poetry

1391a "Stafford Number." *MPS*, 6 (1975), 1 – 38.

1392 *Collected Poems*. New York: Alfred Knopf, 1955.

1393 *Poems: Wallace Stevens*, selected by Samuel French Morse. New York: Vintage, 1959.

1394 *The Palm at the End of the Mind: Selected Poems and a Play*, ed. Holly Stevens. New York: Vintage, 1972. [Random]

Other Relevant Primary Materials

1395 *The Letters of Wallace Stevens*, ed. Holly Stevens. New York: Alfred Knopf, 1966.

1396 *The Necessary Angel*. New York: Alfred Knopf, 1951. [Basic essays.] [Random]

1397 *Opus Posthumus*, ed. Samuel French Morse. New York: Alfred Knopf, 1957. [Essays, plays, and uncollected poems.]

Biography, Bibliography, and Other Reference Materials

1397a *Souvenirs and Prophecies: The Young Wallace Stevens*. Ed. Holly Bright Stevens. New York: Knopf, 1977. [Journals.]

1398 EDELSTEIN, J. M. *Wallace Stevens: A Descriptive Bibliography.* Pittsburgh: Univ. of Pittsburgh Press, 1973.

1399 HUGUELET, Theodore L. *Checklist of Wallace Stevens.* Columbus, Ohio: C. E. Merrill, 1970.

1400 MORSE, Samuel French. *Wallace Stevens: Poetry as Life.* New York: Pegasus, 1970.

1401 WALSH, Thomas F. *Concordance to the Poetry of Wallace Stevens.* University Park: Pennsylvania State Univ. Press, 1963.

Collections of Critical Essays

1401a WILLARD, Abbie F. *Wallace Stevens: The Poet and His Critics.* Chicago: American Library Association, 1978.

1402 BORROFF, Marie, ed. *Wallace Stevens; A Collection of Critical Essays.* Englewood Cliffs, N.J.: Prentice-Hall, 1963. [P-H]

1403 BROWN, Ashley, and Robert S. HALLER, eds. *The Achievement of Wallace Stevens.* Philadelphia: Lippincott, 1962.

1404 EHRENPREIS, Irvin, ed. *Wallace Stevens: A Critical Anthology.* Baltimore: Penguin, 1972. [Very interesting combination of selected Stevens letters and reprinted essays about his work.]

1405 MCNAMARA, Peter L., ed. *Critics on Wallace Stevens.* Coral Gables: Univ. of Miami Press, 1972.

1406 PEARCE, Roy Harvey, and J. Hillis MILLER, eds. *The Act of the Mind, Essays on the Poetry of Wallace Stevens.* Baltimore: Johns Hopkins Univ. Press, 1965.

1407 STANFORD, Donald E., ed. "Wallace Stevens and the Romantic Heritage." *SoR*, 7, 3 (1971). [Issue devoted to Stevens.]

Critical Books and Essays

1408 ADAMS, Richard P. " 'The Comedian as the Letter C': A Somewhat Literal Reading." *TSE*, 18 (1970), 95 – 114.

1409 ALVAREZ, A. "Wallace Stevens: Platonic Poetry." See **38a.**

1410 BAIRD, James. *The Dome and the Rock: Structures in the Poetry of Wallace Stevens.* Baltimore: Johns Hopkins Univ. Press, 1968.*

1411 BENAMOU, Michael. *Wallace Stevens and the Symbolist Imagination.* Princeton: Princeton Univ. Press, 1972.*

1412 BEVIS, William W. "The Arrangement of *Harmonium.*" *ELH*, 37 (1970), 456 – 73. Reprinted in **1405.**

1413 BLESSING, Richard Allen. *Wallace Stevens' "Whole Harmonium."* Syracuse: Syracuse Univ. Press, 1970.

1414 BLOOM, Harold. "The Central Man: Emerson, Whitman, Wallace Stevens." *MassR*, 7 (Winter 1966), 23 – 42. Reprinted in **223.**

1415   BLOOM, Harold. "Notes Toward a Supreme Fiction: A Commentary." See **1402.**

1415a   BLOOM, Harold. *Wallace Stevens: The Poems of Our Climate.* Ithaca: Cornell Univ. Press, 1977.*

1416   BROWN, Merle Elliott. *Wallace Stevens: The Poem as Act.* Detroit: Wayne State Univ. Press, 1970.

1417   BUTTEL, Robert. *Wallace Stevens: The Making of Harmonium.* Princeton: Princeton Univ. Press, 1967.

1418   CUNNINGHAM, J. V. "Tradition and Modernity: Wallace Stevens." *Tradition and Poetic Structure.* Denver: Swallow, 1966. Reprinted in **1403.**

1419   DEMBO, L. S. "Wallace Stevens: Meta-Men and Para-Things." See **45.**

1420   DOGGETT, Frank A. *Stevens' Poetry of Thought.* Baltimore: Johns Hopkins Univ. Press, 1966. [Johns Hopkins]*

1421   DOGGETT, Frank A. "The Transition from *Harmonium*: Factors in the Development of Stevens' Later Poetry." *PMLA*, 88 (1973), 122 – 31.

1422   DONOGHUE, Denis. "Nuances of a Theme by Stevens." See **1406.**

1423   DONOGHUE, Denis. "On Notes *Toward a Supreme Fiction*." See **48.**

1424   EBERHART, Richard. "Emerson and Wallace Stevens." *LitR*, 7 (Autumn 1963), 51 – 71.

1425   ENCK, John J. *Wallace Stevens: Images and Judgments.* Carbondale: Southern Illinois Univ. Press, 1964.

1426   FRYE, Northrop. "The Realistic Oriole." *HudR*, 10 (Autumn 1957), 353 – 70. Reprinted in **1402.** *

1426a   FRYE, Northrop. "Wallace Stevens and the Variation Form." *Literary Theory and Structure: Essays in Honor of W. K. Wimsatt,* ed. Frank Brady, John Palmer, and Martin Price. New Haven: Yale Univ. Press, 1973.

1427   FUCHS, Daniel. *The Comic Spirit of Wallace Stevens.* Durham, N.C.: Duke Univ. Press, 1963.

1428   KERMODE, Frank. "Notes Toward a Supreme Fiction." *AION-SG*, 4 (1961), 173 – 201.

1429   KERMODE, Frank. *Wallace Stevens.* New York: Grove, 1961.

1430   KESSLER, Edward. *Images of Wallace Stevens.* New Brunswick, N.J.: Rutgers Univ. Press, 1972.

1431   LENTRICCHIA, Frank. *The Gaiety of Language: An Essay on the Radical Poetics of Yeats and Wallace Stevens.* Berkeley: Univ. of California Press, 1968.

1432   LITZ, A. Walton. *Introspective Voyager: The Poetic Development of Wallace Stevens.* New York: Oxford Univ. Press, 1972.

1433   MACCAFFREY, Isabel. "The Other Side of Silence: 'Credences of Summer' as an Example." *MLQ*, 30 (1969), 417 – 38.

1434   MACKSEY, Richard. "The Climates of Wallace Stevens." See **1406.**

1435   MARTZ, Louis. "Wallace Stevens: The World as Meditation." *YR*, 47 (1958), 517 – 36. Reprinted in **73.**

1436   MILLER, J. H. "Wallace Stevens." See **77.** *

1436a   MILLER, J. Hillis. "Stevens' Rock and Criticism as Cure." *Ga R*, 30 (1976), 5 – 31, 330 – 48.

1437   MILLS, Ralph. "Wallace Stevens: The Image of the Rock." *Accent*, 48 (Spring 1958), 75—89. Reprinted in **1402.**

1438   MORRIS, Adelaide. *Wallace Stevens: Imagination and Faith*. Princeton: Princeton Univ. Press, 1974.

1439   MORSE, Samuel French. "Wallace Stevens, Bergson, Pater." See **1406.**

1440   NASSAR, Eugene Paul. *Wallace Stevens: An Anatomy of Figuration*. Philadelphia: Univ. of Pennsylvania Press, 1965.

1441   PEARCE, Roy H. "Wallace Stevens and the Ultimate Poem." See **80.***

1442   POULIN, A., Jr. "Crispin as Everyman as Adam: 'The Comedian as the Letter C'." *CP*, 1 (1972), 5—23.

1443   POWELL, Grosvenor E. "Of Heroes and Nobility: The Personae of Wallace Stevens." *SoR*, 7 (1971), 727—48.

1444   RIDDEL, Joseph N. *The Clairvoyant Eye: The Poetry and Poetics of Wallace Stevens*. Baton Rouge: Louisiana State Univ. Press, 1965. [La State U Pr]*

1445   RIDDEL, Joseph N. "Interpreting Stevens: An Essay on Poetry and Thinking." *Bnd2*, 1 (Fall 1972), 79—97.*

1446   RIDDEL, Joseph N. "Stevens on Imagination—The Point of Departure." *The Quest for Imagaination, Essays on Twentieth Century Aesthetic Criticism*, ed. O. B. Hardison, Jr. Cleveland: Press of Case Western Reserve Univ., 1971.

1447   SHEEHAN, Donald. "Stevens' Theory of Metaphor." *PLL*, 2 (1966), 57—66. Reprinted in **1405.**

1448   SIMON, Hi. " 'The Comedian as the Letter C': Its Sense and Significance." *SoR*, 5 (1940), 453—68. Reprinted in **1403.***

1449   SIMON, Hi. "The Genre of Wallace Stevens." *SewR*, 53 (1945), 566—79. Reprinted in **1402.**

1450   STALLKNECHT, Newton. "Absence in Reality." *KenR*, 21 (1959), 545—62.

1451   STERN, Herbert J. *Wallace Stevens: Art of Uncertainty*. Ann Arbor: Univ. of Michigan Press, 1966.

1451a SUKENICK, Ronald. *Wallace Stevens: Musing the Obscure: Readings and Interpretation, and a Guide to the Collected Poetry*. New York: New York Univ. Press, 1967. [NYU Pr]

1452   TURCO, Lewis. "The Agonism and the Existentity: Stevens." *CP*, 6, 1 (1973), 32—44.

1452a VENDLER, Helen Hennessy. *On Extended Wings: Wallace Stevens' Longer Poems*. Cambridge: Harvard Univ. Press, 1969.*

1453   VENDLER, Helen Hennessey. "The Qualified Assertions of Wallace Stevens." See **1406.**

1453a VENDLER, Helen Hennessey. "Wallace Stevens: The False and True Sublime." *SoR*, 7 (1971), 683—98.

1454   WHITAKER, Thomas. "On Speaking Humanly." *The Philosopher-Critic*, ed. Robert Scholes. Tulsa: Univ. of Tulsa Press, 1970.

Allen Tate

Works of Poetry

1455 *Collected Poems: 1919– 1976.* New York: Farrar, Straus, and Giroux, 1977.

1455a *Poems.* New York: Scribner's 1960. [Swallow]

1456 *The Swimmers and Other Selected Poems.* London: Oxford Univ. Press, 1970.

Other Relevant Primary Materials

1457 *Essays of Four Decades.* Chicago: Swallow, 1968. [Apollo Eds]

1458 *The Fathers.* New York: Putnam, 1938. [Novel.] [Swallow]

1458a *Memoirs and Opinions: Nineteen-Twenty-Six to Nineteen-Seventy-Four.* Santa Barbara: Swallow, 1975.

1459 "Narcissius as Narcissius." In **1457.** [On his own "Ode to the Confederate Dead."]

1460 *The Literary Correspondence of Donald Davidson and Allen Tate*, ed. John T. Fain and Thomas D. Young. Athens: Univ. of Georgia Press, 1974.

Biography, Bibliography, and Other Reference Materials

1461 FALLWELL, Marshall, Jr. *Allen Tate: A Bibliography.* New York: David Lewis, 1969.

1462 SQUIRES, Radcliffe. *Allen Tate: A Literary Biography.* New York: Pegasus, 1971.

Collections of Critical Essays

1463 SQUIRES, Radcliffe, ed. *Allen Tate and His Work: Critical Evaluations.* Minneapolis: Univ. of Minnesota Press, 1972. [Sections on "The Man," "The Essayist," "The Novelist," "The Poet," and bibliography.]

1463a "A Special Section on Allen Tate." *So R,* 12 (1976), 685– 97.

Critical Books and Essays

1464 ARNOLD, Willard B. *The Social Ideas of Allen Tate*. Boston: Bruce Humphries, 1955.

1465 BISHOP, Ferman. *Allen Tate*. New York: Twayne, 1967.*

1466 BROOKS, Cleanth. "The Modern Southern Poet." *VQR*, 11 (1935), 304–20. See **40**.

1467 DUPREE, Robert. "The Mirrors of Analogy: Three Poems of Allen Tate." *SoR*, 8 (1972), 774–91. ["The Crow," "The Last Days of Alice," "The Mediterranean."]

1468 FEDER, Lillian. "Allen Tate's Use of Classical Literature." See **1463**.

1469 FLEMING, Rudd. "Dramatic Involution: Tate, Husserl, and Joyce." *SewR*, 60 (1952), 445–64.

1470 MEINERS, R. K. *The Last Alternatives: A Study of the Works of Allen Tate*. Denver: Swallow, 1962.*

1471 NEMEROV, Howard. "The Current of the Frozen Stream: An Essay on the Poetry of Allen Tate." *SewR*, 67 (1959), 585–97. Reprinted in **1463**.

1472 RANSOM, John Crowe. "In Amicitia." *SewR*, 67 (1959), 528–39.

1473 RUBIN, Louis. "The Serpent in the Mulberry Bush." Reprinted in Rubin, ed., *Southern Renaissance: The Literature of the Modern South*. Baltimore: Johns Hopkins Univ. Press, 1953. Reprinted in **1463**.

1474 SQUIRES, Radcliffe. "Mr. Tate: Whose Wreath Should be a Moral." See **173**.

Dylan Thomas

Works of Poetry

1475 *The Collected Poems of Dylan Thomas*. New York: New Directions, 1953. [New Directions]

Other Relevant Primary Materials

1476 *The Notebooks of Dylan Thomas*, ed. Ralph Maud. New York: New Directions, 1966.

1477 *Quite Early One Morning*. London: Dent, 1954. [New Directions]

1478 *Selected Letters of Dylan Thomas*, ed. Constantine Fitzgibbon. New York: New Directions, 1967.

Biography, Bibliography, and Other Reference Materials

1479 ACKERMAN, John. *Dylan Thomas, His Life and Work*. London: Oxford Univ. Press, 1964.

1480 BRINNIN, John Malcolm. *Dylan Thomas in America: An Intimate Journal*. Boston:Q Little, Brown, 1955.

1480a FERRIS, Paul. *Dylan Thomas*. New York: Dial, 1977.

1481 FITZGIBBON, Constantine. *Life of Dylan Thomas*. Boston: Little, Brown, 1965. [Little]

1481a KERSCHNER, R. B. *Dylan Thomas: The Poet and His Critics*. Chicago: American Library Association, 1976.

1481b LANE, Gary. *A Concordance to the Poems of Dylan Thomas*. Metuchen, N.J.: Scarecrow, 1976.

1482 MAUD, Ralph, and Albert GLOVER. *Dylan Thomas in Print: A Bibliographical History*. Pittsburgh: Univ. of Pittsburgh Press, 1970.

Collections of Critical Essays

1483 BRINNIN, John Malcolm, ed. *A Casebook on Dylan Thomas*. New York: Crowell, 1960. [Interesting collection of early critical materials, biographical materials and recent essays.]

1484 COX, C. B., ed. *Dylan Thomas, A Collection of Critical Essays*. Englewood Cliffs, N.J.: Prentice-Hall, 1966.

1485 DAVIES, Wilford, ed. *Dylan Thomas: New Critical Essays*. London: Dent, 1972. [Includes important reconsideration of their earlier essays by Wain, Bayley and Rawson.]

1486 TEDLOCK, Ernest Warnock, ed. *Dylan Thomas: The Legend and the Poet, a Collection of Biographical and Critical Essays*. London: Heinemann, 1961. [Reprints many biographical materials along with critical essays.]

Critical Books and Essays

1487 ADAMS, Robert M. "Crashaw and Dylan Thomas: Devotional Aesthetics." See **1484.**

1488 BAYLEY, John. "Dylan Thomas." See **39.** Reprinted in **1484.**

1489 DAICHES, David. "The Poetry of Dylan Thomas." *Literary Essays.* London: Oliver and Boyd, 1956. Reprinted in **1484.**

1490 DAVIES, Aneirin Talfan. *Dylan: Druid of the Broken Body*. London: Dent, 1964.

1491 DODSWORTH, Martin. "The Concept of Mind and the Poetry of Dylan Thomas." See **1485**.*

1492 FOWLER, Alastair. "Adder's Tongue on Maiden Hair: Early Stages in Reading 'Fern Hill'." See **1485**.

1493 HOLBROOK, David. *Dylan Thomas, The Code of Night.* London: Athlone, 1972.*

1494 HOLBROOK, David. *Llareggub revisited: Dylan Thomas and the State of Modern Poetry.* London: Bowes and Bowes, 1962. [The classic attack on Thomas.]*

1495 JONES, Thomas Henry. *Dylan Thomas.* New York: Grove, 1963.

1496 KIDDER, Rushworth M. *Dylan Thomas: The Country of the Spirit.* Princeton: Princeton Univ. Press, 1973.

1497 KLEINMAN, Hyman H. *The Religious Sonnets of Dylan Thomas: A Study in Imagery and Meaning.* Berkeley: Univ. of California Press, 1963.

1498 MAUD, Ralph. *Entrances to Dylan Thomas' Poetry.* Pittsburgh: Univ. of Pittsburgh Press, 1963. [Univ of Pittsburgh Pr]*

1499 MAYOUX, J. J. "Dylan Thomas au bois lacte." *Critique*, 27 (1971), 675–87.

1500 MERWIN, W. S. "The Religious Poet." See **1483**. Reprinted in **1486**.

1501 MILLER, J. H. "Dylan Thomas." See **77**.*

1502 MOYNIHAN, William T. *The Craft and Art of Dylan Thomas.* Ithaca: Cornell Univ. Press, 1966. [Cornell U Pr]

1503 NEMEROV, Howard. "The Generation of Violence." *KenR*, 15 (1953), 477–83.

1504 OLSON, Elder. *The Poetry of Dylan Thomas.* Chicago: Univ. of Chicago Press, 1954. [Univ of Chicago Pr]

1505 PRATT, Annis. *Dylan Thomas' Early Prose; A Study in Creative Mythology.* Pittsburgh: Univ. of Pittsburgh Press, 1970.

1506 SHAPIRO, Karl. "Dylan Thomas." *In Defense of Ignorance.* New York: Random House, 1960. Reprinted in **1483, 1484,** and **1486**.*

1507 STANFORD, Derek. "Dylan Thomas: A Literary Post-Mortem." *QQ*, 71 (1964), 405–18.

1508 STEPHENS, Raymond. "Self and World: The Earlier Poems." See **1485**.

1509 TINDALL, William York. *A Reader's Guide to Dylan Thomas.* New York: Farrar, Straus and Cudahy, 1962. [FS & G]

1510 TREECE, Henry. *Dylan Thomas, "Dog Among the Fairies,"* 2nd ed. London: E. Benn, 1956.*

1511 TRITSCHLER, Donald. "The Metaphoric Stop of Time in 'A Winter's Tale'." *PMLA*, 78 (1963), 422–30.

1512 WEST, Paul. "Thomas: The Position in Calamity." *SoR*, 3 (1967), 922–43.

Charles Tomlinson

Works of Poetry

1513 *America West Southwest.* n.p.: San Marcos Press, 1970.

1514 *American Scenes.* London: Oxford Univ. Press, 1966.

1515 *The Necklace.* New York: Oxford Univ. Press, 1966. [Reprint of a 1955 volume.]

1516 *A Peopled Landscape.* London: Oxford Univ. Press, 1963. [Oxford U Pr]

1517 *Relations and Contraries.* Aldington: Hand and Flower, 1951.

1518 *Seeing is Believing.* New York: McDowell, Obolensky, 1958. [Revised ed., London: Oxford Univ. Press, 1960.]

1519 *The Way of a World.* London: Oxford Univ. Press, 1969.

1519a *Way In and Other Poems.* New York: Oxford Univ. Press, 1974.

1520 *Words and Images.* London: Covent Garden, 1972. [Poems and graphics; almost all the poems are in *Written on Water.*]

1521 *Written on Water.* London: Oxford Univ. Press, 1972.

Other Relevant Primary Materials

1522 *Castilian Ilexes: Versions from Antonio Machado, 1875– 1939* [by Tomlinson and Henry Gifford]. London: Oxford Univ. Press, 1963.

1522a "An Interview with Charles Tomlinson." *Con Lit*, 16 (1975), 405 – 16.

1523 "Introduction" to *Marianne Moore: A Collection of Critical Essays.* See **1037.**

1524 "Introduction" to *A New Kind of Tie: Poems 1965– 68*, by Simon Cutts. Nottingham: Taresque, 1972.

1525 "Introduction" to *William Carlos Williams: A Critical Anthology*, ed. Tomlinson. Harmondsworth, England: Penguin, 1972.

1526 *The Poem as Initiation.* Hamilton, N.Y.: Colgate Univ. Press, 1968.

Critical Books and Essays

1527 BEDIENT, Calvin. "Calvin Bedient on Charles Tomlinson." *IR*, 1, 2 (Spring 1970), 83 – 100. Reprinted in **100.**

1528 BRIAN, John. "The Poetry of Charles Tomlinson." *FP*, no. 3 (Fall/Winter 1969), 50 – 61.

1529 DAVIE, Donald. "Introduction" to **1515.** [1966 ed.]

1530 EDWARDS, Michael. "Charles Tomlinson: Notes on Tradition and Impersonality." *CritQ*, 15, 2 (Summer 1973), 133 — 44.

1531 EDWARDS, Michael. "Poems and Drawings. An Essay on Tomlinson." *Agenda*, 9, 2 — 3 (Spring/Summer 1971), 126 — 41.

1532 GITZEN, Julian. "Charles Tomlinson and the Plenitude of Fact." *CritQ*, 13 (1971), 355 — 62.

1533 HARVEY, Arthur. " 'Naked Nature' and 'Negotiations': The Poetry of Charles Tomlinson." *New Poetry*, 1, 2 (April 1971), 3 — 8.

1534 SPEARS, Monroe K. "Shapes and Surfaces: David Jones, with a Glance at Charles Tomlinson." *ConLit*, 12 (1971), 402 — 19.

1534a WEATHERHEAD, A. K. "Charles Tomlinson: With Respect to Flux." *IR*, 7, 4 (1976), 120 — 34.

Robert Penn Warren

Works of Poetry

1535 *Audobon: A Vision.* New York: Random House, 1969.

1536 *Incarnations: Poems 1966 — 68.* New York: Random House, 1968.

1537 *Or Else: Poems 1968 — 1974.* New York: Random House, 1974.

1538 *Selected Poems, 1923 — 1943.* New York: Harcourt, Brace, 1944. [A larger selection of earlier poems than in the later *Selected Poems.*]

1539 *Selected Poems: New and Old, 1923 — 1975.* New York: Random House, 1976. [Random]

Other Relevant Primary Materials

1540 "The Briar Patch." See **144.**

1540a *Democracy and Poetry.* Cambridge: Harvard Univ. Press, 1974. [Harvard]

1540b "Interview," with Peter Stitt. *Sew R*, 85 (1977), 467 — 77.

1541 *John Greenleaf Whittier's Poetry: an Appraisal and a Selection.* Minneapolis: Univ. of Minnesota Press, 1971. [Univ of Minn Pr]

1542 *Selected Essays.* New York: Random House, 1958. [Random]

1543 *Who Speaks for the Negro.* New York: Random House, 1965. [Random]

Biography, Bibliography, and Other Reference Materials

1544 HUFF, Mary Nance. *Robert Penn Warren: A Bibliography*. New York: David Lewis, 1968.

Collections of Critical Essays

1545 LONGLEY, John Lewis, Jr., ed. *Robert Penn Warren: A Collection of Critical Essays*. New York: New York Univ. Press, 1965. [NYU Pr]

1545a "Robert Penn Warren." *Oh R*, 18, 1 (1977). [Special issue on Warren.]

Critical Books and Essays

1546 BRANTLEY, Frederick. "The Achievement of Robert Penn Warren." *Modern American Poetry*, ed. B. Rajan. New York: Roy, 1952.

1547 CASPER, Leonard. *Robert Penn Warren: The Dark and Bloody Ground*. Seattle: Univ. of Washington Press, 1960.*

1548 CORE, George. "In the Heart's Ambiguity: Robert Penn Warren as a Poet." *MissQ*, 22 (1969), 313—26.

1549 GARRET, George P. "Warren's Later Poetry." See **1545**.*

1550 MCDOWELL, Frederick P. "Robert Penn Warren's Criticism." *Accent*, 15 (1955), 173—96.

1551 QUINN, Sister Mary Bernetta. "Robert Penn Warren's Promised Land." *SoR*, 8 (1972), 329—58.

1552 RANSOM, John Crowe. "Hearts and Heads." *American Review*, 2 (1934), 554—71.*

1553 SPEARS, Monroe K. "The Latest Poetry of Robert Penn Warren." *SewR*, 78 (1970), 348—57.

1554 STRANDBERG, Victor. *A Colder Fire: The Poetry of Robert Penn Warren*. Lexington: Univ. of Kentucky Press, 1977.

Richard Wilbur

Works of Poetry

1554a *The Mind-Reader*. New York: Harcourt, Brace, Jovanovich, 1977. [Har-Brace J]

1554b *Opposites.* New York: Harcourt, Brace, Jovanovich, 1973.

1555 *The Poems of Richard Wilbur.* New York: Harcourt, Brace and World, 1963. [Har Brace J]

1556 *Walking to Sleep: New Poems and Translations.* New York: Harcourt, Brace and World, 1969.

Other Relevant Primary Materials

1556a "A Conversation with Richard Wilbur," by Edward Honig. *MLR,* 91 (1976), 1084–98.

1557 "The Genie in the Bottle." *Mid Century American Poets,* ed. John Ciardi. New York: Twayne, 1950, 1–7.

1557a "The Image and the Object: An Interview with Richard Wilbur," by David Dillon. *SewR,* 58 (1973), 240–51.

1558 "An Interview with Richard Wilbur," ed. David Curry. *Trinity Review,* 17 (December 1962), 21–32.

1559 "Interview with Richard Wilbur," ed. Willard Pate. *South Carolina Review,* 3 (1970), 5–23.

1560 "Poetry and Happiness." *Shen,* 20 (Summer 1969), 3–23.

1561 "Poetry's Debt to Poetry." *HudR,* 26 (1973), 273–94.

1561a *Responses: Prose Pieces, 1948–1976.* New York: Harcourt, Brace, Jovanovich, 1976.

1562 "Richard Wilbur: An Interview," ed. Robert Frank and Stephen Mitchell. *Amherst Literary Magazine,* 10 (Summer 1965), 54–72.

1563 "Richard Wilbur Talking to Joan Hutton." *Transatlantic Review,* no. 29 (Summer 1968), 58–67.

1564 HALL, Donald. "Method in Poetic Composition." *ParR,* no. 3 (Autumn 1953), 113–19. [Wilbur and Eberhart contrasted with respect to methods of composition; hence some interview information.]

Biography, Bibliography, and Other Reference Materials

1565 FIELD, John P. *Richard Wilbur: A Bibliographical Checklist.* Kent, Ohio: Kent State Univ. Press, 1971.

Critical Books and Essays

1566 CUMMINS, Paul F. *Richard Wilbur: A Critical Essay.* Grand Rapids: Eerdmans, 1971.

1567 FARRELL, John P. "The Beautiful Changes in Richard Wilbur's Poetry."
      ConLit, 12 (1971), 74 – 87.*

1568 FAVERTY, Frederic. "Well-Open Eyes; or the Poetry of Richard Wilbur."
      See **172.**

1569 HALL, Donald. "Ah Love Let us be True: Domesticity and History in Con-
      temporary Poetry." *ASch*, 28 (1959), 310 – 19.

1570 HEYEN, William. "On Richard Wilbur." *SoR*, 9 (1973), 617 – 34.

1571 HILL, Donald L. *Richard Wilbur.* New Haven: College and Univ. Press,
      1967.

1572 LERNER, L. D. "Baroque Rationalist." *Listen*, 2 (Summer – Autumn
      1957), 23 – 26.

1573 MCGUINESS, Arthur E. "A Question of Consciousness: Richard Wilbur's
      Things of this World." *ArQ*, 23 (1967), 313 – 26.

1574 TAYLOR, Henry. "Two Worlds Taken as they Come: Richard Wilbur's
      'Walking to Sleep'." *HC*, 6 (July 1969), 1 – 12.

1575 WARLOW, Francis W. "Richard Wilbur." *BuR*, 7 (1959), 217 – 33.

1576 WEATHERHEAD, A. K. "Richard Wilbur: Poetry of Things." *ELH*, 35
      (1968), 606 – 17.*

William Carlos Williams

Works of Poetry

1577 *Collected Earlier Poems of William Carlos Williams.* New York: New Direc-
      tions, 1951.

1578 *Collected Later Poems of William Carlos Williams: Revised Edition.* New
      York: New Directions, 1963.

1579 *Imaginations*, ed. Webster Schott. New York: New Directions, 1970.
      [Contains *Spring and All* and three early prose works.] [New Directions]

1580 *Paterson: Books I– V.* New York: New Directions, 1963. [New Directions]

1581 *Pictures From Breughel.* New York: New Directions, 1962. [New
      Directions]

1582 *The William Carlos Williams Reader*, ed. M. L. Rosenthal. New York: New
      Directions, 1966. [New Directions]

Other Relevant Primary Materials

1583 "The Art of Poetry VI: William Carlos Williams." *ParR*, 32 (1964), 110 – 51.
      Reprinted in **162,** vol. 3.

1584   *The Autobiography of William Carlos Williams.* New York: New Directions, 1951. [New Directions]

1585   *The Build-Up.* New York: Random House, 1952. [New Directions]

1586   *The Embodiment of Knowledge*, ed. Ron Loewinsohn. New York: New Directions, 1974. [Mostly on education.]

1587   *The Farmer's Daughter.* New York: New Directions, 1961. [Collected stories.] [New Directions]

1588   *In the American Grain: Essays by William Carlos Williams.* New York: New Directions, 1966. [First published in 1925.] [New Directions]

1589   *In the Money.* New York: New Directions, 1940. [New Directions]

1589a *Interviews with William Carlos Williams: 'Speaking Straight Ahead,'* ed. Linda Wagner. New York: New Directions, 1976.

1590   *I Wanted to Write a Poem*, ed. Edith Heal. Boston: Beacon, 1958. [Collection of remarks on specific poems.] [Beacon]

1591   *Many Loves and Other Plays.* New York: New Directions, 1961. [New Directions]

1591a *A Recognizable Image: William Carlos Williams on Art and Artists*, ed. Bram Dijkstra. New York: New Directions, 1978.

1592   *Selected Essays of William Carlos Williams.* New York: Random House, 1954. [New Directions]

1593   *The Selected Letters of William Carlos Williams*, ed. John Thirlwall. New York: McDowell, Obolensky, 1957.

1594   *Voyage to Pagany.* New York: Macaulay, 1928.

1595   *White Mule.* New York: New Directions, 1937. [New Directions]

1596   "A Visit with William Carlos Williams," by Walter Sutton. *MinnR*, 1 (1961), 309—24.

Biography, Bibliography, and Other Reference Materials

1597   HARDIE, Jack. "A Celebration of the Light: Selected Checklist of Writings about William Carlos Williams." *JML*, 1 (1971), 593—642.

1597a MARIANI, Paul. *William Carlos Williams: The Poet and His Critics.* Chicago: American Library Association, 1975.

1598   WALLACE, Emily Mitchell. *A Bibliography of William Carlos Williams.* Middletown, Conn.: Wesleyan Univ. Press, 1968.

1599   WEAVER, Mike. *William Carlos Williams: The American Background.* New York: Cambridge Univ. Press, 1971. [An experiment in biography.]*

1599a WHITTEMORE, Reed. *William Carlos Williams: Poet From Jersey.* Boston: Houghton-Mifflin, 1975.

Collections of Critical Essays

1600 ENGELS, John, ed. *Studies in Paterson.* Columbus, Ohio: C. E. Merrill, 1971. [Merrill]

1601 "William Carlos Williams: A Special Number." *JML*, 1, 4 (May 1971).

1602 MAZZARO, Jerome, ed. *Profile of William Carlos Williams.* Columbus, Ohio: C. E. Merrill, 1971. [Merrill]

1603 MILLER, J. Hillis, ed. *William Carlos Williams, A Collection of Critical Essays.* Englewood Cliffs, N.J.: Prentice-Hall, 1966. [P-H]

1604 TOMLINSON, Charles, ed. *William Carlos Williams: A Critical Anthology.* Harmondsworth, England: Penguin, 1972.

Critical Books and Essays

1605 BRESLIN, James E. *William Carlos Williams, an American Artist.* New York: Oxford Univ. Press, 1970.*

1605a BRESLIN, James. "William Carlos Williams and Charles Demuth: Cross-Fertilization in the Arts." *JML*, 6 (1977), 248–63.

1606 BRINNIN, John Malcolm. *William Carlos Williams.* Minneapolis: Univ. of Minnesota Press, 1963.

1607 BURKE, Kenneth. "William Carlos Williams: Two Judgments." See **1603**. ["Heaven's First Law" and "William Carlos Williams, 1883–1963."]

1608 CONARROE, Joel. *William Carlos Williams' Paterson: Language and Landscape.* Philadelphia: Univ. of Pennsylvania Press, 1970.

1609 DEMBO, L. S. "William Carlos Williams: Objectivist Mathematics." See **45**.

1610 DIJKSTRA, Bram. *The Hieroglyphics of a New Speech: Cubism, Steiglitz, and the Early Poetry of William Carlos Williams.* Princeton: Princeton Univ. Press, 1969.

1611 DONOGHUE, Denis. "Williams, a Redeeming Language." See **48**. Reprinted in **1603**.*

1612 DUFFEY, Bernard. "Williams: *Paterson* and the Measure of Art." *Essays on American Literature in Honor of Jay B. Hubbell,* ed. Clarence Godhes. Durham, N.C.: Duke Univ. Press, 1967.

1613 GREEN, Jesse D. "Williams' *Kora in Hell:* The Opening of the Poem as 'Field of Action'." *ConLit,* 13 (1972), 295–314.

1614 GROGAN, Ruth. "Swaying Form in Williams 'Asphodel'." See **1604**.

1615 GUIMOND, James. *The Art of William Carlos Williams: A Discovery and Possession of America.* Urbana: Univ. of Illinois Press, 1968.

1616 JUHASZ, Suzanne. *Metaphor and the Poetry of Williams, Pound, and Stevens.* See **65**.

1617 LEVIN, Harry. "William Carlos Williams and the Old World." *YR,* 59 (1970), 520–31.

1618 LIEBER, Todd M. "Paterson: The Poet as Tragic Hero." *Endless Experiments: Essays on the Heroic Experience in American Romanticism.* Columbus: Ohio State Univ. Press, 1973.

1619 LOWELL, Robert. "William Carlos Williams." *HudR*, 14 (1961 – 62), 530 – 36. Reprinted in **1603** and **1604.**

1620 MACKSEY, Richard. " 'A Certainty of Music': Williams' Changes." See **1603.**

1620a MARIANI, Paul. "The Satyr's Defense: Williams' 'Asphodel'." *ConLit*, 14 (1973), 1 – 18.

1621 MARIANI, Paul. "Toward the Canonization of William Carlos Williams." *MassR*, 13 (1972), 661 – 75.

1622 MARTZ, Louis L. "Paterson: A Plan for Action." *JML*, 1 (1971), 512 – 22.

1623 MARTZ, Louis L. "The Unicorn in *Paterson*: William Carlos Williams." *Thought*, 35 (Winter 1960), 537 – 54. Reprinted in **73.**

1624 MARTZ, Louis L. "William Carlos Williams: On the Road to *Paterson*." *Poetry New York*, 4 (1951), 18 – 32. Reprinted in **73.**

1625 MAZZARO, Jerome. *William Carlos Williams: The Later Poems.* Ithaca: Cornell Univ. Press, 1973.

1626 MEYERS, Neil. "Williams' Imitation of Nature in 'The Desert Music'." *Crit*, 12 (1970), 38 – 50.

1627 MILLER, J. Hillis. "William Carlos Williams." See **77.***

1628 MILLER, J. Hillis. "Williams *Spring and All* and the Progress of Poetry." *Daedalus*, 99 (1970), 405 – 34.

1629 MOORE, Marianne. "Three Essays on Williams." See **1603.** [Includes "Kora in Hell," "A Poet of the Quattrocento," and "Things Others Never Notice."]

1630 MOTTRAM, Eric. "The Making of Paterson." *Strand*, 7, 3 (Fall 1965), 17 – 34.

1631 PAUL, Sherman. *The Music of Survival: A Biography of a Poem by William Carlos Williams.* Urbana: Univ. of Illinois Press, 1968. [On "The Desert Music."]*

1632 PAUL, Sherman. "A Sketchbook of the Artist in His Thirty-Fourth Year: William Carlos Williams; *Kora in Hell: Improvisations*." *The Shaken Realist*, ed. Melvin Friedman and John B. Vickery. Baton Rouge: Louisiana State Univ. Press, 1970.

1633 PETERSON, Walter Scott. *An Approach to Paterson.* New Haven: Yale Univ. Press, 1967.

1634 POUND, Ezra. "Dr. Williams' Position." See **1161.** Reprinted in **1603** and **1604.**

1635 RIDDEL, Joseph. *The Inverted Bell: Modernism and the Counterpoetics of William Carlos Williams.* Baton Rouge: Louisiana State Univ. Press, 1974.*

1636 RIDDEL, Joseph. "The Wanderer and the Dance: William Carlos Williams' Early Poetics." See **1632.**

1637 SANKEY, Benjamin. *A Companion to William Carlos Williams' Paterson.* Berkeley: Univ. of California Press, 1971.

1638 THIRLWALL, John. "William Carlos Williams' 'Paterson'." *New Directions 17*. Norfolk, Conn.: New Directions, 1961.

1639 WAGNER, Linda Welshimer. *The Poems of William Carlos Williams: A Critical Study*. Middletown, Conn.: Wesleyan Univ. Press, 1964.

1640 WAGNER, Linda Welshimer. *The Prose of William Carlos Williams*. Middletown, Conn.: Wesleyan Univ. Press, 1970.

1641 WEATHERHEAD, Kingsley. *The Edge of the Image: Marianne Moore, William Carlos Williams, and Some Other Poets*. Seattle: Univ. of Washington Press, 1967.

1642 WHITAKER, Thomas R. *William Carlos Williams*. New York: Twayne, 1968.

1643 WILLARD, Nancy. *Testimony of the Invisible Man: William Carlos Williams, Francis Pongé, Ranier Maria Rilke, Pablo Neruda*. Columbia: Univ. of Missouri Press, 1970.

1644 WOODS, Powell. "William Carlos Williams: The Poet as Engineer." *MPS*, 1 (1970), 127–40. Reprinted in **1602**.

James Wright

Works of Poetry

1645 *Collected Poems*. Middletown, Conn.: Wesleyan Univ. Press, 1971. [Wesleyan U Pr]

1645a *To A Blossoming Pear Tree*. New York: Farrar, Straus, and Giroux, 1977. [Noonday]

1646 *Two Citizens*. New York: Farrar, Straus and Giroux, 1973. [FS & G]

Other Relevant Primary Materials

1647 "The Comic Imagination of Young Dickens." *Dissertation Abstracts*, 20 (1959), no. 1, 294.

1648 "An Interview with James Wright," with Michael André. *Unmuzzled Ox*, 1, 2 (February 1972), 3–8.

1648a "Letters From Europe, Two Notes From Venice, Remarks on Two Poems, and Other Occasional Prose." See **150a**.

1649 "Something to be Said for the Light: A Conversation with James Wright," with Joseph McElrath. *SHR*, 6 (1972), 134–53.

Critical Books and Essays

1650 BUTSCHER, Edward. "The Rise and Fall of James Wright." *GaR*, 28 (1974), 257 – 68.

1651 CARROLL, Paul. "James Wright," "As I Step Over a Puddle in the End of Winter, I Think of an Ancient Chinese Governor." See **102.**

1651a COLES, Robert. "James Wright: One of those Messengers." *APR*, 2, 4 (August 1973), 36 – 37.

1652 DEFREES, Madeleine. "James Wright's Early Poems: A Study in 'Convulsive' Form." *MPS*, 2 (1972), 241 – 51.

1653 DITSKY, John. "James Wright Collected: Alterations on the Monument." *MPS*, 2, 6 (1972), 252 – 59.

1654 HOWARD, Richard. "James Wright: 'The Body Wakes to Burial'." See **108.**

1655 JANSSENS, G. A. M. "The Present State of American Poetry: Robert Bly and James Wright." *ES*, 51 (1970), 112 – 37.*

1656 LACEY, Paul. "That Scarred Truth of Wretchedness." See **111.**

1656a MATTHEWS, William. "The Centrality of James Wright's Poems." *Oh R*, 18, 2 (1977), 44 – 57.

1657 MOLESWORTH, Charles. "James Wright and the Dissolving Self." *Sal*, 22 – 23 (Spring – Summer 1973), 222 – 33.

1657a SEAY, James. "A World Immeasurably Alive and Good: A Look at James Wright's *Collected Poems*." *GaR*, 27 (1973), 71 – 81.

1658 STITT, Peter A. "The Poetry of James Wright." *MinnR*, 2 (New Series) (Spring 1972), 13 – 32.

William Butler Yeats

Works of Poetry

1659 *Collected Poems.* New York: Macmillan, 1956.

1660 *Selected Poems and Two Plays of William Butler Yeats*, ed. M. L. Rosenthal. New York: Macmillan, 1962. [Macmillan]

1661 *The Variorum Edition of the Poems of W. B. Yeats*, ed. Peter Allt and Russell K. Alspach. New York: Macmillan, 1957.

Other Relevant Primary Materials

1662 *The Autobiography of William Butler Yeats.* New York: Collier Books, 1969. [Macmillan]

1663 *Collected Plays.* New York: Macmillan, 1956. [Macmillan]

1664 *Essays and Introductions.* New York: Macmillan, 1961. [Macmillan]

1665 *Explorations.* New York: Macmillan, 1962. [Important essays.]

1666 *William Butler Yeats: John Sherman & Dhoya*, ed. Richard J. Finneran. Detroit: Wayne State Univ. Press, 1969. [Early fiction.]

1667 *The Letters of W. B. Yeats*, ed. Allan Wade. New York: Macmillan, 1958.

1668 *Letters on Poetry from W. B. Yeats to Dorothy Wellesley.* New York: Oxford Univ. Press, 1940.

1668a *Letters to W. B. Yeats*, ed. Richard Finneran, et al. New York: Columbia Univ. Press, 1977.

1669 *Irish Fairy and Folk Tales*, ed. W. B. Yeats. New York: Random House, n.d. [G & D]

1670 *Mythologies.* New York: Macmillan, 1962. [Early fiction and some essays, especially "Per Amica Silentia Lunae."] [Macmillan]

1671 *The Oxford Book of Modern Verse*, ed. W. B. Yeats. Oxford: Clarendon, 1936. [His "Introduction" is important.]

1672 *The Poems of William Blake*, ed. W. B. Yeats. London: Routledge, 1905. Reprinted, Cambridge: Harvard Univ. Press, 1969.

1673 *The Speckled Bird*, ed. William O'Donnell. Dublin: Cuala, 1974. [Early fiction.]

1674 *Uncollected Prose by W. B. Yeats, Vol. I*, ed. J. P. Frayne. New York: Columbia Univ. Press, 1970 [1886–96.]

1674a *Uncollected Prose II: Reviews, Articles and Other Miscellaneous Prose 1897–1939*, Ed. J. P. Frayne and Colton Johnson. New York: Columbia Univ. Press, 1976.

1675 *A Vision: A Reissue with the Author's Final Revisions.* New York: Macmillan, 1962.

1676 *W. B. Yeats Memoirs*, ed. Denis Donoghue. London: Macmillan, 1972. [First draft of *Autobiography.*]

Biography, Bibliography, and Other Reference Materials

1677 CROSS, K. G. W., and R. T. DUNLOP. *A Bibliography of Yeats Criticism 1887–1965.* London: Macmillan, 1971. [Lists reviews.]

1678 ELLMANN, Richard. *Yeats: The Man and the Masks.* London and New York: Macmillan, 1948. [Dutton]

1679 HONE, Joseph M. *W. B. Yeats 1865–1939*, rev. 2nd ed. New York: St. Martin's, 1962.

1680 JEFFARES, A. Norman. *W. B. Yeats: Man and Poet*, 2nd ed. with corrections. London : Routledge & Kegan Paul, 1962.

1680a JOCHUM, K. P. S. *W. B. Yeats: A Classified Bibliography of Criticism.* Urbana: Univ. of Illinois Press, 1978.

1681 PARRISH, Stephen, and James PAINTER. *A Concordance to the Poems of W. B. Yeats*. Ithaca: Cornell Univ. Press, 1963.

1682 STOLL, John E. *The Great Deluge: A Yeats Bibliography*. Troy, N.Y.: Whitston, 1971. [Up to 1970.]

1683 WADE, Allan. *A Bibliography of the Writings of W. B. Yeats*, 3rd ed., rev. and ed. by Russell Alspach. London: Hart-Davis, 1968.

Collections of Critical Essays

1684 DONOGHUE, Denis, and J. R. MULRYNE, eds. *An Honoured Guest: New Essays on W. B. Yeats*. New York: St. Martin's, 1965.*

1685 FINNERAN, Richard J., ed. *The Byzantium Poems*. Columbus, Ohio: C. E. Merrill, 1970. [Merrill]

1686 HALL, James, and Martin STEINMAN, eds. *The Permanence of Yeats: Selected Criticism*. New York: Macmillan, 1950. [Classic essays exemplifying the reception of Yeats in the 1940s.] [Macmillan]

1687 JEFFARES, A. Norman, and K. G. W. CROSS, eds. *In Excited Reverie: A Centenary Tribute to William Butler Yeats*. New York: Macmillan, 1965.

1688 KEANE, Patrick J., ed. *William Butler Yeats: A Collection of Criticism*. New York: McGraw-Hill, 1973. [Mostly good selections from books.] [McGraw]

1689 SKELTON, Robin, and Ann SADDLEMEYER, eds. *The World of W. B. Yeats: Essays in Perspective*. Dublin: Dolmen, 1965. [U of Wash Press]

1690 STALLWORTHY, John, ed. *Yeats' Last Poems*. London: Macmillan, 1968. [Aurora]

1691 UNTERECKER, John E., ed. *Yeats: A Collection of Critical Essays*. Englewood Cliffs, N.J.: Prentice-Hall, 1963. [P-H]

1691a "Yeats Number." *JML*, 4, 3 (1975).

Critical Books and Essays

1692 ADAMS, Hazard. *Blake and Yeats: The Contrary Vision*. Ithaca: Cornell Univ. Press, 1955.

1693 ADAMS, Hazard. "Yeats, Dialectic, and Criticism." *Crit*, 10 (1968), 185–99.

1694 ALBRIGHT, Daniel. *The Myth Against Myth: A Study of Yeats' Imagination in Old Age*. New York: Oxford Univ. Press, 1972. [See especially the chapter on "The Tower."]

1695 ALTIERI, Charles. "From a Comic to a Tragic Sense of Language in Yeats's Mature Poetry." *MLQ*, 33 (1972), 156–71.

1696 ARCHIBALD, Douglas. "Yeats's Encounters: Observations on Literary Influence and Literary History." *NLH*, 1 (1970), 439–69.*

1697   AUDEN, W. H. "Yeats as an Example." *KenR*, 10 (1948), 187 – 95.*

1697a BELL, Michael. "The Assimilation of Doubt in Yeats's Visionary Poems." *QQ*, 80 (1973), 383 – 97.

1698   BEUM, Robert. *The Poetic Art of William Butler Yeats.* New York: Frederic Ungar, 1969.

1699   BLOOM, Harold. *Yeats.* New York: Oxford Univ. Press, 1970. [Oxford U Pr]

1700   BORNSTEIN, George. *Yeats and Shelley.* Chicago: Univ. of Chicago Press, 1970.

1701   BRADFORD, Curtis. *Yeats at Work.* Carbondale: Southern Illinois Univ. Press, 1965.

1702   BRADFORD, Curtis. "Yeats's Byzantium Poems: A Study of their Development." *PMLA*, 75 (1960), 110 – 25. Reprinted in **1691.**

1703   BRADFORD, Curtis. "Yeats's Last Poems Again." *Yeats Centenary Papers*, ed. Liam Miller. Chester Springs, Pa.: Dufour Editions, 1968. [On the order of *Last Poems.*]*

1704   BURKE, Kenneth. "On Motivation in Yeats." *SewR*, 7 (1942), 547 – 61. Reprinted in **1686.**

1705   DAVIE, Donald. "Michael Robartes and the Dancer." See **1684.**

1706   DAVIE, Donald. "Yeats, Berkeley, and Romanticism." Reprinted in *English Literature and British Philosophy: A Collection of Essays*, ed. S. P. Rosenbaum. Chicago: Univ. of Chicago Press, 1971.

1707   DE MAN, Paul. "Symbolic Landscape in Wordsworth and Yeats." *In Defense of Reading*, ed. Reuben Brower and Richard Poirier. New York: Dutton, 1962.

1708   DONOGHUE, Denis. "The Human Image in Yeats." See **48.**

1709   DONOGHUE, Denis. "On 'The Winding Stair'." See **1684.**

1709a DONOGHUE, Denis. *Yeats.* New York: Viking, 1971. [Viking]

1710   DUNSEATH, T. K. "Yeats and the Genesis of Supernatural Song." *ELH*, 28 (1961), 248 – 60.

1711   EAGLETON, Terry. "History and Myth in Yeats's 'Easter 1916'." *EIC*, 21 (1871), 248 – 60.

1712   ELIOT, T. S. "Yeats." See **576.** Reprinted in **1686.**

1713   ELLMANN, Richard. *Eminent Domain: Yeats among Wilde, Joyce, Pound, Eliot, and Auden.* New York: Oxford Univ. Press, 1967. [Oxford U Pr]

1714   ELLMANN, Richard. *The Identity of Yeats.* London: Macmillan; New York: Oxford Univ. Press, 1954. [Oxford U Pr]*

1715   ENGELBERG, Edward. "He Too Was in Arcadia: Yeats and the Paradox of the Fortunate Fall." See **1687.**

1716   ENGELBERG, Edward. *The Vast Design: Patterns in W. B. Yeats's Aesthetic.* Toronto: Univ. of Toronto Press, 1964.*

1716a EPSTEIN, Michael. "Yeats' Experiments with Syntax in the Treatment of Time." *Modern Irish Literature: Essays in Honor of William York Tindall*, ed. Raymond Porter and James Brophy. New York: Twayne, 1972.

1717   FRYE, Northrop. "The Rising of the Moon: A Study of *A Vision.*" See **1684.***

1718 FRYE, Northrop. "The Top of the Tower: A Study of the Imagery of Yeats." *SoR*, 5 (1969), 850 – 71.*

1719 FRYE, Northrop. "Yeats and the Language of Symbolism." *Fables of Identity: Studies in Poetic Mythology*. New York: Harcourt, Brace and World, 1963.

1720 GARAB, Arra M. *Beyond Byzantium: The Last Phase of Yeats's Career*. DeKalb: Northern Illinois Univ. Press, 1969.

1721 GROSSMAN, Allen R. *Poetic Knowledge in the Early Yeats: A Study of the Wind among the Reeds*. Charlottesville: Univ. of Virginia Press, 1969.*

1722 HARPER, George M. *Yeats's Golden Dawn*. London: Macmillan, 1974.

1723 HARRIS, Daniel A. *Yeats: Coole Park and BallyLee*. Baltimore: Johns Hopkins Univ. Press, 1974.

1724 HELLER, Erich. "Yeats and Nietzsche: Reflections on a Poet's Marginal Notes." *Encounter*, 33 (December 1969), 64 – 72.

1725 HENN, T. R. "The Accent of Yeats's Last Poems." See **1690**.

1726 HENN, T. R. "The Rhetoric of Yeats." See **1687**.

1727 HENN, T. R. *The Lonely Tower: Studies in the Poetry of W. B. Yeats*, rev. 2nd ed. New York: Barnes and Noble, 1965. [B & N]

1728 HOLLOWAY, John. "Style and World in 'The Tower'." See **1684**.*

1729 HOUGHTON, Walter. "Yeats and Crazy Jane: The Hero in Old Age." *MP*, 40 (1943), 316 – 29. Reprinted in **1686**.

1730 JEFFARES, A. Norman. *A Commentary on the Collected Poetry of W. B. Yeats*. Stanford: Stanford Univ. Press, 1968. [Contains most of the necessary background information for each of Yeats's poems.] [Stanford U Pr]*

1731 KENNER, Hugh. "The Sacred Book of the Arts." [The unity of *Wild Swans at Coole*.] Reprinted in **1691**.*

1732 KNIGHTS, L. C. "Poetry and Social Criticism: The Work of W. B. Yeats." *Explorations*. New York: Stewart, 1947.

1733 LEVINE, Bernard. *The Dissolving Image: The Spiritual-Esthetic Development of W. B. Yeats*. Detroit: Wayne State Univ. Press, 1970.*

1734 MACLEISH, Archibald. "Public Speech and Private Speech in Poetry." *Time to Speak*. Boston: Houghton-Mifflin, 1940. [See Yeats, *LDW*, p. 163 for a reference to this essay.]

1735 MARSH, Derick. "The Artist and the Tragic Vision: Themes in the Late Poetry of W. B. Yeats." *QQ*, 74 (1967), 104 – 18.

1736 MELCHIORI, Giorgio. *The Whole Mystery of Art: Pattern into Poetry in the Work of W. B. Yeats*. London: Routledge & Kegan Paul, 1960.

1737 MILLER, J. Hillis. "W. B. Yeats." See **77**.

1738 MOORE, Virginia. *The Unicorn: William Butler Yeats' Search for Reality*. New York: Macmillan, 1954. [Information on Yeats's interests in Hermetic thought.]

1739 MULRYNE, J. R. "The 'Last Poems'." See **1684**.

1740 OATES, Joyce Carol. *The Edge of Impossibility: Tragic Forms in Literature*. New York: Vanguard, 1972. [Includes two essays on Yeats.]

1741 O'BRIEN, Conor Cruise. "Passion and Cunning: The Politics of W. B. Yeats." *TriQ*, 23 – 24 (1972), 142 – 203.

1742 OLSON, Elder. " 'Sailing to Byzantium': Prolegomenon to a Poetics of the Lyric." *The University Review*, 8 (1942), 209 — 19. Reprinted in **1686.**

1743 PARKINSON, Thomas. "The Modernity of Yeats." *SoR*, 5 (1969), 922 — 34.

1744 PARKINSON, Thomas. *W. B. Yeats: The Later Poetry*. Berkeley: Univ. of California Press, 1965.

1745 PARKINSON, Thomas. *W. B. Yeats, Self-Critic: A Study of His Early Verse*. Berkeley and Los Angeles: Univ. of California Press, 1951.

1746 PERLOFF, Marjorie. " 'Heart Mysteries': The Later Love Lyrics of W. B. Yeats." *ConLit*, 10 (1969), 266 — 83.*

1747 PERLOFF, Marjorie. *Rhyme and Meaning in the Poetry of Yeats*. The Hague: Mouton, 1970.

1748 PRITCHARD, William. "The Uses of Yeats's Poetry." See **161.**

1749 RAINE, Kathleen. "Yeats, the Tarot, and the Golden Dawn." *SewR*, 27 (1969), 112 — 48.

1750 RONSLEY, Joseph. *Yeats's Autobiography: Life as Symbolic Pattern*. Cambridge: Harvard Univ. Press, 1968.

1751 SEIDEN, Morton Irving. *William Butler Yeats: The Poet as Mythmaker 1865— 1939*. East Lansing: Michigan State Univ. Press, 1962.*

1752 SHAPIRO, Karl. "W. B. Yeats: Trial by Culture." *In Defence of Ignorance*. New York: Random House, 1960.

1753 SHAW, Priscilla Washburn. "William Butler Yeats: A Balance of Forces." *Rilke, Valery and Yeats: The Domain of the Self*. New Brunswick, N.J.: Rutgers Univ. Press, 1964.

1754 SNUKAL, Robert. *High Talk: The Philosophical Poetry of W. B. Yeats*. Cambridge: Cambridge Univ. Press, 1973.*

1755 SPITZER, Leo. "On Yeats's Poem 'Leda and the Swan'." *MP*, 51 (1953— 54), 271 — 76.

1756 STALLWORTHY, Jon. "Yeats as Anthologist." See **1687.**

1757 UNTERECKER, John. *A Reader's Guide to William Butler Yeats*. New York: Noonday, 1959. [FS & G]

1757a URE, Peter. *Yeats and Anglo-Irish Literature*, ed. J. C. Rawson. Liverpool: Liverpool Univ. Press, 1974.

1758 VEEDER, William R. *W. B. Yeats and the Rhetoric of Repetition*. Berkeley: Univ. of California Press, 1968.

1758a VENDLER, Helen. "Sacred and Profane Perfection in Yeats." *SoR*, 9 (1973), 105 — 16.

1759 VENDLER, Helen. *Yeats's Vision and the Later Plays*. Cambridge: Harvard Univ. Press, 1963.

1760 WEBSTER, Brenda. *Yeats: A Psychoanalytic Study*. Stanford: Stanford Univ. Press, 1973.

1761 WHITAKER, Thomas R. *Swan and Shadow: Yeats's Dialogue with History*. Chapel Hill: Univ. of North Carolina Press, 1964.*

1762 WILSON, F. A. C. *W. B. Yeats and Tradition*. New York: Macmillan, 1958.

1763 WINTERS, Yvor. *The Poetry of William Butler Yeats*. Denver: Swallow, The Swallow Pamphlets No. 10, 1960.

1764 ZWERDLING, Alex. *Yeats and the Heroic Ideal*. New York: New York Univ. Press, 1965. [NYU Pr]

Louis Zukofsky

Works of Poetry

1764a   *A*. Berkeley: Univ. of California Press, 1978.

1765   *"A" 1— 12*, introduction by Robert Creeley. Garden City: Doubleday, 1967.

1766   *"A" 13— 21*. London: Jonathan Cape, 1969.

1767   *"A" 24*. New York: Grossman, 1972.

1768   *All: Collected Shorter Poems 1923— 1958*. New York: Norton, 1965. [Norton]

1769   *All: Collected Shorter Poems 1956— 1964*. New York: Norton, 1966. [Norton]

1770   *Found Objects 1926— 1962*. Georgetown, Kentucky: H. B. Chapin, 1964.

1771   *The Gas Age*. Newcastle upon Tyne: Ultima Thule, 1969.

Other Relevant Primary Materials

1771a   "Addenda to *Prepositions*." *JML*, (1974), 91 — 108.

1772   *Arise, Arise*. New York: Grossman, 1973. [Play: companion piece to 1767.] [Grossman]

1773   *Autobiography*. New York: Grossman, 1970.

1774   *Bottom: On Shakespeare*. Austin: Univ. of Texas Press, 1963.

1775   *Ferdinand*. London: Jonathan Cape, 1965. [Stories.] [Grossman]

1776   "Interview." *ConLit*, 10 (1969), 203 — 19.

1777   *Little: For Careenagers*. New York: Grossman, 1970. [Novel.]

1777a   *An Objectivist Anthology*. Folcroft, N.H.: Folcroft, 1975. [Reprint of anthology Zukofsky edited in 1932.]

1778   *Prepositions: Collected Critical Essays of Louis Zukofsky*. London: Rapp and Carroll, 1957.

1779   *A Test of Poetry*. New York: Corinth, 1948.

Biography, Bibliography, and Other Reference Materials

1780   ZUKOFSKY, Celia. *A Bibliography of Louis Zukofsky*. Los Angeles: Black Sparrow, 1969.

Collections of Critical Essays

1781   Catullus/Zukofsky Issue, *Grossteste Review*, 3, 4 (Winter 1970). [Considers the versions of *Catullus* by Celia and Louis Zukofsky. Essays on these versions and the issues they raise.]

Critical Books and Essays

1781a   CHARTERS, Samuel. "Essay Beginning 'All'." *MPS*, 3 (1973), 241 – 50.

1782   COX, Kenneth. "The Poetry of Louis Zukofsky: *A*." *Agenda*, 9 – 10 (1971 – 72), 80 – 89.

1783   DEMBO, L. S. "Louis Zukofsky: Objectivist Poetics and the Quest for Form." *AL*, 44 (1972), 74 – 96.

1784   DUDDY, Thomas. "The Measure of Louis Zukofsky." *MPS*, 3 (1973), 250 – 56.

1785   KELLY, Robert. "Song?/After Bread: Notes on Zukofsky's *A 1 – 12*." *Kulchur*, 3, 12 (Winter 1963), 33 – 63.*

1785a   KENNER, Hugh. *A Homemade World*. See **67a**.*

1786   KENNER, Hugh. "Of Notes and Horses." *Poetry*, 3, 2 (November 1967), 112 – 21.*

1787   RAFFEL, Burton. "No Tidbit Love You Outdoors Far as a Bier: Zukofsky's *Catullus*." *Arion*, 8 (1969), 435 – 45.

1788   WILLIAMS, Jonathan. "Zou-cough's Key's Nest of Poultry." *Kulchur*, 4, 14 (Summer 1964), 4 – 13.

1788a   YANELLA, Philip. "On Louis Zukofsky." *JML*, 4 (1974), 74 – 87.

INDEX

INDEX

INDEX

INDEX

INDEX

INDEX

INDEX

INDEX

INDEX

INDEX

INDEX

NOTES

NOTES

NOTES

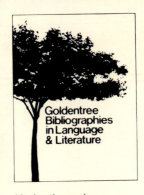

Goldentree
Bibliographies
in Language
& Literature

Under the series
editorship of
O.B. Hardison, Jr.

Afro-American Writers • *Darwin T. Turner*
The Age of Dryden • *Donald F. Bond*
American Drama from its Beginnings to the Present • *E. Hudson Long*
The American Indian: Language and Literature • *Jack W. Marken*
American Literature: Poe Through Garland • *Harry Hayden Clark*
American Literature Through Bryant • *Richard Beale Davis*
The American Novel: Sinclair Lewis to the Present • *Blake Nevius*
The American Novel Through Henry James, Second Edition • *C. Hugh Holman*
The British Novel: Conrad to the Present • *Paul J. Wiley*
The British Novel: Scott Through Hardy • *Ian Watt*
Chaucer, Second Edition • *Albert C. Baugh*
The Eighteenth Century • *Donald F. Bond*
Linguistics and English Linguistics, Second Edition • *Harold B. Allen*
Literary Criticism: Plato Through Johnson • *Vernon Hall*
Milton, Second Edition • *James Holly Hanford and William A. McQueen*
Modern British Drama • *Charles A. Carpenter*
Modern Poetry • *Charles F. Altieri*
Old and Middle English Literature • *William Matthews*
Romantic Poets and Prose Writers • *Richard Harter Fogle*
The Seventeenth Century: Bacon Through Marvell • *Arthur E. Barker*
Shakespeare • *David Bevington*
The Sixteenth Century: Skelton Through Hooker • *John L. Lievsay*
Tudor and Stuart Drama, Second Edition • *Irving Ribner and Clifford C. Huffman*
Victorian Poets and Prose Writers, Second Edition • *Jerome H. Buckley*

FORTHCOMING TITLES
The British Novel Through Jane Austen • *Wayne C. Booth and Gwin J. Kolb*
Women Writers in Britain and the United States • *Florence Howe and
    Deborah S. Rosenfelt*

AHM Publishing Corporation   **ISBN 0-88295-550-0**

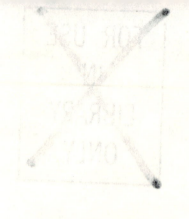

Oil and Water

Oil and Water

Cooperative Security
in the Persian Gulf

Edited by
Bjørn Møller

I.B. Tauris *Publishers*
LONDON • NEW YORK

Published in 2001 by I.B.Tauris & Co Ltd
6 Salem Road, London W2 4BU
175 Fifth Avenue, New York NY 10010
www.ibtauris.com

In the United States of America and in Canada distributed by
St Martins Press, 175 Fifth Avenue, New York NY 10010

ISBN 1 86064 625 5

A full CIP record for this book is available from the British Library
A full CIP record for this book is available from the Library of Congress

Library of Congress catalog card: available

Printed and bound in Great Britain by MPG Books Ltd, Bodmin
from camera-ready copy supplied by the author

CONTENTS

ACKNOWLEDGEMENTS

The present volume is the product of an author's symposium held in Elsinore, near Copenhagen, in March 1999. For the smooth preparation and management of this event, the editor is grateful to his assistant, Ms. Sidsel Westi-Kragh, and other staff at his home institution, the Copenhagen Peace Research Institute (COPRI). He is also grateful to Director Jamal al-Suwaidi of the Emirates Center for Strategic Studies and Research in Abu Dhabi, United Arab Emirates, who agreed to contribute a chapter to the book, even though he was unable to attend the symposium. For financial support not merely for this event, but for a the entire five-year project on the Global Non-Offensive Defence Network of which this event formed a part, he is grateful to the Ford Foundation.

Bjørn Møller
December 2000

INTRODUCTION

Regional Security: From Conflict Formation to Security Community

Bjørn Møller[1]

The Concept of 'Region'

After the end of the Cold War, regions and regionalism have received considerable attention, but the topic remains curiously underdeveloped theoretically.[2] Most studies simply take the concept as given and proceed to analyse regions one by one.[3]

All would agree that a region is a subset of the international system. However, the appropriate delimitation of such a subset is far from self-evident, if only because several criteria might be applied, each yielding a different result. None of them is, of course, more 'correct' than the others.

The most obvious criterion of 'regionness' is probably that of geographical proximity, as a region is usually held to consist of contiguous states. This does, however, beg the question of where to draw the outer limit, unless there happens to be clear natural boundaries (such as oceans). Do Afghanistan or Yemen, for instance, belong to the Persian Gulf region? Also, in the world of international relations 'proximity' is not so much a matter of distance as a function of topography, infrastructure and technology. What used to be insurmountable barriers may, for example, cease to be so as a result of a technological breakthrough. In some cases water divides, while in others—e.g. in the Persian Gulf—it unites, whereas vast deserts tend to divide.[4]

An alternative criterion of delimitation is the geographical distance from a centre, as in the ancient (but recently rediscovered) notion of empires. Conceived in analogy with an empire a region may thus be understood as a set of concentric circles.[5] This does, however, presuppose that there is one centre which is obvious as such to everybody. This may be politically very controversial, and it is entirely possible that there is not one, but several such centres. There is no a priori reason why a region should have the same financial, economic, political, cultural, and religious centre.[6] Some regions may thus have a 'variable geometry' rather than forming concentric circles.

To the extent that the analyst is interested in environmental issues

(including 'environmental security'), the notion of ecosystem (characterized, e.g., by shared rivers and or other sources of water supplies, etc.) may be the appropriate delimitation criterion.[7]

A convenient political or legal criterion of delimitation might be membership of institutions defined as 'regional', e.g. by the UN.[8] However, in parts of the world such as the Middle East and the Persian Gulf the density of institutions is much lower than in Europe. Furthermore, even in that most thoroughly institutionalized part of the world no institutions are all-inclusive.[9] In the Persian Gulf, moreover, no institutions exist which comprise all states (usually regarded as) belonging to the region, and nobody else (see Table 1 below).

A 'softer' criterion may be that of cultural affinity. Thus conceived, regions would be akin to the 'civilizations' between which Samuel Huntington foresees a clash.[10] However, cultural homogeneity is usually greater seen from the outside (where it is viewed as 'otherness') than from the inside. Cultural differences between islamic states such as Turkey, Saudi Arabia, Iran and Indonesia are, for instance, no less significant that those between, say, Denmark, Greece and the United States.[11] Furthermore, 'culture' has many aspects (e.g. religious, ideological, and ethnic) which do not automatically yield the same delimitation.

Related to this notion of cultural community is that of regions as 'imagined communities', in analogy with nations. Like the latter they may be constituted by the members 'imagining' themselves as belonging together, and the rest of the world acknowledging them as such, regardless of whether either has any 'objective' foundation.[12] In some parts of the world, however, a prevailing cosmopolitan orientation may cast doubt on such 'attitudinal regionness'.

Regions might also be identified as such by a greater-than-average intensity of trade and/or other forms of economic interaction. This would, however, lead to a disregard of not only rather autarchic states, but also of states producing mostly for the world market, i.e. which are not economically oriented towards any region, like the oil-exporting countries in the Persian Gulf.

Regions might also be conceptualized as 'zones'. While the term is usually applied to parts of states, it is also sometimes used of groups of states, where special and more peaceful 'rules' apply—i.e. in analogy with 'security communities'.[13]

Finally, regions might be defined by an above-average intensity of security political and military interaction—either benign, as in

alliances or regional collective security systems, or malign, as in arms races or wars. Barry Buzan has suggested the term 'security complexes' for such regions, defined as 'groups of states whose primary security concerns link together sufficiently closely that their national securities cannot realistically be considered apart from one another'.[14]

I shall take this latter criterion as my point of departure as it has the merit of singling out that particular aspect of interaction with which I am concerned on this occasion. The concept of security complexes does, however, have three odd implications, and it seems to require modification in one respect:

First of all, it either presupposes a narrow (i.e. 'traditional') concept of security, or it implies that the borders of a security complex depend on which issues are 'securitized' and 'desecuritized' in the dominant discourse. This may differ both between regions, and within regions over time.[15] Secondly, 'security communities' (between the members of which war has ceased to be regarded as a possibility, and where the attitude to military matters is one of benign neglect) cannot count as regions in this sense—even though a security community is usually seen as the starting point for regional integration.[16] Thirdly, in some parts of the world states may be so preoccupied with domestic ('security') matters, and have so insignificant power projection capabilities that states can constitute neither friends nor enemies to each other. Parts of Africa surely fall into this 'security complex-free' category.[17] Finally, it does not appear sensible to draw (as Barry Buzan does) fixed borders between security complexes so as to rule out the inclusion of certain states in more than one security complex. This presupposes defining those states that seemingly straddle the regional divides (the United States, Russia, Turkey, and China, for instance) as 'buffers', where the term 'transmission cords' seems a much more appropriate metaphor.

We have thus seen that the very concept of 'region' is not as clear as one might wish. The following analysis of the Persian Gulf region will only underline this lack of clarity, thereby pointing to the need for further research, both theoretical and empirical.

The Persian Gulf Region

Just as is the case for many of the world's other regions, the borders of the Persian Gulf region are not easily drawn, regardless of which criterion one applies. The situation is further complicated by the fact

that the name itself is
hotly disputed: the Arab
states resent the use of
the term 'Persian' which
they see as reflecting
Iranian hegemonical
aspirations, whereas both
the Iranians and most of
the rest of the world are
quite comfortable with
the term, underlining that
'Persian' is not the same
as 'Iranian'. In the
following, I shall prefer
the term 'Persian', but
without prejudice with
regard to Arab-Iranian
territorial disputes.

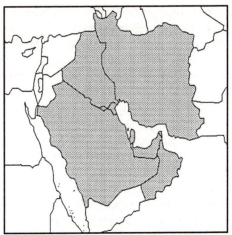

Fig. 1: *The Persian Gulf Region*

Almost inevitably one has to acknowledge a certain overlap
between the Persian Gulf region and, at least, four adjacent regional
systems, namely the Middle East, Central Asia, South Asia and the Red
Sea/Horn of Africa region—as illustrated in Table 1. An alternative
would be to collapse the Middle East and Persian Gulf (with parts of
Central and South Asia as well as the Maghreb) into a larger region
called the 'Greater Middle East', as argued in the chapter by Gulshan
Dietl in the present work.

Even though there is thus no 'correct' delimitation of the region,
borders nevertheless have to be drawn, both for political and analytical
purposes. In the following I shall therefore, rather arbitrarily, define
'The Persian Gulf Region' as encompassing the states marked in Figure
1: Iran and Iraq plus the states belonging to the Gulf Cooperation
Council (GCC), i.e. Bahrain, Kuwait, Oman, Qatar, Saudi Arabia and
the United Arab Emirates (UAE).

As the following analysis will, hopefully, bring out, all of these
states interact with each other in security matters more than they do
with other states (except the United States, more about which later).
Yemen is, of course, part of the picture, but its main security concerns
do not relate directly to the Gulf. Hence I have chosen not to count it
as part of the region.

Thus defined the Persian Gulf region not only qualifies as a

security complex, but it also constitutes a region according to several of the other possible criteria listed above: the 'contiguity', 'centre', and ecological criteria as well as that of 'imagination and recognition'.

TABLE 1: OVER-LAPPING REGIONS	Persian Gulf	Middle East	Other regions
Iran	C	p	Central Asia (South Asia)
Iraq	C	C	(Central Asia)
Bahrain, Kuwait, Oman, Qatar, UAE	C	p	(Red Sea)
Saudi Arabia	C	C	Red Sea
Yemen	p	p	Red Sea
Egypt	p	C	Maghreb (Red Sea)
Syria	p	C	-
Turkey	p	p	(Europe) (Central Asia)
Others	(Central Asian States) (Afghanistan) Pakistan (India)	Israel Palestine Jordan Lebanon Syria Egypt (Turkey)	**Legend:** C: Central member p or (): peripheral

Units and Structure

One might, of course, limit one's perspective to inter-state relations (in conformity with 'Realism'),[18] but one thereby risks missing important pieces of the puzzle. It is simply impossible to understand regional dynamics in the security sphere as exclusively state-centred and endogenous, i.e. without taking into account both internal and external actors, only some of which are states. Moreover, as a result of these dynamics, states definitely do not behave as 'like units', and to treat

them as such would seriously distort the picture.

One may subdivide the *dramatis personae* into at least six categories of relevant actors. Firstly, three sets of state actors:

1. Regional great powers, above all Iraq and Iran, but in certain respects also Saudi Arabia.
2. Regional small powers: Bahrain, Kuwait, Oman, Qatar and the UAE. For the reasons set out above, I have excluded Yemen.
3. External powers, above all the United States and, until recently, the Soviet Union. While Russia no longer plays much of a role, some of the other successors to the USSR do, albeit only as peripheral actors. The same is the case, in certain respects, for countries such as Britain and France, India and Turkey. Egypt and Syria have also recently played a role, albeit only a passing and secondary one.

Secondly, at least three categories of non-state actors have to be taken into account:

4. Substate and 'nonstate' collective actors such as ethnic and religious groups (e.g. Kurds, Palestinians and Shi'ites), ruling elites, clans, religious communities and leaders, and the militaries.
5. Regional organizations such as the GCC and the Arab League (*vide infra*). The EU also plays a role as an external regional organization, as does the Commonwealth of Independent States (CIS).
6. Global organizations, such as the United Nations and its subsidiaries, among which the IAEA (the International Atomic Energy Agency, responsible for monitoring compliance with the NPT, Non-Proliferation Treaty) and both UNSCOM (United Nations Special Commission, monitoring Iraq) and its successor, UNMOVIC (UN Monitoring, Verification and Inspections Commission). Economic organizations such as the World Bank and the IMF (International Monetary Fund) and, more recently, the World Trade Organization (WTO) also play a role, e.g. by significantly affecting the economies of the Gulf states (hence also their ability to purchase military hardware), as does OPEC (Organization of Petroleum Exporting Countries) and its Arab counterpart, OAPEC (Organization of Arab Petroleum Exporting Countries).

We would thus have to step beyond the 'parsimonious' theoretical framework of the 'Realists' in order to get a realistic picture of regional dynamics: by looking both *inside* states to comprehend the motivational factors underlying their international behaviour, and *beyond* states to take into account the growing role of international and supranational organizations.[19] In the following I shall nevertheless, place the focus on the interaction among states.

In trying to come to grips with a region such as the Persian Gulf, the following questions are central, which represent a mixture of such questions as commonly asked by Realists and those emphasized by authors of a more liberalist persuasion: Are the states constituting the region strong or weak states? Is the region dominated by endogenous dynamics, or is it 'overlaid' by external conflicts? Is it anarchical or hierarchical? If the former, does it nevertheless contain elements of order beyond that of self-help? What is the nature of its polarity? Is it unipolar, bipolar, multipolar or perhaps 'non-polar'? What is the predominant pattern of behaviour: balancing (if so: against power or threat?) or bandwagoning? What role, if any, do international organizations play?

On the following pages I shall venture some inevitably brief, superficial and tentative answers to these questions.

Strong or Weak States?

Stable regional dynamics presuppose strong states. Not in the 'traditional' sense of being strong military powers, but in the sense of possessing an internal socio-political cohesion, based on a well-defined 'idea' of the state, as well as the appropriate physical basis and institutional expression.[20] Without such foundations, states tend to be driven by a 'securitization' of domestic political agendas (ethnic or religious cleavages, for instance), which often spread to neighbouring states, thereby destabilizing the region as a whole, perhaps even to the point of war.[21]

Unfortunately for the stability of the Persian Gulf region, all its states fall into the category of 'weak states', even though some are weaker than others: All of them are new states (with the partial exception of Iran); most of them have religious or ethnic minority problems; most have unresolved border disputes with their neighbours; none of them have come anywhere near the standard of 'stable democracies', and none of them thus possess what might be called 'procedural legitimacy'. As far as 'performance legitimacy' is

concerned (which is sometimes held to be an alternative source of legitimacy), this may also be in jeopardy. The 'social contract' upon which this legitimacy (if so it is) has been based is endangered by two coinciding developments: high birth rates in all countries and stagnating oil prices. This will inevitably produce more mouths to feed with a smaller total 'cake', which is bound to create social trouble, perhaps upheavals and maybe even revolutions.[22]

It is beyond the scope of the present chapter to pursue this matter any further, even though I shall return briefly to it below. Suffice it at this stage to say that it would be foolhardy to count on domestic political stability in any of the region's member states, or to assume that such domestic instability will not affect inter-state relations and thereby regional stability.

External Penetration and/or Overlay?
During the Cold War, the bipolar rivalry between the two superpowers resulted in a certain involvement by both the United States and the USSR in regional security matters, i.e. a certain 'penetration', or 'external transformation' in the terminology of Barry Buzan. The question is whether the effect thereof was strong enough to count as 'overlay', under which the external dynamics displace region-internal ones, as was the case in Europe during the Cold War.[23] A brief account of the history of superpower involvement in the Persian Gulf region may shed some light on this question.

The first instance of competition had to do with the Soviet reluctance to withdraw from Iranian Azerbaijan in 1945/46, which developed into something of a crisis, yet without any major US involvement.[24] Indeed, no countries in the Middle East or Persian Gulf were on the list of the sixteen countries deemed to be of the greatest importance to US national security in 1947, even though Iran ranked as number four on the list of countries in urgent need of assistance.[25] The spread of 'domino beliefs' in the USA,[26] however, resulted in a perceived need to 'contain' the USSR anywhere.[27] Hence, a relentless quest for alliances from the late 1940s through the 1950s, partly justified in the name of the 'Eisenhower Doctrine': NATO, OAS, ANZUS, etc.—as well as an increasingly firm alignment with Israel.[28] The Persian Gulf manifestation thereof was the Baghdad Treaty. However, it proved very short-lived (1955-58), and after the Ba'ath revolution in Iraq, it effectively ceased to be.[29] In its place came a set of bilateral relations between the western powers and individual states

in the region.

The British withdrawal from east of the Suez by 1971 was followed by a growing US involvement. This involvement was guided, as elsewhere, by what one might call 'the four cardinal rules of amity and enmity': (1) a friend's friends are friends; (2) a friend's enemies are enemies; (3) an enemy's friends are enemies; and (4) an enemy's enemies are friends.[30]

The only qualification was that the Soviet Union did not have many friends in the region or its immediate neighbourhood. Moreover, the few it had were either too insignificant (South Yemen and Somalia, subsequently 'exchanged' with Ethiopia)[31] or too unreliable (Syria, Iraq and, until around 1972, Egypt), or both to really count for much. What the USSR achieved was little more than some port access rights and temporary access to airfields (in South Yemen, Syria, Iraq and, for a while, Egypt), a certain political influence, and the 'right' to provide arms to selected clients, above all Iraq and Syria.[32] The US policy nevertheless followed the logic that the USSR's friend Iraq was an enemy (according to rule 3), whereas Iraq's enemy Iran was a friend of the US (rule 4). There was, however, a significant anomaly, as the USSR's other friend in the region, Syria, was Iraq's enemy and a partial friend of Iran.

From the late 1960s through the 1970s, US policy toward the region was guided by the so-called 'Nixon doctrine' which envisaged a semi-hierarchical world order: At the pinnacle would, needless to say, be the USA. As an alternative to direct intervention (viz. the Vietnam syndrome), however, the USA would rely on 'regional policemen' (or 'subordinate regional hegemons') whom it would entrust to uphold regional 'order' and assist and equip for the job. Iran under the Pahlavi rule was cast in this role,[33] which, among other benefits, gained Tehran free access to US military technology—with nuclear weapons as the only exception. In a context where steeply rising oil revenues boosted Iran's purchasing power, this 'license to buy' resulted in an unprecedented arms build-up.[34]

After the 1979 revolution in Iran the United States was, of course, forced to reconsider this strategy. The revolution nearly coincided with the Soviet invasion of Afghanistan which, it was believed in Washington, presaged a Soviet 'quest for the warm waters' and a future threat to the oil supplies of the West.[35] Hence, to disengage was not regarded as an option. The review resulted in a renewed emphasis on direct intervention with the so-called Carter Doctrine, e.g. by means of

the Rapid Deployment Force, subsequently renamed CENTCOM (Central Command).[36] The ill-fated 1980 attempt to rescue the US hostages in Tehran, however, tempered this interventionist impulse considerably.[37]

During the 1980-88 Iran-Iraq war, the United States remained officially neutral, yet leaned more to the Iraqi than the Iranian side and supported the 1988 cease-fire, which was generally regarded as an Iranian defeat.[38] The USSR, in its turn, was too preoccupied in Afghanistan to really play much of a role in (the rest of) the region,[39] apart from continuing arms supplies to Iraq—interrupted only by a short-lived embargo imposed in the immediate wake of Baghdad's attack.[40]

The 1990 Iraqi invasion of Kuwait, of course, changed everything. It elevated Iraq from the status of a 'proxy enemy' of the West to an enemy in its own right (an image that was underpinned with rather far-fetched analogies with Nazi Germany)[41]—a position which Iraq continues to enjoy. A corollary thereof has been increased Western (and especially US) support for the GCC, including a (not particularly successful) quest for basing rights[42] and massive arms sales. However, Iran has not (yet) been accepted by the West, as one might have expected. The Islamic Republic remains in the category of 'rogues', hence the US strategy of 'dual containment' of both Iran and Iraq.[43] As a logical consequence thereof one might expect a rapprochement between these two former enemies, but this has yet to materialize.

Throughout the post-war period there was thus a significant penetration of the Persian Gulf region by the two rival superpowers. However, at no point did the bipolar logic determine regional 'patterns of amity and enmity' to anywhere near the extent it did in Europe, hence it would be overshooting the mark to label it 'overlay'. Security dynamics were primarily endogenous, leading us to the question of how to characterize these endogenous dynamics and the regional structure.

Anarchy and/or Order?
The Persian Gulf region is definitely anarchic in the sense that there is no political authority over and above the states. Such anarchy, however, may assume several different forms, some of which are more orderly than others as set out in Table 2.[44]

Along a spectrum of 'maturity' or 'modernity', the Persian Gulf clearly ranks quite low, as argued above. Most states are of very recent vintage and the State as an institution has yet to fully establish itself as

the supreme authority. State-building has yet to be completed, leaving all states as 'weak states', lacking in internal cohesion. Hence the predominance of domestic threats to state security—even though some of these have an inherent propensity to transcend borders, i.e. to become internationalized—the Kurdish problem being merely the most serious among a plethora of such problems.[45] In some cases, militarization and war may even be integral parts of the very state-building process.[46]

TABLE 2: PHASES OF ANARCHY					
	Structure	Pol. relations	Mitigating factors	Interaction	War?
Pre-anarchic Pre-modern	Unsettled	State building Non-recognition	Limited power projection	Low	Internal Small-scale
Anarchic Modern	Westphalian	Sovereignty Non-interference	Balance-of-power	Higher	Frequent Conflict formation
	Mature	State-centred Intern. society	Regimes Intern. Organizations	Interdependence	Rare Cold War
	Security Community	Governance	Cooperation	Very High	Inconceivable
Post-anarchic Post-modern	Integration	Transfer of legitimate authority	Growing together	Domestic	Inapplicable

The global spread of democracy has also not quite reached the Persian Gulf yet—not least because of the weakness of civil societies and persistent conflict between 'secularizers' and 'islamizers'. Hence, even though there are some encouraging signs, the presumed peace-promoting effect of democracy is not to be relied upon.[47]

As a regional system, the Persian Gulf has just entered the 'Westphalian stage', where mutual recognition of sovereignty is not yet

all-encompassing.[48] The region thus remains a 'conflict formation'[49] where war is entirely conceivable (perhaps even likely) between states—as evidenced by the recent wars and other armed conflicts in which regional states have been involved: The Iran-Iraq war (1980-88), the 1990 Iraqi invasion of Kuwait, followed by the UN coalition's war against Iraq for the liberation of Kuwait (January-February 1991), the US and British war against Iraq in December 1998, repeated US air strikes against Iraq (1993, 1996, 1998-2000), repeated Turkish incursions into Iraq in pursuit of Kurdish insurgents, the Yemen secessionist war of 1994, and the Yemen-Saudi Arabian clashes in 1995.

There are no immediate prospects of the region's developing into a security community, defined as a group of states among which war has ceased to be regarded as an option.[50] Part of the explanation is that there are so many outstanding territorial claims and ill-defined borders, reflecting the recent emergence of most of the states of the region.[51]

There are, on the other hand, certain factors that mitigate the rivalry among the states, i.e. certain patterns of restraint, including a certain cultural, religious and linguistic affinity among most states—with the partial exception of Iran. They thus share a commitment to important values, to which comes a certain commitment among all states to the survival of all; and an embryonic institutional framework. While this may arguably make the label 'international society' appropriate, it would surely be overstating the point to claim that the implicit restraints amount to a genuine 'security regime'.[52]

Forms of Polarity

There are different types of polarity.[53] Systems may thus be either unipolar (where states differ mainly according to the closeness of their relations with a hegemonic power); bipolar (where states tend, more or less consistently and tightly, to divide into two opposing camps); or multipolar, as in 'classical' balance-of-power systems. An instance of the latter is tripolarity, where the system comprises three competing poles, each having the option of joining forces with either one of the others against the third.[54] Finally, there may be no polarity to speak of, say when states are largely self-contained and interact only little with each other. This might be called a 'diffused' or 'nonpolar' system, or it may not even deserve the label 'system' at all.

It is difficult to envision a stable balance-of-power among the states of the Persian Gulf region, in either of these traditional forms. The region is definitely not unipolar in the sense of having one internal

pole, even though it may be under the influence of global unipolarity, i.e. the alleged *Pax Americana*—as argued by Birthe Hansen in her chapter in the present work. However, not only is this unipolarity questionable and, almost certainly, of a passing nature, at best; it is also too weak to produce a similar structure on a regional scale.[55]

A reimposition of some new form of global bipolarity on the Persian Gulf region also seems unlikely. So far the apparently most successful attempt at conjuring up a new global divide has been Samuel Huntington's infamous theorem of 'the West against the rest' (*vide supra*). However, even if Huntington should be right (which he, almost certainly, is not) this would tend to pit all of the Persian Gulf region against the West, i.e. serve as a unifying factor that might even supersede the Sh'ia/Sunni division. This is, however, a very unlikely prospect—which may, however, become increasingly conceivable the longer the US-British 'war of attrition' against Iraq lasts and is viewed by the population of the Arab (or Muslim) states as an anti-Arabic or anti-Islamic crusade.

Regional bipolarity does not seem at all likely either. Even though the region has several dividing lines, it lacks a single over-riding fault-line. While the division between Shi'a and Sunni is salient enough to produce frequent clashes between adherents of the two branches of Islam, it is much too weak to serve as a rallying point for alignment within either. Even if it were, the two islamic groupings are far too intermingled for this criterion to produce a bipolar pattern among states. Much more likely is an alignment of Shi'ite minorities in Sunni-dominated states with the main Shi'a-governed state, i.e. Iran.

The division between democratic and dictatorial regimes is too weak to divide the region, if only because of the predominance of shades of grey: No regimes are really totalitarian (even though Saddam Hussein's Iraq comes close)[56] and none are perfect democracies. A rich-versus-poor division might also make sense, but it strains the imagination to envision the poor lining up against the prosperous, at the state level at least.

A tripolar structure seems more likely, as the region has three obvious poles: Iran, Iraq and Saudi-Arabia. However, not only is the balance of power between these three regional great powers 'delicate', it is also highly asymmetrical. Rank-ordering Iran, Iraq and Saudi Arabia according to different yardsticks (all of which are surely important) thus yields quite different results (see Table 3).

While Iran is clearly in the lead with regard to population (i.e.

mobilizable military manpower), Saudi Arabia leads in terms of wealth (i.e. ability to purchase military hardware), and friends, i.e. allies. Iraq is in a tenuous position, the military balance-of-strength vis-à-vis Iran being 'delicate'. Perhaps paradoxically, such an asymmetric balance may be *more* stable than a symmetrical one (in which the disparities are not very large) as the various strengths may even out each other without being truly commensurable. On the other hand, it might also be *less* stable because it could produce such miscalculations of strength as have a well-documented propensity to lead to war.[57] In due course, I shall try to identify the military prerequisites of stable tripolarity.

TABLE 3: RANK ORDER	Population	Wealth	Military power	Friends
Iraq	2	3	2	3
Iran	1	2	1	2
Saudi Arabia	3	1	3	1

While temporary alignments between either two of these three powers against the third do not seem unlikely (in a medium-to-long term perspective at least), such alignments will probably prove fragile—as in a 'classical' balance-of-power system. The fragility of possible alignments may be illustrated by the options available to the regional great powers.

Saudi Arabia certainly fears Iraq, but not quite enough to produce any stable alignment with Iraq's enemies: Iran is also a threat (albeit of a different nature) and Syria too distant as well as too unreliable to really count.[58] Iraq fears Iran and its partial ally Syria[59] as well as Turkey[60] (and almost everybody else) but not quite enough to make alignments with anybody else seem worthwhile. Iran fears everybody else, but perhaps especially Iraq. However, not only does Iran's partial ostracism preclude its alignment with states that are not in a similar situation; Iran is also on a collision course with Saudi Arabia and the smaller oil-producing countries with regard to oil pricing. Furthermore, all the small Gulf states seem fearful of a resurgent Iran, hence they are unlikely to join forces with it—as argued by Jamal al-Suwaidi in his contribution to the present work. Even if they did, they would be too small to make much of a difference.

Tripolarity thus neither seems likely to evolve into bipolarity, nor

to assume the stable form that some scholars have claimed it might. Rather, it will probably produce shifting patterns of ad hoc alignments which may well be interrupted by hot wars. Furthermore, the regional balance-of-power will almost certainly be open-ended rather than self-contained, inter alia because all three states also have to guard against threats from other directions. What might, for instance, push Iraq towards Saudi Arabia would be a Syrian resurgence—say after a peace treaty with Israel that left Damascus with most of its military might intact, now available for use against Iraq. What might tilt Iran towards Iraq would be a more aggressive form of US 'containment' (vide infra); and what might effect a temporary Iran-Saudi Arabian alignment would be a lifting of UN constraints on Iraq, that might produce a resurgent as well as revengeful Iraq seeking regional hegemony. Other uncertainties stem from the rather unpredictable involvement of Israel and Turkey in the region's affairs[61]—which are analysed in the chapters by Gawdat Baghat, Wolfango Piccoli and Dietrich Jung in the present work.

Balancing or Bandwagoning?
What form the regional balance-of-power will assume to a large extent hinges on assumptions about state behaviour. Most analysts seem to agree with Kenneth Waltz and other neorealists that 'balancing' is a stronger inclination for states that 'bandwagoning', i.e. that states tend to join forces *against* a rising great power before the latter becomes predominant, rather than joining forces *with* it.[62]

On the other hand, this needs to be qualified somewhat, in order to account for anomalies such as the small Gulf states' teaming up in the GCC with their larger neighbour, Saudi Arabia, rather than balancing against it. The balance-of-threat analysis developed by Stephen Walt may thus be better at explaining state behaviour in the Gulf than traditional balance-of-power theory. The small states in the Gulf obviously bandwagoned with Saudi Arabia for the simple reason that they have feared the Iranian and/or Iraqi threat much more than that of Saudi Arabia growing too strong, as the latter was obviously more congenial and presumably benign.[63]

The Role of Organizations
A possible manifestation of both balancing and bandwagoning is the establishment of international organizations. The existence, growth and strengthening of international organizations may, furthermore, be the

key to transform regional systems from conflict formations to mature anarchies or security communities.[64] However, the record of the Gulf region is far from impressive in this respect.

TABLE 4: MEMBERSHIP OF INTERNATIONAL ORGANIZATIONS	B	In	Iq	K	O	Q	SA	UAE	Others
Arab League[65]	Y	N	Y	Y	Y	Y	Y	Y	Y
GCC	Y	N	N	Y	Y	Y	Y	Y	N
OAPEC	Y	N	Y	Y	N	Y	Y	Y	Y
OIC	Y	Y	Y	Y	Y	Y	Y	Y	Y
OPEC	N	Y	Y	Y	N	Y	Y	Y	Y

Legend:
B:Bahrain, In: Iran, Iq: Iraq, K: Kuwait, O: Oman, Q: Qatar,
SA: Saudi Arabia; UAE: United Arab Emirates;
GCC: Gulf Cooperation Council,
OAPEC: Organization of Arab Petroleum Exporting Countries,
OIC: Organization of the Islamic Conference,
OPEC: Organization of Petroleum Exporting Countries

First of all, there are no organizations which are truly regional in the sense of comprising all states in the region and nobody else. Membership is either too broad or too narrow, or both (see Table 4).

Secondly, most institutions are either too weak to really matter, or they only deal with security matters indirectly, or not at all. In principle, of course, security might be attained by indirect means, say by weaving a web of peace-furthering economic and other ties, constituting a genuine web of interdependence that might even point in the direction of actual integration (as was the case with the European institutions). However, neither the record of the region's past nor the prospects for its future are encouraging in this respect, as the economies in the region are far too similar to be complementary. Hence, institutions would probably have to deal with security directly for them to have an impact on it.

There has, to be sure, been one noteworthy attempt at institutionalized security cooperation, namely the GCC. Unfortunately, however, rather than seeking to involve the adversaries Iran and Iraq, the GCC has (so far) merely sought to provide defence and deterrence

against them. This is, moreover, a task for which the GCC (rightly or wrongly) considers itself inadequate. Hence the organization's main rationale may actually be to serve as a vehicle for ensuring the desired US support.[66] As I shall try to show below, however, this is probably both too pessimistic (with regard to the regional balance of power) and too optimistic in the implicit hopes for US commitments.

The Security Dilemma in the Persian Gulf

The preliminary assumption that the Persian Gulf region is unstable thus seems to have been confirmed by the above analysis—even without taking military developments into account. This is the topic to which I shall now turn.

One of the most striking features about the Persian Gulf has been the general arms build-up through the 1990s until quite recently (See Table 5). This has set the region apart from most of the rest of the world, where military expenditures have been steadily declining.

The war between Iraq and the UN coalition for the liberation of Kuwait (henceforth 'the Gulf War' for short) dramatically affected the regional balance-of-power by reducing and neutralizing Iraq's military strength. This, in turn, may have raised the ambitions of other states in the region, including Iran,[67] which bodes ill for stability. While it is questionable whether 'balance' is stabilizing if understood as 'rough equality', it is generally agreed that rapid and profound changes in the balance of power have a negative impact on stability. Not only do they hamper a realistic assessment of strength; they also provide declining powers with a motive for preventive war and rising ones with incentives to accelerate their ascent by means of war.[68]

Iraq

Iraq has since 1990 been cast in the role as the main threat to the stability of the Persian Gulf, and its military potential may certainly have warranted this view, at least until recently.

During the Cold War, Iraq benefitted from the Soviet desire for a counterweight to US influence in the region and was a major recipient of Soviet weapons of all kinds: tanks, artillery, combat aircraft and SCUD ballistic missiles. This provided Baghdad with a considerable offensive striking power, which Iraq sought to further enhance by the development of WMD (weapons of mass destruction). While it did assemble a large stockpile of chemical weapons, and actually used some against its own Kurdish population during the war

with Iran,[69] it did not succeed in building nuclear weapons. However, thanks to a concerted clandestine effort, it was a close shot, as evidence uncovered after Iraq's 1991 defeat has made clear.[70] Saddam Hussein also launched a biological weapons programme, producing both anthrax and botulinum toxin.[71]

The motives behind this build-up are not quite as obvious as they might seem. In retrospect, one might be tempted to take the 1980 Iraqi attack against Iran and that against Kuwait a decade later as incontrovertible evidence of inherent aggressiveness, but this may be too simplistic. The 1980 attack may, on closer analysis, have been produced by a combination of 'windows of threat and opportunity' which may have appeared all the more tempting as well as imperative because of the dictatorial form of government. Dictatorships are notoriously prone to both paranoic fears and illusions of grandeur, i.e. they tend to exaggerate both threats to their rule (i.e. 'windows of vulnerability') and their own ability to redress the situation, hence are more likely than other states to jump through presumed 'windows of opportunity'.[72]

On the one hand, Iraq had clearly been surpassed by the US-sponsored Iranian arms build-up during the 1970s (*vide infra*) and may have been worried about a possible Iranian aggression, or at least about Iran's assuming a hegemonic role entailing a 'right' to intervene in the internal affairs of other regional states. The prospects of the latter must have appeared frightening in view of Iraq's Shi'ite majority and 'Kurdish problem'. On the other hand, the 1979 Islamic Revolution and the accompanying severance of the US-Iran link produced a temporary weakening of Iran, which Iraq may have wanted to exploit by means of a war that was supposed to have been short and decisive.[73]

This, of course, proved to be a monumental miscalculation, and the ensuing war depleted Iraq's resources, militarily, financially and otherwise—while its neutral neighbours prospered. Hence perhaps the perceived need to 'redress the balance' with the invasion of Kuwait in 1990, which Saddam Hussein may have regarded as a rather trivial venture, unlikely to attract much attention.[74] This, too, proved to be a miscalculation of gargantuan proportions, as it incurred the wrath of the rest of the world (with a few exceptions) and especially of the USA. Hence Operation Desert Shield which averted a hypothetical further Iraqi expansion, and the subsequent Operation Desert Storm inflicting a crushing defeat on Iraq.[75]

In the aftermath of the war, with UNSCR (United Nations

Security Council Resolution) 687 Iraq has been subjected to the most intrusive and rigid constraints ever imposed on a sovereign state since those imposed on the vanquished after the Second World War. Not only has Iraq lost its 'right' to entire categories of weaponry that were regarded by its adversaries as particularly threatening (WMD and ballistic missiles).[76] It has also temporarily lost control over part of its national territory by the (*not* UN mandated) imposition of 'no fly zones' in the northern and southern parts of the country by the United States, the UK and France. They encompass a total of around sixty percent of Iraq's territory, which the US and the UK have been bombing from the air on an approximately twice-weekly basis since the attack against Iraq in December 1998 (see the chapters by myself, Jalil Roshandel and Anthony McDermott in the present work). Even though Iraq is thus currently being treated by the two Western powers as almost a 'no man's land', nobody (else) seems to want the elimination of Iraq as a state. Hence, it is bound to reemerge, at some stage, as a major player, also in military terms.

Regardless of what motives Iraq may have had for its arms build-up and aggressions, however, they are rightly seen by its neighbours as a threat that can only be ignored at their peril.[77] Hence, Iraq's military strength inevitably spurs a similar build-up in neighbouring states.

Iran
As mentioned above, Iran was the Third World's number one spender on arms in the 1970s, partly as a consequence of the role as a regional hegemon which was envisioned for it by the USA. The Pahlavi regime bought just about everything, with WMD as the only exception. Another explanation of this massive arms build-up was, of course, Iran's vastly expanded purchasing power as a result of its rising oil revenues.

After the 1979 revolution, however, sources of supply rapidly dried out. The war with Iraq, furthermore, rapidly exhausted the stocks (a strengthened indigenous production and some clandestine supplies notwithstanding) with the result that Iran by 1988 had a much depleted military arsenal as well as a severely damaged economy and a weakened political basis. Iranian military planners may also have drawn the lesson from the lost war that their strategy simply did not work, hence that their military posture (or what was left of it) was obsolete.[78] The 1988 cease-fire was thus, understandably, followed by a build-up which some observers regard as excessive, others even take

as evidence of aggressive intentions.[79]

However, while one cannot entirely discount the hypothesis of Iranian expansionist designs, the facts also lend themselves to a more 'innocent' interpretation. First of all, Iran has yet to make up for its wartime losses, and its military strength remains inferior to what it was at a time when it was regarded (by the United States at least) as a stabilizing factor. Secondly, the arms acquisitions of the Islamic Republic as well as its military expenditures remain well below those of the GCC (See Table 5). Thirdly, most of Iran's arms acquisitions have been entirely consistent with defensive intentions. In such an evaluation, one must, in all fairness, take into account that the country must remain fearful of an eventually resurgent Iraq; that it has long borders facing unstable countries such as Afghanistan and some former Soviet republics; and that it must be worried about the new American assertiveness that might even lead to intervention (say, in the name of 'counter-proliferation').[80]

With the possible partial exception of the alleged nuclear weapons programme and the ballistic missiles, the 'Iranian threat' is thus probably not so much a military threat[81] as something *sui generis*, namely a threat of terrorism (to which all countries are vulnerable) and one of 'ideological contagion'. Serious though they may certainly be, neither of these threats warrants a reciprocal arms build-up that will not help at all. Also, there are many indications that Iranian foreign and defence policy have entered, since around 1988 or 1989, a more pragmatic phase, and that the terrorist element has been down-played considerably or abandoned for good. The continued containment of Iran may thus have become counterproductive.[82]

The GCC States
Both Saudi Arabia and the smaller GCC countries have embarked upon an intense arms build-up, that has included the purchase of both armoured vehicles (main battle tanks and armoured personnel carriers), artillery, surface-to-air missiles and Patriot anti-tactical ballistic missiles, as well as an array of warships (frigates, corvettes, patrol craft, etc.), to which may perhaps be added submarines (contemplated by the UAE). Above all, however, the GCC states have bought sophisticated aircraft in large batches (see Tables 5 and 6).

The arms purchases are probably spurred by two different sets of motives: A desire to enhance indigenous defence capabilities, yet not so much that the US would feel that it could disengage completely; and

a wish to please the US by appearing to do whatever could reasonably be expected from them, and do so by buying weaponry 'Made in the USA'. Arms deals may thus be just as much a reflection of 'burden-sharing' concerns as of actual defence planning—as was the case with much of NATO-Europe's planning during the Cold War. Nevertheless, arms acquisitions produce military options, especially when pooled as in the GCC.[83] They may therefore lead to reciprocal steps by the GCC's adversaries, *in casu* both Iran and Iraq, regardless of the 'innocent' motives behind them.

Table 5: Balance of Power[84]										
	Mil. Expend. (Constant 1997 US$)				Armed Forces (1000)				Arms Imports (Constant 1997 US$)	
	1987	%	1997	%	1987	%	1997	%	'87-90	%	'91-97	%
Iran	9,350	13	4,730	13	350	24	575	43	10,044	14	6,226	7
Iraq	35,000	48	1,250	4	900	63	450	33	21,212	30	0	0
GCC	28,644	39	29,515	83	186	13	326	24	40,734	57	88,956	94
Bahr.	214	0	533	2	4	0	9	1	969	1	687	1
Kuwait	1,630	2	2,760	8	20	1	28	2	1,032	1	8,049	9
Oman	2,020	3	1,820	5	27	2	38	3	280	0	1,496	2
Qatar	1,060	2	992	3	11	1	11	1	374	1	3,643	4
S.A.	21,600	30	21,100	59	80	6	180	13	34,353	48	68,197	72
UAE	2,120	3	2,310	7	44	3	60	4	3,726	5	6,884	7

An Arms Race in Progress?
Even though the present level of armament in the Persian Gulf does not warrant the kind of alarmist response from the (much more heavily armed) North that one frequently encounters, it may nevertheless be a cause of concern for the countries in the region themselves. The latter is especially the case if the present build-up continues, which depends on whether we are witnessing an arms race without saturation point, or merely a replenishment of depleted stocks and 'business-as-usual' modernization that will reach a saturation point sooner or later.

If the build-up continues, the region may end up in a situation of fragile balance, i.e. a situation where everybody (at least the three great powers) is in a position to hurt everybody else (including the small powers), but where neither side is capable of defending itself against a determined surprise attack. One might label this a 'mutual offensive

superiority' stance. This would indeed, by an instance of tripolar *in*stability. All three major states may thus be able to retaliate after any attack, which may provide a stability of sorts, like that of the closing scene of the movie *Pulp Fiction*, where the two couples hold each other at gunpoint.

Such a stalemated situation is only stable up to a point, namely when one of the actors moves (in either direction), in which case even a very small move may well produce a chain reaction: If one of the three states lowers its guard (say, by a partial demobilization), the incentive of (one or both of) the others to exploit the window of opportunity may prove irresistible. If either one steps up (say, by a mobilization or just a large-scale military exercise) one or both of the others may fear an impending surprise attack, hence strike preemptively.[85]

The US Role

As described above, the United States has been deeply involved in the Persian Gulf region since the 1950s—both economically and militarily, via shifting alliances, and plans for direct intervention, most recently in the war against Iraq for the liberation of Kuwait. This has been followed by a forging of ties with individual GCC countries and support for the GCC as a combined anti-Iraqi and anti-Iranian alliance.[86]

However, it has also been followed by contingency plans for new (if need be unilateral) interventions, for instance in the name of 'counter-proliferation'. While the latter programme involves mainly arms control initiatives and the provision of incentives to possible proliferators, the possibility of 'pre-emptive' strikes against nuclear facilities has also been contemplated, and actually carried out, as happened in Operation Desert Fox in December 1998.[87]

While the United States might thus play the traditional (stabilizing) role as 'balancer' in the future, it is presently doing the exact opposite, with inevitably detrimental implications for regional stability. A precondition for playing the role of the 'external stabilizer' is a certain impartiality, which is incompatible with singling out, rather arbitrarily, some states as 'rogues' that are dangerous because of their very nature rather than because of their actual behaviour.

To some extent, the United States' allies in Europe have simply 'followed their leader', by providing some support to US-led ventures. To the extent that the Europeans have had their own policies towards

the region, however, they have tended to act as a tempering factor. As a general rule, European states have placed a lesser emphasis on military strength, have been more prepared for a dialogue with the 'rogues' (see the chapter by Lars Erslev Andersen), and less inclined to contain them by military or economic means.[88] However, in view of the fact that the European countries do not, so far at least, play any central role in the region, I shall largely disregard their effect in the following.

Resolving the Security Dilemma?
Having thus painted a far from rosy picture of the security political situation prevailing in the Persian Gulf region, I shall in this section advance some suggestions for an improvement, i.e. stabilization. Not because stability and order is always a good thing, but because changes of the status quo by violent means are nearly always worse. Ideally, the situation should be stabilized and relaxed to such an extent that modifications of the status quo (politically, economically, perhaps even territorially) become possible by peaceful means.

The Philosophy of Common Security
The theory (or even philosophy) of Common Security was developed in the early 1980s against the background of a severe, systemic, ideological and seemingly enduring conflict, *in casu* that between East and West. The regional features of the conflict(s) in the Persian Gulf region bear a striking resemblance to this. Hence, if Common Security was a valid approach to the East-West conflict, it seems reasonable to assume that it might, *mutatis mutandis*, also be relevant to the Gulf.

As formulated by the Palme Commission in its 1982 report,[89] the 'Common Security approach' implies an acknowledgement of the conflict as genuine (contrary to certain peace research theories), and merely suggests alternative means to the same ends, i.e. national security in a hostile environment. The point of departure in the development of a political strategy of Common Security was the interactive nature of international relations: States respond to each other's moves, as they see each other as opponents, hence are predisposed to view their opponent's actions as (potentially) hostile. What states do in response, moreover, becomes a stimulus for response, i.e. it spurs a counter-reaction on the part of their adversaries. This can easily develop into a spiral of malign interaction, as defensive reactions tend to be interpreted as proactive offensive moves.

A consequence of this action-reaction phenomenon is that states find themselves in a 'security dilemma', the two 'horns' of which are not to respond at all (thereby risking vulnerability to whatever the other side might do), or to respond with (re)actions which the other side may find threatening, thereby perhaps provoking the other side to do precisely what the defensive response was intended to avert, or something even worse.[90] Common Security may simply be understood as a strategy for escaping (or at least circumventing and/or mitigating) the security dilemma, i.e. as an admonition to always consider how the respective other side may view the actions one is contemplating. It is thus based on the acknowledgement that neither side can achieve security at the respective other's expense, but that a precondition for the security of either side is that the respective other also feels secure.

This general rule seems perfectly applicable to the Persian Gulf, where it is probably unwise and shortsighted of the smaller states to seek unilateral security at the expense of either Iraq or Iran (or both), if only because the potential of these two regional great powers may eventually manifest itself in military superiority. It is more likely to do so, the more either state feels threatened by its neighbours or others. Should it do so, it will surely be to the smaller states' advantage to have a peaceful rather than a revengeful Iran or Iraq in their vicinity.

Common Security in its original formulation did not presuppose actual negotiations or agreements, but might be implemented in a 'tacit coordination mode', i.e. as a form of 'cooperation among adversaries'.[91] However, if security can only be obtained by two adversaries simultaneously, it will surely facilitate matters if they can actually exchange views and reach agreements—and even more so if there are institutional frameworks ready at hand for such direct collaboration. This was envisaged by the reinvigorated concept of 'common security for the nineties and beyond', namely 'Cooperative Security'.[92]

A cooperative security approach to the regional conflict(s) in the Persian Gulf would have to involve both Iran and Iraq as directly as possible, i.e. integrate rather than contain the two perceived main threats to regional stability (*vide infra*).[93] One possible means to this end might be the forging of economic ties, preferably promoting a multi-dimensional mutual interdependence that would give all states a stake in maintaining peace.[94] An obstacle to this is, however, the above-mentioned lack of complementarity between the economies of the region.

Another approach would entail discussions on security-related matters, which may or may not take the form of actual negotiations. It may be more realistic for such discussions to assume a form similar to that of the consultations held under the auspices of the ASEAN (Association of South-East Asian Nations) Regional Forum, i.e. informal, non-binding discussions. This would allow participants to deal with a comprehensive agenda, including all aspects of an expanded concept of security—which will be particularly useful if it is true that the 'Iranian threat' is primarily an ideological one. Such discussions (in the form of 'track two diplomacy') have taken place for the Middle East, e.g. under the auspices of UNIDIR (United Nations Institute for Disarmament Research), and a similar process (albeit 'track three') pertaining to the Persian Gulf has been launched and is described by Majid Tehranian in his contribution to the present volume. The present author has enjoyed the privilege of being involved in both projects.[95]

Cooperative security, however, would also have to deal directly with military matters. One implication thereof might be a series of regional seminars on military doctrines, similar to those held in Europe under the auspices of the CSCE (Conference on Security and Cooperation in Europe), but which also have their (less formal or official) counterparts in the ASEAN.[96] They might provide a venue for a frank and open, yet in no way binding, exchange of opinions on reciprocal threat perceptions, hence of dismantling unwarranted threat misperceptions. However, divulging military doctrines and strategies and illuminating military postures obviously only have such a benign effect if what is being revealed is actually non-threatening.

Defensive Restructuring

To thus make strategies and military postures non-threatening is precisely what non-offensive defence (NOD) is all about, a concept which is also known as 'structural inability to attack' (SIA), 'defensive defence' (DD), 'non-provocative defence' (NPD) or 'confidence-building defence' (CBD).

While all these terms refer to a (more or less hypothetical) end-point where states have enough defensive strength, but a minimum of offensive capabilities, 'defensive restructuring' refers to the path leading in this direction, i.e. a simultaneous build-down of offensive and upgrading of defensive capabilities.[97] It is beyond the scope of the present paper to elaborate much on this. Suffice it to say that it is *not* a matter of outlawing 'offensive weapons' in favour of 'defensive

weapons', but of changing total military postures and strategies; and that it is not a matter of absolutes but of degrees.[98]

Applied to the Persian Gulf region the aim-point would be a stance where each corner of the Iran-Iraq-GCC triangle would feel secure in its ability to defend itself, preferably even without external assistance, i.e. one of 'mutual defensive superiority'. This notion has traditionally been applied only to bipolar settings and, admittedly, becomes much more complicated and demanding under conditions of multipolarity.[99] In its most demanding version this would require each of the three parties to be able to successfully defend itself against an attack by the other two combined.

Fortunately, living up to this is almost prohibitively demanding standard is probably not required, as it seems extremely unlikely that Iran and Iraq would team up against the GCC states, or that the latter (individually or jointly) would 'bandwagon' with either Iran or Iraq as a putative aggressor against the respective other, however much they might disapprove of the victim. More likely is the, much less demanding, situation where an aggressor would risk having to fight the two others, i.e. where the combined strength of the two should surpass the offensive strength of the third. Such a situation might be described as a 'collective security scenario', where 'balancing behaviour' would predominate, as it was argued above that it generally tends to do. States would team up, but only for defensive purposes, whereas an aggressor would be on his own. The reason why this scenario is more likely than the other is that neither Iran nor Iraq would be comfortable with the other's establishment of a hegemony through aggression—in view of their long history of rivalry.

At worst, either the GCC, Iran or Iraq would try to remain neutral (as Iran did during the Gulf War) in a war between the respective two other sides of the triangle. It further seems likely that the rest of the world would get involved in a renewed war of aggression (as in the Gulf War), regardless of who would start it—albeit most likely with either of the two 'rogues' cast in the role as aggressor. This involvement would not necessarily take the form of military intervention, but arms embargoes and economic sanctions would also help tilt the balance against an aggressor.

The figures in Table 6 seem to provide some support for this rather sanguine view of the prospects for stability through defensive superiority in the region. In most weapons categories as well with regard to military manpower, neither Iran or Iraq nor the combined

GCC possess anything approaching a crushing war-winning superiority.

This optimism however, needs to be qualified with the following considerations. It presupposes that the GCC remains in force and that it will withstand the strains of a war. The assistance of the smaller GCC states may not be decisive for Saudi Arabia, but the opposite is certainly the case, especially on the pessimistic assumption that no outside help will be available. It also presupposes that aggressors will not gang up against victims. Even though this seems a realistic assumption, unlikely events sometimes happen.

Table 6: The Iran-Iraq-GCC Military Balance[100]				
Ground Forces				
Troops (1000)	**Tanks**	**APC/ AFV**	**Artil- lery**	**Heli- copters**
Iran	518	1,520	11,235	2,640	293
% of total	42	28	12	45	28
Iraq	433	2,000	2,000	2,050	370
% of total	35	37	19	35	35
GCC	284	1,870	7,387	1,142	389
% of total	23	35	70	20	37

	Air and Naval Forces				
	SS Missiles	**Combat Aircraft**	**Transport Aircraft**	**Combat Vessels**	**Patrol Craft**
Iran	400	205	91	31	139
% of total	86	22	39	30	33
Iraq	25	210	0	370	2
% of total	5	23	0	35	2
GCC	40	504	145	69	284
% of total	9	55	61	68	67

Legend:
APC/AFV: Armoured Personnel Carriers/Armoured Fighting Vehicles; SS: Surface-to-Surface

Stability trough defensive restructuring obviously presupposes that analytical distinctions can be made between offensive and defensive strength—not only *in abstracto* but also concretely. Should concrete analysis reveal that, say Kuwait's tanks are defensive, but those of Iraq

offensive, then whatever arms control packages might be negotiated would have to be very asymmetrical in order to address the problem. A compelling argument has, for instance, been made (by Eric Arnett) that a build-up of Iranian ground forces is defensive (a shield against Iraq), but that a build-up of the same size in air and naval forces is more offensive.[101] Furthermore, as deterrence is only in the mind of a potential aggressor, perceptions have to be factored into the equations. What matters for war prevention is not whether, say, the GCC could actually defend itself against Iraq or Iran, but whether either of the latter believe so or not. If not, an aggressor would stand to lose the war initiated by itself, but this would be rather cold comfort for the victims.

A final complication may be that both Iran and Iraq probably fear a US attack, especially one undertaken with regional support from (all or some of) the GCC states (such as Operation Desert Fox). It is true that the United States has contingency plans to wage two (or even two-and-a-half) MRCs (major regional conflicts) simultaneously, and to do so offensively with a view to winning swiftly and decisively. However, it is also true that the American public is unlikely to allow the Pentagon to get its way with this—especially not in the case of an unprovoked US attacks that would cost (more than a few) American lives.[102] By implication, both Iran and Iraq should be relatively safe if they were to combine non-provocation with the ability to exact a significant price (in the form of body-bags) from an aggressor, e.g. the United States.

Defensive Restructuring in the Gulf
Having thus sketched the rationale for a defensive restructuring and the standards to which it should live up, what remains is to concretize the implications, both as far as possible arms control endeavours and unilateral defence planning are concerned.

WMD Arms Control
One might, of course, argue (as some self-proclaimed Realists do) that a certain nuclear proliferation would improve stability by virtue of the caution-installing effects of the possession of nuclear weapons. However, even if one were to welcome, say German or Japanese nuclear weapons,[103] virtually nobody would prefer a nuclear-armed Iraq or Iran to the same countries with 'only' conventional weapons.

Relevant safeguards against the regional proliferation of WMD

would, as a minimum, require a strengthening of existing non-proliferation regimes—the NPT (Non-Proliferation Treaty), the CTBT (Comprehensive Test Ban Treaty), and the conventions banning biological and chemical weapons as well as the various export regulations under the Zangger Committee and the NSG (Nuclear Suppliers Group).[104] Rather than addressing WMD proliferation risks one by one, it may be more realistic to 'lump them all together' in a zone free of WMDs, as stipulated as a goal in the 1991 cease-fire resolution alongside the more specific demand for a nuclear-weapons-free zone (NWFZ).[105] This would take account of the fact that whatever chemical and biological weapons Iran or Iraq may have or acquire in the future are probably partly motivated by (or at least justified with reference to) Israel's nuclear weapons, just as the opposite is also the case.[106]

Considering that WMD without suitable means of delivery are of little use, it may also help to deny prospective proliferators access to such means of delivery. The MTCR (Missile Technology Control Regime) falls into this category of indirect supply-side anti-proliferation measures with its restrictions on the transfer of both assembled missiles and various technologies for producing missiles with ranges exceeding 300 kilometres and payloads of more than 150 kilos.[107]

What is conspicuous by is complete absence is, however, any set of restrictions on the acquisition of the most suitable means of delivery of all, namely aircraft—probably for two reasons: First of all, contrary to ballistic missiles aircraft are very effective for conventional as well as for nuclear missions; hence to deny states access to aircraft is seen as tantamount to denying them means of national defence. Applying an offensive-defence distinction, however, will reduce the strength of this argument considerably. Secondly, the global airframe industry is in severe crisis, hence the strong economic motives for continuing to sell to whoever is able to pay.[108]

Confidence-Building Measures
Confidence-building measures (CBMs) are intended to mitigate the security dilemma by reducing misperceptions, i.e. by enhancing transparency of military affairs. Not only does this relieve states of unwarranted concerns about their opponents; it also allows genuinely peaceful states to demonstrate their benign intentions to their adversaries.[109] While such transparency-enhancing CBMs usually

pertain merely to military activities, it would merely be a small step to expand then to military planning and holdings.

Relevant measures might include pre-notification of military manoeuvres above a certain size (for instance in the form of an annual calender) and invitation of observers to these manoeuvres. Contrary to what has been the case in Europe, however, in the Persian Gulf region such measures should preferably not be confined to those on land, but extended to the maritime domain.[110] Also, in order to allay Iranian and Iraqi fears they should also pertain to US forces, at least in so far as they are collaborating with those of the GCC states.

The aforementioned seminars on military doctrines (and strategies) would be the ideal forum for exchanging information on military planning in general. Full compliance with the UN Register of Conventional Arms would also be very helpful.[111] Ideally, it should be supplemented with a more detailed register of a regional scope that should also provide data on military holdings and indigenous arms production. Most of these measures would also have the added advantage of acquainting military personnel with each other—which might contribute to dismantling enemy images.

None of the above, however, would require states to change their practices, as transparency-enhancing measures merely illuminate what is already happening. One might, however, also want to modify practices via confidence and security-building measures (CSBMs) which proscribe or regulate certain activities. Relevant CSBMs would include a prohibition against exercises not listed in the annual calender; a prohibition against military manoeuvres above a certain size, either in general or merely in border areas; and limits on the annual number of exercises, inter alia in order to prevent circumvention of the size constraints (e.g. by a substitution of many small for fewer large manoeuvres). Such regulations should, among other things, rule out the (real or imagined) possibility that a state might conceal attack preparations as large-scale manoeuvres, thus providing some insurance against surprise attacks.

Even though the literature tends to focus on negotiated and bi- or multilateral CBMs and CSBMs, nothing speaks against unilateral confidence-building. A state with merely defensive intentions may find it to be in its own best interest to allay its neighbours' unfounded fears by simply divulging its military plans and activities, even without formal reciprocity. To do so would, moreover, put some indirect pressure on the others to emulate unilateral C(S)BMs, so that the end

result would be a general enhancement of mutual transparency.

Conventional Military Restructuring
The same logic would seem to apply to military restructuring, *in casu* a defensive restructuring. The best solution would, of course, be that everybody undertook such restructuring, but it may also serve the national interests of a state to do so unilaterally—presupposing, of course, that it is defensively motivated, i.e. has no plans to alter the status quo by military means.

For such a state to specialize on defence of the national territory at the expense of offensive capabilities would not have to be seen as a unilateral concession to 'undeserving' adversaries, but might just as well be viewed as simple prudence. Moreover, it would have the added advantage of allaying unfounded fears on the part of that state's neighbours, who may well choose to reciprocate if they are, likewise, defensively motivated. If they do not, they thereby confirm the suspicions of their neighbour, who will thus be better informed than before. There is thus no *a priori* reason why states should make defensive restructuring conditional on negotiations and reciprocity.[112]

Such unilateralism is only rarely a matter of investing in an entirely different military posture, which would indeed by prohibitively expensive, even for wealthy states. Rather, it is a matter of amending strategic conceptions and drawing the consequences thereof in terms of deployments and weapons acquisitions. This might, for instance, entail redeploying certain forces and/or refraining from the acquisition of certain types of weapons, neither of which is expensive, certainly not in comparison with the sums currently being spent on arms.

However, neither is this article the right place, nor is its author the right person, to advance concrete suggestions for modified defence plans for each and every state in the Gulf region. Suffice it therefore to address a few question in abstract terms: how to structure the ground forces; what kind of air force; how to deal with maritime threats; and what to do about the ballistic missile problem.

For the ground forces, an appropriate guideline might be the 'spider-and-web' model developed by the international Study Group on Alternative Defence Policy, entailing a deliberate integration of mobile forces ('spiders') with a stationary web, thereby enhancing their mobility on their home ground, but severely hampering it beyond this.[113] Such a scheme would also appear suitable for integrating the United States. Local forces of the GCC states might be deployed as a

web, within which US (or, even better, United Nations) forces could operate in an emergency, either in a (Desert Shield-type) preventive deployment or in a mission to liberate conquered territory.

Such a web would not necessarily have to cover all of the vast territory of a country such as Saudi Arabia, but might take the form of a 'stronghold defence', where only the essential parts are defended. In any case, they should emphasize anti-tank defence, e.g. be heavy on anti-tank weapons and artillery, but light on tanks and other heavy armoured vehicles. There would surely also be a need for tanks, armed helicopters and other 'indigenous spiders' providing some mobility between fronts—if only because Saudi Arabia might feel the need for a defensive shield vis-à-vis both Iran or Iraq and against Yemen. The fielding of such mobile forces would not, however, inevitably be tantamount to an offensive capability vis-à-vis either, especially not if they were made dependent on a more stationary web.

Countries in a more exposed position, such as Kuwait, would probably be well-advised to explore barrier-type technologies, combined with ordinary artillery or MLRS (Multiple-Launch Rocket Systems), while there would be little need for mobile forces such as tanks.

The situation is a little more complicated for both Iran and Iraq, since neither state has any outside support to rely on, and as both may have to defend themselves against extra-regional states, including the United States. This is both a matter of preventing small-scale armed incursions (like the ones undertaken by Turkey against Iraq) and of being able to deter and defend themselves against fully-fledged invasions—not because the present author believes that such an invasion is likely to ever occur, but because both Iran and Iraq may nevertheless fear such an eventuality, and because they have the same right as other sovereign states to field a defence against it.

While it may not be feasible to prevent small-scale incursions entirely, much can be done to make them costly (militarily as well as, just as important, politically) by means of a good surveillance system and a sufficient number of (lightly armed) border guards combined with some light agile forces. The best defence against large-scale attack would seem to be to make the country difficult to invade (by means of forward defence) as well as 'hard to digest' by means of an ability to wage a protracted war on one's own territory.[114]

Making an invasion costly, especially in terms of human lives, is much more effective vis-a-vis the 'US threat' than to have counter-

attack capabilities that would only make the US Congress and public more casualty-tolerant. These consideration would, once again, seem to point towards a 'spider-and-web' posture, with the highest priority given to light and only tactically mobile forces, yet with a certain internal reinforcement capability in terms of armoured forces (but much fewer than today), helicopters and CAS (Conventional Air Support) aircraft.

As far as seawards threats to their national territories are concerned, only Bahrain, the UAE, Iran and Iraq seem to have much to worry about: Bahrain and the UAE must be concerned about a possible attack by the growing (yet still predominantly defensive) Iranian navy, that has also exercised amphibious landings. The two others mainly have to be concerned about US 'from the sea' operations, *inter alia* by means of 'Tomahawk' cruise missiles.[115] The oil-exporting countries would further have grounds for concern about their SLOCs (Sea Lines of Communication), for instance about a possible blocking of the strait of Hormuz.

The former task of defence against seaward attack is primarily a matter of defence against aircraft as well as ballistic missiles. While the former can be accomplished by means of capable SAMs (surface-to-air missiles), the latter is probably infeasible, hence had better not be attempted at all. The SLOC defence task will be complicated, as it is almost entirely a question of defence against, very unlikely, US SLOC severance attempts. In the present author's opinion, the alleged Iranian submarine threat is not particularly serious (also because Iran is more vulnerable to SLOC severance that the other states around the Gulf).

Should a defence against it nevertheless be deemed indispensable, it is probably best done by means of a convoy-with-escorts system, featuring frigate-size escorting vessels optimized for anti-submarine tasks. Another possibility is that of a temporary blocking of seaways by means of mines (as happened during the Gulf War), which calls for a mine-clearing capability. As demonstrated after the Gulf War, however, this does not necessarily have to be a national one, as international help will undoubtedly be forthcoming. The oil-importing West is definitely not interested in having the oil flows interrupted with inevitable negative repercussions on prices.

Much of the air defence task may be performed by means of SAMs, but a fleet of interceptor aircraft is probably also required. However, just as important as the performance and sophistication of the aircraft may be the availability of dispersal airstrips and/or the

possession of VSTOL (vertical/short take-off/landing) aircraft. The worst type of air force would seem to be one with substantial offensive capabilities that makes the destruction of the aircraft imperative, combined with a high concentration that makes it easy, as illustrated by the swift wiping out of Iraq's air force, during the 1991 war.

Even though the ballistic missile threat seems exaggerated, this does not mean that it can be ignored. It may, however, be addressed in two ways: by fielding a ATBM (anti-tactical ballistic missile) defence, or via arms control. The performance of 'Patriot' in the Gulf War was questionable as far as SCUDs were concerned,[116] albeit not against aircraft. Hence it seems ill-advised to invest much effort in an ATBM defence which may anyhow not work—or the success rate of which is such as to invite the respective opponent to raise the stakes in the measure-countermeasure context, say by arming the missiles with chemical, biological or even nuclear warheads. A much better way of dealing with the TBM (tactical ballistic missile) threat, however, is to make the missiles go away by means of arms control, to which I shall now turn.

Arms Control
Arms control tends to be easier the smaller the number of participants, the more symmetrical their military postures, and the shorter the list of items on the agenda.

The multipolar setting in the Gulf thus complicates matters, especially because of the region's 'open-endedness'. For instance, would parity between Iraq and Saudi Arabia be fair, considering Iraq's need to also defend itself against Turkey and Iran? On the other hand, if all states accept that they have nothing to gain from war, they may also come to realize that an arms race does not serve their national interests, hence be willing to opt out of if, if only the terms are right.

In Table 7 I have sketched the contours of a hypothetical 'package deal', combining measures from various categories as they would seem to best address the main security concerns of the primary protagonists in the region. As these concerns are highly asymmetrical, any package will have to be so as well in order to be mutually beneficial.

Conclusion
We have thus seen that the Persian Gulf region is far from stable, but also that a number of measures are conceivable which would tend to stabilize it, including military restructuring and arms control.

Even more important, however, is a political reorientation, both among the states in the region and in the United States as well as Europe. For a set of proposals to this effect the reader is referred to the present volume's conclusion.

Table 7: 'Package Deal'			
Category	**Iran**	**Iraq**	**GCC**	**USA**
---	---	---	---	---
Political	No state terrorism Associate status in the GCC	Renunciation of territorial claims Observer status in the GCC	No permanent US bases Opening up of GCC	Abandon contain-ment
Economic	Agreement on oil pricing Free trade arrangements			
Military	Non-aggression treaties			Security guarantees
WMD	WMD-Free Zone			
Ground forces	Tank reductions	Tank reductions	None	Export restraint
Air forces	Ceiling on long-range fighter-bombers			Export regulations
Ballistic Missiles	Prohibition on missiles with range > 100 km			Export regulations
Navies	Abandonment of submarines	No acquisition of submarines		Export regulations
C(S)BMs	Regional arms transfer and holdings register Seminar(s) on military doctrines No manoeuvres in border areas Crisis Prevention Centre			No ma-noeuvres in border areas

Notes
1. This is a shortened and updated version of 'Resolving the Security Dilemma in the Gulf Region', *The Emirates Occasional Papers*, no. 9 (Abu Dhabi, UAE: The Emirates Center for Strategic Studies and Research, 1997).

2. Among the modern classics, one might mention Cantori, Louis J. & Steven L. Spiegel (eds.): *The International Politics of Regions: A Comparative Approach* (Englewood Cliffs, NJ: Prentice-Hall, 1970); Haas, Ernst B.: *International Political Communities* (New York: Anchor Books, 1966); Nye, Joseph S.: *Peace in Parts: Integration and Conflict in Regional Organization* (Boston: Little, Brown & Co., 1971); and Russett, Bruce: *International Regions and the International System* (Chicago: Rand McNally, 1967). More recent studies which pay some attention to theory include Wriggins, Howard (ed.): *Dynamics of Regional Politics. Four Systems on the Indian Ocean Rim* (New York: Columbia University Press, 1992); Fawcett, Louise & Andrew Hurrell (eds.): *Regionalism in World Politics* (Oxford: Oxford University Press, 1995), *passim*; Lake, David A. & Patrick M. Morgan (eds.): *Regional Orders. Building Security in a New World* (University Park, PA: Pennsylvania State University Press, 1997); Buzan, Barry: *People, States and Fear. An Agenda for International Security Studies in the Post-Cold War Era*, Second Edition (Boulder, CO: Lynne Rienner, 1991), pp. 186-229; idem, Ole Wæver & Jaap de Wilde: *The New Security Studies: A Framework for Analysis* (Boulder, CO: Lynne Rienner, 1998), pp. 9-20, 42-45 & *passim*; and Adler, Emmanuel & Michael Barnett (eds.): *Security Communities* (Cambridge: Cambridge University Press, 1998). See also Mansfield, Edward D. & Helen V. Milner: 'The New Wave of Regionalism', *International Organization*, vol. 53, no. 3 (Summer 1999), pp. 589-628.

3. Daase, Christopher, Susanne Feske, Bernhard Moltmann & Claudia Schmid (eds.): *Regionalisierung der Sicherheitspolitik. Tendenzen in den internationalen Beziehungen nach dem Ost-West-Konflikt* (Baden-Baden: Nomos Verlagsgesellschaft, 1993); Lawrence, Robert Z.: *Regionalism, Multilateralism, and Deeper Integration* (Washington, DC: The Brookings Institution, 1996); Tow, William T.: *Subregional Security Cooperation in the Third World* (Boulder, CO: Lynne Rienner, 1990); Keating, Michael & John Loughlin (eds.): *The Political Economy of Regionalism* (Newbury Park: Frank Cass, 1997); Coleman, William D. & Geoffrey R. D. Underhill (eds.): *Regionalism and Global Economic Integration* (London: Routledge, 1998); Grugel, Jean & Wil Hout (eds.): *Regionalism across the North/South Divide. State Strategies in the Semi-Periphery* (London: Routledge, 1999); Storper, Michael: *The Regional World. Territorial Development in a Global Economy* (New York: The Guilford Press, 1997); Fukasaku, Kiichiro, Fukanari Kimura & Shujiro Urata (eds.): *Asia and Europe. Beyond Competing Regionalism* (Brighton: Sussex Academic Press, 1998); Aggarwal, Vinod K. & Charles E. Morrison (eds.): *Asia-Pacific Crossroads. Regime Creation and the Future of APEC* (New York: St. Martin's Press, 1998); Solingen, Etel: *Regional Orders at Century's Dawn. Global and Domestic Influences on Grand Strategy* (Princeton, NJ: Princeton University Press, 1998); Calleya, Stephen C. (ed.): *Regionalism in the Post-Cold War World* (Aldershot: Ashgate, 2000).

4. See Ward, Michael Don (ed.): *The New Geopolitics* (Philadelphia: Gordon and Breach, 1992), especially Diehl, Paul F.: 'Geography and War: A Review and Assessment of the Empirical Literature' (pp. 121-137); and Gichman, Charles S.: 'Interstate Metrics: Conceptualizing, Operationalizing, and Measuring the Geographic Proximity of States Since the Congress of Vienna' (pp. 139-158). On the importance of proximity for war-proneness see Goertz, Gary & Paul F. Diehl: *Territorial Changes and International Conflict* (London: Routledge, 1992); Siverson, Randolph & Harvey Starr: *The Diffusion of War. A Study of Opportunity and Willingness* (Ann Arbor: University of Michigan Press, 1991).

5. Wæver, Ole: 'Imperial Metaphors: Emerging European Analogies to Pre-Nation-State Imperial Systems', in Ola Tunander, Pavel Baev & Victoria Einagel (eds.): *Geopolitics in Post-Wall Europe* (London: Sage, 1997), pp. 59-93; idem: 'Europe's Three Empires: A Watsonian Interpretation of Post-Wall European Security', in Rick Fawn & Jeremy Larkins (eds.): *International Society after the Cold War. Anarchy and Order Reconsidered* (Houndsmills, Basingstoke: Macmillan, 1996), pp. 220-260. See also Watson, Adam: *The Evolution of International Society* (London: Routledge, 1992), pp. 3-4 & *passim*.

6. On the Islamic conception of 'religious geopolitics' see, for instance, Fuller, Graham E. & Ian O. Lessler: *A Sense of Siege. The Geopolitics of Islam and the West* (Boulder, CO: Westview, 1995), pp. 137-149 & *passim*. See also Charnay, Jean-Paul: *Représentation stratégique de l'Islam* (Paris: Centre d'Études et de Prospective, 1996), pp. 7-18.

7. Elhance, Arun P.: *Hydropolitics in the 3rd World. Conflict and Cooperation in International River Basins* (Washington, DC: United States Institute of Peace Press, 1999).

8. On the role of regional organizations within the UN, see Weiss, Thomas G., David P. Forsythe & Roger A. Coate (eds.): *The United Nations and Changing World Politics* (Boulder, CO: Westview Press, 1994), pp. 33-36; Alagappa, Muthiah: 'Introduction', in idem & Takashi Inoguchi (eds.): *International Security Management and the United Nations* (Tokyo: United Nations University Press, 1999), pp. 269-294.

9. Rotfeld, Adam Daniel: 'Europe: the Transition to Inclusive Security' (with appendices), *SIPRI Yearbook 1998*, pp. 141-182; and for the present state of affairs *SIPRI Yearbook 2000*, p. 182.

10. Huntington, Samuel: *The Clash of Civilizations and the Remaking of World Order* (New York: Simon & Schuster, 1996), pp. 26-27 & *passim*. The nine civilizations are the Western, Latin American, African, Islamic, Sinic, Hindu, Orthodox, Buddhist and Japanese. See also idem: '"The Clash of Civilizations"—a Response', *Millennium*, vol. 26, no. 1 (1997), pp. 141-142.

11. A good overview is Said, Abdul Aziz: 'Beyond Geopolitics: Ethnic and Sectarian Conflict Elimination in the Middle East and North Africa', in Phebe Marr & William Lewis (eds.): *Riding the Tiger: the Middle East*

Challenge After the Cold War (Boulder, CO: Westview, 1993), pp. 163-186.

12. Adler, Emanuel: 'Imagined (Security) Communities: Cognitive Regions in International Relations', *Millennium*, vol. 26, no. 2 (1997), pp. 249-278; idem & Michael Barnett: 'Security Communities in Theoretical Perspective', in idem & idem: *op. cit.* (note 2), pp. 3-28; idem & idem: 'A Framework for the Study of Security Communities', *ibid.*, pp. 29-65. On nations as imagined communities see Anderson, Benedict: *Imagined Communities. Reflections on the Origins and Spread of Nationalism* (London: Verso, 1991).

13. Singer, Max & Aaron Wildawsky: *The Real World Order. Zones of Peace/Zones of Turmoil* (Chatham, NJ: Chatham House, 1993); Kacowicz, Arie M.: 'Explaining Zones of Peace: Democracies as Satisfied Powers', *Journal of Peace Research*, vol. 32, no. 3 (August 1995), pp. 265-276; idem: 'Third World Zones of Peace', *Peace Review*, vol. 9, no. 2 (June 1997), pp. 169-176; idem: *Zones of Peace in the Third World. South America and West Africa in Comparative Perspective* (Albany: State University of New York Press, 1998), pp. 8-11 & *passim*. Related to this are proposals for nuclear-weapons-free and other zones. See, for instance, Redick, John R.: 'Nuclear-Weapon-Free Zones', in Richard Dean Burns (ed.): *Encyclopedia of Arms Control and Disarmament*, vols. I-III (New York: Charles Scribner's Sons, 1993), vol. II, pp. 1079-1091. On security communities see Deutsch, Karl W. et al.: *Political Community and the North Atlantic Area. International Organization in the Light of Historical Experience* (Princeton, N.J.: Princeton University Press, 1957); and Adler & Barnett (eds.): *op. cit.* (note 2), *passim*.

14. Buzan, Barry: 'A Framework for Regional Security Analysis', in idem, Rother Rizwi & al.: *South Asian Insecurity and the Great Powers* (London: Macmillan, 1986), pp. 3-33; idem: *op. cit.* (note 2), pp. 186-229, quotation from p. 190. The delimitation of security complexes is illustrated by the map on p. 210. For an update-*cum*-revision see idem, Wæver & de Wilde: *op. cit.* (note 2), pp. 15-19 & *passim*. For a critique, see Haftendorn, Helga: 'Das Sicherheitspuzzle: Die Suche nach einem tragfähigen Konzept Internationaler Sicherheit', in Daase & al. (eds.): *op. cit.* (note 3), pp. 13-38, especially pp. 29-30. An application of (vintage 1991) security complex theory for a comparative study is Lake & Morgan (eds.): *op. cit.* (note 2), *passim*.

15. On the expansion of the security concept see Buzan: *op. cit.* (note 2), *passim*; Fischer, Dietrich: *Nonmilitary Aspects of Security. A Systems Approach* (Aldershot: Dartmouth, 1993); Krause, Keith & Michael C. Williams (ed.): *Critical Security Studies. Concepts and Cases* (London: UCL Press, 1997); McSweeney, Bill: *Security, Identity and Interests. A Sociology of International Relations* (Cambridge: Cambridge University Press, 1999). On 'securitization' see Wæver, Ole: 'Securitization and Desecuritization', in Ronnie Lipschutz (ed.): *On Security* (New York: Columbia University Press, 1995), pp. 46-86; idem: *Concepts of Security* (Copenhagen: Institute of Political Science, 1997); or Buzan & al.: *op. cit.* (note 2), *passim*.

16. On integration see Haas: *op. cit.* (note 2); Hansen, Roger: 'Regional Integration: Reflections on a Decade of Theoretical Efforts', in Michael Hodges (ed.): *European Integration. Selected Readings* (Harmondsworth: Penguin Books, 1972), pp. 184-199; Kahler, Miles: *International Institutions and the Political Economy of Integration* (Washington, DC: The Brookings Institution, 1995).

17. Ayoob, Mohammed: *The Third World Security Predicament. State Making, Regional Conflict, and the International System* (Boulder, CO: Lynne Rienner, 1995); Holsti, Kalevi J.: *The State, War, and the State of War* (Cambridge: Cambridge University Press, 1996), pp. 82-120 & *passim*; Clapham, Christopher: *Africa and the International System. The Politics of State Survival* (Cambridge: Cambridge University Press, 1996).

18. An example is Waltz, Kenneth N.: *Theory of International Politics* (Reading: Addison-Wesley, 1979), especially pp. 93-97. For a moderately state-centric analysis see Buzan: *op. cit.* (note 2), pp. 146-185 & *passim*; and idem: 'Rethinking System and Structure', in idem, Charles Jones & Richard Little: *The Logic of Anarchy. Neorealism to Structural Realism* (New York: Columbia University Press, 1993), pp. 19-80.

19. An ambitious recent attempt at forging a new paradigm along these lines is Rosenau, James N.: *Along the Domestic-Foreign Frontier. Exploring Governance in a Turbulent World* (Cambridge: Cambridge University Press, 1997).

20. Buzan: *op. cit.* (note 2), pp. 57-111; idem & al.: *op. cit.* (note 2), pp. 141-162. See also Ayoob: *op. cit.* (note 17), *passim*; Holsti: *op. cit.* (note 17), pp. 82-122.

21. See, for instance, Brown, Michael E. (ed.): *The International Dimensions of Internal Conflict* (Cambridge, MA: MIT Press, 1996), *passim*; Lake, David A. & Donald Rothchild (eds.): *The International Spread of Ethnic Conflict. Fear, Diffusion and Escalation* (Princeton, NJ: Princeton University Press, 1998), *passim*; Carment, David & Patrick James (eds.): *Wars in the Midst of Peace. The International Politics of Ethnic Conflict* (Pittsburg, PA: University of Pittsburg Press, 1997), *passim*; Henderson, Errol A.: 'Culture or Contiguity: Ethnic Conflict, the Similarity of States, and the Onset of War, 1820-1989', *The Journal of Conflict Resolution*, vol. 41, no. 5 (October 1997), pp. 649-668.

22. Bromley, Simon: *Rethinking Middle East Politics* (London: Polity Press, 1994); Zahlan, Rosemary Said: *The Making of the Modern Gulf States*. Revised and Updated Edition (Reading: Ithaca Press, 1998); Schofield, Richard: 'Boundaries, Territorial Disputes and the GCC States', in David E. Long & Christian Koch (eds.): *Gulf Security in the Twenty-First Century* (Abu Dhabi: Emirates Center for Strategic Studies and Research, 1997), pp. 133-168; Doran, Charles F.: 'Economics and Security in the Gulf', *ibid.*, pp. 189-207; Crystal, Jill: 'Social Transformation, Changing Expectations and Gulf Security', *ibid.*, pp. 208-225; Bonnie, Michael E.: 'Population Growth, the Labour Market and

Gulf Security', *ibid.*, pp. 226-264; Dadwal, Shebonti Ray: 'Oil Price Crises: Implications for Gulf Producers', *Strategic Analysis*, vol. 23, no. 1 (Delhi: IDSA, April 1999), pp. 151-166. On the role of the military see Brooks, Risa: 'Political-Military Relations and the Stability of Arab Regimes', *Adelphi Papers*, no. 324 (1998).

23. Buzan: *op. cit.* (note 2), pp. 219-221; idem, Morten Kelstrup, Pierre Lemaitre, Elzbieta Tromer & Ole Wæver: *The European Security Order Recast. Scenarios for the Post-Cold War Era* (London: Pinter, 1990), pp. 15-16, 36-41.

24. On the episode and its background see Rubin, Barry: *Paved With Good Intentions. The American Experience and Iran* (Harmondsworth: Penguin Books, 1981), pp. 17-53; or Weisberger, Bernard A.: *Cold War, Cold Peace. The United States and Russia since 1945* (New York: American Heritage, 1984), pp. 53-54.

25. Joint Strategic Survey Committee: 'United States Assistance to Other Countries from the Standpoint of National Security' (JCS 1769/1, 29 April 1997), reprinted in Thomas H. Etzold & John Lewis Gaddis (eds.): *Containment. Documents on American Policy and Strategy, 1945-1950* (New York: Columbia University Press, 1978), pp. 71-84. On the US strategy for the Middle East as a whole see Cohen, Michael J.: *Fighting World War Three from the Middle East. Allied Contingency Plans 1945-1954* (London: Frank Cass, 1997), pp. 29-61.

26. MacDonald, Douglas J.: 'The Truman Administration and Global Responsibilities: The Birth of the Falling Domino Principle', in Robert Jervis & Jack Snyder (eds.): *Dominoes and Bandwagons. Strategic Beliefs and Great Power Competition in the Eurasian Rimland* (New York: Oxford University Press, 1991), pp. 112-144. See also Jervis, Robert: 'Domino Beliefs and Strategic Behaviour', *ibid.*, pp. 20-50. For a critique of the domino image, based on an analysis of Soviet perceptions, see Hopf, Ted: 'Soviet Inferences from the Victories in the Periphery: Visions of Resistance or Cumulating Gains', *ibid.*, pp. 145-189; and idem: *Peripheral Visions. Deterrence Theory and American Foreign Policy in the Third World, 1965-1990* (Ann Arbor: University of Michigan Press, 1994), *passim*.

27. On the birth of containment see Etzold & Gaddis: *op. cit.* (note 25). See also Gaddis, John Lewis: *Strategies of Containment. A Critical Appraisal of Postwar American National Security Policy* (New York: Oxford University Press, 1982), *passim*; Kennan, George F.: 'Reflexions on Containment', in Terry L. Deibel & John Lewis Gaddis (eds.): *Containing the Soviet Union. A Critique of US Policy* (London: Pergamon-Brassey's, 1987), pp. 15-19; Thompson, Kenneth W.: *Cold War Theories, vol. 1: World Polarization, 1943-1953* (Baton Rouge: Louisiana State University Press, 1981), pp. 118-178; Jensen, Kenneth M. (ed.): *Origins of the Cold War. The Novikov, Kennan and Roberts 'Long Telegrams' of 1946*. Revised edition (Washington, DC: United States Institute for Peace, 1994).

28. Gaddis: *op. cit.* (note 27), pp. 127-164. On the search for allies see Deibel, Terry L.: 'Alliances for Containment', in idem & Gaddis (eds.): *op. cit.* (note 27), pp. 100-119. See also Bowie, Robert R. & Richard H. Immerman: *Waging Peace. How Eisenhower Shaped an Enduring Cold War Strategy* (Oxford: Oxford University Press, 1998); Pruden, Caroline: *Conditional Partners. Eisenhower, the United Nations, and the Search for a Permanent Peace* (Baton Rouge: Louisiana State University Press, 1998). On the origins of the US-Israeli alliance see Ben-Zvi, Abraham: *Decade of Transition. Eisenhower, Kennedy, and the Origins of the American-Israeli Alliance* (New York: Columbia University Press, 1998): Lewis, Samuel W.: 'The United States and Israel: Evolution of an Unwritten Alliance', *Middle East Journal*, vol. 53, no. 3 (Summer 1999), pp. 357-378.

29. Walt, Stephen M.: *The Origins of Alliances* (Ithaca: Cornell University Press), pp. 50-103; idem: 'Alliance Formation in Southwest Asia: Balancing and Bandwagoning in Cold War Competition', in Jervis & Snyder (eds.): *op. cit.* (note 26), pp. 51-84. See also Cohen: *op. cit.* (note 25), pp. 298-323.

30. On the general logic see, e.g., Snyder, Glenn: *Alliance Politics* (Ithaca: Cornell University Press, 1997), *passim*; George, Alexander L.: 'Superpower Interests in Third Areas', in Roy Allison & Phil Williams (eds.): *Superpower Competition and Crisis Prevention in the Third World* (Cambridge: Cambridge University Press, 1990), pp. 107-120. On the regional implications see Chubin, Shahram: 'The Superpowers and the Gulf', *ibid.*, pp. 144-165; Allison, Roy: 'The Superpowers and Southwest Asia', *ibid.*, pp. 165-186; Kuniholm, Bruce R.: 'Great Power Rivalry and the Persian Gulf', in Robert F. Helms II & Robert H. Dorff (eds.): *The Persian Gulf Crisis. Power in the Post-Cold War World* (Westport, CT: Praeger, 1993), pp. 39-56; idem: 'The U.S. Experience in the Persian Gulf', *ibid.*, pp. 57-69.

31. On this curious instance of 'ally swapping' see Selassie, Bereket Habte: *Conflict and Intervention in the Horn of Africa* (New York: Monthly Review Press, 1980).

32. On Soviet naval and air force facilities see Harkavy, Robert E.: *Bases Abroad. The Global Foreign Military Presence* (Oxford: Oxford University Press, 1989), pp. 50-59, 88-92. On Soviet arms sales see Pierre, Andrew: *The Global Politics of Arms Sales* (Princeton, N.J.: Princeton University Press, 1982), pp. 142-154; Brzoska, Michael & Thomas Ohlson: *Arms Transfers to the Third World, 1971-85* (Oxford: Oxford University Press, 1987), pp. 38-46, 191-195, 252-255, 275-276. On the (lack of) political influence on Iraq see Chubin, Shahram: *Security in the Persian Gulf, vol. 4: The Role of Outside Powers* (Aldershot: Gower, 1982), pp. 74-109.

33. *ibid.*, pp. 9-36. For critical accounts of the US strategy see Rubin: *op. cit.* (note 24), pp. 124-189 & *passim*; Halliday, Fred: *Iran. Dictatorship and Development*, 2nd edition (Harmondsworth: Penguin Books, 1979), pp. 251-257; Garthoff, Raymond: *Detente and Confrontation. American-Soviet*

Relations from Nixon to Reagan (Washington, DC: The Brookings Institution, 1985), pp. 74-75; Hooglund, Eric: 'Iran', in Peter J. Schraeder (ed.): *Intervention into the 1990s. U.S. Foreign Policy in the Third World*. 2nd Edition (Boulder, CO: Lynne Rienner, 1992), pp. 303-320; idem: 'The Persian Gulf', *ibid.* pp. 321-342; Sherry, Michael S.: *In the Shadow of War. The United States Since the 1930s* (New Haven: Yale University Press, 1995), pp. 307-334. On the Vietnam syndrome see Rodman, Peter W.: *More Precious Than Peace. The Cold War and the Struggle for the Third World* (New York: Charles Scribner's Sons, 1994), pp. 128-140.

34. See, for instance Sampson, Anthony: *The Arms Bazaar* (London: Hodder & Stoughton, 1978), pp. 238-256; Pierre: *op. cit.* (note 32), pp. 142-154; Klare, Michael: *American Arms Supermarket* (Austin: University of Texas Press, 1984), pp. 108-126; Brzoska & Ohlson: *op. cit.* (note 32), pp. 16-19, 187-191.

35. For a critique see Johnson, Robert H.: 'The Persian Gulf in U.S. Strategy: A Skeptical View', *International Security*, vol. 14, no. 1 (Summer 1989), pp. 122-160; Halliday, Fred: *Threat from the East? Soviet Policy from Afghanistan and Iran to the Horn of Africa* (Harmondsworth: Penguin Books, 1982), pp. 63-80. On the strategic importance of the Persian Gulf for the USSR see MccGwire, Michael: *Military Objectives in Soviet Foreign Policy* (Washington, DC: Brookings Institution, 1987), pp. 185-195.

36. Klare, Michael: *Beyond the 'Vietnam Syndrome'. US Interventionism in the 1980s* (Washington DC: Institute for Policy Studies, 1981); Epstein, Joshua M.: 'Soviet Vulnerabilities in Iran and the RDF Deterrent', *International Security*, vol. 6, no. 2 (Fall 1981), pp. 126-158. See also 'President Carter's State of the Union Address, January 23, 1980', in Leila Meo (ed.): *U.S. Strategy in the Gulf: Intervention Against Liberation* (Belmont, MA: Association of Arab-American University Graduates, 1981), pp. 119-126; and Stork, Joe: 'The Carter Doctrine and US Bases', *MERIP Reports*, no. 90 (September 1990), pp. 3-14; Paine, Christopher: 'On the Beach: The RDF and the Arms Race', *ibid.*, no. 111 (January 1983), pp. 3-11.

37. On the rescue attempt see, e.g. Ronzitti, Natalino: *Rescuing Nationals Abroad through Military Coercion and Intervention on Grounds of Humanity* (Dordrecht: Martinus Nijhoff Publishers, 1985), pp. 41-49; Daggett, Stephen: 'Government and the Military Establishment', in Schraeder (ed.): *op. cit.* (note 33), pp. 193-207, especially pp. 203-206.

38. A good account of the international, and especially US and UN, role in the war, written by a US Foreign Service Officer is Hume, Cameron R.: *The United Nations, Iran, and Iraq. How Peacemaking Changed* (Bloomington: Indiana University Press, 1994), *passim*. See also Toussi, Reza Ra'iss: 'Containment and Animosity: The United States and the War', in Farhang Rajaee, (ed.): *Iranian Perspectives on the Iran-Iraq War* (Gainsville: University Press of Florida, 1997), pp. 49-61. On the US subsequent abandonment of Iraq see Francona, Rick: *Ally to Adversary. An Eyewitness*

Account of Iraq's Fall from Grace (Annapolis: Naval Institute Press, 1999).

39. A good account of the Afghanistan War is Urban, Mark: *War in Afghanistan* (New York: St. Martin's Press, 1988). On the eventual withdrawal and its aftermath see Rubin, Barnett R.: *The Search for Peace in Afghanistan. From Buffer State to Failed State* (New Haven: Yale University Press, 1995). On the subsequent Soviet acquiescence in US dominance, see Saivetz, Carol R.: 'Soviet Policy in the Middle East: Gorbachev's Imprint', in Roger E. Kanet, Tamara J. Resler & Deborah N. Miner (eds.): *Soviet Foreign Policy in Transition* (Cambridge: Cambridge University Press, 1992), pp. 196-216. A comparison of the Soviet 'Afghan syndrome' with the US Vietnam syndrome is Borer, Douglas A.: *Superpowers Defeated. A Comparison of Vietnam and Afghanistan* (London: Frank Cass, 1999).

40. Sajjadpour, Kazem: 'Neutral Statements, Committed Practice: The USSR and the War', in Rajaee (ed.): *op. cit.* (note 38), pp. 29-38. See also Brzoska, Michael & Frederic S. Pearson: *Arms and Warfare. Escalation, De-escalation and Negotiation* (Columbia, SC: University of South Carolina Press, 1994), pp. 134-159.

41. Campbell, David: *Politics Without Principle. Sovereignty, Ethics, and the Narratives of the Gulf War* (Boulder, CO: Lynne Rienner, 1994), p. 21 & *passim*. On the representation of the war as one between good and evil see also Baudrillard, Jean: *The Gulf War Did Not Take Place* (Bloomington: Indiana University Press, 1995); Der Derian, James: *Antidiplomacy. Spies, Terror, Speed and War* (Oxford: Polity Press, 1992), pp. 173-202; Norris, Christopher: *Uncritical Theory. Postmodernism, Intellectuals, and the Gulf War* (Amherst: University of Massachusetts Press, 1992). On the psychological need for such an enemy image see Wayne, Stephen J.: 'President Bush Goes to War: A Psychological Interpretation from a Distance', in Stanley A. Renshon (ed.): *The Political Psychology of the Gulf War. Leaders, Publics, and the Process of Conflict* (Pittsburgh: University of Pittsburgh Press, 1993), pp. 29-48; Fiebig-von-Hase, Ragnhild & Ursula Lehmkuhl (eds.): *Enemy Images in American History* (Oxford: Berghahn Books, 1997).

42. See *Jane's Defence Weekly*, vol. 25, no. 3 (17 January 1996), *ibid.*, no. 11 (11 September 1996); *ibid.*, no. 12 (18 September 1996).

43. On the characterization as 'rogues' see Klare, Michael: *Rogue States and Nuclear Outlaws. America's Search for a New Foreign Policy* (New York: Hill and Wang, 1995), pp. 142-146; Tanter, Raymond: *Rogue Regimes. Terrorism and Proliferation* (New York: St. Martin's Press, 1998).

44. The table is inspired by, but differs from, the conceptions of Barry Buzan and Ole Wæver. See Buzan, Barry: *op. cit.* (note 2), pp. 218-219; idem: 'International Society and International Security', in Fawn & Larkins (eds.): *op. cit.* (note 5), pp. 261-287. For a critique of the Waltzian assumption of anarchy see also Vasquez, John: *The Power of Power Politics. From Classical Realism to Neotraditionalism* (Cambridge: Cambridge University Press, 1998), pp. 183-213.

45. Entessar, Nader: *Kurdish Ethnonationalism* (Boulder, CO: Lynne Rienner, 1992).

46. Krause, Keith: 'Insecurity and State Formation in the Global Military Order: The Middle Eastern Case', *European Journal of International Relations*, vol. 2, no. 3 (1996), pp. 319-354. On the general relationship see Tilly, Charles: *Coercion, Capital and European States, AD 990-1990* (Cambridge: Basil Blackwell, 1990); Giddens, Anthony: *The Nation-State and Violence* (Oxford: Polity Press, 1995).

47. On the democracy-peace linkage see Brown, Michael E., Sean Lynn-Jones & Steven E. Miller (eds.): *Debating the Democratic Peace* (Cambridge, MA: MIT Press, 1996); Mansfield, Edward D. & Jack Snyder: 'Democratization and War', *Foreign Affairs*, vol. 74, no. 3 (May/June 1995), pp. 79-97. On the incipient democratization in the Arab world see Garnham, David & Mark Tessler (eds.): *Democracy, War and Peace in the Middle East* (Bloomington: Indiana University Press, 1995), *passim*; Midlarsky, Manus I.: 'Democracy and Islam: Implication for Civilizational Conflict and the Democratic Peace', *International Studies Quarterly*, vol. 42, no. 3 (September 1998), pp. 485-511.

48. Krasner, Stephen D.: *Sovereignty. Organized Hypocrisy* (Princeton, NJ: Princeton University Press, 1999); Watson: *op. cit.* (note 5), pp. 182-213; Spruyt, Hendrik: *The Sovereign State and Its Competitors* (Princeton, NJ: Princeton University Press, 1994).

49. Väyrynen, Raimo: 'Regional Conflict Formations: An Intractable Problem of International Relations', *Journal of Peace Research*, vol. 21, no. 4 (1984), pp. 337-59.

50. Barnett, Michael & F. Gregory Gause III: 'Caravans in Opposite Directions: Society, State and the Development of a Community in the Gulf Cooperation Council', in Adler & Barnett (eds.): *op. cit.* (note 2), pp. 161-197.

51. See, for instance, Blake, Gerald H.: 'International Boundaries of Arabia: The Peaceful Resolution of Disputes', in Nurit Kliot & Stanley Waterman (eds.): *The Political Geography of Conflict and Peace* (London: Belhaven Press, 1991), pp. 153-165; Walker, Julian: 'Boundaries in the Middle East', in M. Jane Davis (ed.): *Politics and International Relations in the Middle East. Continuity and Change* (Aldershot: Edward Elgar, 1995), pp. 61-72; Kemp, Geoffrey & Robert E. Harkavy: *Strategic Geography and the Changing Middle East* (Carnegie Endowment for International Peace and Brooking Institution Press, 1997), pp. 90-101. On the Iraq-Kuwait border see Rahman, H.: *The Making of the Gulf War. Origin's of Kuwait's Long-standing Territorial Dispute with Iraq* (Reading: Ithaca Press, 1997).

52. On 'international society' see Bull, Hedley: *The Anarchical Society. A Study of Order in World Politics*. Second Edition (Houndsmills, Basingstoke: Macmillan, 1995), *passim*; Fawn & Larkins (eds.): *op. cit.* (note 5), *passim*. On security regimes see Jervis, Robert: 'Security Regimes', *International Organization*, vol. 36, no. 2 (Spring 1982), pp. 357-378.

53. The distinctions are inspired by, but differ from, those of Kaplan, Morton A.: *System and Process in International Politics* (New York: Wiley & Sons, 1957).

54. Sheehan, Michael: *The Balance of Power. History and Theory* (London: Routledge, 1996), *passim*.

55. On the fragility of (global) unipolarity see Layne, Christopher: 'The Unipolar Illusion: Why New Great Powers Will Rise', *International Security*, vol. 17, no. 4 (Spring 1993), pp. 5-51; and Waltz, Kenneth N.: 'The Emerging Structure of International Politics', *ibid.*, vol. 18, no. 2 (Fall 1993), pp. 44-79. For a more optimistic view see Kapstein, Ethan B. & Michael Mastanduno (eds.): *Unipolar Politics. Realism and State Strategies after the Cold War* (New York: Columbia University Press, 1999).

56. Makiya, Kanan: *Republic of Fear. The Politics of Modern Iraq* (Berkeley, CA: University of California Press, 1998). On the ideology behind it see also Bengio, Ofra: *Saddam's Word. The Political Discourse in Iraq* (Oxford: Oxford University Press, 1998); Dawisha, Adeed: '"Identity" and Political Survival in Saddam's Iraq', *The Middle East Journal*, vol. 53, no. 4 (Autumn 1999), pp. 553-567.

57. For a similar comparison of strengths in ASEAN, see Emerson, Donald K.: 'Indonesia, Malaysia, Singapore: A Regional Security Core?', in Richard J. Elllings & Sheldon W. Simon (eds.): *Southeast Asian Security in the New Millennium* (Armonk, NY: M.E. Sharpe, 1996), pp. 34-88.

58. Chubin, Shahram & Charles Tripp: 'Iran-Saudi Arabia Relations and Regional Order', *Adelphi Papers*, no. 304 (1996); Al-Mani, Saleh A.: 'Gulf Security and Relations with Our Neighbours. A Rejoinder', *Security Dialogue*, vol. 27, no. 3 (September 1996), pp. 295-301; Bahgat, Gawdat: 'Iranian-Saudi Rapprochement: Prospects and Implications', *World Affairs*, vol. 162, no. 3 (Winter 2000), pp. 108-115; Kechichian, Joseph: 'Trends in Saudi National Security', *The Middle East Journal*, vol. 53, no. 2 (Spring 1999), pp. 232-253.

59. On the fragile alliance see Agha, Hussein & Ahmed Khalidi: *Syria and Iran. Rivalry and Cooperation* (London: Royal Institute of International Affairs, 1995); Ehteshami, Anoushiravan & Raymond A. Hinnebusch: *Syria and Iran. Middle Powers in a Penetrated Regional System* (London: Routledge, 1997).

60. Picard, Elizabeth: 'Relations between Iraq and its Turkish Neighbour: from Ideological to Geostrategic Constraints', in Derek Hopwood, Habib Ishow & Thomas Koszinowski (eds.): *Iraq. Power and Society* (Reading: Ithaca Press, 1993), pp. 341-356. See also Barkey, Henri J.: *Reluctant Neighbour. Turkey's Role in the Middle East* (Washington, DC: United States Institute of Peace Press, 1996); Winrow, Gareth: *Turkey in Post-Soviet Central Asia* (London: Royal Institute of International Affairs, 1995); Sezer, Duyugu Bazoglu: 'Turkey in the New Security Environment in the Balkan and Black Sea Region', in Vojzech Mastny & R. Craig Nation (eds.): *Turkey Between East and West: New Challenges for a Rising Regional Power* (Boulder: Westview Press, 1996),

pp. 71-96; Kramer, Heinz: *A Changing Turkey The Challenge to Europe and the United States* (Washington, DC: Brookings Institution Press, 2000), *passim*.

61. Kemp, Geoffrey (with Shelley A. Stahl): *The Control of the Middle East Arms Race* (New York: The Carnegie Endowment for International Peace, 1991), pp. 15-16. On Israel-Syria see Cobban, Helena: *The Israeli-Syrian Peace Talks. 1991-96 and Beyond* (Washington, DC: United States Institute of Peace Press, 1999); Rabinovich, Itamar: *The Brink of Peace. The Israeli-Syrian Negotiations* (Princeton: Princeton University Press, 1998); Ma'oz, Moshe: 'From Conflict to Peace? Israel's Relations with Syria and the Palestinians', *The Middle East Journal*, vol. 53, no. 3 (Summer 1999), pp. 393-416. On Israel and Turkey see Waxmann, Dov: 'Turkey and Israel: A New Balance of Power in the Middle East?', *The Washington Quarterly*, vol. 22, no. 1 (Winter 1999), pp. 25-32. On Turkey's other options see Criss, Nur Bilge & Serdar Güner: 'Geopolitical Configurations: The Russia-Turkey-Iran Triangle', *Security Dialogue*, vol. 30, no. 3 (September 1999), pp. 365-376; Hunter, Shireen: 'Bridge or Frontier? Turkey's Post-Cold War Geopolitical Posture', *The International Spectator*, vol. 34, no. 1 (Jan-March 1999), pp. 63-78; Lesser, Ian O.: 'Turkey's Strategic Options', *ibid.*, pp. 79-88; Kramer: *op. cit.* (note 60), pp. 97-145.

62. Waltz: *op. cit.* 1979 (note 18), pp. 125-128; Sheehan: *op. cit.* (note 54), pp. 162-167; Lieshout, Robert H.: *Between Anarchy and Hierarchy. A Theory of International Politics and Foreign Policy* (Aldershot: Edward Elgar, 1996), pp. 135-138; Jervis & Snyder (eds.): *op. cit.* (note 26), *passim*; Walt, Stephen M.: 'Alliance Formation and the Balance of World Power', *International Security*, vol. 9, no. 4 (Spring 1985), pp. 3-43; idem: *op. cit.* (note 29), pp. 27-33: Labs, Eric J.: 'Do Weak States Bandwagon?', *Security Studies*, vol. 1, no. 3 (Spring 1992), pp. 283-416; Walt, Stephen M.: 'Alliances, Threats, and U.S. Grand Strategy: A Reply to Kaufman and Labs', *ibid.*, pp. 448-482; Kauppi, Mark V.: 'Strategic Beliefs and Intelligence: Dominoes and Bandwagons in the Early Cold War', *ibid.*, vol. 4, no. 1 (Autumn 1994), pp. 4-39.

63. Priess, David: 'Balance-of-Threat Theory and the Genesis of the Gulf Cooperation Council: An Interpretative Case Study', *Security Studies*, vol. 5, no. 4 (Summer 1996), pp. 143-171; Walt: *op. cit.* (note 29), pp. 269-273. See also O'Reilly, Marc J.: 'Omnibalancing: Oman Confronts an Uncertain Future', *The Middle East Journal*, vol. 52, no. 1 (Winter 1998), pp. 70-84.

64. Keohane, Robert O. & Lisa L. Martin: 'The Promise of Institutionalist Theory', *International Security*, vol. 20, no. 1 (Summer 1995), pp, 39-51. For a sceptical view see Mearsheimer, John J.: 'The False Promise of International Institutions', *ibid.* vol. 19, no. 3 (Winter 1994/95), pp. 5-49.

65. A good historical account of the Arab League is Sela, Avraham: *The Decline of the Arab-Israeli Conflict: Middle East Politics and the Quest for Regional Order* (Albany: State University of New York Press, 1997). See also Barnett, Michael N.: *Dialogues in Arab Politics: Negotiations in Regional*

Order (New York: Columbia University Press, 1998).

66. Graz, Liesl: 'The GCC as Model? Sets and Subsets in the Arab Equation', in Charles Davies (ed.): *After the War: Iran, Iraq and the Arab Gulf* (Chichester: Carden Publications, 1990), pp. 2-24; Nonneman, Gerd: 'Iraq-GCC Relations: Roots of Change and Future Prospects', *ibid.*, pp. 25-76; Faour, Muhammad: *The Arab World After Desert Storm* (Washington, DC: United States Institute for Peace, 1993), pp. 55-97; Perthes, Volker: 'Innerarabische Ordnungsansätze', in Albrecht Zunker (ed.): *Weltordnung oder Chaos? Beiträge zur internationalen Politik* (Baden-Baden: Nomos Verlagsgesellschaft, 1993), pp. 347-360; Awad, Ibrahim: 'The Future of Regional and Subregional Organization in the Arab World', in Dan Tschirgi (ed.): *The Arab World Today* (Boulder: Lynne Rienner, 1994). pp. 147-160; Hollis, Rosemary: '"Whatever Happened to the Damascus Declaration?"': Evolving Security Structures in the Gulf', in Davis (ed.): *op. cit.* (note 51), pp. 37-60; Tow, William T.: *Subregional Security Cooperation in the Third World* (Boulder, CO: Lynne Rienner, 1990), pp. 45-56 & *passim*; Jentleson, Bruce W. & Dalia Dassa Kaye: 'Security Status: Explaining Regional Security Cooperation and Its Limits in the Middle East', *Security Studies*, vol. 8, no. 1 (Autumn 1998), pp. 204-238.

67. Cordesman, Anthony H.: *After the Storm. The Changing Military Balance in the Middle East* (Boulder: Westview, 1993), pp. 386-427; Brom, Schlomo & Yiftah Shapir (eds.): *The Middle East Military Balance 1999-2000* (Cambridge, MA: The MIT Press, 2000), *passim*; Lewis, William: 'The Military Balance: Change or Stasis?', in Marr & Lewis (eds.): *op. cit.* (note 11), pp. 61-89; Ehteshami, Anopushiravan: 'The Arab States and the Middle East Balance of Power', in James Gow (ed.): *Iraq, the Gulf Conflict and the World Community* (London: Brassey's, 1993), pp. 55-73.

68. Levy, Jack S.: 'Declining Power and the Preventive Motivation for War', *World Politics*, vol. 40, no. 1 (October 1987), pp. 82-107; Gilpin, Robert: *War and Change in World Politics* (Cambridge: Cambridge University Press, 1981), *passim*; Kugler, Jacek & Douglas Lemke (eds.): *Parity and War. Evaluations and Extensions of The War Ledger* (Ann Arbor: University of Michigan Press, 1995), *passim*.

69. McNaugher, Thomas L.: 'Ballistic Missiles and Chemical Weapons: The Legacy of the Iran-Iraq War', *International Security*, vol. 15, no. 1 (Fall 1990), pp. 5-34; Swain, Michael: 'Nonproliferation and Iraq: Lessons for the Chemical Weapons Convention', *Working Paper*, no. 120 (Canberra: Peace Research Centre, ANU, 1992); Zanders, Jean Pascal: 'Towards Understanding Chemical Weapons Proliferation', in Efraim Inbar & Shmuel Sandler (eds.): *Middle East Security: Prospects for an Arms Control Regime* (London: Frank Cass, 1995), pp. 84-110.

70. Samore, Gary: 'Iraq', in Mitchell Reiss & Robert S. Litwak (eds.): *Nuclear Proliferation After the Cold War* (Baltimore: John Hopkins University Press, 1994), pp. 15-32; Barnaby, Frank: *How Nuclear Weapons Spread. Nuclear-Weapon Proliferation in the 1990s* (London: Routledge, 1993), pp. 86-

93; Fischer, David: *Stopping the Spread of Nuclear Weapons. The Past and the Prospects* (London: Routledge, 1992), pp. 66-67; idem, Wolfgang Köttner & Harald Müller: *Nuclear Non-Proliferation and Global Order* (Oxford: Oxford University Press, 1994), pp. 132-136; Bailey, Kathleen C.: *Strengthening Nuclear Nonproliferation* (Boulder, CO: Westview, 1993), pp. 28-35; Klare: *op. cit.* 1995 (note 43), pp. 41-51; Kokoski, Richard: *Technology and the Proliferation of Nuclear Weapons* Oxford: Oxford University Press, 1995), pp. 97-146. On the implications see Posen, Barry R.: 'U.S. Security Policy in a Nuclear-Armed World Or What If Iraq Had Had Nuclear Weapons', in Victor A. Utgoff (ed.): *The Coming Crisis. Nuclear Proliferation, U.S. Interests, and World Order* (Cambridge, MA: MIT Press, 2000), pp. 157-190.

71. *Jane's Defence Weekly*, vol. 23, no. 29 (22 July 1995), p. 18, 19 June 1996, p. 28. On the danger of biological weapons see Dando, Malcolm: *Biological Warfare in the 21st Century* (London: Brassey's, 1994); Lederberg, Joshua (ed.): *Biological Weapons. Limiting the Threat* (Cambridge, MA: MIT Press, 1999); Zilinskas, Raymond A. (ed.): *Biological Warfare. Modern Offense and Defense* (Boulder, CO: Lynne Rienner, 2000).

72. Lebow, Richard Ned: 'Windows of Opportunity: Do States Jump Through Them?', *International Security*, vol. 9, no. 1 (Summer 1984), pp. 147-186.

73. Balta, Paul: 'Relations between Iraq and Iran', in Hopwood, Ishow & Koszinowski (eds.): *op. cit.* (note 60), pp. 381-397; Koszinowski, Thomas: 'Iraq as a Regional Power', *ibid.*, pp. 283-301; Cigar, Norman: 'Iraq's Strategic Mindset and the Gulf War: Blueprint for Defeat', *Journal of Strategic Studies*, vol. 15, no. 1 (March 1992), pp. 1-29.

74. On the reasons for the Iraqi invasion and the unsuccessful (or never attempted) deterrence see Stein, Janice Gross: 'Deterrence and Compellence in the Gulf, 1990-1991: A Failed or Impossible Task?', *International Security*, vol. 17, no. 2 (Fall 1992), pp. 147-179; idem: 'Threat-Based Strategies of Conflict Management: Why Did They Fail in the Gulf?', in Renshon (ed.): *op. cit.* (note 41), pp. 121-153; Chatelus, Michael: 'Iraq and its Oil: Sixty-five Years of Ambition and Frustration', in Hopwood, Ishow & Koszinowski (eds.): *op. cit.* (note 60), pp. 141-169; Ishow, Habib: 'Relations between Iraq and Kuwait', *ibid.*, pp. 303-318; Nakhjavani, Mehran: 'Resources, Wealth and Security: The Case of Kuwait', in Baghat Korany, Paul Noble & Rex Brynan (eds.): *The Many Faces of National Security in the Arab World* (London: Macmillan, 1993), pp. 185-204; Hassan, Hamdi A.: *The Iraqi Invasion of Kuwait. Religion, Identity and Otherness in the Analysis of War and Conflict* (London: Pluto Press, 1999).

75. The best analysis is the monumental study by Cordesman, Anthony & Abraham R. Wagner: *The Lessons of Modern War, Vol. 4: The Gulf War* (Boulder, CO: Westview, 1996). More or less official US accounts of the war include Aspin, Les & William Dickinson: *Defense for a New Era. Lessons of the Persian Gulf War* (Washington, DC: Brassey's US, 1992); Friedman,

Norman: *Desert Victory. The War for Kuwait* (Annapolis, ML: Naval Institute Press, 1991); Scales, Robert S. Jr.: *Certain Victory: The U.S. Army in the Gulf War* (Washington, DC: Brassey's, US, 1994); Pokrant, Marvin: *Desert Shield at Sea. What the Navy Really Did* (Westport, CT: Greenwood Press, 1999); Keaney, Thomas A. & Eliot A. Cohen: *Revolution in Warfare? Air Power in the Persian Gulf* (Annapolis, Maryland: Naval Institute Press, 1995); Vuono, Carl E.: 'Desert Storm and the Future of Conventional Forces', *Foreign Affairs*, vol. 70, no. 2 (Spring 1991), pp. 49-68. For a critique see Mueller, John: 'The Perfect Enemy: Assessing the Gulf War', *Security Studies*, vol. 5, no. 1 (Autumn 1995), pp. 77-117; Posen, Barry R.: 'Military Mobilization in the Persian Gulf Conflict', *SIPRI Yearbook 1991*, pp. 640-654; Biddle, Stephen: 'Victory Misunderstood. What the Gulf War Tells Us about the Future of Conflicts', *International Security*, vol. 21, no. 2 (Fall 1996), pp. 139-179.

76. Molander, Johan: 'The United Nations and the Elimination of Iraq's Weapons of Mass Destruction: The Implementation of a Cease-Fire Condition', in Fred Tanner (ed.): *From Versailles to Baghdad: Post-War Armament Control of Defeated States* (Geneva: UNIDIR, 1992), pp. 137-158; Sur, Serge: 'Security Council Resolution 687 of 3 April 1991 in the Gulf Affair: Problems of Restoring and Safeguarding Peace', *Research Papers*, no. 12 (Geneva: UNIDIR); idem (ed.): *Disarmament and Arms Limitation Obligations. Problems of Compliance and Enforcement* (Aldershot: Dartmouth, 1994), pp. 63-80; Weller, M. (ed.): *Iraq and Kuwait: The Hostilities and their Aftermath*. Cambridge International Documents, vol. 3 (Cambridge: Grotius Publications, 1993), pp. 8-12, 494-536.

77. See Bruce, James: 'Iraq Will Invade Again, Warns Crown Prince', *Jane's Defence Weekly*, vol. 23, no. 40 (7 October 1995); or the interview with the Commander-in-Chief of CENTCOM, *ibid.*, vol. 24, no. 47 (22 May 1996). For a more sanguine view see the report by the UN arms inspector Rolf Ekeus, referred *ibid.*, vol. 23, no. 36 (2 September 1995).

78. Mofid, Kamram: 'Iran: War, Destruction and Reconstruction', in Charles Davies (ed.): *After the War: Iran, Iraq and the Arab Gulf* (Chichester: Carden Publications, 1990), pp. 117-142.

79. Chubin, Shahram: 'Iran and the Lessons of the War with Iraq: Implications for Future Defense Policies', in Shelley A. Stahl & Geoffrey Kemp (eds.): *Arms Control and Weapons Proliferation in the Middle East and South Asia* (New York: St. Martin's Press, 1992), pp. 95-112; Karsh, Efraim: 'Lessons of the Iran-Iraq War', in Daniel Pipes (ed.): *Sandstorm. Middle East Conflicts and America* (Lanham: University Press of America, 1993), pp. 219-240; Cordesman, Anthony D.: *Iran's Military Forces in Transition. Conventional Threats and Weapons of Mass Destruction* (Westport, CT: Praeger, 1999), *passim*.

80. Arnett, Eric: 'Beyond Threat Perception: Assessing Military Capability and Reducing the Risk of War in Southern Asia', in idem (ed.): *Military Capacity and the Risk of War. China, India, Pakistan and Iran*

(Oxford: Oxford University Press, 1997), pp. 1-24, especially pp. 5-6 and 16-20; Loftian, Saideh: 'Threat Perception and Military Planning in Iran: Credible Scenarios of Conflict and Opportunities for Confidence Building', *ibid.*, pp. 195-222. On possible US 'counter-proliferation strikes' see Schneider, Barry R.: *Future War and Counterproliferation.U.S. MilitaryResponsesto NBC Proliferation Threats* (Westport, CT: Praeger, 1999), pp. 147-170.

81. For an excellent analysis, see Chubin, Sharam: *Iran's National Security Policy. Capabilities, Intentions and Impact* (Washington, DC: The Carnegie Endowment for International Peace, 1994). See also Ehteshami, Anopushiravan: 'Iran's National Strategy. Striving for Regional Parity or Supremacy?', *International Defense Review*, vol. 27, no. 4 (April 1994), pp. 29-37; Katzman, Kenneth: 'The Politico-Military Threat from Iran', in Jamal S. al-Suwaidi (ed.): *Iran and the Gulf. A Search for Stability* (London: I.B. Tauris, 1996), pp. 195-210; Cordesman, Anthony H.: 'Threats and Non-Threats from Iran', *ibid.*, pp. 211-286; idem: *op. cit.* (note 79), pp. 20-30; Arnett, Eric: 'Iran is not Iraq', *Bulletin of the Atomic Scientists*, vol. 64, no. 1 (January 1998), pp. 12-14.

82. Gerges, Fawaz A.: 'Washington's Misguided Iran Policy', *Survival*, vol. 38, no. 4 (Winter 1996-97), pp. 5-15; Chubin, Sharam: 'US Policy Towards Iran Should Change—But It Probably Won't', *ibid.*, pp. 16-19; al-Suwaidi, Jamal S.: 'Gulf Security and the Iranian Challenge', *Security Dialogue*, vol. 27, no. 3 (September 1996), pp. 277-294.

83. Kramer, Mark: 'The Global Arms Trade After the Persian Gulf War', *Security Studies*, vol. 2, no. 2 (Winter 1992), pp. 260-309; Cordesman, Anthony: 'Current Trends in Arms Sales in the Middle East', in Shai Feldman & Ariel Levite (eds.): *Arms Control and the New Middle East Security Environment* (Boulder, CO: Westview Press, 1994), pp. 19-60. See also Steinberg, Gerald: 'The Middle East and the Persian Gulf: An Israeli Perspective', in Andrew J. Pierre (ed.): *Cascade of Arms. Managing Conventional Weapons Proliferation* (Washington, DC: Brookings Institution Press, 1997), pp. 227-252; Aly, Abdyl Monem Said: 'The Middle East and the Persian Gulf: an Arab Perspective', *ibid.*, pp. 263-284.

84. Figures are from *World Military Expenditures and Arms Transfers 1998* (Washington, DC: U.S. Department of State, Bureau of Verification and Compliance, 2000). Expenditure figures for Oman are for 1991 and 1996, respectively.

85. The classical work on 'The Reciprocal Fear of Surprise Attack' is Schelling, Thomas: *The Strategy of Conflict* (Cambridge, MA: Harvard University Press, 1960), pp. 207-229. On the general linkage between arms races and war see Wiberg, Håkan: 'Arms Races—Why Worry?', in Nils Petter Gleditsch & Olav Njølstad (eds.): *Arms Races. Technological and Political Dynamics* (London: Sage, 1990), pp. 352-375. For an empirical as well as theoretical analysis, see Hammond, Grant T.: *Plowshares into Swords. Arms Races in International Politics, 1840-1991* (Columbia, SC: University of South

Carolina Press, 1993).

86. Khalilzad, Zalmay: 'The United States and the Persian Gulf: Preventing Regional Hegemony', *Survival*, vol. 37, no. 2 (Summer 1995), pp. 95-120. On the forging of ties during the Gulf crisis see Freedman, Lawrence & Efraim Karsh: *The Gulf Conflict 1990-1991. Diplomacy and War in the New World Order* (Princeton, NJ: Princeton University Press, 1993), pp. 95-109; Gebhard, Paul R.S.: 'Not by Diplomacy or Defense Alone: The Role of Regional Security Strategies in U.S. Proliferation Policy', in Brad Roberts (ed.): *Weapons Proliferation in the 1990s* (Cambridge, MA: The MIT Press, 1995), pp. 199-211; Schneider: *op. cit.* (note 80), pp. 147-190.

87. Roberts, Brad: 'From Nonproliferation to Antiproliferation', *International Security*, vol. 18, no. 1 (Summer 1993), pp. 139-173; Spector, Leonard S.: 'Neo-Nonproliferation', *Survival*, vol. 37, no. 1 (Spring 1995), pp. 66-85.

88. Reissner, Johannes: 'Europe, the United States, and the Persian Gulf', in Robert D. Blackwill & Michael Stürmer (eds.): *Allies Divided. Transatlantic Policies for the Greater Middle East* (Cambridge, MA: MIT Press, 1997), pp. 123-142.

89. Palme Commission (Independent Commission on Disarmament and Security Issues): *Common Security. A Blueprint for Survival. With a Prologue by Cyrus Vance* (New York: Simon & Schuster, 1982).

90. Collins, Alan: *The Security Dilemma and the End of the Cold War* (Edinburg: Keele University Press, 1997).

91. Milner, Helen: 'Review Article: International Theories of Cooperation Among Nations: Strengths and Weaknesses', *World Politics*, vol. 44, no. 3 (April 1992), pp. 466-496; Axelrod, Robert: *The Evolution of Cooperation* (New York: Basic Books, 1984); Stein, Arthur A.: *Why Nations Cooperate. Circumstance and Choice in International Relations* (Ithaca: Cornell University Press, 1990); idem & Robert A. Keohane: 'Achieving Cooperation Under Anarchy: Strategies and Institutions', in David A. Baldwin (ed.): *Neorealism and Neoliberalism. The Contemporary Debate* (New York: Columbia University Press, 1993), pp. 85-115.

92. Nolan, Janne E. et al.: 'The Concept of Cooperative Security', in idem (ed.): *Global Engagement. Cooperation and Security in the 21st Century* (Washington, DC: The Brookings Institution, 1994), pp. 3-18.

93. Kemp, Geoffrey: 'Cooperative Security in the Middle East', *ibid.*, pp. 391-418. See also Jones, Peter: *Towards a Regional Security Regime for the Middle East: Issues and Options* (Stockholm: SIPRI, 1998).

94. Keohane, Robert O. & Joseph S. Nye: *Power and Interdependence. World Politics in Transition* (Boston: Little Brown, 1977); Wilde, Jaap de: *Saved From Oblivion: Interdependence Theory in the First Half of the 20th Century. A Study on the Causality Between War and Complex Interdependence* (Aldershot: Dartmouth, 1991).

95. Balakrishnan, K.S.: 'Asian-Pacific Security and the ASEAN Regional Forum: Lessons for the GCC', *The Emirates Occasional Papers*, no. 25 (1998). On the UNIDIR project see Leonard, James et al.: 'National Threat Perceptions in the Middle East', *Research Papers*, no. 37 (Geneva: UNIDIR, 1995); and Møller, Bjørn, Gustav Däniker, Shmuel Limione & Ioannis A. Stivachtis: *Non-Offensive Defense in the Middle East* (Geneva: UNIDIR, 1998).

96. Krohn, Axel: 'The Vienna Military Doctrine Seminar', *SIPRI Yearbook 1991*, pp. 501-511; Lachowski, Zdzislaw: 'The Second Vienna Seminar on Military Doctrine', *SIPRI Yearbook 1992*, pp. 496-505; Hamm, Manfred R. & Hartmut Pohlman: 'Military Strategy and Doctrine: Why They Matter to Conventional Arms Control', *The Washington Quarterly*, vol. 13, no. 1 (Winter 1990), pp. 185-198.

97. The most comprehensive works on the topic are Møller, Bjørn: *Resolving the Security Dilemma in Europe. The German Debate on Non-Offensive Defence* (London: Brassey's, 1991); idem: *Common Security and Nonoffensive Defense. A Neorealist Perspective* (Boulder, CO: Lynne Rienner, 1992); idem: *Dictionary of Alternative Defense* (Boulder, CO: Lynne Rienner, 1995).

98. Lynn-Jones, Sean M.: 'Offense-Defense Theory and Its Critics', *Security Studies*, vol. 4, no. 4 (Summer 1995), pp. 660-691.

99. On the bipolar version see Boserup, Anders: 'Non-offensive Defence in Europe', in Derek Paul (ed.): *Defending Europe. Options for Security* (London: Taylor & Francis, 1985), pp. 194-209; Møller: *op. cit.* 1992 (note 97), pp. 84-89. On the implications of multipolarity see Huber, Reiner K. & Rudolf Avenhaus: 'Problems of Multipolar International Stability', in idem & idem (eds.): *International Stability in a Multipolar World: Issues and Models for Analysis* (Baden-Baden: Nomos Verlagsgesellschaft, 1993), pp. 11-20.

100. Figures from Brom & Shapir: *op. cit.* (note 67), pp. 151-402. In cases of estimates the median value has been used. In addition to the warships listed, Iran possesses three submarines.

101. Arnett: *loc. cit.* (note 80), pp. 16-18.

102. See, for instance, Luttwak, Edward N.: 'A Post-Heroic Military Policy', *Foreign Affairs*, vol. 75, no. 4 (July-August 1996), pp. 33-44; Gentry, John A.: 'Military Force in an Age of National Cowardice', *The Washington Quarterly*, vol. 21, no. 4 (Autumn 1998), pp. 179-191.

103. An advocate of such controlled proliferation is Mearsheimer, John J.: 'Back to the Future: Instability in Europe After the Cold War', *International Security*, vol. 15, no. 1 (Summer 1990), pp. 5-52. His views are based on Waltz, Kenneth N.: 'The Spread of Nuclear Weapons: More May Be Better', *Adelphi Papers*, no. 171 (1981). For a debate on the pros and cons see Sagan, Scott D. & idem: *The Spread of Nuclear Weapons. A Debate* (New York: W.W. Norton, 1995).

104. See, for instance, Simpson, John: 'The Nuclear Non-Proliferation regime after the NPT Review and Extension Conference', in *SIPRI Yearbook 1996*, pp. 561-589; Kile, Shannon & Eric Arnett: 'Nuclear Arms Control', *ibid.*, pp. 611-655; Anthony, Ian & Thomas Stock: 'Multilateral Military-Related Export Control Measures', *ibid.*, pp. 537-551, esp. pp. 537-542; Robinson, Julian Perry & *al.*: 'The Chemical Weapons Convention: the Success of Chemical Disarmament Negotiations', *SIPRI Yearbook 1993*, pp. 705-734.

105. Prawitz, Jan & Jim Leonard: *A Zone Free of Weapons of Mass Destruction in the Middle East* (Geneva: UNIDIR, 1996).

106. See, for instance, Aronson, Shlomo (with Oded Brosh): *The Politics and Strategy of Nuclear Weapons in the Middle East. Opacity, Theory, and Reality, 1960-1991. An Israeli Perspective* (Albany: State University of New York, 1992); Evron, Yair: *Israel's Nuclear Dilemma* (London: Routledge, 1994); Shahak, Israel: *Open Secrets. Israeli Foreign and Nuclear Policies* (London: Pluto Press, 1997); Cohen, Avner: *Israel and the Bomb* (New York: Columbia University Press, 1998).

107. Anthony, Ian: 'The Missile Technology Control Regime', in idem (ed.): *Arms Export Regulations* (Oxford: Oxford University Press, 1991), pp. 219-227; Karp, Aaron: 'Ballistic Missile Proliferation and the MTCR', in Götz Neuneck & Otfried Ischebeck (eds.): *Missile Proliferation, Missile Defence, and Arms Control* (Baden-Baden: Nomos Verlagsgesellschaft, 1992), pp. 171-184; Kniest, N.: 'Export Controls and the Missile Technology Control Regime', *ibid.*, pp. 185-196.

108. Pike, John & Christopher Bolckom: 'Prospects for an International Control Regime for Attack Aircraft', in Hans Günter Brauch, Henny J. van der Graaf, John Grin & Wim A. Smit (eds.): *Controlling the Development and Spread of Military Technology. Lessons from the Past and Challenges for the 1990s* (Amsterdam: VU University Press, 1992), pp. 313-328; Forsberg, Randall (ed.): *The Arms Production Dilemma. Contraction and Restraint in the World Aircraft Industry* (Cambridge, MA: The MIT Press, 1994).

109. Alford, Jonathan: 'Confidence-Building Measures in Europe: The Military Aspects', *Adelphi Papers*, no. 149 (1979), pp. 4-13; and Holst, Johan Jørgen: 'Confidence-Building Measures: A Conceptual Framework', *Survival*, vol. 25, no. 1 (Jan-Feb. 1983), pp. 2-15.

110. Arnett, Eric: 'Reassurance versus Deterrence: Expanding Iranian Participation in Confidence-Building Measures', *Security Dialogue*, vol. 29, no. 4 (December 1998), pp. 435-448. On naval CBMs in general see Lodgaard, Sverre & John P. Holdren: 'Naval Arms Control', in Sverre Lodgaard (ed.): *Naval Arms Control* (London: Sage, 1990), pp. 1-41; Goldblat, Josef (ed.): 'Maritime Security: The Building of Confidence' (Geneva: UNIDIR, 1992).

111. Anthony, Ian: 'Assessing the UN Register of Conventional Arms', *Survival*, vol. 35, no. 4 (Winter 1993), pp. 113-129; Chalmers, Malcolm & Owen Greene: *Taking Stock. The UN Register After Two Years* (Boulder, CO: Westview, 1994).

112. For a general analysis see Ramberg, Bennett (ed.): *Arms Control Without Negotiation. From the Cold War to the New World Order* (Boulder, CO: Lynne Rienner, 1993), *passim*.

113. See, for instance, Unterseher, Lutz: 'Defending Europe: Toward a Stable Conventional Deterrent', in Henry Shue (ed.): *Nuclear Deterrence and Moral Restraint, Critical Choices for American Strategy* (Cambridge: Cambridge University Press, 1989), pp. 293-342; Grin, John & idem: 'The Spiderweb Defense', *Bulletin of the Atomic Scientists*, vol. 44, no. 7 (August 1988), pp. 28-31. An application to the Middle East is Conetta, Carl, Charles Knight & Lutz Unterseher: 'Toward Defensive Restructuring in the Middle East', *Bulletin of Peace Proposals*, vol. 22, no. 2 (June 1991), pp. 115-134.

114. On the deterrent effect of the ability to wage protracted war see Mearsheimer, John J.: *Conventional Deterrence* (Ithaca: Cornell University Press, 1983).

115. See, for instance, '...From the Sea. Preparing the Naval Service for the 21st Century' (US Navy, September 1992); and Breemer, Jan S.: 'Naval Strategy Is Dead', *US Naval Institute Proceedings*, vol. 120, no. 2 (February 1994), pp. 49-53.

116. On the pros and cons see Postol, Theodore A.: 'Lessons of the Gulf War Experience with Patriot', *International Security*, vol. 16, no. 3 (Winter 1991/92), pp. 119-171; Stein, Robert M.: 'Patriot Experience in the Gulf War', *ibid.* vol. 17, no. 1 (Summer 1992), pp. 199-225; Postol, Theodore A.: 'Correspondence: The Author Replies', *ibid.*, pp. 225-240.

1 IRAN IN THE EMERGING GREATER MIDDLE EAST

Gulshan Dietl

After the disintegration of the Soviet Union, it was generally assumed that the European areas of the Union together with the East European states would eventually reintegrate into the European state system and its Asian territories would revert back to the Third World. A new term 'the Greater Middle East' heralded the integration of five former Soviet republics in Central Asia into the Middle East. Around the same time, the revolution in Iran had stabilized, Iran-Iraq war had ended and Khomeini had died. Each of these developments left an imprint on the Iranian foreign policy.

The paper proposes to examine the prospects of the Greater Middle East as a cogent spatial conception and to bring out the role and relevance of Iran in this enlarged context. The Iranian policies in the Gulf and Central Asia—both in its immediate neighbourhood and the primary arenas of its direct involvement—are closely scrutinized to that end. The Fertile Crescent, an integral part of the Middle East, has been left out of analysis on the plea that Iran is once-removed from that subregion and on the grounds of securing a better focus and brevity.

Middle East: The Term

The term Middle East was invented by actors outside the region. Captain Alfred Thayer Mahan, US naval officer and strategist, identified the geographical area stretching from China to the Mediterranean which lay between thirty and forty degrees latitudes as the 'Debated and Debatable Middle Strip'. According to him, it had been and would be in the future a geopolitical no man's land and was destined to be a disputed area between Russia and the maritime powers. Writing at the turn of the century, he said

> In the relation of land power to the future of Middle Asia—between the parallels of thirty and forty north—natural conditions have bestowed upon Russia a preeminence which approaches exclusiveness .... This

predominance will enable Russia to put forth her strength unopposed, directly, by any other of the same nature, in quarters outside of the extreme range than can with any probability be predicated of sea power.[1]

The state which was perceived to have the naval power to counteract this geopolitical advantage was Great Britain. Even as he appreciated that the application of naval power to prevent Russian expansionism would be difficult, Mahan advocated that Britain should take up the responsibility of maintaining security in the Gulf in order to secure the route to India and to hold Russia in check.

Mahan's theory of spatial relations and historical causation did mould, to an extent, the perceptions and actions of policy-makers in Britain. By 1912, oil had begun to replace coal in the British navy, and Britain was obviously anxious to find dependable supplies of oil. Winston Churchill, the First Lord of Admiralty, was supposed to have delivered one of his first quotable quotes, when he declared during the World War I that 'We are prepared to shed a drop of blood for every drop of oil.' At the end of the War, Britain had secured the League of Nations mandates over the former Ottoman territories of Palestine, Transjordan and Iraq. Churchill, by then the Secretary of States for Colonies, set up in the Foreign Office a Middle Eastern Department to supervise the same.

During the World War II, the British began to use the term 'Middle East' with reference to all Asian and North African lands to the west of India. No definite boundaries were ever set to the term. The Middle East Command and the Middle East Supply Centre were established and the Minister of State in the Middle East was appointed during the war, nonetheless. In 1957, the US proclaimed the Eisenhower Doctrine promising to provide US military and economic aid to 'any nation or a group of nations in the general area of the Middle East'.[2] The acceptance of the term was universal by then.

A 'colonial relic', the term is Euro-centric or British-centric or Churchill-centric. Whereas 'Middle Asia' used by Mahan was a geographical description, the terms like the 'Middle East' or 'Far East' located the territories in relation to the person who termed them so. In other words, looked at from the centre of the world—London—these areas were far, not so far etc. Moreover, the naming of land has often implied control of that land throughout history. For example, Rhodesia was named after Cecil Rhodes, the British administrator and financier. The dispute over the Persian/Arab Gulf amply demonstrates the validity of the argument.

Very often, strategic considerations have contributed to the invention of an area. One such was a short-lived attempt at coining the term 'Southwest Asia' in early eighties. The Iranian revolution had knocked down one of the two pillars and the Soviet presence in Afghanistan had created an eyeball-to-eyeball situation with the Soviet Union. In the circumstances, the Pentagon—the birthplace of the modern discipline of area studies—added the term Southwest Asia to its vocabulary. It served three distinct purposes: it delinked the oil-rich countries from the rest of the Middle East, where the Arab-Israel problem was the major regional issue; it placed the Afghanistan problem squarely in the context of the Gulf; and it accorded a special status and gave specific assignments to Pakistan in the Gulf region. Similarly, locating a state within a region could be a strategic/political decision. Daniel Pipes and Patrick Clawson make a strong case for moving Turkey administratively from the State Department bureau handling Europe to the one handling the Middle East.[3]

Only two leaders in the post-colonial world found the terms offensive. Each reacted in his own characteristic way: Jawaharlal Nehru with a righteous assertion; Mao Tse Tung with a mocking question. Nehru coined the word 'West Asia', which is the official term used by India today. It is a correct description geographically, but is not used, and at times not understood, outside of India. As for Mao, an apocryphal story goes like this. Once, when a journalist used the term 'Far East' in the course of his interview with Mao, the latter-day Emperor of the Middle Kingdom reportedly asked him, almost in a whisper, 'Far for whom?'. As a result thereof, or for some unknown reason, the term Far East is almost extinct; whereas the Middle East is almost the only term used for the region, whose precise borders have remained fluid so that the inhabitant or the observer draws them to suit his purposes.

From within the region, two alternative nomenclatures have been offered; one reflecting a secular nationalist perspective; the other Islamic. Thus, Ali Eddin Hillal Dessouki and Jamil Matar have coined the term the 'Arab regional order' to replace the term 'Middle East', which according to them is a 'euphemism for secure spheres of influence'. The arguments they advance in support of their nomenclature is that the term Middle East 'tears up the Arab homeland as a distinct unit since it has always included non-Arab states' and that the term Arab regional order serves better as a key for the analysis of 'interactions among Arab states, with their neighbours and with the international system at large'.[4] These are precisely the arguments that could be addressed from the other end, that is, the new term

overemphasizes the Arab character of the region whilst down-playing the presence of three non-Arab states—Iran, Turkey and Israel- in the region and the non-Arab peoples among the populations of all the states.

A second alternative term offered is the 'Islamic World'. In principle, it includes all lands in which the Muslims live and aims at Islamic revival and unity. Used as such, it would expand the definition of the region much beyond its present confines; and would challenge the legitimacy of the territorial states. More realistically, however, the term defines the Middle East, including the Arab states, Iran and Turkey, but excludes Israel. In fact, the very rationale of the term is to unite the rest of the region against the presence of Israel in its midst. In this restricted sense, it omits the three states with largest muslim populations—Indonesia, India and Bangladesh.

The Emerging Greater Middle East

The term 'The Greater Middle East' is still being evolved. After the disintegration of the Soviet Union, it was generally assumed that the European areas of the Union together with the East European states would eventually reintegrate into the European state system and the Asian territories would revert back to the Third World. How else could the disappearance of the Second World be accounted for? The most explicit formulation in this regard came from Mohammed Ayoob, who noted that

> In terms of their colonial background, the arbitrary construction of their boundaries by external powers, the lack of societal cohesion, their recent emergence into juridical statehood, and their stage of development, the states of the Caucasus and Central Asia as well as of the Balkans demonstrate political, economic and social characteristics that are in many ways akin to Asian, African, and Latin American states that have been traditionally considered as constituting the Third World.[5]

Only a single book exists so far with the term in its title. It is, Robert D. Blackwill and Michael Stürmer (eds.): *Allies Divided: Transatlantic Policies for the Greater Middle East* (Cambridge, MA: The MIT Press, 1997). As can be clearly seen, the term appears in the subtitle as the book studies the US–European relations in the light of their varied policies towards the region. Most of the contributions deal with themes like the policies vis-à-vis the peace process, the Gulf region etc, with no attempt at examining the policies in a new context, in a larger area;

the area named in the title of the book itself. The introduction defines and delineates the term to mean the 'area from North Africa through Egypt, Israel and the Tigris-Euphrates valley, through the Persian Gulf region into Turkey and on to the Caspian basin.'[6] It is not considered necessary to explain the rationale behind treating the area as a cogent space for a book-length study.

An edited volume by David Menashri: *Central Asia Meets the Middle East* (London: Frank Cass, 1998) seeks to examine 'the impact of the emergence of the new independent republics and its implications for the Middle East.' Special attention is given to Iran and Turkey—the two countries 'closest to, most interested in, and most actively involved in' the area that the book refers to as 'New Middle East'. It is interesting to note that *The New Middle East* is the title of a book by the former Israeli Prime Minister Shimon Peres in which he has called for an increase in regionalism in the Middle East as a complementary path towards establishing peace in the region.[7] The two usages of the term are different however. For Menashri, it is the Middle East plus, but for Peres, it is the Middle East post (the Oslo Accords.)

Like the term 'the Greater Middle East', the region itself is in a state of evolution. Its prospects as a cogent entity will depend on the three attributes of contiguity, commonality and connectedness that are the defining attributes of any region. Whereas contiguity refers to spatial unity; commonality suggests historical, ethno-national, cultural, linguistic, etc. affinity; and connectedness presumes the movement of people, goods, money, ideas and information through the length and breadth of this entity. An examination of the following variables may yield a preliminary assessment.

History
Historically, the Silk Road criss-crossed the entire region, enabling a reciprocal east-west, north-south traffic of goods. One of the chief branches of the Silk Road traversed western China, then followed the oasis route (Khotan, Kashgar, Samarkand, Bukhara, Merv) across south Central Asia into northern Iran, and thence westward on to the Black Sea or the Mediterranean Sea.[8] Along the Silk Road travelled Buddhists, Zoroastrians, Manicheans and Nestorian Christians, and they all left their mark on Central Asia.[9]

Islam came to the region from the southwest, arriving from the Middle East in the seventh century. Central Asia made two significant contributions to the Islamic world. One, the paper was developed and refined, especially in Samarkand, and the paper mills were then exported to the Middle East. Because of its ease of manufacture, the

availability of the raw materials, and the inherent advantages it possessed for bureaucratic needs; the paper was a technological advance with profound effects on the development and universality of a literary culture in the Middle East and throughout Islamdom. Two, the Turkish slaves destined for military and administrative posts. The Abbasid caliphs of the eight and ninth centuries made extensive use of praetorian units composed of Turks imported through Central Asia.[10]

The Russians, first as adventurous Cossack fur hunters and later as agricultural settlers, began to expand eastward from the sixteenth century onwards. The Czars of Russia pursued the twin policy of spatial extension and access to warm water ports through Central Asia to the Black Sea and Persian Gulf. Ivan the Terrible and Peter the Great undertook vigorous expansion in these areas; for example, the Treaty of Gulistan in 1813 and the Treaty of Turkomanchai in 1828 snatched away vast chunks of territory from Iran.

Over time, the Russian advancement came into inevitable confrontation with the British, who in their attachment to their great possession of India, could not relax for a moment from the fear that avaricious foreigners wanted to take it away from them. They reacted to the Russians very much as the Cold War Americans did. They opted to set up buffer zones and client states, in Persia and Afghanistan, to protect their own heartland by a *cordon sanitaire*.[11] In the circumstances, the officials of the British East India sent two military officers—Captain Arthur Conolly and Colonel Charles Stoddart—to Bukhara to forge an alliance with its Emir against the Russians. The vast chess-board on which the struggle for empire in Central Asia took place between London and Moscow stretched from the Caucasus in the West along the great deserts and mountain ranges to Tibet in the East. The Great Game, as it has come to be called, involved espionage and adventure in equal measure. The end result of the game was a historic compromise between them, under which the Russians were given a free hand in Central Asia, and India remained a jewel in the British Crown.

The October Revolution in Russia stirred the region into seeking independence and declaring a new state of Turkestan Independent Islamic Republic. It was soon crushed. What followed was the life within the Soviet Union for the next seventy years.

Ethnicity
The ethnic factor not only binds Central Asia to the Middle East, it remoulds the ethnic contours of the larger entity in a significant way. Under the multi-ethnic state of the Soviet Union with its preponderous population of Russians and under the universalistic doctrine of

Marxism, the local ethnicities in this area had been lying dormant. With independence and the consequent search for their roots, ethnic identities have now come to the fore.

Four observations in this regard are in order. One, during the Soviet period, the introduction of Russians into these far-flung areas was encouraged to serve as the cementing block in the Soviet power structure. It was they who were at the top echelons of the Communist Party and wielded considerable power in the governance of the region. In addition, they also manned the industrial complexes and developmental projects imparting specialized skills and technological know-how. Their role in the services like education, health, etc., was of critical importance. Today, some 25 million Russians are still resident in these states, constituting 36 percent of the population in Kazakhstan, 25 percent in Kyrgyzstan, ten percent in Uzbekistan, eight percent in Turkmenistan and nine percent in Tajikistan. Their well-being is an important issue in bilateral relations between Russia and these states. For instant, the Kazakh government has agreed to retain the use of the Russian language along with Kazakh as a gesture of goodwill towards the Russians; and the Constitution permits every citizen who is 'fluent in Kazakh' to become the president, holding out the possibility of an ethnic Slav occupying the office.

Two, nearly seventy percent of the Central Asian population is of Turkish origin. The increased interest of Turkey in the fate of the so-called 'Outside Turks' (*Dis Turkler*) is a product of the end of the Cold War. Attention, in particular, has focused on the well-being of the Turks in the Balkans— mainly in Bulgaria and Western Thrace in Greece. The Balkans were part of the Ottoman Empire and the Turks there constitute national minorities. The Central Asian Turks, on the other hand, need to be examined separately. Not having been part of the Empire, their historic links with Turkey are distant. Second, they are not minorities in their respective states, but are in the process of nation-building themselves. Third, their mixed racial stock—including Mongol and Persian elements—is generally more pronounced than in the case of Turks in Turkey.[12] Fourth, Turkey is geographically separated from Central Asian territory by the Caspian Sea, which puts it at a disadvantage in its drive towards fostering a Turkish cultural area.

The third observation on the ethnicity relates to its ties to Iran. As noted earlier, large areas of southern Central Asia had been within the orbit of the Iranian world for a long period. Iran gradually lost them to advances of Imperial Russia in the sixteenth, seventeenth and eighteenth centuries. Today, Tajikistan is the only Persian-speaking

state in Central Asia. Among a population of six million in the country, Tajiks constitute about 65 percent. Within Uzbekistan, the cities of Samarkand and Bukhara are Tajik-majority areas and have always been the centres of Persian culture and learning.

The fourth observation on ethnicity relates to the Arabs. In the early Islamic period, the Arabs called it *Ma wara' al-Nahr*, i.e. what lies beyond the river. In English, it would translate as Transoxania. The Muslim Arab armies found the river a dividing line beyond which it proved difficult to establish their authority at first. The Middle East today is routinely defined as the Arab world, Iran, Turkey and Israel. With the inclusion of Central Asia, the Turkish and the Iranian components in the ethnic mosaic would be strengthened and the Arab component, in relative terms, would be weakened.

Islam

Contrary to popular perceptions, Islam was not in captivity during the Soviet era and has not suddenly been liberated in its aftermath. Central Asian Islam is coloured and moulded by its entire history—the Soviet period included. In fact, Russia itself has had an Islamic period of history. From the thirteenth to the sixteenth centuries, Russia was under Tatar domination and to this day it is the only Christian nation, besides Spain, to have been under prolonged Muslim rule.[13]

In 1942, by an agreement with Abdurrahman Rasulaev, one of the few surviving Tatar ulamas, Stalin bestowed upon Soviet muslims an official religious organization. Four Muslim spiritual directorates were set up with headquarters and jurisdiction at Tashkent for Central Asia and Turkestan; at Ufa for European Russia and Siberia; at Makhach Qala for North Caucasus and Dagestan; and at Baku for Shi'a of the USSR and Sunnis of Transcaucasia. The most active of the directorates was the one at Tashkent. It published the quarterly journal *Muslims of Soviet East* in six languages: Arabic, Dari, Uzbek, English, French and Russian. It also brought out several editions of Quran and two collections of the Hadith.[14]

The Soviet establishment brooked no criticism from official Islam against its doctrine, nor did it permit a single Islamic political entity of Turkestan, which was the dream of national Communists like Sultan Galiev. The official Islamic establishment, on its part, was content to belong to the Soviet 'Nomenklatura' and represent the Soviet version of Islam at cultural, religious and diplomatic gatherings the world over. It was a mutually beneficial coexistence. Alongside official Islam, existed a parallel Islam. It was mainly organized in Sufi tariqas: the Naqshbandi in entire Central Asia, the Qadariya in South Kazakhstan,

and the Yusawiya in Kyrgystan and Fargana Valley. The Sufi orders operated on the plane of private piety and not of political activism.

At personal and family levels, Islam survived. Even Communist party leaders in the area observed Islamic rites and duties in the privacy of their homes. It was not easy to reconcile secular Marxism and religion; nor did the Soviet social ethos blend unobtrusively in the Muslim milieu. 'Why is it Communist to be buried in a coffin, but not in a shroud?' or 'As is well-known, pork is socialist, while pilaf (a Central Asian rice dish) is not.'[15] Questions, complaints and doubts persisted.

Since independence, Islam has come into its own. Initially, it manifested itself in such outward signs as rites and rituals associated with births, the Islamic greeting of *Salaam*, attending mosques, fasting in Ramadan, going to Makkah for pilgrimage, dropping the suffixes 'ov' and 'ova' from their names etc. More gradually, there have been more serious efforts at individual and national levels to examine, imbibe and come to terms with the Islamic legacy.

Resurrecting history and harnessing it to the present in order to create an identity and relate to the world is a natural tendency in a collective psyche. Especially in conditions of drastic change, man tends to return to his roots even if his search is highly selective and subjective, and the end result often fictitious. A tenacious grip over tradition ensures internal cohesion, which is expected to lead to a common better future. Islam is a powerful ingredient in this process of search for identity.

States: Demarcation and Formation
The states in the Greater Middle East have a commonality running through their historical experiences. The state borders in the Middle East are of relatively recent origin and, at times, arbitrary. According to Simon Bromley, the victorious European allies in the First World War—the British and the French—stumbled into creating a state system in the Middle East for want of a better alternative, not out of belief or design. And once the state-building strategy had been fixed upon, it was prosecuted with indecent haste and with little or no attention to the realities on the ground.[16]

Thus, it was the British High Commissioner in Baghdad, Sir Percy Cox, who drew the borders of Iraq, Saudi Arabia and Kuwait in a desert camp in Uqair one night in late November 1922. Iraq itself was put together out of the three Ottoman provinces of Baghdad, Basra and Mosul. The seven small sheikhdoms were motivated to merge together to form the United Arab Emirates (UAE). The British

arrogated upon themselves the tasks of 'drawing lines on the map, appointing rulers, elaborating structures of bureaucratic administration and taxation, even training and equipping armies.'[17]

The process of state-formation began, according to Bromley, only after the British ceased to exercise control and conferred formal independence on these entities. Ilia Harik contests the thesis and asserts that 'colonialism affected the boundaries of the Arab states, but it did not, with the exception of the Fertile Crescent case, create those states.'[18] He does concede that the colonial powers affected the structures of many governments, especially by creating a modern civil service and sometimes the nucleus of a modern standing army, and by leaving a major mark on the local political elites.

The Russian involvement in Central Asia is even older than the Anglo-French presence in the Middle East although it had taken the form of a sovereign, ideological state structure only in the past seven decades. The short-lived and ill-fated state of Turkestan Independent Islamic Republic was declared in the immediate aftermath of the Communist revolution. As the Soviet Union consolidated its independence and territorial integrity, it was brought firmly under Soviet sway. As an insurance against bourgeois nationalism, the Soviets drew lines cutting across tribes and hordes to create five distinct entities: Kazakhstan, Kyrgyzstan, Tajikistan, Turkmenistan and Uzbekistan.

The Central Asian states, like the ones in the Middle East, are divided by artificial, manmade borders. However, unlike the British and French, who drew similar international borders in their colonial territories in Africa and Asia towards the end of their rule and then left in a huff, the Central Asian states lived within their Soviet-demarcated spaces all through Soviet rule. To that extent, the independent states of today have inherited political systems, stakes and cultures dating back decades.

Strangely, there were no stirrings of independence when the Soviet Union began to collapse. In early 1991, when a referendum was conducted at Union level, 93.7 percent Uzbeks, 94.1 percent Kazakhs, 94.6 percent Kyrgyz, 96.2 percent Tajiks and 79.9 percent Turkmens voted in favour of preserving the Union. It was the Minsk Agreement of 8 December 1991, under which Russia, Belarus and Ukraine formed themselves into a Commonwealth of Independence States that made the Central Asian Republics realize the irrevocable process of independence, and join the same two weeks later. Independence, in a sense, was dumped upon them.

Political Systems

An oft-quoted story bears repetition once more. After staging a successful referendum to approve/disapprove his leadership, the ruler announces the results, '99.9 percent have voted in favour.' Applause. 'There are, however, 66 negative votes cast.' A palpable sense of fear runs through the crowd as someone asks, 'Who are they?' 'Well, the 60 were cast in our embassies abroad.' 'And the rest?' 'We are looking for them,' assures the ruler. The scene could have been enacted in most of the Middle Eastern as well as Central Asian states. In the former, the leader would have been a former army officer; in the latter, a former boss of the state communist party. The result is the politics of manoeuvring rather than the politics of the masses. An individual seeks his own linkage to the source of power and masters a nimble footwork to chalk out his own route to it through the ever-shifting alliance of power-brokers.

The non-participatory nature of the political systems in the Middle East has meant that the rulers´ legitimacy rests on a blend of ethnic, sectarian and temporal props. The Alawis in Syria, the Takritis in Iraq, the Maronites in Lebanon and so on. The temporal legitimacy is exclusively that of performance rather than that of representation. In the Gulf region, in addition, it is also hereditary. With the exceptions of Brunei and Bhutan, the ruling monarchies of the world today are located in the Arab world, and apart from Morocco and Jordan, all of them are situated on the Western shore of the Gulf. There are twelve of them in all: al-Khalifah in Bahrain, al-Sabah in Kuwait, Qaboos in Oman, al-Thani in Qatar, al-Saud in Saudi Arabia, al-Nayhan in Abu Dhabi, al-Maktoum in Dubai, al-Qasimi in Sharjah, al-Naimi in Ajman, al-Mualla in Umm al-Qaiwan, al-Qasimi in Ras al-Khaima, and as-Sharqi in Fujaira. The Kingdom of Saudi Arabia or al-Mamalik al-Arabiyya as-Saudiyya has the dubious distinction of being named after its ruling dynasty.

As noted earlier, the communist party bosses in Central Asia were extremely reluctant to break away from the Soviet state till the very end. Two weeks after its final dissolution, they declared independence for their countries. Once it was done, the leaders proved themselves extremely adept at changing gears to suit changed circumstances. Communist ideology was quickly discarded in favour of a nationalist one. Unlike in the Baltic states, Armenia and Georgia, the partocrats in Central Asia held firmly on to the reins of power—providing continuity and stability in a turbulent time. Askar Akaev, the president of Kyrgyzstan, is the only ruler without a communist background in the whole region. He together with Nursultan Nazarbaev in Kazakhstan,

Saparmurad Niazov in Turkmenistan and Islam Karimov in Uzbekistan wield enormous power. Each one of them has successfully contested an unopposed presidential election, securing a term of office till the year 2000 and beyond. It was only in January 1999 that the first ever multi-candidate presidential election was organized in Kazakhstan; although the outcome was no different.

In the meanwhile, the political processes are slowly stirring to life. With the Gulf War over, Kuwait liberated, and foreign forces packing up to leave, the whispers of democratic expression grew louder across the Gulf region. The battle of the ballot was won in Kuwait with the successful completion of a free election in October 1992. The other states made tentative moves in that direction, but stopped short of a decisive action. The Saudis issued two major laws: The Basic Law of Government and the Consultative Council Law.[19] They did not promise democracy and did not permit elections. But they did confer a Bill of Rights on the Saudi citizens—however limited and incomplete.[20] Even Iraq went through the motions of presidential referendum and parliamentary elections.

People at the grass-roots level are organizing themselves into human rights movements, environment groups, professional associations, women's organizations and so on. In the Arab world, the civil societal formations are active enough to make 'the coercive impulses of ruling Arab elite increasingly difficult to act out', according to Saad Eddin Ibrahim.[21] In Central Asia, the people's movements are particularly vocal in evoking national historical memories and articulating national concerns. For example, the Nevada-Semipalatinsk movement in Kazakhstan seeks to stop all nuclear weapons testing, convert military industries to environmentally-related activities and shut down Semipalatinsk nuclear testing sites. The Adilet movement represents a political and social activist group seeking to preserve the memory of the martyrs of Stalinist repression who perished in Kazakhstan. The *Birlik* (unity) movement in Uzbekistan calls for the preservation of Uzbekistan's natural, material and spiritual riches.[22]

Weapons and Wars

As the Bush administration heralded a New World Order, its National Security Council formulated a strategic doctrine that would replace the Cold War doctrine of 'Containment'. Anthony Lake, Assistant to the President for National Security Affairs, envisaged an enlargement of the family of nations 'committed to the pursuit of democratic institutions, the expansion of free markets, the peaceful settlement of

conflict and the promotion of collective security.'[23] Whereas containment aimed at exclusion, enlargement aimed at inclusion.

With a few exceptions. Lake cautioned against the recalcitrant and outlaw states that not only chose to remain outside the family but also assaulted its basic values. They lacked the resources of a super power, which would have enabled them to seriously threaten the democratic order being created around them; nevertheless, their behaviour was often aggressive and defiant, he wrote. The ties between them were growing as they sought to thwart or quarantine themselves from a global trend to which they seemed incapable of adapting. Lake chose to call them the 'backlash' states and named them to be Cuba, North Korea, Libya, Iraq and Iran. Variously also called the rogue states, the pariah states and the outlaw states, three of the five of them are in the Middle East. Since August 1996, Iran and Libya are subjected to a unilateral US embargo which threatens any country or company investing more than $20 million in their oil and gas sectors with various forms of penalization. Iraq has been under a UN-imposed embargo for more than eight years. Among others, these states have been accused of clandestine efforts to acquire nuclear weapons.

Central Asia has been an area of nuclear anxiety as well. Soviet strategic forces were located in Russia, Belarus, Ukraine and Kazakhstan. Kazakhstan's strategic nuclear stockpile consisted of 1,410 warheads, 370 of them heavy bombers and the rest on SS-18s. Its Semipalatinsk nuclear test site was prepared in 1948, where the first Soviet nuclear test was conducted in August 1949.

After independence, Kazakhstan showed extreme reluctance to denuclearize itself and a deep resentment to regard Russia as the sole inheritor of the Soviet nuclear legacy. At first, Nazarbaev pointed out that his country was sandwiched between two nuclear powers—Russia and China—both having territorial claims on it. In February 1992, he linked denuclearization with the elimination of American, Russian and Chinese nuclear weapons. On another occasion, he even mentioned that because a nuclear test was conducted on Kazakh territory before the Nonproliferation Treaty (NPT) came into force, Kazakhstan was entitled to be a member of the exclusive nuclear club. Under extreme American pressure, Kazakhstan finally agreed to sign the Lisbon Protocol on 23 May 1992, under which it accepted the schedule of force reductions covering a seven year period and made a commitment to accede to the NPT as a non-nuclear state.[24] The Kazakh parliament, accordingly, ratified the NPT in December 1993.

The Nuclear Threat Reduction Act passed by the US Congress in 1991 provides for financial and technical assistance for the transport,

storage and dismantling of nuclear weapons of the former Soviet Union in accordance with the arms control agreements. Under this Act, the US has promised assistance to the tune of $85 million. Approximately 600 kg of weapons-grade enriched uranium—enough for twenty-four nuclear weapons—was picked up from Kazakhstan under this provision by an American team of experts in 1994 and transported to the United States. There, it was to be blended down for use as low-enriched uranium fuel for consumption in commercial nuclear power stations.[25] Even if every trace of nuclear–bomb grade material is taken away from Central Asia, there are nuclear scientists who remain. In fact, there have been disputed figures of the number of nuclear scientists who have already been employed by the nuclear-ambitious regimes. Some of them in the Middle East.

Related to weapons proliferation is the issue of wars which are expected to engulf the region. Diethelm Weidemann, in an ambitiously titled paper,[26] predicts it with assurance. Ted Robert Gurr places Central Asia and the Caucasus in the category of those regions that are likely to experience civil war, rebellion and deadly intercommunal conflicts in future.[27] Blackwill and Sturmer see 'virtually no chance' that this area will be stable during the next decade. The threats arise, according to them, from the domestic fragility of many of the regimes; the endemic instability in Egypt and Algeria; the challenge of political Islam; rivalries among moderate and radical Arab nations; an enduring threat from Iran and perhaps from a revived Iraq; the continuing struggle between Israel and the Palestinians; the vast oil wealth of the Persian Gulf and Caspian basin; the persisting large-scale conventional arms transfers into the region; any further acquisition of the Weapons of Mass Destruction (WMD) by one or more states in the area; and the uncertain future foreign policy orientation of Russia. For these factors and for events and variables still unknown, they foresee the Greater Middle East as the most precarious region in the world.[28]

Economies

The resource base and development potential of each state in the Greater Middle East is different. The Middle East is divided right down the centre between the oil-rich and the no-oil states. Sudan is the poorest of them all. In Central Asia, Kazakhstan has the most developed infrastructure; Turkmenistan and Uzbekistan are among the largest exporters of natural gas; Tajikistan and Uzbekistan have vast cotton-growing areas; Kyrgystan is the poorest of them all.

There are some strikingly common characteristics between the economies of the Gulf and Central Asian states. One, they have been

shaped and developed in view of the requirements from the outside. The Central Asian states still suffer from the Soviet legacy of the centre-periphery system under which the economic structures there had been contingent upon the requirement of Russia.[29] The oil sector in the Gulf economies has, similarly, been contingent upon the requirement of the industrialized world.

Two, the oil, gas and cotton monoculture economies have made the countries excessively dependent on imports from the outside world, mainly for their food requirements. For example, Saudi Arabia ranked the highest in terms of imports per head in the early eighties. The country was entirely dependent on imports in agricultural sector with the exceptions of dates and melons.

Three, the economies are based on non-renewable resources, which will be used up and will eventually be finished. The cotton, although theoretically a renewable resource, would suffer the same fate in Tajikistan and Uzbekistan in view of the exorbitant demands it has made on river systems through irrigation and reduced water flows into the Aral Sea, which is fast turning into a salt marsh.

Four, their sectoral specialization has translated into a high ratio of exports and imports to the GDP. The economies are highly vulnerable to global trade patterns in terms of price, production, investments and exchange-rates. Economic planning and development are hazardous exercises in the circumstances.

Five, the State is the principal recipient of the rent from oil and gas. It is thus the determining economic agent. It is the state monopoly that keeps the entire economic cycle in motion—awarding contracts, sanctioning incentives, granting subsidies.

Iran in the Gulf

The Iranian foreign policy in the Gulf marked a drastic change with the inception of the Islamic Republic in 1979. The relations between the Arab rulers on the western shore of the Gulf and the Shah on the eastern shore were never entirely devoid of rivalry and suspicion. However, maintaining the status quo was the common broad aim within which the rivalries were contained. With the Shah's departure from the scene, the situation changed completely. Preservation of the status quo was thrown overboard as the revolutionary concept of the struggle of the *mustazafeen* (the exploited) against the *mustaqbareen* (the exploiters) was articulated and actively promoted. A decade later, the revolution had stabilized, the Iran-Iraq war had ended, and Khomeini had died. Each of these developments had left an imprint on the Iranian foreign policy. Iran's response to the Gulf War evolved in this context.

The Gulf War: A Fresh Beginning

The Iraqi occupation of Kuwait sent shivers down the spines of the Iranians, and the subsequent US determination to punish Saddam Hussein thrilled their hearts. These circumstances helped Iran break out of the old foreign policy straitjacket of exporting the revolution. Its stand on the issue stemmed from its smugness at having proved correct in its assessment of Saddam Hussein. 'We told you so' was the consistent Iranian refrain every time an accusation was levelled against him. He had finally proved that Iran had fought its own war against him on moral grounds for a just cause. He himself confirmed this when he agreed to return Iranian territory and Iranian Prisoners of War (PoWs) and retreat to the Thalweg demarcation of the Shatt al-Arab River between the two.

The evolving Iranian policy on the issue marked a radical departure from its earlier Islamic revolutionary ideology on many points. In sharp contrast with its consistent position of keeping the Gulf out of bounds for foreign military presence, President Ali Akbar Hashemi Rafsanjani came close to accepting it as a necessary evil in the circumstances. 'We have no objection to them obstructing aggression; anybody may help in any way. However, it would have been better if the regional countries had done so', he said at a Friday sermon as the multinational forces started landing in the area.[30] An equally radical departure from the earlier Iranian position of one, indivisible Islamic *umma* and the artificiality of nation-states was its concern over even a slight change in the political map of the region. In an interview with the French daily *Le Monde*, Rafsanjani opposed any territorial compromise. 'If Kuwait were to go ahead and cede Bubian to Saddam all the same, we would act within our means to stop it', he warned.[31] Iran's earlier defiance of the United Nations and its questioning of its very legitimacy gave way to its acceptance and enforcement of all UN resolutions on the crisis. Its UN envoy, Kamal Kharrazi, went out of his way to underscore Iran's compliance with the UN resolutions. 'No Iraqi oil was exported through Iran and the Iranian authorities had arrested 430 persons on the charge of attempted smuggling of food to Iraq', he declared.[32]

When Saddam sought to woo the Iranians by his peace offer, the Gulf Cooperation Council (GCC) rushed in to outbid him. The Kuwaiti Foreign Minister, Sheikh Sabah, visited Tehran on 22 August 1990 and met his counterpart, Ali Akbar Velayeti, with a message for Rafsanjani. He expressed his regrets for the 'past mistakes' of Kuwaiti support to Iraq during the Iran-Iraq war, which the Iranians accepted.[33] In the following month, there was a constant one-way traffic of high-level

GCC dignitaries paying visits to Tehran. The culmination came on 29 September 1990, when the Foreign Ministers of the GCC countries met Velayeti in the Iranian office at UN Headquarters in New York. On 19 November 1990, Fawzi al-Jasii presented his credentials in Tehran as the new Kuwaiti Ambassador.

Beginning 12 December 1990, Iran launched a big air, sea and military exercise involving nine thousand troops, fifty warships, several helicopters, and hundreds of speedboats in the Gulf and the Gulf of Oman. Codenamed Piroozi, it lasted ten days. Velayeti then set off on his tour of the GCC capitals. Firepower and diplomacy were both geared to securing a role for Iran in the security arrangement in the Gulf. His visit took place on the eve of the next GCC Summit. And he used his visit to stress the need to convene a seven-member GCC session. He wanted such sessions to be held regularly.[34]

The GCC Summit met at Doha, Qatar, from 22 to 25 December 1990. In an unusual move the Iranian Ambassador to Qatar, Nasrollah Mirzaiee Nasir, was invited to attend one of its sessions. The Summit communique contained a special section on 'Relations with Iran' in which the GCC welcomed the Iranain desire to improve its relations with all GCC countries and stressed its own desire to establish relations with Iran on the basis of 'good neighbourliness, noninterference in domestic affairs and respect for sovereignty, independence, and peaceful coexistence deriving from the bonds of religion and heritage that link the countries of the region'. Further, it underlined the importance of serious and realistic action to settle all outstanding differences between Iran and the GCC.[35]

The Doha Summit marked the high point of Iran's reconciliation with the GCC. The differences inherent in the worldview of Iran and the GCC countries and their mutual suspicions of the roles they aspired to play in the regional power game were irreconcilable. In any case, Iran simply stayed out of the war. It kept up its search for a rapprochement with individual GCC states in the aftermath of the war.

Iran and the GCC since the Gulf War
Iran and Saudi Arabia were the chief protagonists across the Gulf in the 1980s. At the level of rhetoric, the two questioned each other's Islamic credentials; at the level of specifics, the major issue was the *hajj* (the pilgrimage to Makkah made as prescribed in Islam). Whereas Iran charged Saudi Arabia with grave neglect of the holy places and ill-treatment of the *hajj* pilgrims, the Saudis alleged that Iranian pilgrims engaged in political propaganda and demonstrations which disrupted *hajj* rituals and violated their sanctity. In 1987 the *hajj* was marred by

violence and ended in an unprecedented tragedy: Saudi security guards and Iranian demonstrators engaged in a confrontation that, according to Iran, left more than six hundred dead as a result of the fifty thousand bullets fired on them.

Early next year Saudi Arabia declared at the annual meeting of the Foreign Ministers of the Organization of the Islamic Conference (OIC) that it would assign a quota to each country on the basis of the principle of one thousand pilgrims for each million of its Muslim population. The proposal was accepted with one dissenting voice—that of Iran. After that, Iran stopped sending pilgrims in protest. The Saudis on their part made doubly sure that the Iranians did not reach Makkah by abruptly breaking off diplomatic relations with Iran in April 1988. It was only in the context of the cordiality generated between the two countries in the wake of the war in Kuwait that Iranian pilgrims performed the *hajj* in 1991.

Next year, Ayatollah Ali Khamenei himself issued a fatwa (religious edict) that the performance of any ritual by the Shi'ites which created discord among the Muslims or weakened Islam was *haram* (evil).[36] Ayatollah Reyshahri, his representative, led pilgrims from Iran with a message of 'friendship, unity, and brotherhood under the banner of monotheism'. Thus, after many years, the *hajj* season passed off in an atmosphere of cordiality rather than tight security.

Gholam Ali Nadjafabadi was appointed the new Iranian Ambassador to Riyadh in June 1992. Presenting his credentials he said, 'The Islamic world has two wings, and it is not possible to fly without its two wings of the Islamic Republic of Iran and the Kingdom of Saudi Arabia. Both have their weight and place in the Islamic world.'[37] The statement marked a 180 degree turn in the official Iranian attitude to Saudi Arabia and went a long way in facilitating the process of reconciliation between the two.

In November 1992 the Islamic Development Bank, which is financed mainly by Saudi Arabia, held its annual meeting for the first time in Tehran. Although the Bank had been formed in 1975, Iran joined it only in 1988. Since then, the Bank had cooperated in several projects in Iran totalling more than $130 million. At the Tehran meeting, according to Mohsin Noorbaksh, the then Iranian Minister for Economic Affairs and Finance, it granted a further $8.5 million credit to the Sharif Technical University for the purpose of laboratory equipment.[38]

On Bosnia-Herzegovina, the single most pressing Islamic issue, Iran coordinated its policy with that of Saudi Arabia in spite of its occasional outbursts at Saudi inaction.

The year 1997 witnessed a flurry of visits between the two countries. In March, Velayeti visited Saudi Arabia to invite its leaders to the OIC Summit to be held in Tehran at the end of the year. In April, Rafsanjani visited Saudi Arabia; ostensibly in a private capacity to perform *hajj*. The Saudi Crown Prince Abdullah visited Tehran in June; ostensibly to confirm the Saudi participation at the OIC. He visited again in December to participate at the Summit. The Summit turned out to be the largest gathering of the organization in which fifty-five member-states participated, most of them represented by the heads-of–the-states or the heads-of-the –governments.

After having paid an unofficial visit as the president, Rafsanjani paid an official visit to Saudi Arabia as the former President in February 1998. A path-breaking event in itself, its importance was enhanced when the Ruler of Bahrain, Sheikh Salman al-Khalifa, came to Saudi Arabia and met Rafsanjani. In view of Bahraini accusations of Iranian involvement in its domestic disturbances, the meeting signified a thaw in Iran-Bahrain relations. In May, the Saudi Foreign Minister Prince Saud al-Feisal visited Tehran in order 'to reinforce and expand' bilateral ties.[39] Several agreements, ranging from trade and investments to environment, transport, culture and sports, were signed during the visit.

Iran's relations with Kuwait too went steadily on the upswing. As the Iraqi threat persisted, the Kuwaitis were forced to show deference to the Iranian wishes.[40] In a telling instance, the Kuwaiti Defence Minister, Sheikh Ahmad al-Sabah, made an extraordinary announcement that Kuwait had received and reviewed an Iranian proposal for a joint military manoeuvre with the GCC and had decided to raise it at the forthcoming session of Defence Ministers of the GCC.[41] A border dispute between Saudi Arabia and Qatar provided Iran with a unique opportunity to assume the posture of an honest broker and to send off messages to King Fahd and Sheikh Thani offering to mediate.[42] Saudi-Omani rivalries propelled King Qaboos to adopt a more accommodative policy vis-a-vis Iran and Iraq. The Iranian relations with Bahrain and the UAE remained strained through most of the nineties. Bahrain accused Iran of fomenting domestic troubles; the UAE nourished a justified grievance at the Iranian seizure of the Abu Musa island. Bilateral talks were held with each of the two towards the end of the decade.

Dispute over Abu Musa
Situated 56 kilometres from Sharjah and 70 kilometres from the Iranian coastline, the island of Abu Musa came under the co-sovereignty of the

two in 1971. The Iranians used their side of the island as a base for the naval forces of the Iranian Revolutionary Guard Corps (IRGC). Abu Musa was one of a string of islands in the Gulf that was used for attacks on international shipping during the war between Iran and Iraq. Apart from its military significance, Abu Musa is rich in resources. It contains half a billion barrels of oil in addition to substantial deposits of gas and red iron oxide.

In April 1992 Iran sent back expatriate school teachers, mainly Indian nationals, returning to the Sharjah side of the island after their vacation. It also cancelled the work and residence permits of expatriates who had kept the power and desalination plants running for the benefit of some two thousand Sharjah residents.[43]

The UAE reacted rather belatedly to the development, but when it did, it chose to reopen the issue of the islands of Greater and Lesser Tunbs as well. Although the Shah had occupied all the three islands in one fell swoop, there was a basic difference in the status of Abu Musa. Sharjah came to an agreement with Iran over Abu Musa, but Ras al-Khaimah did not reach such agreement with Iran over the Tunbs. In September 1992 Mustafa Haeri-Fumani, adviser to the Iranian Foreign Minister, visited the UAE for talks, which broke down over the agenda that included the Tunbs.

Subsequently the Supreme National Security Council of Iran issued an eight-point statement expressing its readiness to have talks on the agreement of 1971, but ruled out any discussion on the Tunbs as a precondition for its participation in the talks.[44] As the UAE prepared to take the matter to the International Court of Justice, the Iranian posture hardened. It said that it would in that case make no concession on this matter. In any case its agreement was necessary if the dispute was to be submitted to the International Court of Justice.

In December 1993 the GCC Summit finally endorsed the UAE proposal to refer the dispute to the International Court of Justice and urged Iran to agree to it. Sheikh Muhammad, Chairman of the Ministerial Council of the Summit, took every care to make the request palatable to Iran. He stated, formally: 'We have mutual interests and live in the same region with Iran. There is no dispute other than the occupation..'[45] The dispute has been on the GCC agenda and is routinely included in the GCC resolutions. The communique issued at the end of the Summit held in Kuwait in December 1997 expressed satisfaction at the positive indications of Iranian policy that were demonstrated at the OIC Summit and called for the GCC-Iranian relations to be based on 'peaceful co-existence, good-neighbourliness, non-interference in internal affairs and mutual interest.' It also called

for a negotiated solution between Iran and the UAE.[46]

In May 1998, the new Iranian Foreign Minister, Kamal Kharrazi, went to the UAE to discuss the Abu Musa island among other things. The Iranians claimed that the visit 'opened new avenues for discussion on all issues including an acceptable solution to the islands.' Sheikh Zayed, the Ruler of Abu Dhabi and the President of the UAE, was a little more restrained in his assessment, when he said that the two sides had agreed to continue the talks on the bilateral relations, including the question of the three islands.[47] Abu Musa, nonetheless, is now a bilateral issue between the states concerned.

Iran and Iraq since the Gulf War

On 14 August 1990, a little more than a week after he invaded Kuwait, Saddam Hussein wrote a letter to Rafsanjani in which he appeared to meet all of Iran's conditions for a peace treaty formally ending the Iran-Iraq war. He said that he would begin an unconditional withdrawal of Iraqi troops from Iran's territory within three days, start exchanging PoWs at the same time, and negotiate their boundary in the Shatt al-Arab River on the basis of the Algiers Accord of 1975.[48]

The offer was clearly related to the invasion of Kuwait. He wished to secure his eastern flank, to ensure that Iran did not join in any military offensive against Iraq, and to free his troops for redeployment on the Kuwait-Saudi border. [49]He conceded as much in his letter to Rafsanjani. He was making his offer, he said, 'so as not to keep any of Iraq's potentials disrupted outside the field of the great battle, and to mobilize these potentials in the direction of the objectives on whose correctness honest Muslims and Arabs are unanimous'. In the weeks that followed, Iraq made swift progress in withdrawing troops and releasing Iranian captives.

The pace slackened soon thereafter. Iran showed no inclination to stand up for Iraq. An unconditional Iraqi withdrawal from Kuwait was the consistent Iranian demand throughout the entire crisis. As the war began in mid-January 1991 with an Allied air bombardment of Iraq, Saddam made one last attempt to involve Iran on its side of the conflict: he sent some 165 warplanes to Iran in the hope that they would join the war from Iranian territory at a later date and drag Iran into the fray in the process. Iran did not let that happen. In fact it confiscated the planes 'as part payment' of the war reparations it had demanded from Iraq![50]

Postwar Iraq is an isolated, embargoed state. Its territory is divided along sectarian-ethnic fault-lines. North of the 36th parallel are the Kurds in the Allies' Security Zone and south of the 33rd parallel are

the Iraqi Shi'ites in the Allies' No Fly Zone.[51] It is a highly precarious balance and could easily tilt, undermining the very existence of the state of Iraq.In the event of the balance tilting, however, there would be no immunity for the territorial sanctity of the neighbouring states. Without surrendering its options in case of a breakup, Iran seems to have decided to lend a helping hand in shoring up Iraq's fledgling territorial unity. A brief account of its policies on the Kurdish and Shi'a situations is in order here.

Estimates put the strength of the Kurds at ten to twelve million in Turkey, four million in Iran, three million in Iraq, less than a million in Syria, and a hundred thousand in the former Soviet Union. If the Kurds should unite themselves into a political entity, they could be a regional power incorporating large areas of these states. That explains why nobody wants a Kurdish state. The states concerned have at times coordinated their anti-Kurdish policies. More often, however, each has used its neighbours' Kurds as a cat's-paw for destabilizing them.

In the aftermath of the Kuwaiti war, Iran, Syria and Turkey have tried to coordinate their policies towards the Iraqi Kurds. At their biannual meetings, the Foreign Ministers have reiterated their support for the total sovereignty and integrity of Iraq, respect for the wishes of the majority of its people, opposition to any move towards its disintegration or partition, and right to be consulted on any decision on Iraq.

Since the Revolution, Iran has played host to Islamic dissident groups from most of the Gulf states. The Supreme Assembly of the Islamic Revolution in Iraq (SAIRI) is perhaps the oldest and the largest of them all. It certainly is the best looked after. It has scrupulously kept out of the Iraqi National Congress (INC)—a conglomeration of the anti-Saddam forces. It has declared that to join it would amount to its according its approval to 'factionalism' and to its showing its 'disregard for the rights of other groups'.[52] The Shi'a representative on the three-member Presidential Council of the INC belongs to the Shi'a Independent Islam Party instead. The INC has also not been able to hold a session in Iran although it has held many sessions in several other Gulf states.

As things stand today, there are far too many outstanding contentious issues between the two countries that preclude any possibility of an early rapprochement. Technically they are still in a state of war with each other. The territorial dispute and the issue of the Thalweg demarcation are not yet resolved. The Iranian PoWs are still in Iraq and the Iraqi PoWs in Iran. The Iranians have refused to return

the Iraqi warplanes. In fact, as we have already noted, they have confiscated them in part payment of the war reparations allegedly due from Iraq. The issue of reparations itself is rife with complications. Lastly, Iraq has granted asylum to Iranian dissidents, the *Mujahideen-e Khalq*; Iran on its part has granted asylum to Iraqi dissidents, the SAIRI.

In spite of these outstanding issues, or because of them, the two countries have continued their contacts, albeit at a low level. In October 1993 the Iranian Deputy Foreign Minister Muhammad Javad Zarif visited Baghdad—the first official visit at that level since the Kuwaiti crisis. Ostensibly he met his Iraqi counterpart to discuss the question of exchange of PoWs.[53] Iranian media correctly interpreted the significance of the visit: the daily *Salam* described Iraq as Iran's 'natural ally in the region', and *Tehran Times* urged Iran and Iraq 'to form an anti-US front'.[54]

In October 1994 there was a sudden crisis in the Gulf when Saddam dispatched some 64,000 troops to the Kuwaiti border. The US sent a counterforce, sharply escalating the tensions. The Iranian leader Ali Khamenei took a hard line over the US military buildup when he said, 'It is up to the regional countries to maintain Persian Gulf security, and global arrogance has no right to intervene in this region.'[55] At the United Nations, the Iranians suggested a regional approach to diffuse the escalating tensions in the region and called for special efforts to alleviate the suffering caused to the Iraqis by the UN sanctions. There were reports of the Iranians taking delivery of Iraqi oil over the Baghdad-Tehran highway at Khanaquin or from Iraqi small tankers over the Gulf waters and selling them on Iraq's behalf for a profit and for friendship. In December 1994 the United States accused Iran, in a letter to the UN Security Council's Sanctions Committee, of complicity in the smuggling of Iraqi petroleum through the Gulf ports in violation of UN Security Council resolutions prohibiting such trade. The Iranians promptly denied the charge, accusing the US of ulterior motives in making them.

The relations between the two have registered a steady improvement in the recent past. In April 1997, the two repatriated some 6,000 PoWs in the biggest swap since the end of the Iran-Iraq war. In September, Baghdad announced that the Iranian pilgrims would be allowed to visit the Shi'a shrines in Najaf and Karbala in Iraq for the first time since the Iranian revolution. In November, the Iranian Trade Minister visited Iraq on the occasion of the Baghdad International Trade Fair and made agreements boosting bilateral trade under the UN-organized oil-for-food programme. In December, the Iraqi Vice-

President Taha Yassin Ramadan participated at the OIC Summit in Tehran. The next month, the Iraqi Foreign Minister Mohammad Saeed al-Sahaf paid a visit to Iran.

During the subsequent Iraq-US stand-off towards the end of 1998, Iran's response was along the old lines. It called for an easing of sanctions in order to lessen the hardships of the Iraqi people, stressed that any resort to force brings greater instability and insecurity and called on Baghdad to comply with the UN resolutions. James Rubin, the spokesperson of the US State Department, stated at that time that the US would not object if Iran assisted groups suffering under the Iraqi rule. Asked if Iran might cooperate with the US in toppling Saddam, the naval commander of the Revolutionary Guards said that Iran insisted on maintaining the territorial integrity of Iraq and maintained that the Iraqi people had the right to self-determination without any foreign intervention.[56]

Iran in Central Asia

For more than a century, Iran's geopolitical calculation had been informed by the threat of Russian/Soviet imperialism and its considerable weight against a vulnerable and long Iranian border. Its historical gravitation toward alliance with distant powers like the British Empire up to 1945 and the United States in the postwar years was a result of this historical vulnerability.[57] After the Revolution, Iran dismantled the military-intelligence defence network along the Soviet-Iranian border and revoked its earlier role of the policeman of the Gulf. These were the net gains for the Soviet Union. Beyond these, however, the relations between the two did not make much headway. The anti-Western orientation of the Islamic revolution did not necessarily mean a pro-Soviet orientation. The Iranian suspicions of the Soviet intentions regarding their domestic politics were deep and intense. By early 1983, the atmosphere had been completely ruined as the Iranian regime cracked down upon the leaders of *Tudeh* (the Iranian Communist Party) who made devastating confessions about their anti-state activities and directly implicated the Soviet Union in them. The confessions were repeatedly telecast in Iran as the Soviets helplessly looked on.

In a critical message to Gorbachev a decade after the Revolution, Khomeini predicted that 'from now on communism should only be sought in museums' and advised him 'to turn to truth', to faith, and to study Islam.[58] As events in the Soviet Union marched towards the fulfilment of his prophesy, Iran seemed less than enthusiastic to welcome the final outcome of the process. There were several reasons for this. First, the visit of the Soviet Foreign Minister Edouard

Shevardnadze to Tehran in February and the visit of Rafsanjani in the summer of 1989 had symbolized a new spirit in Soviet-Iranian relations as a result of which 'for the first time in three hundred years Iran could look forward to having quiet and peaceful borders in the north'.[59] Coming as it did, barely two and half weeks after Khomeini's death before the forty-days period of mourning had passed, the timing of Rafsanjani's visit lent it an additional significance. Second, the dramatic developments in the Soviet Union coincided with difficult circumstances in Iran as well. The country was going through the immediate aftermath of a debilitating war and the passing away of Khomeini. The last thing it needed was a major security and foreign policy challenge of the magnitude presented by the collapse of the Soviet Union.[60] Third, the removal of the Soviet Union meant an inevitable increase in the power and reach of the United States.

As Iran began to make contacts with the Central Asian Republics, it was careful to do it with the Russian knowledge and approval. Thus, Velayeti's first visit to the region in November-December 1991 included Russia in the itinerary. Iran has continued to work closely together with Russia in the region ever since. Both share similar anxieties about nationalism and irredentism in the area. Russia guards the external borders of the region, and Iran perceives its security interest in the maintenance and control of existing borders. Russia remains committed to keeping outsiders out of security structures and is likely and able to check the further expansion of US interests and involvement there. Like Russia, Iran also views Turkey's regional ambitions and a possible spread of some form of pan-Turkic ideology with suspicion. And bilaterally, Russia is an important trading partner, a major supplier of arms and a willing collaborator in technical, most notably nuclear, projects.[61]

Oil, Gas and the Pipelines
Most of the Central Asian oil reserves are located in and around the Caspian Sea. The jurisdiction over the Sea and its under-water resources has been stridently contested, as a result. According to the 1921 Treaty of Moscow, which was reaffirmed in 1935, the inland Caspian Sea belonged to Russia and Persia and was referred to as a 'Soviet and Persian Sea.' In the singular relevant precedent concerning joint sovereignty over enclosed or semi-enclosed bodies of water—the case of the Gulf of Fonseca, which formerly belonged to Spain, but is now bordered by El Salvador, Honduras and Nicaragua—the International Court of Justice saw no advantage in disrupting the unity of the body of water after the emergence of successor coastal states.[62]

Today, the Caspian coast is shared by Azerbaijan, Turkmenistan and Kazakhstan besides the original signatories Iran and Russia.

Whereas Iran and Russia favoured the inner sea concept, the rest insisted on treating it like any other sea. Under the first option, the under-water resources would be jointly developed and equally shared among the coastal states; under the second option, the law of the sea would apply according an exclusive economic zone to each. In November 1996, Russia broke ranks with Iran on the issue and joined the rest by proposing a compromise whereby each state would be given exclusive jurisdiction over oil fields lying within 45 miles of a zone extended out from national shorelines.

Iran continues to reject the law of the sea regime for the Caspian Sea. There are several reasons for Iran's insistence on a common strategy for Caspian resources. One, the oil is concentrated more around the Azeri and the Kazakhi coasts and not evenly spread. Two, the joint effort towards exploring and extracting oil would firmly bind the states together for a considerable period of time during which Iran could emerge as the natural leader. Three, the US law prohibiting an investment of more than $20 million dollars in the Iranian oil and gas sectors and threatening any non-complying country or company with various forms of penalization would hamper Iranian attempts to go it alone with the development of its own share of the territory.

As the Azeris and the Kazakhis went on with the development of their sectors, Iran followed suit.[63] Accordingly, the Khazar Exploration and Production Company was formed and affiliated to the National Iranian Oil Company. On 15 December 1998, it entered into a major deal with Anglo-Dutch Shell and the UK Independent Lasmo to carry out a study of 10,000 square kilometres of unexplored waters in the Iranian sector of the Caspian.[64] According to the US Department of Energy, Iran had already explored and identified 40 reservoirs containing as much as three bb of oil in its territorial waters in the Caspian.[65]

The Caspian Sea oil potential has come under a close scrutiny which has deflated the earlier claims suggesting that the region would be the Gulf of the Twenty-first century. According to most estimates, the oil reserves in the region are anywhere between twenty and thirty billion barrels.[66] There have been few new discoveries in the recent years to justify an upward revision of the estimates. Saudi Arabia alone has at least ten times as much, and the Middle East twenty times as much. The Caspian oil may not prove cost-effective given the current low oil prices and the high cost of extraction and transportation in addition to a host of complicated technical, geological, logistical and

political obstacles which block its speedy development.

The pipeline politics continues to remain an intractable problem in the meanwhile. The three possible routes are via Turkey to the Mediterranean,[67] via Georgia and Russia to the Black Sea and via Iran to the Gulf. The US has consistently championed the route through Turkey even though it is the least feasible of the options. And it has equally consistently blocked any move towards the route via Iran, even though it is the shortest and cheapest of the options. The oil companies have sought a compromise by advocating the Georgia-Russia-Black Sea route—without winning the argument so far. The Caspian Pipeline Consortium is, nonetheless, finalizing plans for a private 1.34 million barrels-a-day (mbd) pipeline from the Tengiz field in Kazakhstan to the Russian port of Novorossisk, utilizing an existing Russian line from Tengiz to Grozny. There already is a pipeline from Baku to Novorossisk through Chechenya, which could be updated.

In addition to politics, the issue of pipeline seems to have also become a point of prestige for the advocates of different routes. In view of the fact that the oil market has remained sluggish and the prices have continued to slip, there probably is no need for a grand pipeline project. And it still remains unclear whether there will be large enough flows of oil from the region to the potential markets. Economic rationale should suggest short haul solutions left to the countries concerned. In a few instances, that has been the reality on the ground.

The oil geography and geology in Iran are less than fortunate. Its oil fields are located in the southwest of the country and along the Gulf coast. The main refining centres are in the north of the country in Tabriz, Tehran and Arak. The domestic market for the oil is also more or less concentrated in the north as the urban centres, industries and agro-industries are around the Caspian rim. The country has a large domestic network of pipelines from the source to the consumers, which has to pass through mountain ranges rather than flat terrain. Additionally, the Iranian oil-wells are more distant from water than those in Saudi Arabia, and the 'drive' provided by the water latent under the oil reservoirs is generally not as great in Iran as it is in Saudi Arabia.[68] At present, Iran uses more than a third of its annual gas output to increase pressure in the oilfields to extract petroleum. Moreover, Iran is likely to become an oil-importing nation by the end of the century if the domestic demand for oil increases at the current pace.[69]

Iran has quietly been turning this inconvenience into an opportunity in recent past. In 1997, Iran and Kazakhstan signed an agreement under which the latter will sell two million tons of oil to

Iran annually which will be consumed in the north of the country. In return, Iran will sell an equal amount of oil from its production in the south to the Kazakhi buyers. Towards the end of the year, a 200-kilometre pipeline was inaugurated to carry natural gas from Turkmenistan Korpeye gas field to Kord Kui in northeast Iran. The initial two billion cubic metres (bcm) to be pumped annually are to be raised first to four bcm in 1999 and then to double that amount.[70] A Memorandum of Understanding exists, in the meanwhile, to build a 1,500-kilometre pipeline to carry an annual load of thirty bcm of natural gas from Turkmenistan to Turkey via Iran. The work on it is expected to be finished by 2002.

Diplomacy in the Region

Iran and Turkey are the natural and inevitable rivals for influence in the region. According to an overly optimistic view, Tehran and Ankara are 'more complementary than competitive...an amalgam of pan-Turkish and pan-Islamism together assisting the newly emergent Muslim-majority countries to move away from the legacy of the socialist red star and towards the green crescent (the official Turkish symbol, but in green, the colour of Islam).'[71] The things have developed differently.

With the emergence of independent states in Central Asia, Turkey made vigorous attempts to project itself as their role-model. Islam, democracy, free-market economy and pro-Western orientation were highlighted as the four major components of its identity that needed to be adopted by the republics. In March 1992 the Turkish Foreign Minister, Hikmet Cetin, visited the republics, followed two months later by the official state visit of the Turkish Prime Minister, Sulayman Demirel.

During his visit, Demirel submitted to the Uzbek, Kazakh and Kyrgyz leaders draft Constitutions for their consideration. Alparslan Turkes, the arch-nationalist and Pan-Turkic politician, was a member of Demirel's entourage during his tour, evoking fears regarding Turkey's resurrected ambitions of recreating a political empire. In what was to become an infamous speech, Demirel declared that with the collapse of the Soviet Union there had appeared a 'gigantic Turkish world' stretching from the Adriatic to the Great Wall of China.[72] The area included the Balkans, the Caucasus and Central Asia in this 'Turkish' world.

The Iranians have relied on Islamic solidarity, Persian culture and language, and Shi'a fraternity as diplomatic props; but the primary emphasis of their offensive has been the geopolitical centrality.

'Cooperation should certainly be carried out via Iran. For links between the north and the south, the east and the west, these countries and Europe, Europe and Asia, everything should cross Iran—oil and gas pipelines, railways, communication routes and international airports', Rafsanjani exhorted the Central Asian leaders.[73] Iran reacted swiftly as the republics started opening up. Six new customs checkpoints were constructed in the country's northern border regions to facilitate trade, transit and overland travel. The Turkmenistan railway was integrated into the Iranian railway network at Mashhad along the old Silk Road. The Azeris were promised direct linkage of their railway with the Iranian railway system, bypassing Armenia. Simultaneously, the construction of a bridge over the Aras river secured direct supplies of Iranian oil and other essential goods to Armenia in times of Azeri blockade. Tajikistan was offered overland routes to import and export its goods.

It also devoted considerable energy towards developing its ports. The ports which were damaged during the Iran-Iraq war have been coming back on line. It has seven terminals for exporting crude oil and two for refined products. All of Iran's crude oil exports from its onshore fields are currently shipped from its Kharg Island terminal. The two ports at Bandar Abbas and Bandar Khomeini in the South have handled nearly two-thirds of the entire Iranian imports since early nineties.[74] Efforts are now afoot to develop the Anzali port in the north to handle six million tons of cargo annually, to berth ships weighing 5,000 tons and to provide storage and transit of goods with the least formalities.[75] For the landlocked countries of the region, an easy and secure access to the world has been a matter of topmost priority. It is specially so for the oil and gas-rich countries seeking an outlet to the markets.

In the circumstances, Iran and Turkey resented and resisted each other. Early on, Iran did make a half-hearted attempt to pre-empt potential rivalry with Turkey within a multilateral framework. Both are founder-members of the Economic Cooperation Organization[76] (ECO). Tehran mooted the idea of reviving and expanding the dormant Organization[77] and hosted its enlarged summit in February 1992. But even as the summit was in session, Iran and Turkey went their separate ways. Tehran announced the formation of Caspian Sea Littoral Zone with Azerbaijan, Kazakhstan, Turkmenistan, Russia and Iran as members. Turkey responded by hammering together a Black Sea Group. Two days after the formation of the Caspian Grouping, Iran, Tajikistan and the representatives of the Afghan Mujahideen agreed to establish an Association of Persian Language Speakers.

Mediation in Tajikistan

Tajikistan is the most volatile of the newly independent entities. Its geography and ethnic composition, as well as uneven economic development, are the main causes of strife. The Khojand province in the north and the Kulyab in the south are relatively better developed. Development programmes during the Soviet era were concentrated in the plains of the north and around Dushanbe, the capital. Most of the country's industrial investments were in Khojand, whereas massive irrigation projects on Amu Darya and its tributaries were in the south. The south, therefore, became an important cotton-growing area, producing eleven percent of the Soviet Union's cotton. Most of the Uzbek population, nearly twenty-five percent of the total, lives in this area. All the major communication links also run through Uzbekistan as it is separated by a mountain range from the eastern part of the country. The Garno-Badakhshan province in the east comprises sparsely populated, rugged mountain terrain. Its people, the Pamirs, belonging mainly to the Ismaili sect of Islam, have been underprivileged and isolated.

The upsurge began there once the heavy-handed Soviet administration came to an end. What started out as an ethnic-regional upsurge acquired other powerful strands like Islam, democracy and nationalism. Beginning in 1990, opposition surfaced in the form of various parties. The Rastokhez called for a revival of Tajik culture and language. The Islamic Renaissance Party (IRP)[78] advocated Islamization of society though not an Islamic state or Sharia law. The Democratic Party swore by democratization and called for improved socioeconomic status for the province. The Lal-e Badakhshan sought greater autonomy for the province. The conduct of the presidential election in late 1991, which Rakhmon Nabiev manipulated to get himself elected, disillusioned many more and a loose alliance of organizations, espousing everything from Islam to Tajik nationalism to democracy, came into being.[79] Nabiev was swept away to make place for a Pamiri, Akbarsho Iskandarov, in order to assuage the Pamiri demands. He was soon overthrown by a military coup which put Emamoli Rakhmanov, a Kulyabi, in his place. The Kulyabs have always been the junior partners of the Khojand ruling elite.

Tajikistan occupies a special place in the Iranian policy in the region. It is the only Persian-speaking state and has belonged to the Persian world in terms of culture, literature and way of life. It is the only state that switched its alphabet from Cyrillic to Persian when the rest did it to Latin. It celebrated its first year of independence by unveiling a statue of Ferdowsi, the great Persian epic poet, in the place

previously occupied by a statue of Lenin in the capital city of Dushanbe. Iran feels a sense of responsibility towards this Persian island in a sea of Turkic population.[80]

Tajikistan came in for the most-favoured-nation treatment from the beginning. The Tajik President, Rakhmon Nabiev, visited Tehran in late June 1992. The visit resulted in $50 million credit to buy industrial machinery and the establishment of a joint commission to explore areas of cooperation in oil, gas, banking, etc. The republic was also offered Iranian overland routes to import and export its goods. Tajik diplomats were given training courses at the Iranian Foreign Ministry.

The exodus of Russians from and hostility towards Uzbeks in Tajikistan sucked in Russia and Uzbekistan into the conflict. Afghan involvement on the side of the rebels had continued to expand in the meanwhile. There are about four million Tajiks in Afghanistan. Many of them had left Central Asia as refugees at the height of the anti-Soviet Basmachi Movement (1917-21) and the collectivization campaign in the early 1930s. They were in the forefront of the pro-Pamiri support base. Burhanuddin Rabbani and Ahmad Shah Masood are both Tajiks. Gulbuddin Hikmatyar, a Pashtun, forged links with the IRP on the platform of Islamic solidarity. In April 1992, the opposition forces led by the IRP leader Said Abdulla Nuri declared a Badakhshan Autonomous Republic. After it was brought under Dushanbe control, a Government-in-Exile was formed in Talogan, Afghanistan.

Two years after coming to power, Rakhmanov organized presidential elections in November 1994 and won with a 62 percent majority. A referendum held simultaneously endorsed the draft constitution with a two-thirds majority. The elections for a 181-member parliament (*Majlis-e Oli*) were organized in February 1995. The Government claimed 85 percent turnout in spite of the fact that its writ did not run in much of the state. The opposition remained unimpressed by these popular exercises in legitimacy. In July 1995, the three former prime ministers—Abdumalik Abdullajonov, Jamshed Karimov and Abdulzhalik Samadov—announced the formation of the National Revival Block. In late October 1995, it entered into a coalition with the IRP under the banner of the United Tajik Opposition. As a result, the Rakhmanov regime faced a combined politico-military threat from a majority of regions of Tajikistan.

After five years of civil war that consumed 60,000 lives and three years of tortuous negotiations, the strife was finally put to rest. The deal was solemnized in the Kremlin on 27 June 1997 between the warring parties in the presence of Russian and Iranian leaders and the

UN mediator Dietrich Merren.[81] The Russians and the Iranians had pressurized the secularist president Rahmanov and the Islamist opposition respectively to make that possible; and both had worked with each other sufficiently closely to make it happen. Abdulla Nuri and Akbar Turajanzade, the leader and the deputy leader of the IRP respectively, returned from Tehran to Dushanbe. Nuri is now on the monitoring commission that is entrusted with the task of ensuring a proper implementation of the agreement. Turajanzade is the First Deputy Prime Minister.

Conclusions

Like the term the Greater Middle East, the region itself is in a state of evolution. Its prospects as a cogent spatial entity will depend on the three attributes of contiguity, commonality and connectedness, which are the defining characteristics of any region. Contiguity is self-evident; requiring no belabouring of its validity. Commonalities in terms of history going all the way back to antiquity; ethnicity enlarging Turkic and Persian habitats; and religion have been the constant common characteristics. In addition, the region has passed through similar political experiences of colonial masters who marked their borders by drawing lines on the maps; and then ruled them either directly or through intermediaries in the form of kings or local communist party bosses.

Connectedness is the attribute that will finally decide the feasibility or otherwise of the emergence of the new region. Whenever the third wave of democracy finally reaches this area, it is bound to sweep across its length and breadth, as its proponents watch across their territorial confines, seek allies, compare notes and learn from experiences/mistakes made elsewhere. And whenever oil and gas find a regular outlet from the landlocked Central Asia to the consumers, it is bound to be integrated into the global oil market. And not just the market; but the global oil economy involving operations all the way from exploration and extraction to sale, purchase, refining, transportation, distribution, currency fixation and so on.

The emergence and general acceptance of the Greater Middle East as a region seems certain in the circumstances. At least for some time to come. The areas are not eternal entities. And they definitely are not sacrosanct. They expand, contract and move in different directions with the changing realities. So will the Greater Middle East. At present, though, its contours embrace a space that deserves scholarly scrutiny and policy initiatives.

After the revolution, Iran pursued an almost predictable course of

seeking to export the revolution in order to bring about fundamental changes in the domestic politics and foreign policies of its neighbours. The states in the Gulf, and specially the hereditary kings there, found themselves at the receiving end of the revolutionary rhetoric. A destabilized state system in the region would have been a triumph for the Iranian revolution; though certainly not for the Iranian state. As a natural hegemon in the Gulf, Iran has high stakes in its stability. Today, Iran finds itself in the most comfortable situation in the triangular power balance as the two of its adversaries—Iraq and the Saudi-led GCC—are enemies of each other with almost no prospect of reconciliation in the foreseeable future. There is a pronounced polarization within the GCC itself as Kuwait, Oman and Qatar are seeking better ties with Iran. Would Iran seek a breakup of the GCC by pulling its friends away from it? Or, would it seek an eventual role within, or even membership of, the GCC? Similarly, would Iran build upon the rapprochement with Iraq or would it seek an Islamic Republic of Iraq under the SAIRI?

The Gulf is the most penetrated region in the world, however. The external powers are permanently poised there and have repeatedly resorted to violent shows of their might. The uncertainties are far too many and the consequences too unpredictable. Iran will be directly and drastically affected—for better or worse—with the changing circumstances in its immediate neighbourhood.

The emergence of new states in its northern neighbourhood presented Iran with a major security and foreign policy challenge. At the same time, it provided possibilities for political influence and economic advantage. The Iranians have relied on Islamic solidarity, Shi'a fraternity and Persian language as diplomatic props; but the primary emphasis of their offensive has been the geopolitical centrality. Roads, railways, bridges, ports and customs checkpoints have facilitated trade, transit and overland travel. A short-haul gas-pipeline with Turkmenistan and an oil-swap agreement with Kazakhstan have brought oil and gas to the Iranian refineries and consumers in the north, relieving production in the south for sales overseas, and thereby avoiding long domestic pipelines across mountainous terrain.

Iran has been careful to venture into the area with Russian knowledge and approval and has not challenged its armed presence there. The two countries share common concerns in the area, in addition to mutually beneficial bilateral ties. The resolution of Tajiki civil war, in which the Russian-supported regime and the Iranian-supported rebels agreed to give peace a chance, testify to the strength of their resolve to stay together. Would Iran continue to coordinate its

policies with Russia? Would it also continue to support Islamic political forces? A confrontation may not be inevitable, but not unlikely either.

Located in the extreme eastern corner of the Middle East, Iran is the most strategically situated in the Greater Middle East. Not only does it straddle the two large energy-rich areas of the world; it provides the best access route for the land-locked resources of Central Asia to the global market. The only Persian-speaking state in a predominantly Arab Middle East, Iran along with Tajikistan, Samarkand and Bukhara constitutes a strengthened Persian segment in a multi-ethnic mosaic of the Greater Middle East. Today, Iran seems to be in no hurry to move away from the Islamic causes it has espoused and the Islamic constituencies it has nourished. Tajikistan is a case in point. Nor is it about to renounce its regional ambitions as the takeover of Abu Musa clearly shows. Its active involvement in this emerging geopolitical space is set to influence the regional profile as also the Iranian foreign policy itself.

Notes

1. Mahan, Alfred Thayer: *The Problem of Asia and Its Effect upon Policies* (Boston: Little, Brown & Co., 1900), p. 47.

2. *The President's Proposal on the Middle East*, US Congress 85. Session 1, Hearing before the Committee on Foreign Relations and the Committee on Armed Services (1957), Pt. 1, pp. 23-24.

3. Moving Turkey administratively into the Middle East, according to this argument, would help in coordinating policy on the Kurdish zone in northern Iraq; in ensuring that the 'howl of the Central Asian wolf' does not distract the Turks into thinking they have become a world power; and encouraging Turkey to stay out of the Caucasus imbroglio. See Pipes, Daniel & Patrick Clawson: 'Ambitious Iran, Troubled Neighbors', *Foreign Affairs*, vol. 72, no. 1 (1992-93), p. 137.

4. Dessouki, A. E. H. & G. Matar: *The Arab Regional System: An Examination of Inter-Arab Political Relations* (Centre for Arab Unity Studies, 1979, in Arabic), quoted in Abdel Monem Said Abdel Aal: 'The Super Powers and Regional Security in the Middle East' in Mohammad Ayoob (ed.): *Regional Security in the Third World: Case Studies from Southeast Asia and the Middle East, 1967-91* (London: Croom Helm, 1986), pp. 197-198.

5. Ayoob, Mohammed: 'State Making, State Breaking and State Failure: Explaining the Roots of Third World Insecurity', paper presented at the seminar on 'Conflict and Development: Causes, Effects and Remedies ', The Hague, Netherlands Institute of International Relations, 22-24 March 1994, pp. 2-3.

6. Blackwill, Robert D. & Michael Stürmer (eds.): *Allies Divided: Transatlantic Policies for the Greater Middle East* (Cambridge, MA: MIT Press, 1997), p. 1.

7. Peres, Shimon (with Arye Naor): *The New Middle East* (Dorset: Element, 1993). Peres's call for regional integration did not find an echo in the region. On the contrary, concerns were raised that the economic might of Israel would lead to an Israel-dominated regional economy.

8. Akiner, Shirin: 'Relations between Iran and Central Asia: An Overview', in K. Warikoo (ed.): *Central Asia: An Emerging New Order* (New Delhi: Har Anand Publication, 1995), p. 251.

9. Juergensmeyer, Mark: *Religious Nationalism Confronts the Secular State* (Delhi: Oxford University Press, 1994), p. 126.

10. McChesney, Robert D.: 'Central Asia's Place in the Middle East: Some Historical Considerations', in David Menashri (ed.): *Central Asia Meets the Middle East* (London: Frank Cass, 1998), pp. 32-33.

11. Hitchens, Christopher: 'On the Fringes of Empire', *Guardian Weekly* (17 January 1993).

12. *Cumhuriyet* (Ankara, 24 February 1992); quoted in Winrow, Gareth M.: 'Turkey and the Former Soviet Central Asia: A Turkic Culture Area in the Making?', in Warikoo (ed.): *op. cit.* (note 8), p. 280.

13. Juergensmeyer: *op. cit.* (note 9), p. 127.

14. Palat, Madhavan K.: 'Emergence of Central Asia', unpublished paper presented at a seminar on *Trends in Central Asia*, organized by the Institute for Defence Studies and Analyses (New Delhi) 16 January 1993, p. 3.

15. Wixman, Ronald: 'Ethnic Attitudes and Relations in Modern Uzbek Cities', in William Fierman (ed.): *Soviet Central Asia: The Failed Transformation* (Boulder, CO: Westview, 1991), p. 172.

16. Bromley, Simon: *Rethinking Middle East Politics: State Formation and Development* (Cambridge: Polity Press, 1994) p. 47.

17. *Ibid.*, p. 84.

18. Harik, Ilia: 'The Origins of the Arab State System', in Giacomo Luciani (ed.): *The Arab State* (London: Routledge, 1990), pp. 1-28.

19. For a legal analysis of the Saudi Basic Laws, see Tarazi, A. Michael: 'Saudi Arabia's New Basic Laws: The Struggle for Participatory Islamic Government', *Harvard International Law Journal*, vol. 34 (Winter 1993), pp. 258-275.

20. Aba-Namay, Rashed: 'The Recent Constitutional Reforms in Saudi Arabia', *International and Comparative Law Quarterly*, vol. 42, no. 2 (April 1993), pp. 295-331.

21. Ibrahim, Saad Eddin: 'Arab Elites and Societies After the Gulf Crisis', in Dan Tschirgi (ed.): *The Arab World Today* (Boulder, CO: Lynne Rienner Publishers, 1994), pp. 85-89.

22. For a first-hand account of Birlik in its formative years, see Smith, Hedrick: *The New Russians* (London: Hutchinson, 1990), pp. 297-323.

23. Lake, Anthony: 'Confronting Backlash States', *Foreign Affairs*, vol. 73, no. 2 (1994), p. 45.

24. Zuberi, Matin: 'Kazakhstan's Nuclear Inheritance'. Unpublished paper presented at a seminar on *Central Asia in the Changing World: Trends and Development* (JNU, New Delhi, 22-23 March 1995), p. 2.

25. *Ibid.*, p. 3.

26. Weidemann, Diethelm: 'The Asian Dimension of the Dissolution of the USSR: The Central Asian Conflict Constellation: Origin, Structure, Complexity and Specificity', *Strategic Studies* (Islamabad), vol. 16, no. 3 (Spring 1994), p. 53.

27. Gurr, Ted Robert: 'Communal Conflicts and Global Security', *Current History*, vol. 94, no. 592 (May 1995), pp. 216-217.

28. Blackwill & Stürmer: *op. cit.* (note 6), pp. 303-304.

29. According to a Central Asian scholar, what Lenin wrote about imperialism being the highest state of capitalist robbery of colonial nations was to prove applicable to the reality of Soviet communist power especially in Central Asia. See Tairov, Tair: 'Communism and National Self Determination in Central Asia', in Kumar Rupesinge, Peter King & Olga Vorkunova (eds.): *Ethnicity and Conflict in a Post-Communist World: The Soviet Union, Eastern Europe and China* (New York: St. Martin's Press, 1992), p. 171.

30. *Survey of World Broadcasts—Middle East* (London), 22 August 1990. Cited hereinafter as *SWB-ME*.

31. *Le Monde* (9 October 1990), quoted in *Middle East Economic Digest* (19 October 1990), p. 26.

32. *SWB-ME* (21 December 1990).

33. *SWB-ME* (24 August 1990).

34. Islamic Republic of Iran Radio, quoted in *SWB-ME* (19 December 1990).

35. For the text of the communique, see *SWB-ME* (29 December 1990).

36. The Shi'is kiss the holy shrine in Medina and say their prayers in the Baqi cemetary, where the bodies of several imams are lying buried. See *Tehran Times* (26 May 1992).

37. *Ibid.* (3 June 1992).

38. *SWB Weekly Economic Report* (17 November 1992).

39. *Iran Focus* (Norfolk), vol. 11, no. 6 (June 1998), p. 15.

40. A recent victim of Iraqi expansionism, Kuwait has set up a sand-bank, a trench and an electrified fence to guard its 200-kilometre long border with Iraq. Additionally, 3000 US ground troops are permanently stationed in the country.

41. *Ibid.* (21 August 1994).

42. The Qataris responded enthusiastically: the Qatari ambassador in Tehran said he appreciated Iran's positive attitude. The Deputy Foreign Minister paid a visit. The Sheikh himself replied to say that 'the Arabs should unite with Iran against certain Western powers, which are seeking their own interests in the strategic Persian Gulf region.' (It is highly unlikely that the Qatari King would use the term 'Persian Gulf' even if one concedes the authenticity of the message as reproduced in the Iraninan media.) See *Keyhan*

Havai (Tehran, 7 October 1992).

43. *Middle East* (London, October 1992), pp. 17-18.

44. *Kayhan Havai* (7 October 1992).

45. *Khaleej Times* (Dubai, 22 December 1994).

46. Quoted in Glubb, Faris: 'The GCC: Important Steps Forward', *Middle East International*, no. 566 (16 January 1998), pp. 15-16.

47. *Iran Focus*, vol. 11, no. 6 (June 1998), p. 16.

48. Quoted in Bakhash, Shaul: 'Iran: War Ended, Hostility Continued,' in Amatzia Baram & Barry Rubin (eds.): *Iraq's Road to War* (Basingstoke: Macmillan, 1994), p. 219.

49. *Ibid.*, p. 220.

50. *Iran Focus*, vol. 10, no. 9 (October 1997), p.12; and vol. 11, no. 8 (September 1998), p. 14. The number of planes has varied according to differing estimates. Iran maintains that there are only 22 aircrafts on its soil.

51. Originally drawn across the 32nd parallel, the US expanded the southern zone to the 33rd parallel hugging the outskirts of the Iraqi capital Baghdad. The move was inexplicable as it came as a response to the trouble in the north in September 1996.

52. *SWB-ME* (2 November 1992).

53. *New York Times* (21 October 1993).

54. *Middle East International*, no. 461 (22 October 1993), p. 11.

55. *Middle East Economic Digest* (21 October 1994), p. 22.

56. Quoted in Barzin, Saeed: 'Iran's Dilemma', *Middle East International*, no. 588 (27 November 1998), p. 8.

57. Mesbahi, Mohiaddin: 'Iran and Tajikistan', in Alvin Z. Rubinstein & Oles M. Smolansky (ed.): *Regional Power Rivalries in the New Eurasia: Russia, Turkey, and Iran* (Armonk: M.E. Sharpe, 1995), p. 113.

58. *SWB-ME* (10 January 1989).

59. Hunter, Shireen T.: 'Iran and Transcaucasia in the Post-Soviet Era', in Menashri (ed.): *op. cit.* (note 10), p. 99.

60. *Ibid.*

61. For a detailed discussion of the Iran-Russian collaboration in the region, see Edmund Herzig: *Iran and the Former Soviet South* (London: Royal Institute of International Affairs, 1994).

62. Kemp, Geoffrey & Robert E. Harkavy: *Strategic Geography and the Changing Middle East* (Washington, DC: The Brookings Institution, 1997), p. 134.

63. 'Otherwise, the *nouveau riche* government of Azerbaijan with the help of its American and Zionist allies, will finally gobble up the entire undersea crude.' See *Iran News* (Tehran, 12 December 1998), available at www.irna.com/newshtm/eng/21132258.htm.

64. See http://www.irna.com/newshtm/eng/23173818.htm. The deal is worth $19.8 million, that is, just under the threshold of $20 million permitted under the US-imposed sanctions.

65. Kemp & Harkavy: *op. cit.* (note 62), p. 103.

66. An optimistic estimate puts the proven reserves at 32.5bb, potential reserves at 218bb, production at 4mbd in 2010 and 6mbd in 2020, net exports at 2.3 and 3.6 in 2010 and 2020 respectively. See Wilfred Kohl, http://www.turkestan-n@vm.ege.edu.tr (vol. 98, 183, 28 October 1998).

67. The Turkish option envisions gathering the oil exports at Baku in Azerbaijan, thereafter crossing either Georgia, Armenia or Iran to terminate at Ceyhan in Turkey's Gulf of Iskenderan on the Mediterranean. The British Petroleum-led Azerbaijan International Operating Company has refused to build the 2000-kilometer Baku-Ceyhan pipeline. The Azeris are searching for options including forming their own company to do it. See *ibid.*, vol. 98, 207 (21 December 1998).

68. Rand, Christopher T.: 'The Arabian Oil Fantasy: A Dissenting View of the Oil Crisis', *Harper's* (New York), vol. 284 (January 1974), pp. 43-44.

69. Lotfian, Saideh: 'Threat Perception and Military Planning in Iran: Credible Scenarios of Conflict and Opportunities for Confidence Building' in Eric Arnett (ed.): *Military Capacity and the Risk of War: China, India, Pakistan and Iran* (Oxford: Oxford University Press, 1997), p. 211. The Iranians have been projecting this scenario mainly as a justification for building the Bushehr nuclear reactor, which is expected to provide future energy security.

70. Hiro, Dilip: 'Caspian Gas: New Pipeline Benefits Iran', *Middle East International*, no. 568 (13 February 1998), p. 16.

71. Hiro, Dilip: *Between Marx and Muhammad: The Changing Face of Central Asia* (London: Harper Collins, 1994), p. 324.

72. Winrow: *op. cit.* (note 12), pp. 251. See also Yilmaz, Bahri: 'Turkey's New Role in International Politics', *Aussenpolitik*, vol. 45, no. 1 (1994), pp. 90-98.

73. *FBIS* (18 February 1992).

74. *Middle East Economic Digest* (19 September 1992).

75. http://www.irna.com/newshtm/eng/13112451.htm.

76. The roots of ECO could be traced all the way to the Baghdad Pact in mid-fifties, which was renamed the Central Treaty Organization in late-fifties and the Regional Cooperation for Development (RCD) in 1964. The first two were military pacts, whereas the RCD was formed to provide economic, cultural and technical cooperation. In 1985, the RCD member-states – Iran, Pakistan and Turkey - renamed the group ECO.

77. Interestingly, the Shah had proposed an enlargement of the RCD grouping to include India, Afghanistan and Iraq in the mid-seventies.

78. The Islamic Renaissance Party was formed in Astrakhan in early June 1990 by some 200 Muslims from various parts of the Soviet Union. It advocated religious freedom for all, reform by peaceful means, a restructuring of the economy, taking greater account of the environment, and public recognition of what they saw as women's primary role of home-building and child-rearing. The Tajik branch of the party was formed in October 1990 just outside Dushanbe. See Atkin, Muriel: 'Islamic Assertiveness and the Waning

of the Old Order', *Nationalities Papers* (Agingdon: Oxon), vol. 20, no. 1 (Spring 1992), pp. 63-64, quoted in Anderson, John: *Religion, State and Politics in the Soviet Union and Successor States* (Cambridge: Cambridge University Press, 1994), p. 201.

79. Bonner, Raymond: 'Asian Republics Still Caught in the Web of Communism', *New York Times* (13 October 1993).

80. There is a theory suggesting that the Turkification of the region was more linguistic than ethnic. After the introduction of Turkic elements to the region, many non-Turks came to identify themselves as Turks because of the change in their language. A conscious policy of historic falsification during the Soviet era and its continuance to date has led to a situation where the people are not aware of the Iranian dimension of their origins. See Hunter: *loc. cit.* (note 59), p. 101.

81. For the provisions of the agreement, see Hiro, Dilip: 'Tajikistan: Peace Pact Threatened', *Middle East International*, no. 556 (8 August 1997), pp. 11-12.

2 REGIONAL SECURITY CHALLENGES

A GCC Perspective

Jamal Al-Suwaidi

Despite the sobering events of the Iran-Iraq War, Desert Storm and the conflict over Kuwait, Gulf security remains volatile and the search for a more stable arrangement unsettled. A certain regional balance of power structure exists, constituted by Western military power, primarily the United States.

From Short to Long-Term Security

Despite the inability of the two main antagonists, Iran and Iraq, to effectively challenge this security umbrella, such a framework represents neither a final answer to the problem at hand nor can it be maintained indefinitely. The argument that the present structure has been relatively successful is plausible. This, however, does not mean that regional security in the Gulf has become part of the *Pax Americana* world order. In addition to questions raised regarding its durability, equally strong arguments can be enunciated against the maintenance of an external security umbrella to contain the threats that exist from Iran and Iraq. Recent events have in fact made it clear that military confrontation still remains to a great extent the order of the day—from the almost daily confrontations between Iraq and the US over the respective no-fly zones to military manoeuvres and missile testing from Iran. In such a context, the Gulf region remains on the brink of conflict with the constant danger of a renewed confrontation generating broader instability.

As the search for a more stable and lasting security regime for the Gulf region continues, it is important to focus on the forces and factors which impact on the current situation and its future prospects. Within this framework, it is natural for each of the countries directly involved to have its own view of Gulf security, based on individual interpretations of national interests. A balance of power structure based on a US security umbrella is viable mainly because this policy deals primarily with a military paradigm that in no way reflects the larger issues that determine Gulf security. For example, dual containment has

achieved neither a more cooperative attitude from Iran or Iraq nor has it set the basis for a more long-lasting security arrangement in the region.[1] Primarily, deterrence exists due to overwhelming US strength and the relative weakness of Iran and Iraq, unable to challenge its preeminent position. It is important to realize, however, that there is no substitute for a more long-term strategy centred on the military and political cooperation of the Arab Gulf states. Such a strategy should actively promote a more secure environment and may eventually incorporate a US or Arab role.

Apart from the current US role, the effectiveness of any security structure is determined by whether it tangibly increases security among the participatory nations. A Gulf security framework will not bear fruit unless misperceptions on all sides subside. The existing intra-regional mistrust, a situation fostered by factors of geography, history and demographics, is the main impediment towards the establishment of a more amicable regional environment.[2] Consequently, the region neither practices collective or cooperative security, nor do the regional powers of Iran and Iraq provide each other and the Gulf Cooperation Council (GCC) states with mutual reassurances about their respective intentions. Moreover, an indigenous debate regarding a region-wide outlook for the future remains limited.

As a result, it is important to focus on several fronts when assessing the current security environment in the Gulf region. First, the challenges that Iran and Iraq continue to represent must be highlighted, as well as the factors which contribute to and endanger the establishment of a more cooperative balance of interests among the region's states. It makes little sense to discuss the creation of a regional security regime when the challenges posed by two key actors within that region continue unabated.

Second, it is important to analyse the current security arrangement and determine how to mitigate the tensions so inherent in the system. Ultimately, it will only be through this combination of assessing individual interests and defining the broader context within which security exists that it will be possible to construct a new paradigm which moves beyond the current system of hostility. Gulf security should thus not be solely defined by the triangular relationship between Iran, Iraq and the United States. Rather, it is the active contribution of the GCC states themselves that has to become part of the equation in which these states define their national security and integrate it with regional security requirements.[3]

Finally, the thought processes involved have to be future-oriented and focus on what immediate steps can be taken to allow a more viable

order to emerge. In this context, it is important not to continue living in the shadow of historical legacies that have remained but to channel the available energies forward and capitalize on the determination to foster more positive developments.

Common Challenges from both Iran and Iraq

The main threat to the continued livelihood and security of the Arabian Gulf region stems from its two northern neighbours, Iran and Iraq. At the outset, it is worth mentioning that these two states are not monolithic actors. Each has its own individual policies based on the leadership's assessment of national interest. In response, the Arab Gulf states require a separate policy and agenda to deal with both Iran and Iraq. Nevertheless, there are certain features that are common to both and that pose a direct challenge to the security of the Gulf.

First, it is a fact that both states engage in low-intensity conflicts with the possibility of causing considerable collateral damage throughout the region. For Iran, this includes first, the step-by-step approach in bringing the UAE (United Arab Emirates) islands of Abu Musa and the Greater and Lesser Tunbs under its complete control, trying to establish a *de facto* situation on the ground that will prove difficult to reverse. Iran's continued hard-line and inflexible stance on this issue represents the main hurdle to a more effective relationship with the Arab Gulf states. In addition, Iran's policy of using extremist groups to spread its revolutionary message throughout the region, using methods which are difficult to counter, denotes a deliberate effort by the Iranian leadership to de-legitimize the governments of the Arab Gulf.

Iraq, on the other hand, continues to fight a low-level civil war within its country against various sections of the population and inflames regional tensions by launching verbal attacks against its Gulf neighbours. This includes statements in the first months of 1999 calling for the overthrow of GCC (Gulf Cooperation Council) leaders, the demand for an Arab tribunal to publicly try Kuwaiti and Saudi rulers as well as the threat to withdraw recognition of Iraq's border with Kuwait thereby questioning, once again, the very legitimacy of Kuwait.[4] Meanwhile, Iraq's domestic policies are defined by repression, clan rivalries and military intrigues.

A second common feature of Iran and Iraq is the fact that both harbour regional hegemonic ambitions as well as territorial claims against their neighbours. In the case of Iran, this is illustrated by Iranian occupation of the UAE islands and the Iranian leadership's refusal to consider any of the proposals put forth by the UAE to solve

the crisis peacefully and amicably. Iran's territorial ambitions extend even further, however, and include claims against the state of Bahrain as well as several off-shore resource fields in the Gulf.[5] Iraq's historical intent, meanwhile, to incorporate Kuwait as one of its provinces is deep-rooted. Despite the official acceptance of the current borders, there is little doubt that if given the opportunity, Iraq would once again renew its claims.

Third, Iran and Iraq have significant capabilities to wage war and have gained experience from previous military conflicts. The Iran-Iraq War, the Desert Storm campaign, as well as the use of security forces internally, provides both Iran and Iraq with capabilities considered threatening to the Arab Gulf states. Having attained a military mentality, it will prove difficult for these states to suddenly adapt a more flexible, peaceful and cooperative stance in their foreign policies.

Finally, it is also important to consider that in the past, neither Iran nor Iraq have operated as rational bargainers in terms of their external relations. If strategic considerations had been applied by the respective leaders, neither the Iran-Iraq War nor the 1991 Gulf War would have occurred. This aspect also relates to the specifics of the military campaigns, such as the Iranian human wave attacks against Iraqi positions early in the Iran-Iraq War. As a result of such thinking, it is quite difficult to propose reasonable and effective solutions to the issue of Gulf security. Even with the establishment of a forum for constructive and comprehensive talks, there is little guarantee of how either of these states might react. Rationality is not necessarily a part of their decision-making process.[6]

The fact that there are threats to Gulf security which are common to both Iran and Iraq does not mean, however, that these two states can be treated in exactly the same manner. As such, it is important to look beyond the prevailing features and focus on the more individual threats that endure alongside existing mutual concerns. In this context, it is important to note that while Iraq poses a clear and relatively straight forward threat—being primarily one of military conquest and intimidation—Iran represents a geopolitical and geostrategic challenge that is of far greater magnitude and complexity than a cursory glance would indicate. Iran's ability to strike at the Gulf states, for example, far exceeds the strength of its conventional military forces.

Furthermore, one should distinguish between the existence of direct threats and indirect challenges with which the Arab Gulf states are confronted. While much focus has been directed at identifying ways in which Iran and Iraq can launch attacks on their southern neighbours, equal attention should be paid to the domestic political developments

inside these two states. Intra-state disorder has the potential of causing severe instability throughout the region. A more detailed examination will illustrate this line of thinking further.

Gulf Security and Iran

Even in 1999, the actions and policies of the Islamic Republic of Iran remain a source of concern to the future stability of the Gulf region. There have been some encouraging indications since the appointment of Mohammad Khatami as President in May 1997 that a certain reevaluation of regional policy is underway within political circles. However, numerous developments tend to underline the continuing policy positions of the past. Most worrisome is the determined Iranian effort to upgrade its military preparedness and increase its offensive capabilities, particularly its ballistic missiles and weapons of mass destruction (WMD). Equally troublesome is the inflexible position towards regional issues and the continuing deterioration of Iran's economic and domestic order. These combined factors make Iran an extremely complex partner with which to deal. While on the one hand, it is Iran's foreign policy practices and rhetoric which to a large degree prompted the collective security relationship of the GCC states, the continued isolation of Iran may adversely affect the security and stability of the region.

The Military Threat

To begin with, the continued military acquisition program pursued by Iran is not in line with the strategic and economic realities of the republic. While Iraq has been subject to the stringent inspection campaigns of the UN and under the watchful eye of the international community, Iran has quietly pursued a policy of what has been termed 'creeping proliferation' and which involves substantially increasing its military readiness, both in conventional and unconventional terms.[7]

Iran's build-up includes significant advances in its military production capability, improvements with regard to its missile arsenal and naval capabilities, as well as a sustained effort to upgrade its WMD program. The expansion of the Iranian naval weapons program, for example, includes fast attack craft possibly armed with missiles, submarines with mine-laying capability, and the acquisition of numerous anti-ship weapons, as well as the continued fortification of various islands in the Gulf, including the UAE islands of Abu Musa and the two Tunbs. This gives Iran a sea-denial capability that seriously threatens the security of Gulf shipping.

On the level of WMD, there is a general consensus that Iran does

possess chemical and biological weapon arsenals, and that it has undertaken research to attain a nuclear capability.[8] Anthony Cordesman refers to Iran as having 'some of the largest unconventional warfare capabilities in the world.'[9] The precise nature of these capabilities, however, is difficult to ascertain because, as noted by the Monterey Center for Non-Proliferation Studies, 'most weapons of mass destruction programs remain secret and cannot be verified independently.'[10] Iran has continuously maintained that its research in the nuclear field is solely for civilian purposes, and inspections by the International Atomic Energy Agency (IAEA) have thus far uncovered no evidence of a clandestine program.[11] Still, the fact that Iran has no definite requirement for a civilian nuclear program—given its vast oil and gas energy reserves which adequately cover domestic consumption needs, and because it is spending precious amounts of foreign reserves on a project that is technically dubious at best, and at a time when its economy is in dire need for structural reforms—raises significant doubt.[12] The pursuit of a WMD program is even more worrisome when combined with the significant progress Iran has made in its ballistic missile capability. Iran's demonstration of its ability to deliver WMD agents includes the partially successful test firing of the Shehab-3 missile on July 21, 1998 with a range of between 1,200 and 1,500 kilometres[13] and the subsequent announcement of the development of the Shehab-4 which has an even greater range.[14]

The threat perception is increased by the many military exercises that Iran conducts, many of which are offensive in nature. In a blatant disregard for UAE national rights and sensitivities, Iran conducted such military manoeuvres in the territorial waters of Abu Musa in February of 1999. This action was condemned by the GCC as a 'violation of the UAE's sovereignty and an attempt by Tehran to secure its occupation of the three islands.'[15] As stated during the GCC ministerial meeting held in Abu Dhabi on March 4, 1999, the current Iranian armament program is considered 'more extensive than Iran's legitimate defense needs.' Taken together then, these developments are not in line with Iranian needs for adequate self-defense nor do they correspond to the existing financial realities.[16]

Foreign Policy Duality

Next to its advances in military technology and capability, Iran's foreign policy, which is closely tied to domestic developments, continues to cause concern for the region. Most recently, Iran has made an effort to improve its regional image by opening a far-reaching dialogue with the GCC states, focusing specifically on repairing its

damaged relationship with Saudi Arabia, and pledging to refrain from any interference in the internal affairs of its neighbours. Both President Khatami and Defence Minister Ali Shamkhani have called for more effective coordination between the two countries, even advocating an Arab-Persian NATO-like alliance to police the region. In an extraordinary statement by Iran's Ambassador to Saudi Arabia, Mohammad Reza Nouri, the Ambassador stated:

> Iran's missile capabilities are at the disposal of the Kingdom of Saudi Arabia ... We believe that Iran's power is the Kingdom's power, and the Kingdom's power is Iran's power. Our relations with Saudi Arabia have reached a historical stage where we are complementing one another, and if we have a missile or non-missile capability, it is at the kingdom's disposal.[17]

From this perspective, Khatami's call for a dialogue based on principles of mutual respect and non-interference in the internal affairs of other countries is welcome news to those in the Gulf who are accustomed to a different kind of rhetoric. There can be no doubt, of course, that much of the revolutionary rhetoric has lost its spark, and the Iranian public seems to be less concerned about chanting slogans against the West than they are about ensuring their daily survival. Today, there are 37 million Iranians under the age of 24 who have only scant knowledge of the events of 1979.[18] Yet while the revolutionary rhetoric out of Tehran has been toned down significantly since the election of Khatami, there is no genuine proof that Iran has completely abandoned the practices of exporting its revolutionary ideology, or its support for various extremist and covert groups once and for all. Furthermore, Persian nationalist ideology might be the next driving force behind Iranian foreign policy, replacing the fanaticism of the past. As such, it appears that regardless of which regime is in power in Tehran, Iran will continue its attempt to dominate the Gulf. This should be a major worry to the Arab Gulf states.

While Iran has exerted great effort to present as unified a position as possible in terms of its regional and international relations, there exist mounting differences in opinion, reflected in the continued dualism of Iranian foreign policy, in particular the great divide that exists between its foreign and security policy. Statements that initially appear genuine and well-intentioned are often quickly countered by pronouncements indicative of a much more radical and obstructionist outlook. Such a dichotomy certainly represents its own unique challenges in terms of projecting a genuine and solidly-grounded

national interest strategy. What it does not necessarily indicate is a higher degree of moderation on the part of the Iranian leadership. One challenge from Iran therefore is its unpredictable behaviour. With so many diffused centres of power, it is often unclear where the real authority lies.

Domestic Uncertainties
Even on the domestic front, where President Khatami appears intent on instituting the 'rule of law' as his basis for better government at home and better relations abroad, there are still many influential actors within Iranian power circles who have not given up their radicalism and who seem equally determined to bring Khatami's liberalization experiment to an end. The unprecedented acknowledgment of the involvement of members of the Ministry of Intelligence in the murder and disappearance of a number of Iranian intellectuals and critics in January 1999 serves as a poignant example of the methods that the hard-line forces inside Iran will utilize in order to stop the movement toward greater openness and freedom. Under these conditions, a termination of the reform process of Khatami and consequent increase in domestic turmoil can no longer be discounted.

As stated by a number of specialists, there is a distinct possibility that Iran will encounter a period of heightened instability due to the fact that people's expectations are not being met through government policies. In reference to what dimensions such a conflict could take, Khatami urged the armed forces to stay out of the political rivalries engulfing the country, stating that they should 'focus on beefing up the country's defences and stay above political factionalism.'[19] This call was rejected by Ali Akbar Nateq-Nuri, the Speaker of parliament and conservative competitor to Khatami in the May 1997 presidential election, who indicated that the Islamic Revolutionary Guard Corps was not just a military power but had important internal responsibilities and tasks in order to protect the principles of the revolution.[20]

Finally, the possibility of further economic instability and even the collapse of the Iranian economy has to be taken seriously. It was not by accident that Khatami's successful campaign concentrated almost solely on domestic and economic matters. Since that time, conditions have deteriorated, mostly due to the collapse of oil prices in 1998. Iran now suffers from inflation estimated to hover above twenty percent, a debt burden around US$23 billion, and a budget revenue deficit for the past fiscal year which ended in March 1999 at approximately US$6.5 billion.[21] As far as the more immediate prospect is concerned, the economy as a whole is expected to contract by around

2.6 percent in 1999 with state spending already having experienced a cut of 30 percent and a number of projects being postponed due to respective liquidity problems.[22] All this has been exacerbated by a crisis within the labour market where only fourteen million out of a population of 64 million are actively employed and where up to fifteen million Iranians will enter the workforce within the next decade.[23] President Khatami himself has referred to Iran's economy as 'sick,' stating that it suffers from grave structural problems.[24]

As a result, the possibility of parallel political inconsistency should not be discounted as long as Iran continues to face tremendous economic woes. Conservative forces inside Iran have begun to use the economic situation as a platform to launch an attack on President Khatami saying that political reforms are actually too costly to pursue in the present environment.[25] Yet, if economic reform does not begin to take hold soon, Iran may be confronted with what could be termed a 'new revolution.'[26] Of concern to the Arab Gulf states is the fact that continued economic deterioration could easily lead to domestic discontent, spilling over into the process of foreign policy formation and manifesting itself in the adoption of a more radical foreign policy posture.[27]

Need for Realism

Taken in its entirety, there is little wonder that the GCC states continue to watch developments in Iran with a wary eye. Still, there is a need for realism. First, it must be acknowledged that there are inhibiting factors placed on the Iranian system that constrain its manoeuvring capability. As already pointed out, the multitude of economic and social problems confronting Iran have led to a spread of indifference and cynicism throughout the population. Under such conditions, it is highly unlikely that Iranians would support an adventurous foreign policy that in turn could result in a further degradation of their economic posture. The fact that any military attack would be immediately repulsed is also something that the Iranian leadership is quite conscious of.

Second, it is important to view Iran's security posture from the perspective that Iran does have a number of legitimate security concerns. In that context, to state that Iran is the cause of all instability and insecurity in the region pushes the debate on regional security to a level where it becomes an exercise in futility. Instead, it is important to place current developments in their proper context and focus on the possibilities of enacting a common responsive foreign policy that adequately deals with the present threat environment. For Iran, this

means making a clear break with the interventionist policies of the past and having the political courage to place Arab Gulf — Iran relations on a level of mutual respect and equal footing. For the GCC, it is important to recognize the central regional security role which Iran has to play and to allow for a far-reaching dialogue that takes serious note of Iranian security concerns and threat perceptions.

Gulf Security and Iraq

Events since the end of 1997 once again underlined the threat that Iraq represents for Gulf security. Until that period, the danger from Iraq was somewhat limited due to the fact that a stringent sanctions regime and containment policy ensured that threats and possible attacks from Iraq would remain in check. Operation Desert Fox (the four-day bombing campaign in December 1998) brought an end to these inspections. This, coupled with the renewed determination of Saddam Hussein to break out of his stranglehold—including a more confrontational posture vis-à-vis the GCC states—has revived the threat emerging out of Baghdad.

The WMD Problem

The main obstacle inside Iraq is the fact that Saddam Hussein is still in power. He remains revanchist in nature, meaning that he has not accepted the reality on the ground and will continue to implement his grandiose designs if given the opportunity. As a result, Iraq is more overtly aggressive than Iran and is therefore more likely to take higher risks. Iraq's basic political character remains intact and its military, although depleted and demoralized, still represents a formidable fighting force. Iraq can still mobilize quickly to threaten Saudi Arabia and Kuwait. By rejecting the UN inspection team, Iraq has retained the ability to rebuild a covert arms procurement network that will pose a level of direct military danger towards the Arab Gulf states.

The past eighteen months have witnessed the gradual breakdown of the United Nations Special Commission (UNSCOM) regime inside the country. Throughout all of 1998, inspections were only carried out with interruptions and were therefore only nominal in nature. The four-day bombing campaign in December 1998—launched as a response to Saddam Hussein's delaying tactics—finally caused all UNSCOM work to cease. Since then, the dispute with Iraq has centred on the almost daily altercations with regard to the enforcement of the no-fly zones over northern and southern Iraq. While it is generally acknowledged that UNSCOM did an exceptional job in terms of destroying Iraqi capabilities with regard to WMD, viewed from a threat perspective, the fact is that Saddam Hussein has now had almost two years time in

which to rebuild much of his program and add it to what he was able to originally save and conceal.

As a result, the threat posed by Iraq manifests itself in unaccounted stockpiles of chemical and biological weapons in addition to a significant delivery capability that could be utilized against its Gulf neighbours.[28] While Iraq's nuclear program has been largely disabled, this does not mean that technology and the relevant knowledge connected to a nuclear capability has been erased.[29] Reports about the implementation of a clandestine purchasing system having been put in place underlines the continued effort by the Iraqis to rebuild such a capability.[30] These attempts become more serious if one considers that Iraq has had half a decade in which to improve 'its decoys, dispersal concepts, dedicated command and control links, targeting methods, and strike plans.'[31] Furthermore, as a result of the success by UNSCOM, Iraq may well have increasingly focused on biological weapons rather than a nuclear capability as these are much easier to conceal and can be produced at relatively little cost.

Internal Instability
Apart from its military capabilities, Iraq's internal instability remains acute. The danger exists that even under a post-Saddam regime, general anarchy could spread throughout the country, thus further complicating an already difficult transition period until the establishment of a new government. The current regime has severely damaged the existing political culture where sub-national loyalties continue to be mainly fostered by relying on tribal affiliation. Because of the almost complete destruction of Iraqi civil society and the uncertain nature and direction of any post-Saddam regime, the possibility of a whole new set of factors appearing that might in turn threaten the security of the Arab Gulf states is high. It is in this context that the current sanctions regime in place needs to be evaluated. One could argue that as a result of the tight embargo, new seeds of violence are being planted that could easily grow into threats to Gulf security. This includes the emergence of revisionist and revanchist policies at some point in the future.

Some of the recent data underscore the dilemma being faced as a result of the current UN sanctions. According to the former UN humanitarian coordinator for Iraq, up to 5,000 children die each month due to the effects of malnutrition and disease.[32] The Food and Agricultural Organization (FAO) estimates that one-third of Iraqi children under the age of five as well as a quarter of adults under the age of 26 are said to be suffering from malnourishment, culminating in a total of four million people being on the verge of starvation.[33] In

addition, the infant mortality rate has doubled between 1990 and 1995 and 75 percent of the medical equipment in Iraqi health facilities is said to be not operational. Meanwhile, Iraq's gross domestic product per capita income has fallen from US$2,900 in 1990 to under US$60 at present. Other items include the 'de-education' of an entire Iraqi generation due to the lack of proper educational materials and declining enrolment rates, the high increase in crime and domestic violence, and the crumbling of the country's infrastructure leading to severe interruptions in power and water supplies throughout the country.[34] The doubling of the amount available through the UN Oil-for-Food program to US$5.25 billion has done little to alleviate the situation. For one, the Iraqi government continues to disrupt its operations, seeing the oil-for-food program as an encroachment on its own sovereignty. Second, due to Iraq's crumbling oil infrastructure, it is nearly impossible for Iraq to export the amount of oil that would meet the target revenue. Moreover, only two-thirds of the money actually goes towards the purchase of humanitarian items with the rest being used for war reparations and to offset UN-related expenses.

Furthermore, relatively little discussion has been undertaken about how to properly fill the political vacuum that would result from a respective leadership change. Besides the political problems of the Kurdish and the Shi'a issue, Iraq will still have to deal with the security of its water resources—for example the implications of the Great Anatolia Water Project (GAP) being pursued by Turkey which could reduce the flow of water into Iraq by as much as 50 percent—its access to Gulf waters as an export route for its oil resources, and finally unresolved border disputes which are dormant at the moment but far from settled.[35] All these items combine to make Iraq an uncertain partner in terms of constructing a future indigenous Gulf security environment.

Security Dilemmas

As a result, a certain dilemma presents itself. One the one hand, due to Iraq's ability to retain a covert arms procurement network, the possibility of a direct military threat against the Arab Gulf states is still in effect.[36] As discussed earlier, economic sanctions have done little to negate the threat emanating from Iraq. On the other hand, a weakened and isolated Iraq has very little actual power to challenge the status quo. Rather, it represents a disruptive force, if anything.

In order to counter the more ominous scenarios, it is imperative to develop a plan that reintegrates Iraq into the regional scene following a change of leadership. While it remains relatively futile that

such steps can be effectively implemented with Saddam Hussein still in power, the alternatives available to Iraq following his demise should be articulated and put forth now so as to ensure that whoever follows in Saddam's footsteps will be more likely to engage the Arab Gulf states on a more cooperative basis. The contradiction inherent in the sanctions regime is that its restrictions are weakening the central state at the same time that the integrity of Iraq's territory remains its highest priority. If anything, it needs to be understood that there is a definite need for Iraq to finally reconcile itself with the events of the past, in particular its defeat in the Gulf War, and to start thinking about proper ways of reconciliation and rebuilding its shattered country.

Furthermore, there is the need to discuss the situation inside Iraq within the proper context of overall regional strategic balance. Unfortunately, some countries are using the opportunity of an opening with Iran as a way to further tighten the noose around the neck of Iraq, seeing this as a way and opportunity to completely isolate Saddam Hussein. The faulty thinking at the bottom of this approach is that with Iran being available, why worry about Iraq.[37] Yet, the transition inside the Iranian political establishment from its authoritarian past is far from complete until now and precious little actual policy action has been applied to substantiate the more conciliatory rhetoric coming from Tehran. An objective analysis about the current threats as posed by both Iran and Iraq is essential in this regard as it will be only through the establishment of a working relationship between all the states in the region that one could begin to discuss the creation of a lasting stable balance within the Gulf.

The question therefore arises whether the current containment policy is viable and should continue or whether certain adjustments are essential. The previous discussion should indicate that the status quo cannot continue. Staying indefinitely on the current path of crisis management as has been the case for the past eight years has not only proved ineffective in bringing about a solution but it will also very likely sow the seeds for further instability emanating from the northern Gulf. The imperative is on the development of a differentiated approach that combines regional and international policy vis-à-vis Iraq into one comprehensive viable plan. There are a number of steps that can be taken in this regard. For one, an opening in terms of a political dialogue would be beneficial not only in terms of initiating contact and avoiding the complete isolation of Iraq's ruling elite but also to be able to speak frankly about what it will take to reintegrate Iraq into the Arab regional fold. Second, one could consider starting a second-track channel of communication, for example on the level of academic non-

technical and cultural exchanges. Third, there is the need to approach the sanctions regime with a higher degree of flexibility in order to allow for the further build-up of economic and social infrastructure such as power plants and sewage facilities. In addition, the reparations issue has to be made more conditional on future behaviour so as not to cripple Iraq economically from the outset. Overall, the utility of economic trade can be used as one instrument to facilitate dialogue.[38]

Gulf Security and the GCC

Based on the above discussion concerning Iran and Iraq, the GCC states are faced with a certain dilemma. On the one hand, there is a clear and unequivocal realization that a stable regional security environment can only be implemented through the active participation of all the states that border the Arabian Gulf, namely the GCC countries, Iran and Iraq. On the other hand, the policies pursued by the two northern states have been diametrically opposed to such a unified approach and instead have been based on interference in the internal affairs of the GCC states and the attempt to dominate regional policies.

To be able to integrate these diverging strands, there is a need to put forward a strategic vision, one that is centred around a more serious role played by the Arab Gulf states with regard to their military and political cooperation. For one, there is an urgent need for the GCC states to become more serious with regard to their military cooperation and to implement steps which will significantly boost the GCC's regional deterrent posture. The creation of a rapid deployment force would be one important step that could serve in such a capacity. In addition, increased attention should be paid to ensuring the maritime security of the GCC states with particular emphasis on strengthening the defensive parameter of coastal areas and allowing for uninterrupted maritime traffic on the waters of the Arabian Gulf. By focusing the efforts of a Rapid Deployment Force on coastal security as well as concentrating on anti-mine capabilities, one will begin to deal more effectively with both aspects.

Gulf security will of course not be solved by simply removing the threats emanating from Iran and Iraq. Ultimately, an improved political climate serves as a precondition to any kind of security cooperation.[39] Consequently, the second area of concentration in terms of GCC security policy has to be on the political front. A resolution to the outstanding border disputes that exist among the GCC states would be an important step in the right direction towards overcoming some of the misperceptions of the past. The agreement between the UAE and Oman is, in this sense, an example that should be emulated throughout

the region. There are also other steps that can be taken to increase confidence within the Gulf. The establishment of a regional crisis management centre as an institution based on conflict prevention rather than conflict resolution could serve as an important component in terms of lessening existing threat perceptions. Of equal importance would be the emphasis on intensive track-two type diplomacy and dialogue. All of these steps, however, involve the precondition that the security concerns of the smaller states be treated with the same kind of concern as afforded to the larger states.

Third, it is important to recognize that security maintenance should no longer be viewed solely in terms of its military dimension. Instead, there is an urgent need to focus on comprehensive security involving issues of economic development growth strategies, social change, population growth, health concerns, and the construction of a responsive and flexible public policy. As stated previously: 'The prerogative for the coming decade is not only to prepare for or deter against traditional external military threats but also to ensure that change—economic, political and social—remains evolutionary.'[40] In this context, the establishment of a regional trade zone, one that focuses on the expansion of economic cooperation in such areas as oil, banking, and investment would be a positive initiative.

Fourth, constructive solutions to other regional issues such as the Arab-Israeli conflict need to be sought as a way to eliminate further tension in the region. With linkage being a fact of life in the Middle East, it is absolutely necessary that immediate and substantial progress be achieved in the peace process and that such progress be tied to tangible and direct benefits for the Palestinian people as well as neighbouring states. There is the need, however, to view the Gulf security region as distinct from the greater Middle East, as a means to concentrate more fully on the intricate issues which are at the heart of Gulf security and stability. Such a distinction would allow one to break down the problems into more manageable portions and to more effectively propose solutions on a step-by-step basis.

Finally, there is an urgent need to control missile and WMD proliferation and refocus efforts on arms control including the establishment of WMD-free zones, conventional arms limitations, the establishment of a missile control regime, strengthening verifications measures and various aspects of military restructuring. The nuclear detonations by India and Pakistan, the end to UNSCOM inspections in Iraq, an already existing WMD capability and missile testing by Iran, Israel's continued policy of nuclear ambiguity and the export of WMD-related technology into the region have all significantly increased the

threat that exists connected with proliferation policies. In addition to these items, the particular emphasis of arms control measures for missiles with no defensive utility whatsoever is a policy which the GCC states need to support. Greater transparency and the pre-notification to all military manoeuvres in the Gulf would be another important component worthy of consideration.

Together, these issues will be instrumental in determining the manner in which security will be structured in this region. By assessing individual interests and placing them in the larger security context, it will become possible to construct a new paradigm that moves beyond the current system of hostility. The priority of the GCC will be to structure its security policy in such a fashion that it is able to accommodate the various contradictions which are inherent in the policies of the main actors. Equally imperative is to find a new mechanism that allows for re-constituting of the Arab regional system, including the strengthening of the Arab League and other regional and international organizational institutions.

Concluding Remarks

Having outlined the various challenges to Gulf security as well as the relationship between the GCC and the development of a viable security regime, it is necessary to place the recent events into their proper context and project their implications into the near future with the purpose of providing some alternative suggestion to the problems at hand.

The recent more conciliatory tone coming from Tehran lends a certain aura of hope to a more cooperative and beneficial relationship developing between the Islamic Republic and the Arab Gulf states. Realistically speaking, however, even if his calls for greater cooperation are serious, President Khatami will have to carry out his work under the severe restrictions imposed on him by the Iranian decision-making system. Power and control over issues of foreign policy are clearly limited and overall responsibility remains with the spiritual leader Ayatollah Khameini. Khatami's primary focus in any event will be the domestic economic and social arena, an area of primary importance where improvements could very well add to the overall prospects of Gulf security.

One therefore should be cautious about accepting Iranian statements at face-value. In a way, one is reminded of Ronald Reagan's admonition to then Soviet President Mikhail Gorbachev regarding arms control initiatives and agreements of 'Trust, but verify.' Policy change within a state rarely occurs overnight, and the current calls for a more

cooperative relationship with the Arab Gulf states are grounded in the Iranian realization that its revolutionary rhetoric and oppositional stance is no longer in line with the economic and governing realities that the Islamic Republic is faced with today. The new pragmatism might sound and look like new moderation, but it most certainly is based on age-old structures of Persian hegemony.

Iran can, however, not be isolated. Neither can the bilateral relationship between the Islamic republic and the Arab Gulf states be seen through an American lens. Iran is faced with some very real security threats including the possible hostile intervention of the United States, the lingering conflict with Iraq, various opposition movements, an unstable northern region and domestic turmoil. These issues need to be considered when erecting a new *modus vivendi* for the region. In addition, to refer to amicable relations without considering Iran's domestic policy, its economic agenda or its social structure, would prove irrelevant. It is important for one to focus on efforts that would increase the competitiveness and diversification of the Iranian economy, in turn leading to a more stable and predictable internal climate. At the same time, the Iranian leadership must understand that any type of economic assistance cannot be seriously considered until Iran reduces its revolutionary rhetoric as well as its military modernization and rearmament program. To do otherwise, would be a repeat of mistakes in the past, i.e., Iraq.

With respect to Iraq, the most urgent matter is to establish a blueprint that has at its core the reintegration of the state into the regional structure. Principles need to be set forth that will clear the way for the recognition of any post-Saddam government. Current tensions remain high but manageable. Can we afford to alienate the Iraqi population as a whole for an indeterminate period while suffocating sanctions are kept in place? Underlying such proposals, however, is the need to avoid a repeat of Versailles and the devastating consequences of the treaty on political and economic development on Germany. While possible steps to alleviate the situation have been elaborated upon, how applicable these suggestions are is a matter of debate.

With reference to the subject of Gulf security in general, the role of the United States as filling the security vacuum created by Iraq can only be considered a short-term solution. A new stable security paradigm is absolutely necessary for the establishment of Gulf security, one that involves all countries of the Arabian Gulf. Although effective military security is paramount, continuing on the military paradigm that has been in place over the last few years will begin to create unnecessary instability and extend additional burdens. Economic

prosperity, meanwhile, has shown itself to be a stabilizing factor and every effort should be made to establish strong economic and trade relations between all the countries of the Arabian Gulf. This will not only support the fragile structures that currently exist in Iran and Iraq, but it will also add to the well-being and prosperity of the GCC states.

In conclusion, the various challenges which present themselves currently to the governments of the Arab Gulf states are broad in nature and cannot be confined solely to military-related aspects coming from its two northern neighbours. The development of an effective public policy, the continuing evolvement of economic growth strategies, as well as the broader regional issues such as the Arab-Israeli conflict all have an impact on the Gulf, and thus determine the manner in which security will be structured in this region. One needs to be aware of the danger that both Iran and Iraq pose and accordingly put forth policy alternatives that both counter such threats as well as offer credible future solutions. But one cannot make this the sole focus.

Notes

1. While it has to be acknowledged that dual containment was never conceived as a long-term solution, it was a policy intricately tied to progress on the Arab-Israeli issue. Without substantial progress in this arena, the contentious issues which are intricate to Gulf security became mitigated to a certain degree and the debate shifted to contingencies which are not necessarily tied directly to the furtherance of peace and stability in the Gulf region. The purpose here, however, is not to debate the fallacies of the dual containment approach, something which has already received attention. See, for example, Katzman, Kenneth: 'Beyond Dual Containment', *Emirates Occasional Paper* no. 6 (Abu Dhabi: The Emirates Center for Strategic Studies and Research, 1996); Hisham Melhem: 'Dual Containment: The Demise of a Fallacy', *Occasional Paper Series* (Washington, DC: Center for Contemporary Arab Studies, Georgetown University, 1997); and Sick, Gary 'Rethinking Dual Containment,' *Survival* vol. 40, no. 1 (Spring 1998), pp. 5-32.

2. Gargash, Anwar M.: 'Prospects for Conflict and Cooperation: The Gulf toward the Year 2000,' in Gary G. Sick & Lawrence G. Potter (eds.) *The Persian Gulf at the Millennium: Essays in Politics, Economy, Security and Religion* (New York: St. Martin's Press, 1998), p. 321.

3. This is an argument initially laid out in my chapter 'The Gulf Security Dilemma: The Arab Gulf States, the United States and Iran,' in Al-Suwaidi, Jamal S. (ed.): *Iran and the Gulf: The Search for Stability* (Abu Dhabi: The Emirates Center for Strategic Studies and Research, 1996), pp. 327-351.

4. See, for example, 'Iraq Says Kuwait's Land and Coast Belong to Iraqi People,' *Associated Press* (14 January, 1999); 'Saddam Slams Saudi, Kuwait,' *FBIS* translated text from the Iraqi News Agency, INA (23 January, 1999); 'Iraqi MPs Blast Gulf Leaders over U.S. Attack,' *Reuters* (26 January, 1999);

and 'Iraq Warns Kuwait, Saudi Arabia over Air Bases,' *Reuters* (14 February 1999).

5. For an account of Iranian involvement in domestic GCC affairs see Pelletiere, Stephen: *The Iran-Iraq War: Chaos in a Vacuum* (New York: Praeger Publisher, 1992), especially pp. 60-63.

6. See, for example, Waltz, Kenneth N.: *Man, the State and War: A Theoretical Analysis* (New York: Columbia University Press, 1954), especially pp. 16-41.

7. The term is used by Anthony Cordesman in 'Recent Military Developments in the Persian Gulf: Defense Efforts, the Conventional Balance, Weapons of Mass Destruction, and Terrorism' (Washington, DC: Center for Strategic and International Studies, 12 November 1998), available at http://www.csis.org.

8. For an overview of Iran's nuclear program, see Koch, Andrew & Jeanette Wolf: 'Iran's Nuclear Procurement Program: How Close to the Bomb?,' *The Nonproliferation Review*, vol. 5, no. 1 (Fall 1997), pp. 123-135.

9. Cordesman, Anthony: 'Saudi Arabia, the US and the Structure of Gulf Alliances,' *Middle East Net Assessment Report*, 25 February 1999 (Washington, DC: Center for Strategic and International Studies, CSIS), available on the CSIS website at http://www.csis.org.

10. Refer to a summary of the status of Iran's WMD programs published by the Monterey Institute's Center for Non-Proliferation Studies (Monterey, California) at http://cns.miis.edu/research/wmdme/iran.htm.

11. This was poignantly clear during an interview in December 1997 with Iranian President Rafsanjani on the US television program *60 Minutes* where he replied to the question of whether Iran had a nuclear weapons program with: 'Definitely not. I hate this weapon.'

12. Jones, Peter: 'Iran's Threat Perceptions and Arms Control Policies,' *The Nonproliferation Review*, vol. 6, no. 1 (Fall 1998), especially pp. 46-49. For example, as reported by *Reuters* (12 October 1998), Iran has earmarked US $140 million to build the nuclear power plant in Bushehr with Russian assistance.

13. *New York Times* (23 July 1998); 'Iran provides details on missile,' *Associated Press* (2 August 1998). For a detailed description of the Iranian missile program see Karp, Aaron: 'Lessons of Iranian Missile Programs for U.S. Nonproliferation Policy,' *The Nonproliferation Review*, vol. 5, no. 3 (Spring-Summer 1998).

14. Despite Iranian claims that the Shehab-4 is to be used solely for the purpose of launching satellites into orbit, the fact is that the missile represents a new version of the old SS-4 Soviet missile which does not have the capability to be used as a space launcher. Iran also tested a sea-launch ballistic missile in 1998 as well as a surface-to-air missile in April 1999. Overall, the Iranian inventory in reference to missiles includes 200-300 Scud-Bs with a range of 200 to 310 km, approximately 60-100 Scud-Cs with a range of over 500 km, the already mentioned Shehab-3, although it is unclear how opera-

tional the missile is at this stage, as well as various types of surface-to-surface missiles, anti-ship cruise missiles, surface-to-air missiles, and other long-range cruise missile systems imported from China. In addition, there are concerted efforts on-going to manufacture entire missile systems and warhead packages domestically.

15. The GCC statement is available in the *Emirates Daily Digest of News and Features* (4 March, 1999).

16. The International Monetary Fund (IMF) has noted that Iran in fact devotes more funds to defense spending than it actually admits in its official budgets, since the budget itself does not reflect the heavy subsidies being extended to the domestic arms industry in addition to excluding numerous arms imports. See, *Jane's Defence Weekly*, vol. 29, no. 6 (11 February 1998), p. 18.

17. The statement by Nouri was made on 29 July, 1998 to the *Al-Hayat* newspaper. It is also listed, alongside those by President Khatami and Defense Minister Shamkhani in the *Global Intelligence Update*, put out by Stratfor Systems, Inc. See 'Developments in Russia and the Persian Gulf,' (6 August 1998), available on the organization's website at http://www.stratfor.com.

18. 'One Year on, Iran's Economy Remains Khatami's Biggest Challenge,' *Agence France-Presse* (20 May 1998).

19. As reported by *IRNA* and carried by *Reuters* (1 August 1998).

20. As reported by *Al-Hayat* (18 September 1998).

21. 'Country Report Iran', *Economist Intelligence Unit* (EIU), 1st Quarter 1999; *Reuters* (9 March 1999); *Financial Times* (10 March 1999).

22. 'Iran: Country Update,' *Economist Intelligence Unit* (10 September 1998).

23. Statement by the Deputy Minister for Industry, Akbar Torkan, to the daily *Iran News* as quoted by *Reuters* (25 May 1998).

24. *Emirates News* (16 March 1998). See also, *Reuters* (16 June 1998).

25. Ayatollah Mohammad Yazdi, the head of the judiciary, told worshippers at the weekly Friday prayers that 'today political development is of fourth or fifth degree of importance. Economic problems are of primary importance.' His comments were echoed by Ali Akbar Nateq-Nuri who stated that the real problems were 'inflation, low oil prices, and unemployment.' See 'Conservatives Say Reform too Costly for Iran,' *Reuters* (5 July, 1998).

26. This warning has been mentioned frequently since the rise of President Khatami. See, for example, the article by Sa'id al-Qaysi in *al-Watan al-Arabi* (12 June 1998), pp. 32-33; the *Iranian Press Service* (9 June 1998) warning of a coup against the President; or the *Christian Science Monitor* (23 June 1998).

27. Al-Suwaidi, *op. cit.* (note 3), p. 329.

28. Anthony Cordesman has stated that: 'Iraq retains the technology it acquired before the war and evidence clearly indicates an on-going research and development effort in spite of the UN sanctions regime.' See idem: 'Military Balance in the Middle East XIV: Weapons of Mass Destruction,' *Report* (Washington, DC: CSIS, 16 March, 1999), updated version available on

the CSIS website at http//www.csis.org. Cordesman notes that next to its delivery capability, Iraq has the capability to produce stable, highly lethal VX gas and it retains the capability to manufacture various biological agents including the bacteria which cause anthrax, botulism, tularemia and typhoid. See also Bowman, Steve: 'Iraqi Chemical and Biological Weapons (CBW) Capabilities', *Congressional Research Service*(Washington, DC, April 1998).

    29. For a detailed description of Iraq's systematic attempt to deceive the International Atomic Energy Agency and continue in its quest for a nuclear program see Hamza, Khidhir: 'Inside Saddam's Secret Nuclear Program,' *The Bulletin of the Atomic Scientists*, vol. 54, no. 5 (September/October 1998), pp. 26-33.

    30. See, for example, respective reports in the *New York Times* (20 November, 1998), *Associated Press* (29 November, 1998), *Washington Post* (18 October, 1998), or the *Times of London* (4 August, 1998).

    31. Cordesman: *loc. cit.* (note 28), p. 56.

    32. 'U.N. Aid Chief Resigns over Iraq Sanctions,' *The Independent* (1 October, 1998). See also 'Sanctions Still Take Very Heavy Toll among Iraqis,' *Reuters* (24 April, 1999).

    33. 'Special Report: FAO/WFP Food Supply and Nutrition Assessment Mission to Iraq,' (Rome: FAO, 1997).

    34. See Halliday, Dennis & Jennifer E. Horan: 'A New Policy Needed for Iraq,' *Boston Globe* (22 March, 1999); 'Sanctions Drive 1 Million Iraqis from School' *Reuters* (10 December, 1998); Adebajo, Adekeye: 'Saddam's Bazaar,' *The World Today* (March 1998), pp. 60-63; the special issue of *Middle East Report*, 'The Impact of Sanctions in Iraq' (Spring 1998); and UNICEF: 'Nearly One million Children Malnourished in Iraq' (16 November 1997).

    35. Bahgat, Gawdat: 'Iraq after Saddam—What Lies Ahead?,' *Journal of Social, Political and Economic Studies*, vol. 23, no. 1 (Spring 1998), pp. 39-52.

    36. Important to emphasize in this regard is the fact that such a danger does not translate into unqualified support for U.S. military actions which run counter to many humanitarian principles of the Arab Gulf states and whose concern over the implications are widely shared by the public in the region. In terms of the effort Iraq has put up to deceive U.N. weapon inspectors see Hamza: *loc. cit.* (note 29); and the two part series by Gellman, Barton: 'A Futile Game of Hide and Seek,' and 'Arms Inspectors ''Shake the Tree''. UNSCOM Adds a Covert Tactic,' in *Washington Post* (11 and 12 October, 1998).

    37. This approach was made clear in a recent discussion by Bruce Riedel, Special Assistant to the President and Senior Director for Near East and South Asian Affairs at the National Security Council, Washington, DC on the *World-net* program of the United States Information Agency on 1 October, 1998.

    38. These were some of the conclusions reached during a conference entitled 'The West and the Gulf' organized by Wilton Park and held November 2-6, 1998.

39. Gargash: *loc. cit.* (note 2), p. 325.

40. These are some of the issues dealt with in Long, David & Christian Koch (eds.): *Gulf Security in the Twenty-first Century* (Abu Dhabi: The Emirates Centre for Strategic Studies and Research, 1998), especially pp. 11-12.

3 THE CASPIAN SEA GEO-POLITICAL GAME

The United States Versus Iran

Gawdat Bahgat

The United States is the world's largest energy consumer and net importer. In recent years Washington's crude oil production has fallen from nine million barrels of oil a day (b/d) in 1985 to 5.84 million b/d in 1999.[1] The Department of Energy predicts a continuation of this decline at an average rate of 1.1 percent a year between 1997 and 2020 to a projected level of 5.0 million b/d.[2] This decline in U.S. oil production is largely a result of American major oil companies slashing their spending on exploration and development of oil in the United States (a mature oil region for the most part), and shifting their focus to newer, potentially larger prospects abroad. This declining production in conjunction with rising demand leads to growing dependence on imported oil. In 1998, oil imports represented 52 percent of US oil consumption. The share of petroleum consumption met by net imports will rise to 65 percent in 2020.[3]

Given this increased reliance on foreign suppliers, Washington began to consider the steady flow of oil a matter of national security. Access to cheap energy remains a cornerstone of U.S (indeed, world) economic prosperity. In order to ensure against energy disruptions, the United States has sought to diversify sources of oil supplies. For a long time, the Persian Gulf has been considered the most significant repository for reasonably priced energy. The region contains approximately 65 percent of world's oil reserves and 33.3 percent of its natural gas reserves.[4] Furthermore, these hydrocarbon resources can be extracted from the ground at a relatively low cost and are found along effective and well-developed transport routes.[5] In 1998 the Persian Gulf's shares of net oil imports of the United States, Western Europe, and Japan were 21.9, 50, and 76 percent respectively.[6] These figures are projected to rise further in the foreseeable future. In other words, despite political instability and security challenges, global demand for and dependence on energy supplies from the Persian Gulf will continue to grow.

The end of the Cold War and the collapse of the Soviet Union provided access to another promising energy repository—the Caspian Basin. The region contains some of the largest undeveloped oil and gas reserves in the world. The intense interest shown by the major international oil and gas companies testifies to its potential. Although the area is unlikely to become 'another Persian Gulf', it could become a major oil supplier at the margin, much as the North Sea is today.[7] As such, it could help increase world energy security by diversifying global sources supply. In spite of this promising and, largely untapped, hydrocarbon wealth, the Caspian Basin faces tremendous obstacles. These obstacles are less geological in nature. Rather, the full utilization of the region's resources is a function of several geopolitical issues including questions of sovereignty and regional stability. Important disputes regarding ownership of the resources and financing the exploration, production and transportation of oil and gas supplies need to be resolved. The manner in which these issues are resolved, whether adversarial or cooperative, will determine how quickly Caspian Basin's oil and gas penetrate world markets.

The Islamic Republic of Iran enjoys strategic location between the Persian Gulf and the Caspian Basin. It holds nine percent of the world's oil reserves and fifteen percent of its gas reserves.[8] These vast resources and strategic location make Iran a crucial player in both regions (the Persian Gulf and the Caspian Basin) as well as world energy market. However, for the last two decades Iran has presented the United States government with a difficult dilemma by containing two conflicting pillars of American foreign policy: a desire to promote United States economic interests around the world and a determination to exert pressure on Iran to change its behaviour on certain foreign policy issues.

This paper examines Washington's efforts to contain and slow down the development of Iran's energy sector. In particular the analysis focuses on the United States role in opposing foreign investment to Iran and preventing Tehran from playing a role in the exploration and transportation of oil and gas from the Caspian Basin. The study highlights the recent thaw between the two countries and suggests that in the energy sector, relations between Washington and Tehran should not be seen in zero-sum terms. Rather, both the United States and the Islamic Republic of Iran share a common ground and mutual interests in promoting political stability in the Persian Gulf and the Caspian Basin and the full utilization of hydrocarbon resources from these two regions.

Iran and the United States

Since the early 1990s, the Clinton administration's policy toward Iran has been dominated by three allegations: that Tehran is opposing the Middle East peace process between the Arabs and the Israelis; that it is sponsoring international terrorism against Americans; and that it attempt to acquire and develop weapons of mass destruction (WMD). Iran denies all these accusations.[9] In order to deprive Iran of the financial resources to pursue these objectives, Washington imposed several restrictions on investment in the Islamic Republic's energy sector—the main source of national income. These include the 1995 executive order that made it illegal for American oil companies to operate in Iran and established penalties for any US person or corporation doing business there. Another important step was the 1996 Iran-Libya Sanctions Act (ILSA) which imposed sanctions on any foreign corporation that invested $40 million or more in the Iranian oil and gas sector.[10]

This American policy of trying to limit foreign investment in the Iranian energy sector has been partially successful. Both domestic political chaos in the late 1970s and the war with Iraq in the 1980s left very few resources, if any, to upgrade and expand the economic infrastructure. Consequently, since the early 1990s Tehran has sought to resist the American sanctions and to attract investment from other sources. An important impediment, however, is the fact that the Iranian constitution does not allow giving concession to foreign identities in the energy sector. In response, the government developed arrangement called 'buy-back' which allows firms to finance projects for repayment in produce. These Iranian efforts have recently succeeded in breaking the wall of economic isolation and signing several agreements with non-American oil and gas companies. The list includes France's Total and EIF Aquitaine, Italy's ENI, Canada's Bow Valley, Russia's Gazprom, Malaysia's Petronas, and Britain's Lasmo, among others. Three important reasons explain this global interest in investing in the Iranian energy sector. First, the country's well-known huge oil and gas reserves which means there is low risk involved in the exploration and development of these resources. Second, the fact that with the exception of the United States, the rest of the world does not subscribe to the policy of containing and isolating Iran. Thus, the European Union has pursued a policy of accommodation and dialogue with Iran. It is important to point out that under European pressure the Clinton administration decided in May 1998 to wave the provisions of ILSA against a consortium of French, Russian and Malaysian companies that signed a $2 billion agreement to develop Iranian gas fields.

Finally, the election of President Muhammad Khatami in 1997 and his efforts to introduce economic and political reform have convinced many foreign leaders that the Iran of the late 1990s is different from that of the 1970s and 1980s. A real change is taking place in Tehran and a policy of accommodation might accelerate and consolidate this shift toward moderation. Thus, for the foreseeable future it is likely that Iran will continue to attract foreign investment, particularly if the Khatami administration succeeds in offering more incentives for international oil companies to develop the country's massive energy resources and if the United States continues to show a benign opposition to such investments. In contrast, Washington has expressed strong opposition to Tehran's efforts to become a major player in the Caspian Basin.

The Caspian Basin
Shortly after the collapse of the Soviet Union, the newly-independent central Asian states, particularly Azerbaijan, Kazakhstan and Turkmenistan, invited western oil companies to explore and develop their energy resources. They wanted to be economically independent from Moscow. In the following years, Washington has articulated several strategic interests in the Caucasus and central Asia. These include the removal of nuclear weapons from the region, solving regional conflicts, formation of democratic political institutions and preventing any single country from establishing hegemony over the region. These last two objectives have direct impact on the development of energy resources from the region and the potential role Iran might play.

Since the early 1990s, Washington has sought to promote the democratic transformation of these central Asian states. The assumption is that political freedom and economic markets are the long-term guarantors of stability and prosperity. A milestone in this direction is the Silk Road Strategy Act, enacted by the United States Congress in 1999. The Act specifies five American objectives: 1) promote sovereignty, independence, democracy and respect for human rights; 2) assist in the resolution of regional conflicts and facilitate the removal of impediments to cross-border commerce; 3) promote economic cooperation and market-oriented principles; 4) assist in the development of infrastructure necessary for communications, transportation, education, health, and energy and trade on an East-West axis in order to build strong relations and commerce between those countries and the democratic, market-oriented countries of the Euro-Atlantic community; and 5) support U.S. business interests and investments in the region.[11]

In spite of these stated goals of promoting democratic transformation, it is important to point out that, to a large extent, United States policy toward these central Asian states has been based on winning the personal favour of the leader currently in power. In other words, for most of the 1990s, the United States has chosen stability (i.e. supporting authoritarian leaders) over taking risk by pressuring the regimes in power to introduce political reform. In short, Washington has achieved little success in promoting democratic institutions in the Caucasus and Central Asia.

By contrast, American foreign policy has been, relatively speaking, more successful in achieving the second goal—containing the Iranian involvement in the region. In the early 1990s, Washington showed considerable worry over the spread of 'fundamentalist Islam', sponsored by Tehran, in these newly-independent states. For example, in 1995 direct American pressure resulted in the removal of the National Iranian Oil Company (NIOC) from the list of companies with shares in the Azerbaijan International Operating Company (AIOC). However, the exclusion is by no means complete, with NIOC receiving a ten percent share in the May 1996 Production Sharing Agreement (PSA) for the Shah Deniz Field.[12] Still, the American concern over a massive Iranian penetration of these central Asian states has not materialized.

Several reasons explain this limited Iranian role. First, several cultural, religious and linguistic differences have restrained the expansion of Iranian influence in the region. Second, Tehran lacks the financial and economic resources necessary to play a leading role in the geopolitical game in the Caucasus. Indeed, for the last several years the Islamic regime has been more interested in economic reconstruction at home than pursuing foreign adventures abroad. Third, the Iranian leaders realize that a high profile role in central Asia would heighten Western and Russian concerns and increase the suspicion of the Central Asian states themselves with regard to Iran's intentions.

Thus, instead of trying to penetrate and destabilize the region, the Iranian policy can be described as pragmatic, cautious and moderate. This can be illustrated by examining two specific issues: the legal status of the Caspian Basin and transportation routes.

The Legal Status of the Caspian Basin

Before 1991, the Soviet Union and Iran treated the Caspian Sea as a shared lake, in which they alone held any rights. They based their relationship on the Treaty of Friendship of 1921, which extended equal sailing rights to both parties. The treaty of Commerce and Navigation

in 1940 established exclusive fishing zones ten miles out from the respective coastlines.

The collapse of the Soviet Union introduced new dynamics into these legal arrangements for the Caspian. Instead of two littoral states (Russia and Iran) three sovereign states were added (Azerbaijan, Kazakhstan and Turkmenistan). Equally important, each country has approached the question of the legal status of the Caspian Sea in a different way. The experience since 1991 suggests that the old regime is not relevant any more and that a new one is slowly emerging.

The legal status of the Caspian Basin effectively came onto the international agenda in April 1991 when the Russian Ministry of Foreign Affairs sent a diplomatic note to the British embassy in Moscow warning that the issue of ownership of Caspian resources 'remained to be settled'.[13] The Russian government raised the issue in the context of an investment agreement that had just been signed with the Azeri government by a British Petroleum-led consortium. Later, Kazakhstan and Turkmenistan also announced international tenders on prospecting the seabed along their coasts and developing hydrocarbon resources.

In November 1996, at a meeting of foreign ministers of the five Caspian states Russia camp up with a compromise solution. It said that within the 45-mile coastal zone each country exercised exclusive, or sovereign, rights of the seabed mineral resources. The central part was to remain common property with its hydrocarbon resources developed by a joint stock company of the five states.[14] This compromise solution was immediately rejected by Azerbaijan and Kazakhstan and later by Turkmenistan as well. In 1998 Russia and Kazakhstan suggested dividing the seabed while keeping the sea surface as a common property. Azerbaijan hailed Russia's agreement to delimitate the seabed yet insisted on delimitation of the sea surface as well. While favouring the previous Russian proposal of 45-mile coastal zones Turkmenistan was prepared to go along if other states agreed.[15] Tehran voiced its agreement, in principle, on dividing the Caspian Basin among the five states on an equal basis. Following a tour of the littoral states in August 1998, Iranian Foreign Minister Kamal Kharrazi had been quoted as saying that the five Caspian states should operate on the basis of 'divide all equally or divide nothing'—a remark that was interpreted as an Iranian assertion that each state should possess exactly twenty percent of the Caspian's surface area.[16]

In line with this new Iranian attitude, in December 1998 the National Iranian Oil Company signed a $19 million exploration deal with the Royal Dutch/Shell and London Independent Lasmo to conduct

a seismic survey of Iran's Caspian Sea coast.[17] The deal enraged neighbouring Azerbaijan, which accused Iran of encroaching on what Baku sees as its sector of the Caspian. Tehran rejected the Azeri protest as lacking legal basis. Similarly, Azerbaijan and Turkmenistan have considerable overlapping claims, notably concerning one oilfield in the centre of their disputed section named Serdar-Independence by the latter and known as Kyapaz by the former.[18]

Two conclusions can be drawn from this discussion of the legal status of the Caspian Basin. First, the legal uncertainties do not appear to have significantly slowed investment in the Caspian Basin. Favourable geological prospects provide significant incentives for companies to be present in this important producing region. Moreover, since companies have few indications as to how long a final settlement of these issues would take, they apparently prefer not to delay their plans indefinitely. Foreign investors seem to be confident that because agreements have been signed with a large number of companies from different nationalities, these agreements will be honoured. Second, for all their official posturing, all the five littoral states now accept the principle that the Caspian should be divided into national sectors. They may not agree on how big those sectors should be, or whether the boundary lines should be sited on the surface of the sea or on the seabed, but each now wants the right to develop for itself the hydrocarbon resources lying under the seabed and adjacent to its Caspian coastline. This emerging consensus, however, does not put an end to the disputes over the region's promising resources. An agreement has yet to be found on the most appropriate routes to transport the Caspian's oil and gas to the international market.

Pipeline Diplomacy

The oil and gas pipeline systems of central Asia and the Caucasus were originally designed and built to serve the needs of the Soviet Union. As such, they often cross the borders of its successor states. All oil and gas export pipelines inherited from the Soviet period pass through Russia. Russia's oil and gas operators, facing capacity constraints due to lack of maintenance and other technical problems, have capped exports from the region. In the case of gas, there is also a certain reluctance to share markets. For the region's newly independent states—particularly Azerbaijan, Kazakhstan and Turkmenistan—development of their rich energy resources is seen as the pathway to economic independence and prosperity. On the other side, the countries whose transit routes are eventually chosen will benefit not only from heavy capital inflows in terms of investment and transit fees but, more importantly, will gain

considerable influence throughout the region in particular and tremendous leverage in the global energy market in general. In other words, the choice of export routes has economic and strategic implications. Not surprisingly, many players (transit states, importing countries, international oil companies and the Caspian producers) have proposed a variety of competing routes.

In early 1990s the Azerbaijan International Operating Company (AIOC), a consortium between the Azerbaijani government and 11 international oil companies was created. These foreign firms are: British Petroleum (17.1%, UK); Amoco (17%, US); Unocal (10.05%, US); Lukoil (10%, Russia); Socar (10%, Azerbaijan); Statoil (8.56%, Norway); Exxon (8%, US); Tpao (6.75%, Turkey); Pennzoil (4.82%, US); Itochu (3.92%, Japan); Ramco (2.08%, UK); and Delta oil (1.68%, Saudi Arabia).[19] The presence of a diverse number of nationalities in this consortium reflects the strong global interest in the exploration and development of the Caspian's hydrocarbon resources. Under a 1994 contract between Baku and these eleven foreign companies a decision were to have been made on selecting the direction of the main export pipeline route (MEP).[20] By the end of 1999, these parties had yet to agree on the most appropriate route both from economic and strategic prospects. In addition to the northern pipeline to the Russian port Novorossiysk on the Black Sea, three routes have been under serious considerations: 1) to the Turkish port Ceyhan on the Mediterranean; 2) to the Georgian port Supsa on the Black Sea; and 3) south through Iran.

Since the mid 1990s, the United States has been firmly committed to the pipeline from Baku, Azerbaijan to Ceyhan, Turkey. Bypassing both Russia and Iran, this route would accomplish three American foreign policy goals: strengthen the independence of the Caspian states by reducing their dependence on Russia for energy exports; exclude Iran from any possible financial benefits (i.e. transit fees and foreign investment) as well as from any potential political leverage; and solidify ties with Turkey, a NATO member. An important step in promoting this route was taken during the celebrations marking the 75th anniversary of the Turkish Republic in October 1998. The presidents of Turkey, Azerbaijan, Georgia, Kazakhstan and Uzbekistan signed a declaration in Ankara confirming their determination 'in realizing the Caspian-Mediterranean project as the main export pipeline.'[21] The United States signed as an observer. A year later, October 1999, the scheme received another significant endorsement when BP Amoco said that it would back the construction of an oil export pipeline from Baku to Ceyhan and would take a lead in helping

companies work with other parties to assemble financing. According to a company spokesman, "We have come to the conclusion that the Baku-Ceyhan pipeline is a strategic transportation route that should be built.[22] A giant step in this direction was taken during a summit meeting of the Organization for Security and Cooperation in Europe (OSCE) held in Istanbul, Turkey in November 1999. The presidents of Azerbaijan, Georgia, Kazakhstan and Turkey signed a series of agreements to build the 1,080-mile oil pipeline from Baku to Ceyhan. In addition, another agreement was reached on advancing the construction of a companion pipeline, a 1,250-mile natural gas line from Turkmenistan to the Turkish city of Erzurum.[23] President Clinton, who attended the ceremony, stated that, 'these pipelines will be an insurance policy for the entire world by helping to ensure our energy resources pass through multiple routes instead of a single chokepoint.'[24]

In spite of this strong American support, there are some important obstacles that need to be overcome. First, many industry analysts argue that this proposed pipeline would need to see oil production double to around two million barrels per day (b/d) to make it commercially viable. Put differently, the volume of crude is not yet there. Second, there is the matter of cost. In 1998 the AIOC estimated construction costs at $3.7 billion, but since the consortium officially delayed its decision on Baku-Ceyhan in November 1998, Turkey has insisted that the pipeline could be built for $2.4 billion, and even talked of the possibility that it would cover cost overruns. However, in May 1999 Ankara increased its estimate to $2.7 billion, citing specifications insisted upon by the AIOC.[25] Third, political events within Turkey are becoming increasingly tense, further leading the consortium to question the stability of such a line. Recently, the average tenure for governments in Ankara is about a year. Several political parties have created a fragile and unstable political environment. The list includes Islamist parties, Motherland Party, and the Democratic Left, among others. In addition, the army generals enjoy tremendous leverage in the political process. Furthermore, in spite of the arrest and sentencing to death of Abdullah Öcalan, the leader of the Kurdistan Workers Party (PKK), there is no guarantee that the Kurdish rebellion is over. In short, domestic political instability in Turkey poses an important challenge to huge investment in the Baku-Ceyhan scheme.

Finally, the proposed pipeline travels through two troubled spots in the Caucasus: Abkhazia and Nagorno-Karabakh. The continued presence of separatist movements in the Georgian republic of Abkhazia, a region with an ethnic minority along the Black Sea coastline,

threatens Georgia's stability. A cease-fire to the bloody battle was negotiated in 1993, but tension persists over the likelihood of future fighting. Consortium members are uncertain about the relative security of a pipeline investment through Georgia, fearing that relations with Abkhazia could deteriorate in the future. Likewise, a fragile cease-fire in the Armenian enclave of Nagorno-Karabakh in Azerbaijan also threatens the stability of the pipeline as ethnic Armenians occupy 20 percent of Azerbaijan. Continued disagreement over the territory continues to weigh heavily on pipeline security as the conflict remains largely unsettled.[26]

Given these problems and potential obstacles associated with the Baku-Ceyhan pipeline, the AIOC has considered doubling the capacity of the Baku-Supsa pipeline, which came into operation in April 1999. New emphasis as an export route for Azerbaijani crude has also fallen on Supsa as a result of Russia's decision to close the Chechen section of the Baku-Novorossiysk pipeline. Washington supports the expansion of Baku-Supsa as an integral part of Baku-Ceyhan not as an alternative one. The main advantage of this route is its low cost. Once crude reaches the Georgian port of Supsa, it would be loaded onto tankers and travel through the Turkish straits. The Turkish Straits comprise the Istanbul Strait (Bosphorus), the Sea of Marmara, and the Canakkale Strait (Dardanelles). The nineteen nautical miles of the Istanbul Strait contain four turns of more than 45 degrees and at one point the passage narrows to only 700 meters. The Strait passes through Istanbul (population twelve million) and constitutes one of the busiest waterways in the world.[27] In other words, there is concern that future oil exports from the region could significantly increase tanker traffic through the Straits, thereby raising the risk of a serious accident that could pose environmental and safety threats, as well as disrupt the flow of oil from the region. Consequently, since November 1998 Turkey has implemented new rules that further constrain tanker movement through the Straits. These obstacles associated with both Baku-Ceyhan and Baku-Supsa underscore the significance of another route, the one south through Iran.

Iran is considered an attractive export route for oil and gas between Central Asia on one side and Europe and Southeast Asia on the other side. It already has a well-developed hydrocarbon infrastructure. By almost all estimates, an Iranian route could prove significantly cheaper than other proposed pipelines. Not surprisingly, many sources have expressed interest in transporting Caspian's resources through Iran. According to Michael Stinson, Conoco's senior vice president for government affairs "most energy companies operating

in the Caspian believe trading Caspian crude through Iran could be highly competitive and probably represent the lowest capital costs.'[28]

The major problem preventing the full utilization of the Iranian option is the strong American opposition. In spite of wavering sanctions against foreign companies investing in the Iranian energy sector, the United States has shown strong determination to oppose the transportation of Caspian's oil and gas through Iran. According to US Secretary of State Madeleine Albright 'Washington remains strongly opposed to oil and gas pipelines which transit Iran and, as a policy matter, we will continue to encourage alternative routes for the transport of Caspian energy resources.'[29] Thus, from mid 1997 to mid 1998, when the countries of the Caspian region began to turn their attention toward Iran as an exit route for their oil and gas, the United States invited the presidents of Azerbaijan, Kazakhstan and Turkmenistan to Washington for official visits with President Clinton.[30] Heavy discouragement by the United States of the Iranian option has led these leaders to re-consider alternatives when making transport decisions.

In spite of this strong American opposition, a pipeline has already been constructed from Korpedzhe in southeastern Turkmenistan to Kurt-Kui in north-central Iran. Turkmenistan will see little revenue from this project for several years, since gas deliveries will be used to reimburse Iran for construction costs. In addition, Tehran is also assisting Caspian oil exports by means of swaps. The British Monument Oil and Gas Company already export Caspian crude through Iran under swap arrangements. Under this agreement, Monument supplies crude to northern Iran to be refined and consumed locally. Iran in return supplies crude to Monument at its southern port of Kharg Island on the Persian Gulf, thus effectively allowing crude to transit Iran without the need for a pipeline at all.[31] In spite of Monument's success in exporting the Caspian's crude through Iran under swap arrangement, the Clinton administration rejected applications by two American companies (Optimarket and Mobil) to engage in oil-swap deals with Iran.

Finally, it is important to point out that Iran is seeking finance for a pipeline to carry crude oil from its Caspian Sea port of Neka to Tehran. In late 1999 a partnership of China National Petroleum Company (CNPC) Sinoped and two other Chinese firms have opened negotiations with the National Iranian Oil Company (NIOC) for construction of the pipeline. The talks follow the failure of the local Iran Power Plant Projects Management Company (MAPNA), which had put in the winning bid in December 1998, to raise the necessary

finance.[32]

Three conclusions can be drawn from these intense debates and political manoeuvres over choosing the appropriate pipelines. First, investment in an infrastructure to transport Caspian oil will keep pace with the development of the region's hydrocarbon reserves. In other words, pipeline construction will be gradual. Second, the existence of multiple export routes could increase the energy security of both exporters and importers by making exports less subject to technical or political disruptions on any one route. However, security will have to be balanced by economic feasibility since a larger number of pipelines would mean smaller economies of scale and greater expenses for each project. Third, pipeline routes through Iran should not and would not be ruled out. If geopolitics were not such an important part of the pipeline questions, the preferred route in commercial terms to the growing markets in Asia would be through Iran to the Indian Ocean.

Conclusion

Since the election of President Muhammad Khatami in 1997, the American-Iranian relations have taken different direction from the escalating animosity which characterized their policies toward each other for most of the 1980s and the early 1990s. The outcome can be described as a 'partial thawing, but no breakthrough'.[33]

A close examination of the two countries' policies in regard to the energy sector suggests several lessons which might facilitate and accelerate a rapprochement between Washington and Tehran. First, in spite of the prominent American role in the global energy market, Washington cannot achieve its goals without some level of cooperation with other powers. The United States' efforts to isolate Iran has caused some economic and financial hurt on the regime in Tehran. However, it is hard to describe the policy as a complete success. The record, as has been discussed above, is mixed. Increasingly, the Islamic Republic is able to break the wall of isolation. Meanwhile, the American determination to continue this policy is fading. Second, energy markets have never been driven by economic factors alone, as strategic considerations have always shaped producers and consumers' policies. The Iranian case illustrates the large gap between Washington's economic interests and its geo-strategic objectives.[34] American efforts to isolate Iran have proven costly to the American oil companies. These companies are at a competitive disadvantage with their European competitors. A tangible progress to remove this unfairness is not likely before the Iran-Libya Sanctions Act expires in 2001. Meanwhile, there is a growing feeling in Washington among members of both Congress

and the Administration that unilateral sanctions have probably been used too often and too indiscriminately in the past and are not the most appropriate vehicle to advance U.S. foreign policy interests.

Third, a relaxation of the American sanctions against Iran will serve the long-term American strategic interests. In spite of efforts to diversify the Iranian economy and make it less dependent on oil, oil revenues still constitute the main source of national income. The flourishing of the Iranian energy sector would produce overall economic prosperity, generate jobs, reduce social and political tension and eventually lead to a substantial moderation of both domestic and foreign policies. Put differently, an impoverished Iran is likely to adopt an aggressive attitude at home and in relations with its neighbours and foreign powers. Finally, the Islamic Republic of Iran and the United States need each other. American oil companies have the most advanced technology in the industry and Washington has keen interest in ensuring the non-interruption of supplies to the world oil market. In addition, U.S. plays a dominant role in promoting and preserving regional security in both the Persian Gulf and the Caspian Basin.

On the other side, Iran, with its significant oil and particularly gas reserves inevitably has a major role to play in helping meet future world energy needs. Furthermore, given its size, population and location, Iran is too large and too strategically located to be ignored or isolated. More to the point, Washington and Tehran have many shared interests, particularly in ensuring the unrestricted flow of energy from the Persian Gulf and promoting and maintaining political stability in Central Asia and the Caucasus.

Instead of approaching the energy issue as a zero-sum competition between the two nations, both Washington and Tehran need to coordinate their efforts to develop and promote their mutual interests in this vital sector. This will require a lot of courage from politicians in the two countries, but the stakes are high. The sooner a rapprochement is reached, the better for global economy and world peace.

Notes

1. Energy Information Administration: *Country Profile: United States of America* (Washington, DC: USGPO, 1999) at www.eia.doe.gov/emeu/cabs/usa.html.

2. Energy Information Administration: *Annual Energy Outlook* (Washington, DC: USGPO, 1999), p. 5.

3. *Ibid.*, p. 5.

4. British Petroleum-Amoco: *BP Amoco Statistical Review of World Energy* (London, June 1999), pp. 4, 20.

5. Geoffrey Kemp: *Energy Superbowl* (Washington, DC: Nixon Centre for Peace and Freedom, 1997), p. 19.

6. Energy Information Administration: *Persian Gulf Oil Export Fact Sheet* (Washington DC: USGPO, 1999), at www.eia.doe.gov/emeu.cabs/ pgulf.html.

7. International Energy Agency: *Caspian Oil and Gas* (Paris: OECD Publications, 1998), p. 3.

8. Energy Information Administration: *Country Profile: Iran* (Washington, DC: UNGPO, 1999), at www.eia.doe.gov/emeu/cabs/iran.html.

9. For a detailed discussion of these accusations see Bahgat, Gawdat: 'Beyond Containment: US-Iranian Relations at a Crossroads', *Security Dialogue*, vol. 28, no. 4 (December 1997), pp. 453-464.

10. A year later, the amount was reduced to $20 million.

11. United States Congress: *Bill Summary & Status for the 106th Congress* (Washington: USGPO, 1999), at http://thomas.loc.gov/cgi-bin/bdquery.

12. MacFarlane, Neil: *Western Engagement in the Caucasus and Central Asia* (London: The Royal Institute of International Affairs, 1999), p. 55.

13. International Energy Agency: *loc. cit.* (note 7), p. 147.

14. Merzliakov, I.: 'Legal Status of the Caspian Sea', *International Affairs*, vol. 45, no. 9 (March 1999), p. 35.

15. *Ibid.*, p. 37.

16. Johnston, Daniel: 'Permits—the Value of a Word', *Energy Economist*, no. 204 (October 1998), p. 20.

17. 'Iran Says Shell, Lasmo Started Caspian Exploration', *Reuters* (15 September 1999).

18. Roberts, John: 'Caspian Conundrum', *Energy Economist*, no. 209 (March 1999), p. 9.

19. 'Turkey Chastises BP and Amoco for Lack of Baku-Ceyhan Enthusiasm', *Middle East Economic Survey*, vol. 41, no. 47 (23 November, 1998), at www.mees.com.

20. Kinzer, Stephen: 'Decision on Pipeline in Caspian is Delayed', *New York Times* (14 November 1998), p. A4.

21. 'Turkey, US, Caspian Countries Sign Declaration Backing Oil Pipeline', *Associated Press* (29 October 1999).

22. "BP Amoco Says Backs Baku-Ceyhan Oil Pipeline', *Reuters* (19 October, 1999).

23. LeVine, Steve: 'A Cocktail of Oil and Politics: US Seeks to End Russian Domination of the Caspian', *New York Times* (20 November 1999), p. 2.

24. Kinzer, Stephen: 'Caspian Lands Back a Pipeline Pushed by West', *New York Times*, 19 November, 1999, p. A12.

25. 'Richardson Pursues "Endgame" For Baku-Ceyhan and TransCaspian Pipelines', *Middle East Economic Survey*, vol. 42, no. 34 (23 August, 1999), at www.mees.com.

26. Miles, Carolyn: 'The Caspian Pipeline Debate Continues: Why Not Iran?', *Journal of International Affairs*, vol. 53, no. 1 (Fall 1999), p. 338.

27. International Energy Agency: *loc. cit.* (note 7), p. 133.

28. 'Long Wait for US Oil Investment in Iran Warns a New York Conference', *Middle East Monitor*, vol. 29, no.3 (March 1999), p. 23.

29. 'US Waives Sanctions on South Pars Fields', *Oil and Gas Journal*, vol. 96, no. 21 (25 May, 1998), p. 18.

30. Nanay, Julia: 'The U.S. in the Caspian: The Divergence of Political and Commercial Interests', *Middle East Policy*, vol. 6, no. 2 (October 1998), p. 150.

31. 'Total May Export Caspian Oil through Iran', *Reuters* (7 December 1998).

32. 'Chinese Team Offered Neka-Tehran Pipeline', *Middle East Economic Digest*, vol. 43, no. 39 (1 October, 1999), p. 18.

33. Sick, Gary: 'The Future Of US-Iran Relations', *Middle East Economic Survey*, vol. 42, no. 25 (21 June, 1999), at www.mees.com.

34. For a detailed discussion of this issue see Bahgat, Gawdat: 'Oil Security in the New Millennium: Geo-Economy vs. Geo-Strategy', *Strategic Review*, vol. 14, no. 4 (Fall 1998), pp. 22-30.

4 THE 'SÈVRES SYNDROME'

Turkish Foreign Policy and its Historical Legacy

Dietrich Jung

Introduction: Whither Turkey?

With the demise of the Soviet Union and the subsequent end of bipolarity many states and their respective foreign policy experts are confronted with the uncertainties of a 'new world order' in the making and the question where to find an adequate place in this emerging new order.

This scenario fits particularly for Turkey that is often characterised for its uniqueness, both with regard to its geographic dimension 'overlapping Europe and Asia',[1] and its combination of Western with Turkish and Muslim orientations.[2] Under the catch-phrase of an 'identity crisis' Turkey's political identity and future role in world politics is widely discussed both inside and outside the country. However, despite the apparent necessity and shared opinion that Turkey has to redefine her strategic role in the post-Cold-War era, extreme differences occur in the judgements made about Turkey's future role.

Some authors consider Turkey as a "successful democracy",[3] and as a regional power poised to play a central role not only in the region but also in world politics.[4] Others come to the conclusion 'that the Turkish political system is far from being democratic',[5] and that the country represents an 'unwelcome outsider on the margins of both Europe and the Middle East'.[6] Ranging from being described as a 'political and economic model for her neighbours', over the 'bridge between Europe and the Middle East', to being assessed as an 'awkward and uneasy actor in both European and Middle Eastern politics', Turkey is the object of a whole range of positive and negative judgements. But where is Turkey's political future to be sought, in Europe or in the Middle East? Should Turkey play the role of a bridge between the two regions or fall back into isolationist neutrality as in the days of the early Turkish Republic? Or has Turkey to play a more active role in the Middle Eastern security context after the demise of the Soviet Union?

A brief glance at Turkey's military potentials demonstrates the importance of the country for the security environment of the Middle East. Under the impact of the Cold War the Turkish Armed Forces developed into the second largest army in NATO. The permanent staff of 514,000 men includes 72,000 professionals, while more than 900,000 men serve as reserve. With a large tank force (4,300 combat tanks, including 400 Leopard-I), and an Air Force of 750 combat aircraft (of which 240 F-16), the Turkish Armed Forces are certainly among the strongest in this volatile region, both technologically and in terms of manpower. Furthermore, in an ambitious modernisation program Turkey is going to invest 150 billion US Dollars during the next three decades , mainly aiming at an enhancement of the combat power of the Air Force and the Navy with a view to preparing her army for out-of-area operations.[7]

This brief survey clearly shows that in terms of military capabilities the Turkish Armed Forces can hardly be matched by any of its neighbours. Therefore, and because the Turkish army lost its major task to contain the Soviet Union, it is supposed to play a pivotal role in the regional security context. Surprisingly enough, Turkey neither appeared on the agenda of a recent Persian Gulf security conference,[8] nor in a new study about Middle Eastern security.[9] Why has Turkey been ignored in these regional security discussions?

A possible explanation might be that Turkey as a member of NATO and thus involved in the Euro-Atlantic security system simply does not play the above-mentioned pivotal role in the Middle Eastern security context. However, this interpretation is not tenable. Turkey is not at all detached from the regional security environment. On the one hand there is the Kurdish question which represents the major domestic security threat for Turkey and links it to the internal security of Iran, Iraq and Syria. On the other hand there are still territorial disputes between Turkey and Iraq (Mosul) and Turkey and Syria (Hattay). Together with the Kurdish question and the dispute about the waters of the Euphrates and Tigris this can easily cause severe conflicts among these three countries.

This tense situation has been further aggravated by the military agreements between Israel and Turkey,[10] two countries that have repeatedly shown their readiness to use military power against their immediate neighbours regardless of international laws and conventions. Furthermore, there are conflicting interests of Turkey and Iran in the Caucasus and the central Asian states. Last but not least, since the late 1940s Turkey became the backbone of US regional foreign policy. Taking into account that Iran as well as some Arab states consider the

presence of the United States in the Persian Gulf region as a key problem of regional security and stability, the neglect of Turkey as a regional player is not just surprising but almost incomprehensible.

Against this background the article puts forward the assertion that the neglect of Turkey's role for Middle Eastern security from outside mirrors the perceptions of its Kemalist élite that has been trying to deny Turkey's cultural and historical roots in the Middle East. For the republican élite modernisation has been synonymous with westernisation or Europeanisation, and in the course of her republican history Turkey distanced herself increasingly from her Middle Eastern neighbours. The argument is that the Kemalist worldview, which is grounded in the historical legacy of the security situation of the late Ottoman Empire and the early Turkish Republic, continues to shape Turkey's foreign policy. This anachronistic worldview prevents the élite of the country from developing a vision of Turkey's future role in the Middle East. Moreover, given Turkey's economic and military capabilities as well as her interconnection with regional conflicts this situation could lead the country into a dangerous confrontation with its neighbours.

In order to explain the persistence of this anachronism of ideas, the sociological concept of the 'social habitus', as developed by Pierre Bourdieu and Norbert Elias, will be applied. As a set of cognitive schemes and ultimate values, the social habitus represents durably installed generative principles which produce and reproduce the practices of a social group. In the following section the social habitus as a theoretical frame of reference will briefly be presented together with empirical examples of the worldview of some representatives of Turkey's political establishment. It will be shown that the 'Sèvres Syndrome', i.e. the feeling of being encircled by enemies attempting the destruction of the Turkish state, remains a feature of the social habitus of the Kemalist élite.

In the third part of this article the social habitus of Turkey's current Kemalist élite will be discussed in relation to its construction during the historical formation of the Turkish state. The equation of internal and external aspects of security as well as the persistence of conspiracy theories among Turkey's élite are related to this context of social history. The fourth section, then, presents a categorisation of Turkey's foreign policy in four phases. Based on the assumption of a durable social habitus confronted with a changing political and economic environment, these four phases can be interpreted as steps in the direction of more activism in Turkish foreign policy and increasing involvement in Middle Eastern affairs.

In order to explain how domestic security problems are reinterpreted as caused by foreign intervention, the fifth section deals with issues linking Turkey's internal security interests to the Persian Gulf region, mainly to the three littoral states Iran, Iraq and Saudi Arabia. The Kurdish question and the wave of political Islam are the two salient points at hand to further examine how regional and domestic conflicts are related to each other. Finally, the article will conclude with some hypothetical policy options and their constraints.

Encircled by Enemies: Social Habitus and Turkish Foreign Policy Perceptions

The unexpected and unpredicted demise of the Soviet Union is still causing a lot of turmoil in the field of International Relations. With the end of bipolarity major theoretical concepts have been lost, and the hastily announced 'New World Order' has revealed itself as wishful thinking rather than as a new device that might help us explain recent developments in the international system. Moreover, the classical state-centred approach of both Realism and Institutionalism is challenged by the rise of so-called critical approaches in International Relations theory.

Those approaches are united in their focus on how international politics is 'socially constructed', and in their claim that these structures are not made only of a distribution of material capabilities, but are also of social relationships.[11] In accordance with this 'constructivist turn', the foreign policy of a particular state cannot be explained as a pure strategic action in pursuit of national interest.

Both Realists and Institutionalists see states as the principal actors in world politics and state action is explained by rational choice models based on the category of utility maximisation.[12] Foreign policies are thus results of rational choices within constraints that are either imposed by the particular choice situation (decision theories) or by the choices of others (game theories).[13] Constructivists, however, place the emphasis on social structures shaping actor's identities and interests. Ruggie, for instance, divides social structures into three analytically distinct dimensions: material environments (economic relations), strategic behaviour (the matrix of constraints and opportunities for social actors) and 'epistemology' (cognitive and ideological aspects of society).[14] With reference to the last dimension, the social episteme, the conception of the social habitus seems to be an appropriate heuristic tool to show, first, how these cognitive and ideological structures, which are historically rooted social constructions, are influencing the action of concrete actors. Secondly, the conception of the social habitus

can explain how social structures find their way into the mind-set of a specific group of actors.

According to Bourdieu and Elias[15], the social habitus comprises a system of historically and socially constructed generative principles providing a frame within which individuality unfolds. The worldview, which is rooted in the social habitus, provides a general reservoir of cognitive and normative resources to which individual strategies of action correspond.[16] As a 'generative grammar' of patterns of action, the habitus forms the intersection between society and the individual, between structure and action.[17]

These generative principles are the means for social groups to shape their particular ways of action in pursuing their interests. Rationally calculated interests are, therefore, transformed into action in the light of this set of ideas. Whereas the historical and social construction of the social habitus stress its liability to change, it remains also to be a relatively stable disposition of groups and individuals, acquired by socialisation. Its an important point for this study that social change and the change of the social habitus do not necessarily proceed in parallel. Thus, in times of accelerated social change the structures of the social habitus might become anachronistic to a changing environment.[18]

As mentioned above, a part of the social habitus is the general worldview in which the perceptions of groups and individuals are embedded. In order to asses Turkish foreign policy behaviour in the Middle Eastern region, it is therefore necessary to examine first, how Turkey's current political élite perceives the region? One general view about the geographical location of the country is that Turkey is 'encircled by enemies'. The former speaker of parliament Hikmet Cetin, for example, said in 1993, then serving as Foreign Minister: 'Turkey is in the neighbourhood of the most unstable, uncertain and unpredictable region of the world, it has turned into a frontline state faced with multiple fronts'.[19] Even more pronounced was the senior diplomat Shükrü Elekdag who considers 'Turkey as besieged by a veritable ring of evil'.[20] Against this general background of being besieged it comes as no surprise that many of Turkey's current political problems are explained by conspiracy theories.

Especially the extreme right-wing National Action Party (*Milliyetci Hareket Partisi*, MHP) exploited the Kurdish question and the war between the state and the Kurdish Workers Party (PKK) in claiming 'that there is a conspiracy of foreign enemies to use the PKK to destroy the unity of the Turkish state'.[21] President Süleyman Demirel reacted similarly to European instructions to peacefully settle

the Kurdish question. Demirel responded that there is no political solution, but to 'render these people ineffective by force'. He further accused the West of trying 'to invoke the Sèvres Treaty to set up a Kurdish state in the region, (...) and that this was what they meant by political solution'.[22] This standpoint has also been strongly supported by the former leader of the Islamist Welfare Party (*Refah Partisi*), Necmetin Erbakan. In a more recent interview then Interim Prime Minister Bülent Ecevit from the Democratic Left Party (*Democratic Sol Parti*, DSP) confirmed that there is no Kurdish problem in the country, but only PKK terrorism that is supported from outside in order to divide Turkey.[23]

Many representatives of Turkey's state élite associate, like the Kurdish insurgency, the rise of political Islam in Turkey to a conspiracy from outside. General Fevzi Türkeri, the former chief of military intelligence, for example, was pointing out that 'political Islam is working closely with Iran and some other Islamic countries to pull Turkey into an endless darkness'.[24] In a remark on Merve Kavakic, the Islamic Virtue Party's (*Fazilet*) Deputy from Istanbul who appeared in the Turkish Parliament wearing a headscarf, Prime Minister Ecevit said in May 1999: 'Even though Turkey does not meddle in Iranian affairs, Iran is continually trying to export its regime to Turkey'.[25]

Large parts of the Turkish establishment consider Islam as an irrational force. Ali Karaosmanoglu, for instance, is criticising Arab foreign policy as lacking the notion of *realpolitik*. He explains this deficiency as a result of the merger between nationalism and religion in the Arab world, where Islam infuses an irrational element into national politics.[26]

The above described perceptions are best summarised in an article of General Cevik Bir, former Deputy Chief of Turkey's General Staff and former Commander of the Turkish First Army Corps in Istanbul.[27] In criticising the position of the European Union towards Turkey, Bir accused the EU of excluding Turkey from the new map of Europe, pointing out that Turkey's soldiers and members of the U.S. Army have always been comrades-in-arms with shared visions and a common destiny. Located at the epicentre of regions fraught with crises, Turkey, as a front state, has to be considered as a centre of power that can affect delicate balances of power in the region. While Turkey wants to enhance regional security and stability, some neighbouring states would still lay claim to Turkish territory and some of them support terrorism. Moreover, some states are even trying to export their regime contrary to Turkey's constitutional order and the moral values of the modern

world. Against these threats, says General Bir, Turkey will find the right answer, and he ends with the following warning: 'Turkey hopes to see its European friends come to the realisation that excluding Turkey from Europe will have extremely high costs which might be vital for all members of the Alliance in the future'.

Generally speaking, Turkey's élite perceives the country to be in a situation in which her neighbours are permanently threatening her security and stability. Furthermore, many of Turkey's domestic problems are put down to the interference of neighbouring states and the distinction between internal and external conflicts becomes blurred. Like in the late Ottoman Empire and the Early Republic internal and external security are equated and the army considers itself as the essential institution to safeguard the Turkish state.

This standpoint was clearly expressed in a statement of Turkey's current General Chief of Staff, Hüseyin Kivrikoglu. In the spring of 1998, as then Commander of the Land Forces, he criticized Prime Minister Yilmaz for not implementing the security measures suggested by the generals in the National Security Council. Kivrikoglu assured "that the Turkish Armed Forces are prepared to fight against all kinds of terrorism and fundamentalism as well as against internal and external threats regardless what it costs'.[28]

Behind the perceptions expressed in these quotations—of being besieged, facing multiple fronts, being encircled by forces aiming at the destruction of the Turkish State—one can easily detect the historical legacy of the security context in which the Turkish Republic was founded: a radicalisation of the security context, which was also the driving force behind the Ottoman reforms in the nineteenth century.

Both the Ottoman and Kemalist reforms were initiated and sustained by the military-bureaucratic élite aiming at securing the State against external and internal threats. Furthermore, they were attempts to stabilise the power positions of the army and the bureaucracy representing the authoritarian state. The social relations and historical experiences of this state élite can still be discerned as the 'Sèvres Syndrome' in the social habitus of Turkey's current élite. The historical and social background for the construction of this habitus will be addressed now.

The Ottoman and Kemalist Heritage
Contrary to its revolutionary appearance, the 'Kemalist revolution' was in many aspects rather a continuation of than a clear break with the Ottoman past.

Like the early Ottoman reforms under Selim III (1789-1807) and

Mahmud II (1808-1839), and the reform epoch of the late Ottoman Empire, the Tanzimat era (1839-1878), the Kemalist reforms of the 1920s and 1930s followed the same route of imposing modernity from above. Behind the Ottoman reform movement was not an economically self-confident bourgeoisie, calling for political participation, but the particular interests of the Ottoman court and the higher echelons of the administration and the army.[29] Their common point of reference was the internal and external security of the Ottoman State. It was an attempt to sustain the integrity of the Empire and the social position of its élite by means of an instrumental adaptation of modern forms of organisation and scientific knowledge.

Concerning the threats from outside, the beginning of the decline of the Ottoman Empire can be located in the second half of the seventeenth century. The Ottoman defeat at Vienna 1683, the formation of the so-called 'Holy Alliance' against the Ottomans in 1684 and the advance of Hapsburg troops in Serbia 1687 are cases in point. After the 1774 peace treaty of Kücük Kaynarca, which ended the Ottoman-Russian war (1768-1774), the Empire did not only lose its sovereignty over the Crimea, but was increasingly dragged into the ongoing power struggle among the European pentarchy.[30] In changing alliances and confrontations with the European powers, the former challenger of Europe was in the nineteenth century at the mercy of European states. While engaged in warfare with European powers, internal forces started also to rebel against Istanbul.

In the Arab territories of the Empire, the expansion of the Saudi kingdom at the turn of the century, the factual independence of Egypt under Muhammad Ali (1805-1848), the search for autonomy of the Lebanese emirate of Emir Bashir Shihab II (1788-1840), and the modernisation and formation of an independent Tunesia under Ahmad Bey (1837-1855) are examples for the dissolution of the Ottoman state from within. Even more dramatic were the events happening in the European provinces of the Empire. The Serbian revolts of 1804-1806 and 1815-1817, the Greek war of independence 1821-1830 or the rebellions in Bosnia and Hercegovina in 1857 are cases in point, which indicate how precarious the situation for the political élite of the Ottoman Empire was. Moreover, in their struggle with the Ottoman state internal and external forces were joining sides and the Ottoman élite in Istanbul saw itself in an atmosphere of outside conspiracy and inside betrayal.

Against this background it comes as no surprise that the reform efforts of the Ottoman Empire were not guided by any long-term strategy to modernise society, but rather determined by the political

events of the day. Confronted with a deteriorating security situation and with the integrity and sovereignty of the state at stake, the Ottoman reforms were a classical example of a modernisation imposed from above. Although the reforms could not stop the decline, they led to remarkable changes in the social structure of the Empire. As a result of the reforms in the army and in the bureaucratic and educational system, new social groups emerged who played a major role in the foundation of the Turkish Republic. Furthermore, many of the structural changes and political discussions of the Tanzimat became a platform for the Turkish nation-state. In terms of worldview and social background, the republican élite was a clear continuation of the military-bureaucratic élite of the late Ottoman Empire. This continuation applies in an even more radical version to the security context in which the Turkish Republic was founded.

After heavy territorial losses in the Balkan wars between 1912 and 1913 and the subsequent First World War, a delegation of the Ottoman Sultan signed the treaty of Sèvres in August 1920. This treaty provided for a partition of the Ottoman Empire leaving only parts of Anatolia with Istanbul as capital for the Turks. At the same time Turkey's republican forces were fighting against Greek occupation forces which landed in May 1919 in Izmir with the consent of the Allies. After almost ten years of warfare, Turkey was about to disappear from the political map due to territorial claims of Russia, Britain, France, Italy, Greece and Armenia. The new republican state itself emerged out of the Turco-Greek war that ended with the victory of the republican forces in 1922. In July 1923 the treaty of Lausanne abolished Sèvres and the sovereignty of the Turkish Republic was acknowledged. However, the Sèvres experience was not forgotten and the integrity, sovereignty and consolidation of the new state continued to be at the centre of the Kemalist reforms.

With respect to the internal situation of Turkey's formative period, the new Turkish political forces also inherited the complex structure of political actors from the Ottoman past. The leadership of the 'Young Turks', the so-called triumvirate of Cemal, Enver and Talat Pasha, as well as the republican forces under Mustafa Kemal had to defend their position not only against foreign threats, but also against domestic ones. Thus the republican leaders were from the beginning confronted with the power aspirations of traditional local notables, of ethnic and religious groups, and of circles wanting to restore Ottoman rule. Moreover, the internal fragmentation of the republican military-bureaucratic élite, which was mainly derived out of the members of the Young Turk 'Committee for Unity and Progress', created an increasing

potential for the internal conflicts of the newly established republic. The foundation of the oppositional Progressive Republican Party 1924, the Kurdish rebellion under the Naqshbandia Sheik Said 1925, or the assassination attempt against Mustafa Kemal in Izmir 1926 are cases in point.[31] It is this structural setting of external and internal threats and the political theory and action of Mustafa Kemal Atatürk that had been blended into the foundational myth of the Turkish Republic and in its ideological form, Kemalism or Atatürkism, is still an influential pattern of Turkish politics.[32]

The foundational myth of the republic and the political culture of modern Turkey resulted out of this violent struggle with internal and external foes. This experience reinforced the Ottoman heritage of conspiracy and betrayal that had already become a part of the social habitus of the republican élite and which has been sustained till now. Thus, it comes as no surprise that in the eyes of the military-bureaucratic establishment of Turkey the Turkish State is permanently endangered. The Turkish military considers itself as the guardian of this endangered state, a task given to the army by Atatürk and their elders.[33] Therefore, any attempt to change the basic principles of Atatürkism is seen as a direct threat for the state.

It was against this historical and sociological background that the Turkish foreign policy evolved. However, while Turkish foreign policy can be explained in the light of this background, it is not determined by it. The Sèvres Syndrome works as a constraint and the following section shows how rational choices have been made within this inherited constraint of the Kemalist social habitus.

From Isolationism to Activism: Four Phases of Turkish Foreign Policy

Phase One: Isolationism
During the first two decades of the Turkish Republic the republican regime was preoccupied with the internal and external consolidation of the new territorial Turkish nation-state. The internal policy of de-Arabisation and de-Islamisation, in which the new élite identified Islamic traditions with the 'other', was extended to the external otherness of the Arab world.[34] Thus, the Kemalist modernisation project directly detached the Turkish Republic from its Arab neighbours.

In order to secure the territorial and political integrity of Turkey, Atatürk concluded a series of treaties of friendship. In March 1921 the so-called 'national government' signed a treaty with the Soviet Union

that was extended in 1925. In June 1926 Ankara accepted that the area around Mosul became Iraqi territory. The treaty of friendship with Greece 1930 and the Balkan Pact 1934 among Turkey, Yugoslavia, Bulgaria, Romania and Greece was aimed at a normalisation of Turkey's relations with the former European provinces of the Ottoman Empire. In 1934, Reza Shah of Iran visited Ankara and a number of agreements on tariffs and trade, borders and security were signed between Iran and Turkey in the 1930s. Finally the two countries signed together with Afghanistan and Iraq a non-aggression pact, the Saadabad Treaty of 1937, which later proved to be ineffective during the Second World War.[35]

The territorial consolidation of the Turkish Republic ended eight months after the death of Mustafa Kemal Atatürk, as in July 1939 the then independent republic of Hatay decided for its integration into the Turkish State—a decision which Syria has never accepted.[36] Although Atatürk in domestic politics was following a clear policy of westernisation, his foreign policy remained indifferent in terms of integration. The normalisation of foreign relations was accompanied by the will to keep the country neutral.

His immediate successor, Ismet Inönü, was basically following this line and 'insisted on balanced budgets in order not to be dependent on foreign aid'.[37] Furthermore, he tried to keep Turkey neutral during the Second World War, before Turkey eventually declared war against Germany in February 1945. On the basis of the described social habitus of the republican élite, it seems obvious that Atatürk and Inönü were suspicious towards both the intentions of the European powers and the emerging Arab states. As leaders of a state with scarce power resources, however, the Sévres Syndrome led them to pursue a cautious foreign policy which was guided by détente without engagement,[38] by a deliberate neutrality without being isolated from outside.

Phase Two: Western Integration
The second phase of Turkish foreign policy began after the Second World War. This phase was characterised by Turkey's integration into the western system. With Moscow's abrogation of the Turkish-Soviet friendship pact in 1945 and Stalin's demands to return the Kars and Ardahan provinces as well as the establishment of Soviet military bases along the Bosphorus and the Dardanelles, Turkey began to seek full affiliation with the West.[39] The security and integrity of the Turkish State could now no longer be guaranteed by neutrality and the deep-rooted suspicions against the West had to be overcome.

From its previous neutrality Turkey switched to the other extreme

and was 'acting as if she was a cold war warrior'.[40] Between 1946 and
1959 the development of her alignment with the West to a large extent
took place in the form of relations with the United States.[41] The
decisions to recognise Israel in 1949, to send troops to Korea in 1950,
and to join NATO in 1952 are cases in point. The Cold war pushed
Turkey back in a role that the Ottoman Empire already had played. The
Ottoman challenge to counterbalance Russia's power in the Eastern
Mediterranean was thus inherited by the Turkish Republic. As the
Ottoman Empire had played for Great Britain, the Turkish Republic
played a key role in the US-containment policy against the USSR.

Since then, the historical and political integration of Turkey with
Europe and the US has been materialised in a number of institutional
relations. Turkey was a founding member of the Organisation of
European Economic Cooperation in 1948, and is a member of the
Council of Europe since 1949 and of NATO since 1952. In 1963 the
Ankara association agreement with the European Community was
concluded and a customs union with the European Union was signed
in 1996. Hence, the internal westernisation of Turkey was completed
with the westernisation of her foreign relations.

Turkey began also to play a new role in the Middle Eastern
policies of western powers. She joined the so-called Middle East
Command (MEC) together with the U.S., Britain and France in October
1951, in the face of Arab suspicion. In June 1952 Turkey supported the
Middle East Defence Organisation (MEDO) between the United
Kingdom and the United States. Starting with the 'Northern Tier',
Turkey under Prime Minister Menderes became the leading regional
force to forge the Baghdad Pact among Iran, Iraq, Pakistan and Turkey.
The Menderes government was thereby not only pushing for the
Baghdad Pact, but also tried to intimidate anti-western regimes. In both
the Syrian crisis of 1957 and the Iraqi crisis of 1958 the West had to
discourage the Turkish government from taking any kind of unilateral
military action against her neighbours.[42] Not only were the politics of
neutrality abolished, but there was also a first sign of activism in
Turkish foreign policy, although restricted by western interests.

The ten years under the rule of the Democratic Party (1950-1960)
were characterised by an almost complete westernisation of Turkey's
foreign policy. This westernisation brought Turkey back into Middle
Eastern affairs, but as an ally of the West and therefore at the expense
of an increased alienation from her Arab neighbours. In contradiction
to his western attitude in foreign policy, however, Menderes started
domestically a 're-Islamisation' of the Turkish society in order to get
support for his populist government. His Democratic Party promised

respect for Islamic traditions and presented itself as the voice of the marginalised Anatolian majority.[43]

Both the increasing signs of activism in foreign policy and the weakening of secularism in domestic politics, were followed with suspicion by the generals. In May 1960 the Turkish army, the guardian of the state and its Kemalist principles, toppled the civilian government and Prime Minister Menderes was executed in 1961. This second phase of Turkish foreign policy brought about Turkey's institutional integration into the western world and her increasing isolation in the Middle East. However, the new course of western integration was not due to a change in the worldview of Turkey's élite, but was rather triggered by security threats from outside and by Turkey's increasing economic dependency on the West as a political rent-seeker in the Cold War.

Phase Three: Middle Eastern Rapprochement

The third phase, which can be described as a move towards rapprochement with the Arab world, was also a reaction to the changing political and economic environment. The deep-rooted suspicions against the West never disappeared and were strongly reconfirmed during the developments of the 1960s and 1970s. The Jupiter missile crisis 1962, the Cyprus crises 1964 and 1974, and the EU's 1997 rejection of Turkey's candidacy for full membership, were events during which the Sèvres Syndrome with its conspiracy theories re-emerged.[44] Especially the letter of U.S. President Johnson to Ismet Inönü, written during the Cyprus Crisis of 1964 seemed to confirm Turkish suspicion and stirred anti-American and neutralist sentiments. In this letter, Johnson was 'cautioning Inönü that if Turkish action on the island would invite a Soviet attack, then NATO was not obliged to defend Turkey'.[45] Another proof was provided by the arms embargo the American government placed on Turkey after her military intervention in Cyprus 1974.

The attempt to normalise relations with the Arab world was a response to these disappointments with western policies. The Turkish decision not to allow the U.S. to use its military base in Incirlik during the Arab-Israeli wars in 1967 and 1973 and Turkey's recognition of the Palestinian Liberation Organisation (PLO), whose formal representation in Ankara began in 1979,[46] are examples of her willingness to act against western interests.

While rooted in political problems, Turkey's rapprochement with her Middle Eastern neighbours was also due to economic problems and to rising Islamic sentiments in her populace. The 1973 oil crisis,

Turkish supplies of manpower to Arab states and later the search for new markets in the Middle East were economic aspects of Turkey's change in foreign policy.[47] In 1973 the Islamic National Salvation Party (*Milli Selamet Partisi*), founded in 1972 by Necmettin Erbakan, joined a coalition government and favoured a withdrawal from the 'Western Club'.[48] Although the Democratic Party was instrumentalising religious sentiments in domestic politics during the 1950s, its leadership was still following the Kemalist way. It was not until the rise of Erbakan during the 1970s that the Islamic politics entered Turkey's political scene.[49] However, the change in Turkish foreign policy was still reactive, an attempt to adjust to the changing international and regional environment under the dominant principles of the Kemalist habitus.

Phase Four: Activism
The fourth phase, characterised by a new quality of activism, began after the military coup in 1980 and was to a large extent related to political decisions made by Prime Minister (1983-1989) and later President (1989-1993) Turgut Özal. His domestic policy of economic liberalisation and gradual Islamisation was accompanied by an active export strategy especially towards Middle Eastern countries. Between 1980 and 1985 Turkish exports to the Middle East increased fivefold, in 1985 64 percent of total exports went to neighbouring Iran and Iraq.[50] Turkish exports to Iran rose from twelve million US Dollars in 1979 to a peak of 1.1 billion in 1985.[51] In the mid-1980s Özal opened the country also for Saudi capital and Turkish-Saudi joint ventures.[52] While the economic ties with the Arab world and Iran steadily improved, the relations with Israel deteriorated further after the coup of September 1980. Ankara recalled its ambassador from Tel Aviv and relations were not restored to the ambassadorial level until December 1991.[53]

Whereas in the 1980s Özal's new activism was following the pattern of rapprochement with Turkey's neighbours, the Iraqi invasion of Kuwait in August 1990 marked a radical turning point. Meanwhile Turkey's economic boom with her neighbours had proved to be a passing fancy. Turkey's export rate with Arab countries was falling, reaching a marginal percentage of twelve percent of her total exports in 1994.[54] The export boom to Iraq and Iran in the 1980s was not due to the establishment of solid trade relations, but a result of the First Gulf War 1980-1988 and Turkey's neutral stand and willingness to trade with both sides. In the run-up to the Second Gulf War (1991) the Turkish president had changed his mind. Özal now saw a chance for a

reorientation in Turkish foreign policy. While his diplomats and the army rather advocated a neutral policy, he was eager to play a major role in the US-led coalition against Iraq. Uninformed about Özal's decision to close the Iraqi oil pipelines, and under the President's pressures to adopt a more active military stance, then General Chief of Staff, Necip Torumtay, resigned in December 1990.[55]

The degree of activism and boldness, that characterised the fourth phase of Turkish foreign policy introduced by Turgut Özal, has remained visible after his death. The new Turkish-Israeli axis, re-emerging dreams of pan-Turkism, Turkish military operations in Iraq and the threat of force against Syria in October 1998 are clear examples that Turkey adopted a more active role in Middle Eastern politics. Whereas the reconciliation with the Middle Eastern neighbours was triggered by the dissatisfaction with Europe and the US, the reorientation in the fourth phase was due to the volatile decisions of a strong political leader. Although the army and parts of the Kemalist establishment were critical to Özal's policies, they did not escape his impact. They are now proponents of a more activist foreign policy.

Since the end of the Second World War, Turkey has increasingly been dragged into regional politics, without accepting herself as a part of the Middle East. The powerless threatened state of Atatürk's time is now a regional power with the intention to use its capabilities in a more active and independent way. However, this regional activism is not guided by any new vision of Turkey's role in Middle Eastern politics, but remains under the impact of the traditionalist Kemalist worldview. This is, on the one hand, visible in the still existent mistrust towards both the West and the Middle Eastern neighbours.[56] On the other hand it is incarnated in the political structure of the Turkish State and the inherited narrow notion of security, limited to the sovereignty and territorial integrity of the state. A brief glance at the problems of Kurdish separatism and religious fundamentalism with regard to Turkey's relations with Syria, Iraq, Iran and Saudi Arabia makes this more transparent.

Kurdish Nationalism, Islamism and Turkey's Foreign Policy

Domestic Roots
In a recently published statement, the Turkish Armed Forces reiterated that they will preserve their image 'as the Turkish people's stronghold against all domestic and foreign threats' and will therefore continue their fight against separatism and religious reactionaries.[57]

With respect to both targets, Kurdish nationalism and political

Islam, issues of domestic security are indeed linked with regional foreign policy. While the Kurdish question and Turkey's war with the PKK transcends her borders with Iran, Iraq and Syria, the confrontation between the secularist Kemalist state and Islamist forces brings Iran and Saudi Arabia in, both known as supporters of Islamist groups. Thus, the three most important littoral states of the Persian Gulf region, Iran, Iraq and Saudi Arabia play important roles in the Turkish security complex. Moreover, Turkey, Iran and Saudi Arabia are also competitors in Central Asia, supporting different political and social forces. This factual overlap of internal and external security concerns has the potential to cause severe conflicts in the region, involving the Middle East as a whole.

The Kurdish question and political Islam are not recent phenomena, but were two major sources of internal conflict of the Turkish Republic since its outset. Therefore, Kurdish nationalism and political Islam are almost by nature interpreted through the prism of the Sèvres Syndrome. In the foundation phase of the modern Turkish state between 1924 and 1938 eighteen rebellions against the republican regime were reported, of which seventeen took place in eastern Anatolia and sixteen of them involved Kurdish groups.[58]

The crucial date for the eruption of these series of rebellions was the abolition of the caliphate in March 1924. The famous Sheikh Said rebellion of 1925 clearly shows that no clear distinction between Kurdish and Islamic aspects of the east-Anatolian resistance against the republican regime can be made. The Kurdish Naqshbandi Sheikh Said mobilised his followers by denouncing the republican government for its godless policies and claimed to have come to restore religion.[59] What characterised the leadership was even more true for the participants, of whom it has been said that 'religious and nationalist loyalties cannot be separated: they coincided and were virtually identical'.[60] It was the modernisation of Turkish society under republican rule itself that resulted in the separation of Kurdish and religious opposition against Kemalism. Therefore, secular Kurdish nationalism is a product of the Kemalist reforms themselves and not the result of foreign intervention.

The close connection between the rise of Kurdish nationalism and the modernisation process in Turkey is also proved by the change in its leadership. Whereas the revolts in the 1920s and 1930s were led by traditional tribal and religious leaders, from 1945 onwards modern forces within the Kurdish society have become more relevant. The extension of state bureaucracy, the spread of modern education and the growing integration in the world market have contributed to the

emergence of a modern stratum of Kurdish society.

Until the 1970s Turkey was rather successful in containing the national aspirations of these new social actors. This had happened either through integration into the modern political and economic sectors of Turkish society or through the repressive subordination of radical forces. During the intensification of the economic and political crisis in the 1970s, when violent clashes among radical right- and left-wing groups, and between them and the state authorities, claimed almost daily victims, the Kurdish movement likewise became radicalised.[61] In 1978 the PKK was founded, based on Marxist-Leninist ideology. In combining nationalists and social revolutionaries, the PKK called for armed struggle against the state and for the establishment of a socialist Kurdish state. The PKK was later the only Kurdish political organisation that managed to reorganise itself after the military coup in 1980. In 1984 the PKK launched its guerrilla war in the south-east of Turkey and became a political tool in the hands of Turkey's neighbours.

Like the Kurdish question, political Islam developed within the country and was not stirred from outside. It was Mustafa Kemal Atatürk himself who needed Islam as a component of a definition of the Turkish nation in order to form a people out of the ethnically and religiously fragmented Anatolian society. Even the war of independence against Greek occupation forces was sometimes called a holy war. Since the inception of the multi-party system after the Second World War, Turkish politicians have been instrumentalising religious sentiments for political gains to the extent that 'political patronage became the basic strategy of obtaining votes, in which religion was frequently used for political purposes'.[62] In Turkish politics a double discourse was adopted: 'Islam was disestablished as the state religion while religious language was incorporated into the nationalist discourse, without making its conceptual grammar essentially Islamic'.[63] The development of political parties like the National Salvation Party, *Refah* or *Fazilet* is therefore nothing more than a logical outcome of both the use of religious language in politics and the existence of strong religious sentiments in Turkey's population.

Not only politicians, but also the generals tried to instrumentalise Islam. After the civil unrest in the 1970s and the subsequent military coup, Islam seemed to be the means at hand to discipline and stabilise society. In the aftermath of the coup, 'the State Planning Organisation prepared a report for the leaders of the 1980 coup suggesting the reintegration of Islamic ethics into public education as a means of consolidating national unity'.[64]

In order to achieve a new social consensus it was the state élite itself that politicised religion under the official banner of a 'Turkish-Islamic synthesis'.[65] Turgut Özal further strengthened this new discourse and thus both the generals and leading politicians of the 1980s paved the way for the relative success of *Refah* and its successor *Fazilet*. With the decision of the National Security Council on February 28, 1997, which led to the resignation of Prime Minister Erbakan and to the closure of *Refah*, the military tried to get rid of a 'monster' they had themselves helped creating.

Meanwhile, however, this Islamic political identity has been rooted in a new urban and modern context, brought about by the same forces of social change that are behind the rise of Kurdish nationalism.[66] With the accelerated modernisation of Turkish society, especially during the last two decades, a new modern segment of society has emerged which has challenged the position of the Kemalist élite with new patterns of Islamic and Kurdish identity.[67]

Regional Implications

Under the traditional Kemalist perception, however, the Kurdish insurgency and the rise of religious parties are attributed to conspiracies from outside. Domestic conflicts caused by social change are thus associated with attempts at foreign political interference. This is clearly visible in Turkey's relations with her neighbours, in which fields of possible cooperation tend to become battle-fields of confrontation.

Although it is true that Syria hosted PKK-leader Abdullah Öcalan for more than fifteen years, it was not Syria which created the PKK and the national sentiments among Turkey's Kurdish population. Syrian support for the PKK was a means of extortion in the conflict about the waters of the Euphrates rather than an attempt to destroy the territorial integrity of the Turkish State. It was used as a tool in the foreign relations between two states that were historically suspicious of each other, contributing to increased tension between the two states. The same situation, although in a more complex way, applies to Turkish-Iraqi relations.

Since the PKK began its war against the Turkish state in 1984, the Turkish army intervened in northern Iraq no less than 57 times, according to official Turkish accounts.[68] After the Second Gulf War and the Kurdish refugee crisis in Iraq in April and May 1991, northern Iraq became the theatre for major Turkish military operations. In August 1991, almost 5,000 Turkish troops entered northern Iraq to create a buffer zone along the border. More than 20,000 troops backed by tanks and the Turkish air force crossed the border area to Iran and

Iraq in October 1992. In the aftermath of a military operation in March 1995, in which 35,000 Turkish troops went forty kilometres deep and 220 kilometres wide into Iraqi territory, Turkey's president Süleyman Demirel publicly spoke about a change in the Turkish-Iraqi border in favour of Turkey.[69] This statement together with operation Murad, during which more than 50,000 Turkish soldiers entered northern Iraq in May 1997, raised suspicions in the Arab world that Turkey could have territorial claims and might want to revoke the Mosul decision of 1926.[70]

Operation Provide Comfort, which created a Kurdish sanctuary in northern Iraq, brought Turkey in a paradoxical situation. While denying a Kurdish question at home and claiming the preservation of the integrity of the Iraqi state as a major objective of her foreign policy, Turkey is now fully embroiled in the Kurdish struggle in northern Iraq and participates in the upholding of its *de facto* division. On the one side Turkey wants to avoid a Kurdish 'buffer state' in northern Iraq and the possible spill-over of Kurdish self-determination into Turkey itself. On the other side her war against the PKK aligns Turkey with Barzani's Kurdish Democratic Party (KDP), which for decades has been a major force in the Kurdish struggle with Iraqi regimes in Baghdad. [71] In March 1991 representatives of the KDP and of its Kurdish adversary, Talabani's Patriotic Union of Kurdistan (PUK) were invited to visit Ankara—a U-turn of the previous policy of not contacting the Kurdish groups in northern Iraq.[72] Meanwhile Barzani and his KDP, who was in the 1970s fighting the Baathist regime in Baghdad, supported by the CIA and Iran, became the main ally in Turkey's fight against the PKK in northern Iraq, receiving military and logistic support.

The results of the Second Gulf War and Özal's reorientation turned out to be not a new chance, but a new predicament for Turkey's foreign policy. There is now the permanent danger of a complete disintegration of the Iraqi State, which would have a tremendous impact on the Kurdish question in Turkey. Furthermore, Turkey's military interventions in northern Iraq evoked new suspicions in Baghdad and the Arab world over Turkish irredentist claims to the Mosul province. Both issues became confused with the water issue and the question about the reopening of the two oil pipelines between Iraq and Turkey. In addition to this climate of increasing mistrust and suspicion, Turkey is confronted with huge economic losses due to the embargo against Iraq. According to senior officials in the Turkish ministry of foreign affairs the Turkish economy had to bear a loss of around forty billion U.S. Dollars since the end of the Second Gulf

War.[73] This negative economic situation has been further aggravated by the U.S. containment policy against Iran.

Contrary to Iraq, whose current problems are mainly linked to its lack of a tradition of statehood, Turkey and Iran have the historical background of patrimonial and imperial rule. Their current frontiers were established under the Treaty of Zohab in 1639, and although the history of Iranian-Turkish relations has not always been characterised by friendship, territorial claims do not exist. In spite of their cooperation in the Baghdad and CENTO pacts, a mutually shared mistrust towards the other side always exists. Since the Islamic revolution in 1979 the ideological difference between Ankara's secularism and Tehran's Islamism has aggravated Turkish-Iranian tensions over issues such as the Kurdish question, Turkey's alliance with the West, and competing interests in the post-Soviet republics. While Armenia and Iran provide 'physical obstacles' to Turkey's entry into the Caucasus and Central Asia,[74] Turkish nationalism in Azerbaijan poses a threat to the national integrity of Iran. This was especially apparent during the early 1990s, as the then Azeri President Elchibey used a heavy Azeri and pan-Turcic rhetoric and nationalistic political claims to unite 'northern and southern Azerbaijan' became known.[75]

Whereas the pan-Turkic wave has almost faded away,[76] the Kurdish question remains a major source of tension. For a short period from 1992 to 1995, Turkey, Iran and Syria sought to coordinate their policies towards northern Iraq in order to prevent a Kurdish state.[77] However, the common ground of those Tripartite conferences was dissolved with the outbreak of warfare in northern Iraq between the KDP and PUK in 1996. Since then the three states are again supporting their respective Kurdish clients: Turkey the KDP, Iran the PUK and Syria the PKK.[78] Besides Iranian support for Talabani's PUK, there is an rather unsubstantiated support for the PKK from Iran. Turkish sources are talking about an estimated number of 35 PKK camps on Iranian territory.[79] Moreover, Iran is suspected of supporting *Hizbullah*, a terrorist organisation operating in Turkey and aiming at the establishment of an Islamic state in the Kurdish areas.[80] These Turkish accusations are countered by Iranian allegations that Turkey harbours opponents of the regime in Tehran and supports the *Mujaheddin-e Khalq*.[81]

While Pan-Turksim and Kurdish nationalism have always been possible sources of tension between Turkey and Iran, the ideological conflict has further increased them. Right after the revolution, Khomeini condemned Kemalism and Iranian representatives have

frequently refused to visit the mausoleum of Atatürk during official visits to Ankara. Furthermore, the Iranian regime has produced anti-secular propaganda material that has been smuggled into Turkey.[82] The domestic rise of Islamist political forces could therefore easily be attributed to foreign intervention.

How this situation affects the bilateral relationship between Turkey and Iran was clearly shown by the 'Jerusalem incident' in Sincan, a small town in the vicinity of Ankara. On 1 February 1997, the mayor of Sincan, who was a member of the Islamist *Refah* party, organised a rally to protest the Israeli occupation of East Jerusalem. During the event, posters supporting Hizballah and Hamas were displayed and the Israeli-Turkish agreements were denounced in the presence of the Iranian ambassador. Three days later tanks turned up in Sincan, the mayor was arrested and the ambassadors were mutually withdrawn from Ankara and Tehran.[83]

Although the support of Islamist groups in Turkey is mainly attributed to Iran, Saudi money, rather than political influence also plays a role. With the economic opening for Saudi capital in the 1980s, Turkey also attracted the influx of 'ideological money' from non-governmental organisations in Saudi Arabia. At this time even Turkish imams in Europe were financed by Saudi money with the consent of the Turkish government.[84] It is apparent that Saudi money contributed to the Islamisation of the Turkish society, although Saudi Arabia has no interest in destabilising Turkey. However, both countries are competitors in the Middle East and Central Asia, where Saudi Arabia is using its monetary resources as well as Sunni Islam as a means to boost its influence.[85] That Turkish-Saudi relations still bear the imprints of historically rooted mistrust and suspicion between Turks and Arabs was proved by the 'cool reception given by Saudi Arabian officials to Turkey's offer to send troops during the Gulf War'.[86]

To sum up: although there are apparent links between Turkey's domestic conflicts and the above-mentioned neighbours, the roots of the Kurdish question and of political Islam are to be found within Turkish society. The neighbours merely capitalise on Turkey's unresolved social conflicts. In these conflicts the traditional Kemalist establishment is confronted with the claims of a 'counter-elite' to participate in the political and economic sectors of society. The exclusiveness of 'Kemalist enlightenment', a legacy of Turkey's top-down modernisation and its conservation in the social habitus, is losing its legitimacy. Under the dominant Kemalist worldview this domestic conflict is perceived as an attempt to destroy the integrity of the Turkish state. Again internal and external threats are equated, internal

social conflicts interpreted as a result of external interference that has to be countered by force.

The factual overlapping of domestic causes and foreign support of terrorism, especially in the Kurdish question, seems to provide evidence for this conspiracy theory. With regard to the reaction of Turkey's Kemalist élite and the quotations in section two of this article, it is hard to distinguish between conviction and instrumentalisation. Most likely it is both. On the one hand, the instrumental usage of threat perceptions attached to the Sèvres Syndrome to legitimise the endangered position of a privileged élite; on the other hand the expression of a social habitus still guiding the political action of an élite which has lost the pace of social change it once has initiated.

Conclusions

This article set out to shed light on the question of the future of Turkish foreign policy and whether the country should play a more active role in the Middle Eastern context. The question has been partly answered by the factual development of the Turkish Republic.

From the Menderes era onwards, Turkish politicians became gradually more activist in their foreign policies and more involved in Middle Eastern affairs. The demise of the Soviet Union added new challenges and opportunities to this general development and at the same time Turgut Özal introduced previously unknown patterns of activist behaviour into Turkish foreign policy. Adding Turkey's economic interests and her security concerns related to the Kurdish question and political Islam, there can be no doubt that the country is already highly involved in the Middle Eastern scene. Furthermore, the economic and military agreements between Israel and Turkey introduced a new power axis into Middle Eastern politics which will have a major impact on regional security. Thus, factual developments in the international system and the region forced Turkey to become a regional player and to confront her Ottoman legacy.[87]

This confrontation with the Ottoman legacy and Turkey's historical and cultural roots in the Middle East brings us back to the social habitus of the Kemalist élite. Although the structural environment of the region and the social and economic structure of Turkey's society have changed, the Turkish establishment is still inclined to perceive the region and Turkey's position in categories of the 1920s. This applies not only to foreign policy perceptions, but also to the way the Kemalist élite is dealing with domestic problems.

These problems are not due to the fact that the country is a 'torn state' in the sense of Huntington's analysis,[88] but grow out of a society

with a high proportion of uneven developments. The coexistence of an individualised urban society in the western cities with tribal societies in the east, the blend of modern and traditional values among its youth,[89] the mushrooming of nepotism and corruption under the impact of an accelerated neo-liberal reconstruction of the economy, these are side-effects of modernization when traditional forms of social integration give way without being sufficiently replaced by modern ones.

Like in its reaction to the changing regional environment, the Kemalist establishment reacts to the domestic challenges according to the same anachronistic patterns of interpretation. The attempt, however, to stop this process of social disintegration by the means of authoritarian corporatism is bound to fail. The unitarian idea of a corporatist society of the 1920s has to give way to a pluralistic approach to reintegrate Turkey's population, based on a consensus of identity as diversity. The major threat to the integrity of the Turkish state is not posed by foreign powers with territorial ambitions as it was at Sèvres, but is caused by centripetal societal forces that are themselves a result of the Kemalist modernisation project. Although the process of redefining Turkey's social identity is in full process, the uncompromising reaction against Kurdish nationalism and political Islam and their association with foreign intervention could lead to destructive political decisions, making Turkey a predicament for regional stability.

The future role of Turkey depends on the ability of her élite to come to terms with its own history and its Ottoman and Kemalist legacy. To assume an appropriate regional role, Turkey has to overcome the Sèvres Syndrome so that feelings of suspicion and encirclement could give way to a new self-confidence based on the material capabilities the country has achieved. A self-confident, pluralistic and democratic Turkey would have a major impact on the region. It could spearhead the forces of economic and political integration and play a decisive role in pacifying the conflictive Eastern Mediterranean and the Persian Gulf. Turkey, then, could develop into a cornerstone of stability and security in the Middle East. The contentious issues of Central Asia, the Kurds, water etc., need not necessarily lead to confrontation. On the contrary, once escaped from the Sèvres trap, they could provide opportunities for cooperation between a strong and self-confident Turkey and her neighbours.

However, Turkey will not be able to shake off its historical ballast and to develop a post-Kemalist vision without assistance from outside. On the one hand, the European Union had to revoke the Luxembourg

decision of 1997, which many observers now see as a historical mistake.[90] The solution of the critical domestic situation in Turkey needs the strait-jacket for reforms that only by an accession strategy to the EU can provide. The revitalisation of Turkey's European track would support her civil society in its fight against a new stream of nationalist isolationism within the state élite. On the other hand one has to understand that in the current situation any attempt at confidence-building in the region that bypasses Turkey can be counterproductive as any such regional security regime could be perceived by the Turkish élite as a direct threat to the Turkish State.

Ironically, from the Turkish perspective, a cooperative security arrangement among the countries of the Persian Gulf region or the Middle East could then lose its cooperative character. It could be perceived as a collective security arrangement of Iran and the Arab world targeting Turkey as their mutual foe. Neither Turkey nor their neighbours should deny the Ottoman legacy and the strong impact the decline of the Ottoman Empire had on both the modernisation of Turkey and the formation of states in the region. Therefore, any security regime concluded in the 'Greater Middle East' that does not include Turkey to some extent, could swing to the other extreme and increase instability in the region.[91] If cooperative security stresses informal cooperation and dialogue between regional states as well as the development and implementation of agreed principles among theses states,[92] the inclusion of Turkey in this process seems to be a must.

Notes

1. Carley, Patricia: 'Turkey's Place in the World', in Henri J. Barkey (ed.): *Reluctant Neighbor. Turkey's Role in the Middle East* (Washington, DC: United States Institute of Peace Press, 1996), p. 3.

2. Eralp, Atila: 'Facing the Challenge. Post-Revolutionary Relations with Iran', *ibid.*, p. 93.

3. Göle, Nilüfer: 'Secularism and Islamism in Turkey: The Making of Elites and Counter-Elites', *Middle Eastern Journal*, vol. 51, no. 1 (Winter 1997), p. 47.

4. Fuller, Graham E. & Lesser, Ian O.: *Turkey's New Geopolitics. From the Balkans to Western China* (Boulder, CO: Westview, 1993), p. 163.

5. Türsan, Huri: 'Ersatz Democracy: Turkey in the 1990s', in Richard Gillespie (ed.): *Mediterranean Politics*, Volume 2 (1996), p. 216.

6. Robins, Philip: *Turkey and the Middle East* (London: Royal Institute of International Affairs, 1991), p. 16.

7. Korkisch, Friedrich: 'Die amerikanisch-türkischen Beziehungen', *Österreichische Militärische Zeitschrift*, vol. 37, no. 2 (1999), p. 140; and *NATO's Sixteen Nations & Partners for Peace*, Special Supplement, edited by

Manfred Sadlowski on 'Defence and Economics in Turkey; Pillar of Regional Stability" (1998).

8. *The Ninth International Seminar on Persian Gulf: Present Realities and Future Perspectives* (Institute for Political and International Studies, Tehran, 22-23 February, 1999).

9. Although Turkey is mentioned as particular important, only one of the participants/experts came from Turkey. Furthermore, Turkey is excluded from the Middle East by definition. See Jones, Peter: *Towards a Regional Security regime for the Middle East: Issues and Options* (Stockholm: SIPRI, 1998), pp. 19, 22.

10. For the Turkish-Israeli agreements see the article of Wolfango Piccoli in this book.

11. Wendt, Alexander: Constructing International Politics, *International Security*, vol. 20, no. 1 (Summer 1995), pp. 71-81.

12. See, for instance, Keohane, Robert: 'Institutional Theory and the Realist Challenge after the Cold War', in David A. Baldwin (ed.): *Neorealism and Neoliberalism. The Contemporary Debate* (New York: Columbia University Press, 1993), p. 288.

13. Bohman, James: *New Philosophie of Social Science. Problems of Indeterminacy* (Cambridge: Polity Press, 1991).

14. Wendt: *loc. cit.* (note 11), p. 72; Ruggie, John Gerald: 'Territoriality and Beyond: Problematizing Modernity in International Relations', *International Organization*, vol. 47, no. 1 (1993), pp. 139-74.

15. See Elias, Norbert: *Die Gesellschaft der Individuen* (Frankfurt a. M.: Suhrkamp, 1988), p. 244.

16. Bourdieu, Pierre: *Die verborgenen Mechanismen der Macht* (Hamburg: VSA Verlag, 1992), p. 33.

17. *ibid.*, p. 33.

18. Müller, Hans-Peter: 'Kultur, Geschmack, Distinktion. Grundzuge der Kultursoziologie Pierre Bourdieus', *Kölner Zeitschrift fur Soziologie und Sozialpsychologie*. Special issue: Kultur und Gesellschaft (1986), p. 164.

19. Quoted in Mufti, Malik: 'Daring and Caution in Turkish Foreign Policy', *Middle East Journal*, vol. 52, no. 1 (Winter 1998), p. 33.

20. Quoted *ibid.*, p. 34.

21. Quoted in Arikan, E. Burak: 'The Programme of the Nationalist Action Party: An Iron Hand in a Velvet Glove?', *Middle Eastern Studies*, vol. 34, no. 4 (1998), p. 127.

22. Quoted in Gözen, Ramazan: 'Two Processes in Turkish Foreign Policy: Intergration and Isolation', *Foreign Policy* (Ankara), vol. 21, no. 1-2 (1997), p. 119.

23. Interview with the Turkish Prime Minister Ecevit in *Die Zeit*, no. 13 (25 March 1999), p. 15.

24. Quoted in Meyer, James H.: 'Politics as Usual: Ciller, Refah and Susurluk: Turkey's Troubled Democracy', *East European Quarterly*, vol. 23, no. 4 (1999), p. 496.

25. So the official Turkish news agency *Anatolia* (9 May 1999).

26. Karaosmanoglu, Ali: 'Islam and Foreign Policy: A Turkish Perspective', *Foreign Policy* (Ankara), vol. 12, no. 1-2 (1985), p. 68.

27. All quotations from Bir, Cevik: 'Turkey's Role in the New World Order', *Strategic Forum*, no. 135 (February 1998), pp. 1-4.

28. *Turkish Daily News* (1 April 1998).

29. Davison, Roderic H.: *Reform in the Ottoman Empire, 1856-1876* (Princeton, NJ: Princeton University Press, 1963), pp. 6-8.

30. Russia, Hapsburg, Prussia, Britain and France.

31. For an detailed description and analysis of these developments, see Zürcher, Erik J.: *The Unionist Factor: The Role of the Committee of Union and Progress in the Turkish National Movement, 1905-1926* (Leiden: Brill, 1984); idem: *Political Opposition in the Early Turkish Republic. The Progressive Republican Party 1924-1925* (Leiden: Brill, 1991).

32. It is worth to mention that one of the last founding members of the Turkish Republic, Ismet Inönü, died in 1973.

33. See Birand, Mehmet Ali: *Shirts of Steel. An Anatomy of the Turkish Armed Forces* (London: I.B. Tauris, 1991), p. 23.

34. Yavuz, Hakan M.: 'Turkish Identity and Foreign Policy in Flux: The Rise of Neo-Ottomanism', *Critique*, no. 12 (Spring 1998), p. 27.

35. Pahlavan, Tschanguiz H.: 'Turkish-Iranian Relations. An Iranian View', in Barkey (ed.): *op. cit.* (note 1), p. 71.

36. The decision was based on the Franco-Turkish agreement of 1921 in which France acknowledged the existence of a Turkish majority in the province inhabited by Turks and Arabs. In 1937 Hatay was supposed to become an independent territory, however, represented by Syria in foreign affairs. Elections in July 1938 resulted in a thin Turkish majority in the newly established parliament that declared the independent Republic of Hatay. See Steinbach, Udo: *Die Türkei im 20. Jahrhundert. Schwieriger Partner Europas* (Bergisch Gladbach: Lübbe Verlag, 1996), pp. 149-150.

37. Heper, Metin & Keyman, Fuat E.: 'Double-Faced State: Political Patronage and the Consolidation of Democracy in Turkey', *Middle Eastern Studies*, vol. 34, no. 4 (1998), p. 260.

38. For relations between Arab nationalists and the Turkish republican movement see: Eppel, Michael: 'Iraqi Politics and Regional Policies', *Middle Eastern Studies*, vol. 28, no. 1 (1992), pp. 108-119; and Tauber, Eliezer: 'Syrian and Iraqi Nationalist Attitudes to the Kemalist and Bolshevik Movements', *ibid.*, vol. 30, no. 4 (1994), pp. 896-915.

39. Mufti: *op. cit.* (note 19), p. 41.

40. Gözen, Ramazan: 'The Turkish-Iraqi Relations: From Cooperation to Uncertainty', *Foreign Policy* (Ankara), vol. 19, no. 3-4 (1995), p. 74.

41. See the introduction of Karpat, Kemal H. (ed.): *Turkey's Foreign Policy in Transition 1950-1974* (Leiden: Brill, 1975), p. 3.

42. Sever, Ayseguel: 'The Compliant Ally? Turkey and the West in the Middle East 1954-1958', *Middle Eastern Studies*, vol. 34, no. 2 (1998), pp. 75-85.

43. Yavuz, Hakan M.: 'Turkish-Israeli Relations through the Lens of the Turkish Identity Debate', *Journal of Palestine Studies*, vol. 27, no. 1 (1997), p. 24.

44. An interesting account of this suspicion can be found in Heper, Metin, Ayshe Öncü & Heinz Kramer (eds.): *Turkey and the West. Changing Political and Cultural Identities* (London: I.B. Tauris, 1993). The book comprises a number of articles on structure and mind-set of social groups in Turkey such as the military, journalists, bureaucrats, politicians etc.

45. Criss, Nur Bilge: 'Strategic Nuclear Missiles in Turkey: The Jupiter Affair, 1959-1963', *Journal of Strategic Studies*, vol. 20, no. 3 (1997), p. 119.

46. Gözen: *loc. cit.* (note 40), pp. 74-75. For a detailed account of Turkish policy in the Palestine question see Aykan, Mahmut Bali: 'The Palestinian Question in Turkish Foreign Policy from the 1950s to the 1990s', *International Journal of Middle Eastern Studies*, no. 25 (1993), pp. 91-110.

47. In 1975, for example, Turkey and Libya agreed about 600.000 Turkish workers to be supplied to Libya. See *ibid.*, p. 98.

48. Karaosmanoglu: *loc. cit.* (note 26), p. 76.

49. Erbakan entered the Turkish Parliament as an independent candidate in 1969 and founded the National Order Party (*Milli Nizam Partisi*) in 1970. After the National order Party was closed down for violating the constitution, Erbakan in 1973 formed the National Salvation Party (*Milli Selamet Partisi*) which served in several coalition governments until it was closed down during the coup of 1980. See Gülalp, Haldun: 'Political Islam in Turkey: The Rise and Fall of the Refah Party', *The Muslim World*, vol. 89, no. 1 (1999), pp. 22, 33.

50. Dalacoura, Katerina: 'Turkey and the Middle East in the 1980s, *Millenium*, vol. 19, no. 2 (1990), p. 210.

51. Eralp: *loc. cit.* (note 2), p. 101.

52. Bagis, Ali Ihsan: 'The Beginning and the Development of Economic Relations Between Turkey and Middle Eastern Countries', *Foreign Policy* (Ankara), vol. 12, no. 1-2 (June 1985), p. 87.

53. Yavuz: *loc. cit.* (note 43), p. 24.

54. *ibid.*

55. Mufti: *op. cit.* (note 19), p. 44. For an account of these events from Torumtay's memoirs, see Heper, Metin & Aylin Günay: 'The Military and Democracy in the Third Turkish Republic', *Armed Forces and Society*, vol. 22, no. 4 (1996), pp. 619-642.

56. The perceptions of encirclement quoted in the second section may be a proof of this insecurity feeling.

57. So in a pamphlet published by the General Chief of Staff on 8 April 1999. See *Turkish Daily News* (9 April 1999).

58. Kirisci, Kemal: 'The Kurdish Question and Turkish Foreign Policy', *PrivatView*, vol. 2, no. 6 (Autumn 1998), pp. 74.

59. Olson, Robert: *The Emergence of Kurdish Nationalism and the Sheikh Said Rebellion, 1880-1925* (Austin: University of Texas Press, 1989), p. 95.

60. Bruinessen, Martin van: *Agha, Shaikh and State. The Social and Political Structures of Kurdistan* (London: Zed Books, 1992), p. 299.

61. For a study about this crucial phase of radicalisation and insurgency in Turkey, see Sayari, Sabri & Hoffman, Bruce: 'Urbanisation and Insurgency: the Turkish Case, 1976-1980', *Small Wars and Insurgencies*, vol. 5, no. 2 (1994), pp. 162-179.

62. Heper & Keyman: *op. cit.* (note 37), p. 259.

63. Cizre-Sakallioglu, Umit: 'Rethinking the Connections between Turkey's "Western" Identity versus Islam', *Critique*, no. 12 (Spring, 1998), p. 16.

64. Yavuz: *loc. cit.* 1998 (note 34), p. 29.

65. *Ibid.*, p. 30.

66. *Ibid.*, p. 25.

67. Cf. Göle: *loc. cit.* (note 3) and her notion of 'counter-elite'.

68. Gunter, Michael: 'Turkey and Iran Face of in Kurdistan', *Middle East Quarterly*, vol. 5, no. 1 (March 1998), p. 40.

69. Former President Özal and the founder of the extreme right-wing MHP, Alparslan Türkesh, are also known for loudly contemplating about the 'Mossul question'.

70. Gözen: *loc. cit.* (note 22); and Gunter: *loc. cit.* (note 68), pp. 36-38.

71. Marr, Phebe: 'Turkey and Iraq', in Barkey: *op. cit.* (note 1), pp. 54-56. Since 1945 the Kurdish organisations in Iraq fought in six wars against the regime in Baghdad. See Jung, Dietrich: 'Das Kriegsgeschehen im Nahen Osten: 43 Kriege und ein Friedensprozess', *Orient*, 38/2 (1997), pp. 340-342.

72. Aykan, Mahmut Bali: 'Turkey's Policy in Northern Iraq, 1991-1995', *Middle Eastern Studies*, vol. 32, no. 4 (October 1996), p. 347.

73. This is the figure mentioned by representatives of the Turkish Foreign Policy Institute in Ankara, interviewed by the author on April 7, 1999.

74. Eralp: *loc. cit.* (note 2), p. 88.

75. *ibid.* p. 106.

76. Bal, Idris: 'The Turkish Model and the Turkic Republics', *Perceptions* (September-November 1998), pp. 105-129.

77. Gunter: *loc. cit.* (note 68), p. 35.

78. For a good account of the intra-Kurdish fighting, see the articles of Gunter, Michael: 'Kurdish Infighting: The PKK-KDP Conflict', in Robert Olson (ed.): *Kurdish Nationalist Movement in the 1990s. Its Impact on Turkey and the Middle East* (Lexington: University Press of Kentucky, 1996), pp. 50-64; idem: 'Civil War in Iraqi Kurdistan: The KDP-PUK Conflict', *The Middle East Journal*, vol. 50, no. 2 (1996), pp. 225-242.

79. Interview with the Foreign Policy Institute (see: endnote 73).

80. So senior officials of the Ministry of Foreign Affairs in Ankara during an interview conducted by the author on April 8,1999. About Hizbullah see the article in *Turkish Daily News*, 2 April 1999.

81. Calabrese, John: 'Turkey and Iran: Limits of a Stable Relationship', *British Journal of Middle Eastern Studies*, vol. 25, no. 1 (1998), p. 76.

82. Dalacoura: *op. cit.* (note 50), pp. 211-218.

83. Yavuz: *loc. cit.* 1997 (note 43), p. 22.

84. Dalacoura: *op. cit.* (note 50), p. 218.

85. Pahlavan: *loc. cit.* (note 35), p. 84.

86. Birand, Mehmet Ali: 'Is There a New Role for Turkey in the Middle East?', in Barkey (ed.): *op. cit.* (note 1), p. 172.

87. Cf. Karpat, Kemal H. (ed.): *Turkish Foreign Policy: Recent Developments* (Madison, Wisconsin: University of Wisconsin, 1996), p. 2.

88. Huntington comes to the conclusion that Turkey as 'a torn country, ..., has a single predominant culture which places it in one civilization but its leaders want to shift it to another civilization.' See Huntington, Samuel: *The Clash of Civilizations and the Remaking of World Order* (New York: Simon & Schuster, 1996), p. 138.

89. Konrad Adenauer Foundation: *Turkish Youth 98. The Silent Majority Highlighted* (Ankara: no publisher, 1998).

90. Bayard, Jean-Francois: 'L'Europe et la laicité contre la democratie en Turquie', *Critique Internationale*, no. 1/1998 (Autumn 1998), pp. 15-22.

91. For the term 'Greater Middle East' see the article of Gulshan Dietl in this book.

92. Jones: *op. cit.* (note 9), p. 9.

5 TURKISH-ISRAELI MILITARY AGREEMENTS

Implications for Regional Security in the Gulf

Wolfango Piccoli

Since the establishment of the Republic in 1923, Turkey's relationship with its Middle Eastern neighbours has been awkward, if not overtly hostile. The collapse of the Ottoman Empire left a legacy of territorial grievances, historic resentments, political tensions and mutual suspicions which neither the Turks nor the Arabs have so far overcome.[1]

Despite its geographical position, Turkey decided to isolate itself from developments in the Middle East and adopted a very cautious and hands-off approach to the region.[2] As Philip Robins points out, its main features have been strict adherence to the principles of non-interference and non-involvement in the domestic politics and interstate conflicts of all countries in the region, and a commitment to the development of bilateral political and economic relations with as many states in the region as possible.[3]

Turkey's reluctance to become involved in the developments of its immediate southern periphery clearly emerged during the Gulf War. Turkish President Turgut Özal's decision to actively support the US-led coalition against Saddam Hussein caught many Turks by surprise and sparked a lively debate within the country. The reaction against Özal's brushing aside Turkey's long-standing policy of non-interference in Middle East disputes was not confined to the Parliament and the press, it also involved the Turkish Armed Forces, the last guardians of the Kemalist orthodoxy. When Özal asked to the Chief of General Staff, General Necip Torumtay, to start the operations for the deployment of a 100,000 men-strong force along the Turkish-Iraqi border, the General, in open conflict with the President, decided to submit his resignation.[4]

Almost a decade after that episode, public opinion in Turkey is still divided on whether Özal was a dangerous adventurist or a visionary, but as Alan Makovsky put it, 'his conviction that Turkey should pursue an activist foreign policy appears to have carried the day'.[5]

Origins of the Israeli-Turkish Relationship

Ankara has been quick to exploit the opportunities offered by a transformed Middle East characterised by the sharp reduction of the military strength of Syria and Iraq and freed from the constraints imposed by the Cold War and by the Arab-Israeli freeze.

On 13 November 1993, exactly two months after the handshake by Yitzhak Rabin and Yasser Arafat at the White House, Hikmet Cetin became the first-ever Turkish Foreign Minister to visit Israel. Since then, Turkish-Israeli relations have developed in unprecedented ways and the extraordinary flurry of high-level visits between the two countries over the past six years has produced agreements covering virtually all sectors: economic, political, cultural, agricultural, intelligence and health.[6] However, the most significant component of the Turkish-Israeli relationship thus far has been the military one, which is tantamount to a proto-alliance between the two countries.

Contrary to what is commonly perceived in the Arab world, the impetus for the military alignment between the two countries did not come from Israel, but from the Turkish side and, more precisely, from the Armed Forces. While in the late 1950s it was Israel which looked to Turkey for a suitable partner in its 'peripheral pact' strategy[7], in the early 1990s the initiative was largely undertaken by Ankara's powerful generals. As Henri Barkey suggests, 'the old courtship game has been reversed'.[8]

Thanks to the prerogatives granted them by the Constitution and to the fact that Turkish politics has been characterized, in recent years, by a succession of weak civilian governments, the military has emerged as a major force in foreign policy-making.[9] A role vigorously asserted by former Deputy Chief of the General Staff, General Cevik Bir, when he stated that 'the Armed Forces are an integral part of Turkey's foreign policy'.[10] Ironically, 'the primary heir to Özal's foreign policy activism today'[11] is none other than the institution that was accused by the late President for status-quo bias and timidity: the Turkish Armed Forces.[12]

The analytical framework best suited to assess the impact of the Turkish-Israeli axis on the security of the Gulf region is Barry Buzan's concept of a 'security complex'.[13] Accordingly, the security complex in our analysis is composed of Iran, Iraq, Israel, Turkey and Syria, a group of states whose 'security concerns link [them] together sufficiently closely that their national securities cannot realistically be considered apart from one another'.[14] However, because the focus of this paper is on Gulf security, Syria will only briefly be taken into account, while the focus is placed on Iran and Iraq. The concept of a

security complex is not just a useful analytical device.[15] It also describes an empirical phenomenon with historical and geopolitical roots which influences the relations between the local states and external actors. Specifically, a relative autonomy notwithstanding, the regional security relations between Turkey, Israel, Iran and Iraq are far from immune from external influence. Rather the security complex mediates the interplay between these states and the only remaining superpower, the United States.

Against this framework, the main purpose of this paper is twofold. First, it is aimed at demonstrating that Ankara's decision to align with Israel was not based on any perceived threat to Turkey from the Middle East, but rather due to Turkey's predominant concerns regarding its relationship with the West, in particular the US. For Israel, on the other hand, the rationale was mainly based on regional security priorities. Secondly, the impact of the Turkish-Israeli military cooperation will be assessed both in terms of a 'internal transformation'[16] of the security complex and its interplay with the US.

Turkish Anxieties

Turkey's strategic posture was dramatically affected by the end of the Cold War, as for the first time in three centuries it no longer shared a border with a Russian empire. Ironically, despite the disappearance of the Soviet threat, the importance attached to NATO by the Turks became even more pronounced, as the end of the Cold war threatened to undermine Turkey's geostrategic role and its principal institutional and symbolic links with the West.

This sense of anxiety was further increased by the attitude of the European Union (EU) toward Ankara's efforts to gain full membership in the EU and in the Western European Union (WEU). Turkish exclusion from full participation in both arrangements was understood in Ankara as a demonstration of Europe's unwillingness to grant Turkey a legitimate security and political role on the old continent. These Turkish suspicions were strengthened by other developments. First and foremost the EU's decision, at the December 1997 summit in Luxembourg, to exclude Ankara from the list of candidates for membership in the Union while it extended invitations to several formerly communist Eastern European countries as well as Cyprus. Turkey's deep dissatisfaction and anger were well summarized by General Cevik Bir, who noted that 'the same West which once described Turkey as a "staunch ally" and a "bastion" is now following a policy of excluding Turkey from the map of Europe'. The

Turkish General continued by stressing that 'today Europe is, on the one hand, keeping Turkey outside the EU, while on the other, adopting an attitude that almost ignores and even complicates Turkey's legitimate security requirements'.[17]

Following the demise of the Soviet threat, Turkey, as a 'security consumer', capitalizing on its geostrategic importance, was worried that its main ally, the US, would no longer be willing to extend unconditional protection, political support and financial contributions to its security.[18] Iraq's invasion of Kuwait provided Ankara with a new trump card that allowed it to reassert its strategic value to Washington. By supporting the US-led coalition against Baghdad, Turkey managed to transform itself into an indispensable partner in a particularly sensitive region, i.e. the Middle East and, in particular, the Gulf area.

The strategy of close cooperation with the Bush administration was primarily designed, as suggested by Sayari, 'to reaffirm Ankara's commitment to US-Turkish bilateral relations and to highlight Turkey's importance to US strategic interests and concerns in the Middle East'.[19] Moreover, the Gulf War showed that Turkey could not count on NATO support against Middle Eastern threats[20], forcing Turkey to become more proactive in its pursuit of security policies in its Middle Eastern neighbourhood while, at the same time, developing a 'new strategic cooperation' with the US.[21]

However, because of Washington's inability to develop an effective policy for the Middle East in the post-Gulf war phase, the strategic cooperation between the US and Turkey never fully materialized. The wartime consensus between the two allies over the policies to be pursued towards Saddam Hussein-led Iraq collapsed with the liberation of Kuwait. In this regard, the repeated extensions by the Turkish Parliament of basing rights related to operation 'Provide Comfort' (renamed 'Northern Watch' in December 1996) appear to have resulted from rational calculations by Turkish statesmen of the benefits accruing to Turkey from keeping this force on Turkish soil, despite the evident disadvantages that made Turkey the main economic victim, after Iraq, of the Gulf War.[22]

Moreover, Ankara fears that the US efforts to topple Saddam Hussein may further destabilize the region and open the way for the creation of an independent Kurdish state in northern Iraq, an event that would represent a dangerous precedent for the Kurds in Turkey. This sense of distrust toward the Clinton administration's initiatives in Iraq has been manifestly expressed by Bülent Ecevit, then Turkish Prime Minister, who said that the US intends to violate Iraq's territorial

integrity by establishing a Kurdish state in the north, a Shi'ite state in the south and a weak Arab state in the central part of Iraq.[23]

The faltering US support was visible across a range of other issues. For instance, despite the inflated US public rhetoric that pointed to Turkey as a model of development for the newly independent states of the Trans-Caucasus and Central Asia, Washington's political and financial support never fully materialized. Rather, by pursing its 'Russian-first' policy the US sanctioned Moscow's 'Near Abroad' doctrine and Russian request to relax the CFE (Conventional Armed Forces in Europe) restrictions on the flanks. In both issues Ankara felt it was being ignored and sidelined about decisions that affected its immediate interests.

Further strains on the Turkish-US relationship were created by the linking by the US Congress of economic and military assistance to the improvement of Turkey's human rights record, a conditionality that was bluntly rejected by Turkey. Ankara has also found the US an increasingly unreliable source of arms. In 1996, pro-human rights groups, together with the pro-Greek and the pro-Armenian lobbies in Congress, were able to block the shipment of ten Super Cobra helicopters and freeze for more than a year the transfer of three frigates to Turkey.[24] As the Director of the Foreign Policy Institute in Ankara, Seyfi Tashan, stresses, 'the anti-Turkish lobbies in the US are capable, from time to time, to cause major setbacks in Turkish-US strategic cooperation'.[25]

Leaning Towards the Middle East

Against this background Turkey has become increasingly involved in the affairs of the Middle East, where its future political and economic role is ambiguous and not easily definable. Ankara has seen in Israel a potential ally that may help it overcome both challenges. By nurturing ties with Israel, the Turkish military-bureaucratic elites have seen the possibility of striking a balance between the need to find 'Middle Eastern solutions to its Middle Eastern problems'[26] and their desire to maintain Turkey's Western-oriented Middle Eastern policy.

What Israel has to offer, seen from Turkey's point of view, is neither limited to a security contribution (*vide infra*) nor to reliable and continuous links to Washington. It also promises significant and advantageous economic relations and cooperation in various fields, such as those of agriculture, science and industry.

Ankara has noted that trade with the Arab world, once the great hope of Turkish economic success, has declined sharply, with Turkey's exports to Arab countries falling from 47 percent of its total exports in

1982 to only twelve percent in 1992. The volume of bilateral trade between Turkey and Israel has, on the other hand, registered a significant increase over the last few years—from $200 million in 1993 to $700 million in 1998. Moreover, the two countries in March 1996 concluded an agreement for the creation of a free-trade area, the goal of which is to reach a bilateral trade volume of $2 billion by the end of the year 2000.

Israel has also opened the US market to Turkish products: Turks sell textiles and other commodities duty-free to Israel, which adds its labour to the product and sells it duty-free to the US. This boosts the Turkish economy, which hires Israeli companies to develop irrigation and agricultural projects in the GAP (the Southeastern Anatolian Project) region. More impressive is the fact that some 300,000 to 400,000 Israeli tourists visit Turkey each year, spending more than $400 million.[27]

In the opinion of a former senior Turkish diplomat, the only country in the Middle East that is 'like us' is Israel.[28] Implicit in this short but meaningful statement is that ideational factors play an important role in Turkish-Israeli cooperation. Both Turkey and Israel share a pro-West and pro-US foreign policy orientation, are committed to democratic and secular values and have large and relatively sophisticated market economies.

Precisely these common characteristics create an additional problem of regional legitimacy for both states, as Makovsky argues: 'Turkey and Israel share a common sense of otherness in a region dominated by Arabs and non-democratic regimes'.[29] The axis with Israel fits politically well with the Kemalist establishment's quest to become a 'European country within the Islamic world', it confirms Turkey's Western orientation and demonstrates its 'secular' credentials.

At a time when the domestic challenges to the homogenizing vision of the Kemalist orthodoxy are growing, the partnership with Israel allows Ankara to assume a greater role in the Middle East without having to fear any interference in its own internal affairs from this involvement that might challenge Turkey's long-pursued westernization project.[30]

In recent years, 'conspiracy theories' have taken an increasing hold in the Turkish bureaucratic-military establishment. Turkish decision-makers seems to be afflicted by the so-called 'Sevres phobia', i.e. to the conviction that the outside world is conspiring to weaken and divide the country. [See the chapter by Dietrich Jung in this volume, *The Editor*]. This phenomenon partly explains Turkey's growing sense of insecurity which pushed Ankara to look for alternatives to safeguard

its national sovereignty and protect its vital interests in the region. A good example of the prevailing 'encirclement syndrome' appears in the preface of the Turkish Ministry of Defence's *White Paper* for 1998: 'As a result of the extreme nationalist, expansionist and aggressive tendencies of her regional neighbours, Turkey lives together with the threats of radical fundamentalist movements, the proliferation of weapons of mass destruction, long range missiles, and terrorism in particular.'[31]

According to Andrew Mango, 'the West, specifically the US, has helped fostering this attitude in Turkey, not only by withholding help and sympathy but, paradoxically, by providing help and allowing a dependency culture to develop in Turkey'.[32]

This sense of dependency clearly emerges from Turkey's tendency to overestimate the willingness of the Jewish lobby to support the Turkish stance on Capitol Hill. Sixteen years ago, the late Prime Minister Özal argued that 'If the Arabs ask for it (i.e. severing ties with Israel) we will always place emphasis on the cost-benefit issue. We know the role of the Israeli lobby in the US'.[33] If historically it was a factor in some Turkish foreign policy decisions to not alienate the pro-Israeli lobby, recently the importance of gaining its support has grown, as a means of balancing the Greek and Armenian American lobbies.

The Evolving Turkish-Israeli Relationship

Before assessing the impact of the Turkish-Israeli military agreements on the security of the Gulf region, a brief look at their contents and later developments might be helpful.

On 23 February 1996, Israel and Turkey signed a military cooperation agreement providing for the exchange of military information, experience and personnel. It called, *inter alia*, for joint training exercises, exchange of military observers at each other's exercises, and reciprocal port access for naval vessels. Each country's planes exercise in the other's airspace for one week four times a year, which has occurred regularly since April 1996. Such visits are mutually beneficial. They enable the Israeli pilots to gain experience flying long-range missions (a skill that would be required for missions over Iran) and over mountainous areas, where visually identifying an enemy aircraft is more difficult than during over-sea flights.[34]

In exchange, Turkish pilots benefit from Israel's systems of training in advanced technology warfare in general, and in particular from access to the air combat manoeuvring range in the Negev. Moreover, such exercises also enable each air force to become familiar

with the procedure and tactics used by the other, which could facilitate wartime cooperation. In January 1998, the navies of Israel, Turkey and the US held a joint naval search and rescue (SAR) exercise in the Eastern Mediterranean. Despite their official 'humanitarian purpose', the SAR manoeuvres were, according to the experts, similar to naval operations aimed at localizing and intercepting enemy vessels.[35]

The military agreements are also believed to have strengthened the long-standing intelligence ties between Turkey and Israel. In April 1996, addressing the Washington Research Institute, General Cevik Bir revealed that Israel had requested Turkey's assistance in collecting information, Israel's first priority target being Syria followed by Iran. The positive reply from Ankara was taken for granted.[36]

Turkey will benefit from Israel's experience from the 'security zone' in Lebanon, which could be applied to the monitoring of its borders with Iraq and to preventing cross-border infiltration by the *Partiya Karkaren Kurdistan* (PKK) terrorists. In this regard, Israel seems to have abandoned its reluctance to become involved in the conflict with the PKK, a change of attitude that can be attributed to Benyamin Netanyahu's election for Israeli Prime Minister (May 1996) and the subsequent freezing of the peace process. Netanyahu has not hesitated to condemn Syria's support for the PKK and has vigorously supported the idea of a joint struggle against terrorism aimed at isolating countries sponsoring terrorist groups.[37]

Finally, a joint forum for strategic research and assessment, which meets every six months, has been institutionalized. In this forum high-ranking people gather to discuss topical strategic issues, which, according to Israeli analyst Efraim Inbar, 'is probably the heart of the relationship'.[38]

The military agreement related to the defence industries, signed on 26 August 1996, has established a legal framework for the transfer of military technology and know-how. This allows the Turkish Army, with the Pentagon's blessing, to obtain weapons and technology which Turkey would not be able to purchase from Europe and/or the US, because of its human rights record and its dispute with Greece.

Its reliability, technological standards and capacity to meet most defence needs has made the Israeli military industry an unique partner for the Turkish armed forces, which are currently engaged in a giant program of investment—a plan of rearmament and modernisation to the amount of $31 billion over five years, which will reach $150 billion in 25 years.[39] The transfer of Israeli technology also furthers the objective of developing the indigenous Turkish arms industry which today covers only 21 percent of the armed forces' needs.[40] The

agreement on military industry cooperation has produced an extraordinary range of actual and possible arms sales, overwhelmingly from Israel to Turkey, but characterized by a significant amount of work given to Turkish firms.[41]

Benefits for Israel

As Ed Blanche argues, 'Israel is now conducting what is probably the broadest and most far-reaching review of its strategic doctrine in history'.[42]

Following recent developments in the region, in particular the proliferation of weapons of mass destruction (WMD) and long-range ballistic missiles, and the shock of the Gulf War (when the country was paralysed for weeks because of the Scud threat)[43], the Israelis have reached the conclusion that regional threats cannot be dealt with unilaterally, especially not when emanating from the more distant countries of the region. This has encouraged Israeli policy-makers to seek tacit or overt alliances with nearby states as well as cooperation with foreign partners. In 1993, former Israeli Foreign Minister, Shimon Peres, suggested that the traditional approach to security based primarily on self-reliance is no longer relevant, but needs to be replaced with a regional approach.[44]

The combination of Turkey's military power, its strategic location bordering Iran, Iraq and Syria and its close ideological affinity with Israel, make Turkey an invaluable ally in the region. Despite the fact that both countries have made clear countless times that their cooperation is not directed against any third country in the region, Israeli officials have not hesitated to stress, whenever possible, the great value that they place on Israel's relationship with Turkey. In a press briefing during his visit to Ankara, on 8 December 1997, the Israeli Minister of Defence, Yitzhak Mordechai, summed up the overall Israeli aim of the relation with Turkey, stating that 'when we lock hands we will form a powerful fist. This relation will help us defend ourselves against any threat and help establish peace in the region.'[45] He added that 'I certainly described the relationship between us and the Turks as the development of a strategic relationship'.[46] Mordechai's remarks were echoed by Israeli Prime Minister, Benjamin Netanyahu, who stated that the new Israeli-Turkish military ties could serve as the 'axis' of a future regional structure.[47]

Facing the threat of long-range missiles that have made the home front more vulnerable, Israel is now focusing more and more on 'over-the-horizon capabilities,' which would allow its Air Force to hit a distant enemy, possibly with a pre-emptive strike. Even without directly

participating in a such a war, Turkey could play an important role. It could, *inter alia*, allow damaged Israeli aircraft to land at Turkish bases, permit Israeli combat SAR crews to rescue downed pilots while operating from its soil, and allow air-refuelling operations in its airspace. This would significantly extend Israel's striking range as well as 'allow the Israeli air force to be more aggressive and take greater risks'.[48] Such a scenario was openly referred to, during the February 1998 crisis with Iraq, by the former Turkish Ambassador to Washington, who mentioned that Turkey would consider allowing Israel to use Turkish airspace to retaliate following a possible Iraqi missile attack on Israel.[49]

Regional Implications

For Iran and Iraq, this Turkish-Israeli military cooperation has brought Israel right up to their borders.

Israel now has a 'window' on the territories of both 'rogue states' through which it can undertake monitoring and electronic listening operations or even launch air strikes against Iran's non-conventional weapons infrastructure. Syria, Iran and Iraq thus now have to take the new strategic reality into account when developing their military-strategic plans, and an 'element of uncertainty'[50] has been introduced into the military calculations of Tehran, Baghdad and Damascus.

Ankara's military activism in the region may have grown out of legitimate strategic concerns, albeit not in response to any serious external military threat to Turkey's security. Neither Syria nor Iran pose any significant military threat to Turkey. There are certainly various sources of tension, such as Teheran's relentless support for Islamic fundamentalist movements in the region, the buildup of its military arsenal, and the prospects of its acquiring nuclear technology. However, Ankara's immediate economic concerns and political interests do not allow it to pursue a policy of confrontation towards Iran. As Aykan suggests, 'Turkey considers the nature of the Iranian threat to be more political than military'.[51]

The Turkish-Israeli military cooperation rather creates a climate of permanent tension in the Middle East which highlights Turkey's strategic importance for the US in the region. Historically, Turkey's strategic significance to Western interests has always been enhanced during periods of tension in the area. Turkey has thus benefited significantly, both in terms of economic and military assistance, from the Iranian Revolution and the later Soviet move into Afghanistan, from the Iran-Iraq war and also from the Gulf War.[52] However, in this last case, the advantages were merely confined to military equipment.

It is possible to argue that the Turkish-Israeli military alignment represents an 'internal transformation' of the security complex[53] by changing the distribution of power among the regional actors. More specifically, it is possible to identify a growing political and strategic polarisation in the regional security system. The Turkish-Israeli axis has provided Iran and Syria with further stimuli to reinforce their long-standing collaboration. Damascus and Teheran have thus launched diplomatic manoeuvres aimed at creating a military-political alignment that would provide a credible countermeasure to the 'threat' posed by Turkey and Israel.

These two countries thus concluded a military cooperation agreement in February 1997 during the visit to Damascus of the Iranian Minister of Defence, Muhammed Foruzandeh.[54] According to this agreement, Iran will provide the required economic guarantees for Syria's rearmament and modernization of its dated, but still considerable, arsenal. Teheran assumed responsibility vis-à-vis Moscow for Damascus's debt in the event of defaults of payments. In the initial phase, the program will include the modernization of Syria's T-72 and T-55 tanks and MIG-29 fighters, but later it will also include the procurement of modern anti-aircraft systems.[55] Syrian President Hafez al-Assad's extremely rare foreign visit to Iran (31 July 1997) well illustrated the importance that Damascus attaches to its ties with Teheran.

In a further attempt to maintain strategic parity with Turkey, Iran has since 1995 been intensifying its contacts with Greece and Armenia, thereby forging what is perceived in Ankara as an antagonist alliance. During his visit recent visit to Iran, Turkish Foreign Minister, Ismail Cem, openly accused Athens of 'hiring Muslim soldiers for the new crusades against Turkey' and warned Iran not to become a 'pawn in Greece's manoeuvres'.[56]

Since 1997 Syria and Iran have, moreover, shown increasing willingness to improve their relations with Iraq, as demonstrated by the reopening, after more than fifteen years, of three border posts between Syria and Iraq and by the meeting between Iranian President Khatami and Iraqi Vice-President Taha Yassin Ramadam during the December 1997 symposium of the Organization of the Islamic Conference—the highest-level Iran-Iraq meeting since the war of 1980-88.

There has also been a certain rapprochement between Syria and Iraq, likewise motivated by the Turkish-Israeli ties. The Israeli Chief of Staff, Amnon Shahak, has thus argued that the improved commercial relations between Iraq and Syria was a clear sign of increasing Syrian concerns over Israel's links with Turkey.[57] Syrian Foreign Minister,

Faruq al-Shar', said that commercial steps 'may be followed by other steps related to the regional and international situation', obliquely referring to the Turkish-Israeli axis.[58]

A Security Complex under Transformation

It thus appears that the security complex composed by Iran, Iraq, Israel, Syria and Turkey is currently characterised by competitive rather than cooperative security. The regional actors, for different reasons, rely on force and explicit balancing mechanisms to maintain interstate stability. The options exercised by the five members of the security complex in their attempts to improve their security and respond to perceived threats include both internal mobilisation (involving domestic mobilization and arms production) and external alignment pointing towards the forging of strategic alliances.[59]

Moreover, one cannot rule out that the endogenous security dynamics of the security complex may in the long run become subordinated to the security orientation and interest of the world's remaining superpower. The development of such as 'overlay' (in the terminology of Barry Buzan)[60] may be accelerated by the military cooperation between Turkey and Israel, two of America's most prominent allies in the region. Fearing a reduced involvement of the US in the region,[61] Ankara and Tel Aviv may decide to conclude an unequal alliance with Washington, which would provide the basis for an American-oriented regional security system.[62]

The Turkish-Israeli alignment holds out the promise of allowing the US to reduce its direct military presence in the region—which would also help allaying suspicions in the Arab world—without any relaxation of its deterrence posture in the Middle East, which could now be based on Turkey (a Muslim country) and Israel, both of which are stable and democratically oriented states.

At the same time, the synergies inherent in the cooperation between Turkey and Israel increase the importance of both regional states to the great power. This is likely to happen because Turkey and Israel's roles within a US-oriented regional security system can be advocated on the basis of both their undeniable strategic importance and with reference to their ideological affinity to the US. Ankara believes that its alignment with Israel is likely to ease its way to the US administration and that it may 'conquer' Congress on its behalf. This is especially important at the present juncture when US-Turkish relations have become inflicted with a certain uneasiness, manifested in the increasing difficulties that the US executive branch faces in defending its political, economic and military support to Turkey before

Congress.[63] As Kemal Kirisci argues, 'Jewish lobby groups are seen by many Turkish officials and commentators as another means with which to counter anti-Turkish influence in the Congress. In these circles there is a belief that this would be a natural outcome of enhanced Israel-Turkish relations.'[64]

The cooperation with Israel serves well another key interest of Turkey's Kemalist elites, as it demonstrates Ankara's continued orientation toward the West and its commitment to secularism. This is especially important at a time when the country is facing a severe identity crisis that has eroded the pillars of Atatürk's doctrine while allowing greater public space to political Islam, nationalism and neo-Ottomanism.[65]

Nowadays, also the islamist Virtue Party (*Fazilet Partisi*), in marked contrast with its predecessor, the Welfare Party (*Refah Partisi*), seems to endorse the close cooperation with Israel. Cemil Cicek, one of the leading figures of the party, declared that '*Fazilet* does not evaluate anything on the bases of ideology and religion. National interest is the determining factor in Turkey's relationship with Israel. (...) Arab reactions were mainly emotional in evaluating these criticisms, national interests comes first. Arabs did not support Turkey vis-à-vis Greece. Their anger is due to misinformation and bias.'[66]

Undoubtedly, while Ankara views Israel as a reliable ally in the region in terms of security, the principal benefit of close relations with Israel is seen in terms of enhancing Turkey's influence and image in the West, most notably in the US.

Conclusion

In conclusion, even though the Israeli-Turkish relationship is not one in which either partner is committed by a mutual defence pact in case of war, it enables Israel to significantly augment its military superiority in the region. The growing military relationship with Turkey has both changed the regional balance of power and introduced a new element into the Israeli military posture, which fits the new defence doctrine perfectly that is currently being implemented.[67]

From a Turkish perspective, doubts about and differences with US policy in the Middle East have motivated Ankara to pursue closer ties with Israel which may bolster Turkey's position in Washington while, at the same time, ensuring that alternatives will be readily available, if needed. Maybe these were the considerations that Özal had in mind in 1986, ten years before Turkey concluded the alignment with Israel, when he explained the necessity of keeping contacts with Israel, which he regarded as 'a window on future events'. For Turkey to play a role

in solving the problems in the Middle East, he maintained, 'that window must remain open'.[68]

Notes

1. As Eric Rouleau put it, 'Seventy years after the collapse of the Ottoman Empire, a mutual suspicion—largely unfounded—persists. The former rulers have not forgotten what they saw as the Arab "betrayal" of rallying to the British during World War I to gain their independence. The former subject peoples have not forgotten the centuries of Ottoman rule and the harsh repression that followed the emergence of their national movements and some Arabs suspects Ankara of harbouring Ottoman ambitions'. See 'The Challenges to Turkey', *Foreign Affairs*, vol. 72, no. 5 (Nov-Dec. 1993), p. 115.

2. The main exception to this trend was in the latter 1950s when Turkey briefly pursued an activist policy in the Middle East which was reflected in its aspirations for a leadership role in regional Western-sponsored alliances such as the Baghdad Pact and the Central Treaty Organization. In this regard see Sever, Aysegul: 'The Compliant Ally? Turkey and the West in the Middle East 1954-58', *Middle Eastern Studies*, vol. 34, no. 2 (April 1998), pp. 73-90

3. Robins, Philip: *Turkey and the Middle East* (London: Pinter, 1991), pp. 65-67.

4. General Torumtay declared that 'I have decided to resign because it is impossible for me to serve the country according to the principles to which I am faithful'. See the long article 'Torumtay's Resignation Seen as a Blow to Özal', *Briefing*, no. 816 (10 December 1990), pp. 4-8.

5. Makovsky, Alan: 'The New Activism in Turkish Foreign Policy', *SAIS Review*, vol. 19, no. 1 (Winter-Spring 1999), p. 94.

6. The nineteen agreements concluded, since 1990, by Turkey and Israel clearly manifest the importance given to their bilateral relations. The total number of the agreements has been indicated by Oguz Celikkol, Deputy Director for Middle Eastern Affairs at the Turkish Ministry of Foreign Affairs, in his speech 'Turkey and the Middle East: Policy and Prospects' given at the Washington Institute for Near East Policy on 6 April 1998.

7. For a detailed analysis on the matter, see Nachmani, Amikam: *Israel, Turkey and Greece. Uneasy Relations in the East Mediterranean* (London: Frank Cass, 1987), especially pp. 43-82.

8. Henri Barkey: 'Turkey and the New Middle East', in idem (ed.): *Reluctant Neighbor. Turkey's Role in the Middle East* (Washington, DC: United States Institute of Peace Press, 1996), p. 38.

9. Between 1989 and 1996 there were eight different governments and twelve Ministers of Foreign Affairs. For some comments, see Cevik, Ilnur: 'Military Emerges a Major Force in Foreign Policy', *Turkish Daily News* (21 April 1998), p. 3; and Demir, Metehan: 'Military Fills Gaps in Turkish Foreign Policy', *ibid.* (11 May 1998), pp. 1-2. For a deeper analysis see Sakallioglu, Umit Cizre: 'The Anatomy of the Turkish Military's Political Autonomy', *Comparative Politics*, vol. 29, no. 2 (January 1997), pp. 151-166.

10. *Summary of World Broadcast* (henceforth: SWB), ME/2634 MED/8 (10 June 1996).

11. Makovsky, *op. cit.* (note 5), p. 106.

12. As Özal put it, 'some Generals are not keeping in step and are acting to preserve the status-quo. While we are taking brave steps forward, they are trying to put the brakes on'. Quoted in Hale, William: 'Turkey, the Middle East and the Gulf Crisis', *International Affairs*, vol. 68, no. 4 (1992), p. 686.

13. Buzan, Barry: *People, States and Fear: An Agenda for International Security Studies in the Post-Cold War Era* (Boulder, CO: Lynne Rienner, 1991), p. 190.

14. *Ibid.*

15. Buzan argues that 'it serves as a perceptual lens designed to bring the regional level of analysis more clearly into focus', *ibid.*, p. 191.

16. *Ibid.*, p. 217.

17. Cevik, Bir: 'Turkey's Role in the New World Order. New Challenges', *Strategic Forum*, no. 135 (1998), p. 4.

18. For a comprehensive and updated analysis of the US-Turkish relationship see Kirisci, Kemal: 'Turkey and the United States: Ambivalent Allies', in Barry Rubin & Thomas Keany (eds.): *Friends of America: US Allies in a Changing World'* (London: Frank Cass, forthcoming).

19. Sayari, Sabri: 'Turkey: The Changing European Security Environment and the Gulf Crisis', *Middle East Journal*, vol. 46, no. 1 (Winter 1992), p. 14.

20. NATO deployed an allied mobile force in Turkey more than a month after Ankara's official request, but most of the forty planes sent were obsolescent F-104s and Alpha-Jets. The move triggered complaints in Germany, where there was strong opposition to any military involvement in the Middle East. This in turn provoked some sharp attacks by Turkish President Özal on the Germans as unreliable allies, see *The Guardian* (25 January 1991).

21. See the interview with President Özal on the concept of 'strategic cooperation' in *Foreign Broadcast Information Service. Western Europe Series* (2 April 1991), p. 32.

22. As Aykan put it, 'the departure of the force would, however, deprive Turkey of an important bargaining chip in contacts made with both the North Iraqi Kurdish leaders and the Western states with a view to discouraging the establishment of an independent Kurdish state in northern Iraq', in Bali Aykan, Mahmut: 'Turkey's Policy in Northern Iraq, 1991-95', *Middle Eastern Studies*, vol. 32, no. 4 (October 1996), p. 356.

23. Cevik, Ilnur: 'Iraq Remains a Source of Concern for Turkey', *Turkish Probe* (10 January 1999), p. 10.

24. Demir, Metehan: 'At Last, Turkey Is Able to Take Delivery of Controversial Frigates from US', *Turkish Daily News* (8 November 1997), p. 1-2; and Akinci, Uguz: 'Turkey Hits US for Double Standard in Arms Sales', *ibid.* (10 December 1997), p. 3.

25. Tashan, Seyfi: 'A Review of Turkish Foreign Policy in the Beginning of 1998', *Foreign Policy* (Ankara), vol. 22, no. 1-2 (1998), p. 2.

26. Makovsky, Alan: 'Israeli-Turkish Relations: A Turkish Periphery Strategy?', in Barkey (ed.): *op. cit.* (note 8), p. 153.

27. Figures indicated by Ekrem Guvendire, President of the joint Turkish-Israeli Council for Economic Cooperation, reported by the *Turkish Daily News* (7 February 1998).

28. Quoted from Robins: *op. cit.* (note 3), p. 82.

29. Makovsky: *loc. cit.* (note 8), p. 169.

30. For an analysis of this point see Yavuz, Hakan: 'Turkish-Israeli Relations Through the Lens of the Turkish Identity Debate', *Journal of PalestineStudies*, vol. 27, no. 1 (Autumn 1997), pp. 22-37. The former Deputy Chief of the General Staff, General Cevik Bir, said Turkey concluded the pact because 'Turkey and Israel are the two democratic countries in the region, and we must show the region that democracies can work together'. See Pomfret, John: 'Nervous Turks tilt to Israel', *International Herald Tribune* (4 June 1996), p. 2.

31. *White Paper-Defense 1998* (Ankara: Ministry of National Defense, 1998). For a deeper analysis see the chapter by Dietrich Jung in this book.

32. Mango, Andrew: 'Testing Time in Turkey', *Washington Quarterly*, vol. 20, no. 1 (Winter 1997), p. 5. Among the several statements by US officials supporting the perception of Turkey as a front-line state, Richard Holbrooke stated that 'Turkey after the Cold War is equivalent to Germany during the Cold War—a pivotal state where diverse strategic interests intersect', quoted in Barkey: *op. cit.* (note 8), p. vii.

33. Quoted in Yavuz, Hakan: 'Turkey's Relations With Israel', *Foreign Policy* (Ankara), vol. 5, no. 3-4 (1991), p. 49.

34. According to the *Jerusalem Post*, in 1997, 'the Israeli fighter jets have carried out 120 sorties in Turkey, many of them practise for long-range missions, since Israeli air space is so limited'. See O'Sullivan, Arieh: 'IAF Jets Fly Long-range Training Sorties in Turkey', *Jerusalem Post* (12 December 1997), p. 3.

35. 'Naval Exercise Will Link Israel, Turkey and USA', *Jane's Defence Weekly*, vol. 28, no. 50 (17 December 1997), p. 6.

36. SWB ME/2581 MED/9 (9 April 1996).

37. In May 1997, the Israeli Premier, in a television interview with a Turkish channel, rejected the idea of a Kurdish state and openly condemned the PKK: 'Turkey has suffered the terrorist attacks from the PKK and we see no difference between the terrorism of the PKK and that which Israel suffers', as reported by Gresh, Alain: 'Turkish-Israeli-Syrian Relations and Their Impact on the Middle East', *Middle East Journal*, vol. 52, no. 2 (Spring 1998), p. 194.

38. Inbar, Efraim: 'The Turkish-Israeli Strategic Partnership', Lecture given at the Woodrow Wilson Center in Washington DC, 16 September 1998.

39. *Turkish Daily News* (7 February 1998).

40. Regarding Ankara's plan to expand its defence industry see 'A Turkish Defence Industry' in *NATO's 16 Nations & Partners for Peace, Special Issue: 'Defence and Economics in Turkey: Pillar of Stability'* (Bonn: Monch, 1998).

41. The largest contract that Israel has won so far is a $630 million agreement to upgrade 54 Turkish F-4 fighters, then an Israeli-Singaporean consortium won a $75 million contract to do the same to 48 F-5. Turkey agreed to buy 100 Popeye-I air-to-ground missiles, larger fuel tanks for its F-16s and to co-produce 200 Popeye-II for the same aircraft. Israel is bidding to have its Merkava chosen as Turkey's new battle tank and has proposed to upgrade Turkey's aging M-60 tanks, to sell unmanned aerial vehicles (UAVs) and early warning aircraft (AEWC). Israel is also participating in a joint venture with the Russian Kamov helicopter company and in a similar arrangement with the competing Italian firm Agusta, both bidding to sell combat helicopters to Turkey. In 1998, Israel and Turkey reportedly agreed to cooperate on the production of a new medium range anti-ballistic missile called 'Delilah' similar to the 'Arrow' missile that Israel has developed with considerable US funding.

42. Blanche, Ed: 'Israel Addresses the Threats of the New Millennium', *Jane's Intelligence Review*, vol. 11, no. 2 (February 1999), p. 24. See also Cohen, Eliot A., Eisenstadt, Michael J. & Bacevich, Andrew J.: 'Israel's Revolution in Security Affairs', *Survival*, vol. 40, no. 1 (Spring 1998), pp. 48-67.

43. As Shimon Naveh points out, 'By employing surface-to-surface ballistic missiles against civilian targets located in depth, a hostile state which does not share a mutual border with Israel managed to inflict strategic terror upon the Jewish state'. See 'The Cult of the Offensive: Preemption and Future Challenges for Israeli Operational Thought', in Efraim Karsh (ed.): *Between War and Peace. Dilemmas of Israeli Security* (London: Frank Cass, 1996), p. 170.

44. Peres, Shimon: *The New Middle East* (New York: Henry Holt, 1993), pp. 61-64.

45. 'Turkey Pledges to Deepen Ties', *Ha-aretz* (9 December 1997).

46. O'Sullivan, Arieh: 'News', *Jerusalem Post* (10 December 1997), p. 7.

47. Esmer, Alparslan: 'PM Yilmaz's Trip to Israel Clouds other Visits', *Turkish Probe* (13 September 1998), p. 12. An Israeli source is 'Bashing, Promising and Whitewashing', *Ha-aretz* (3 September 1998).

48. Eisenstadt, Michael: 'Turkish-Israeli Military Cooperation: An Assessment', *PolicyWatch*, no. 262 (24 July 1997).

49. Akinci, Ugur: 'Kandemir: Turkey May Allow Israel to Retaliate against Iraq', *Turkish Daily News* (21 February 1998), pp. 1-2.

50. Eisenstadt: *op. cit.* (note 48).

51. Bali Aykan, Mahmut: 'Turkish Perspectives on Turkish-US Relations Concerning Persian Gulf Security in the Post-Cold War Era, 1989-95', *Middle East Journal*, vol. 50, no. 3 (Summer 1996), p. 353.

52. The 1980 Defence and Economic Cooperation agreement between the US and Turkey was primarily in response to the Iranian Revolution and the Soviet invasion of Afghanistan. Regarding the Iran-Iraq war, Barkey argues that 'Turkey by dramatically increasing its exports both to Iran and Iraq immeasurably improved the outlook of its crisis-ridden economy. On the other hand, Turkey's strategic importance in the region was clearly enhanced by the war in general and specifically by a once possible Iranian victory'. See Barkey, Henri: 'The Silent Victor: Turkey's Role in the Gulf War', in Efraim Karsh (ed.): *The Iran-Iraq War. Impact and Implications* (London: Macmillan, 1987), pp. 133-153. In return for Ankara's military assistance during the Gulf war, the American aid, in conjunction with a German package, included: 600 M-60 tanks, 400 Leopard tanks, 700 armoured personnel carriers, 40 Phantom fighters, as well as a complement of Cobra helicopters and Roland surface-to-air missiles.

53. Buzan: *op. cit.* (note 13), p. 217.

54. 'Syrian-Iranian Defence Pact', *Gulf Report*, no. 70 (April 1997); and 'Syria and Iran in War Talks', *Intelligence Digest* (February 1997).

55. 'Russian Industry Reaps Benefits of Iran-Syria Past', *Defense News*, vol. 12, no. 13 (31 March-6 April 1997).

56. 'Armenia, Greece and Iran: Towards an Evil Merger?', *Turkish Probe* (20 September 1998), p. 5.

57. Lt. General Amnon Shahak: 'Address to the Foreign Affairs and Defense Committee, the Knesset' (24 June 1997).

58. SWB MED/2952 MED/8 (23 June 1997).

59. Such competitive security arrangements are closely associated with the notorious security dilemma, see Jervis, Robert: 'Cooperation Under the Security Dilemma', *World Politics*, vol. 30, no. 2 (January 1978), pp. 167-214.

60. Buzan: *op. cit.* (note 13), pp. 219-220.

61. Efraim Inbar, the director of the Begin-Sadat Center for Strategic Studies, openly stated that 'Both Israel and Turkey fear abandonment by the West... Israel seems to be in a better position than Turkey in Washington, but both are interested in strengthening their ties with the US, which for various reasons is not sensitive enough to their security needs'. See 'A New Balance of Power', *Jerusalem Post* (15 December 1997), p. 8.

62. The State Department declared in May 1997, 'It has been a strategic objective of the US that Turkey and Israel ought to enhance their military co-operation and their political relations', quoted in Waxman, Dov: 'Turkey and Israel: A New Balance of Power in the Middle East', *Washington Quarterly*, vol. 22, no. 1 (Winter 1999), p. 31.

63. Sukru Elekdag, a former Turkish diplomat and a well-respected commentator, in an article published in *Milliyet* (14 December 1994) wrote: 'The Israeli lobby in the US is far superior to all other ethnic lobbies put to-

gether. Whenever this lobby has worked for us, Turkey's interests have been perfectly protected against the fools in the US. The development of relations between Turkey and Israel and the formalization of their de-facto alliance will place this lobby permanently on our side'.

64. Kirisci: *op. cit.* (note 18).

65. On the identity crisis in Turkey and its impact on Ankara's foreign policy orientation see Sakallioglu, Umit Cizre: 'Rethinking the Connections Between Turkey's "Western" Identity Versus Islam', *Critique*, no. 12 (Spring 1998), pp. 3-18; and Yavuz, Hakan: 'Turkish Identity and Foreign Policy in Flux: The Rise of Neo-Ottomanism', *ibid.*, pp. 19-41.

66. Interview with Cemil Cicek in Ankara on 13 April 1998.

67. Cited in Gresh: *op. cit.* (note 37), p. 189.

68. Cited in Bali Aykan, Mahmut: 'The Palestinian Question in Turkish Foreign Policy from the 1950s to the 1990s', *International Journal of Middle Eastern Studies*, vol. 25 (1993), p. 103.

6 IRAN AND ISRAEL

Prospects for Detente

Gawdat Bahgat

For a long time the Islamic Republic of Iran has occupied a central stage in the international system. With a population approaching seventy million people, Iran is the most populous country in the Middle East and one of the largest. More important, it holds the world's fifth largest proven oil reserves and its second largest natural gas proven reserves. In addition, the country is considered an important gate to the energy-rich Central Asia region. Given all these attributes, Tehran is a central player in any security system in both the Persian Gulf and the Middle East. Since the Islamic Revolution in 1979, Iran has had extremely hostile relations with another important regional power: Israel. The Jewish state was created in 1948 and has become an established part of the Middle East landscape and even evolved into a regional superpower.[1] This can be explained by its technological advances in both military and economic affairs. Israel is the only nuclear power in the region and its gross national economy per capita is approaching those of western Europe.[2]

For more than two decades, each of these two important Middle Eastern powers has seen the other as its main enemy. Iran believes that the struggle with Israel is one of Islam against a western surrogate state which will not end until Palestine is liberated. Tel Aviv, on the other side, perceives the Islamic Republic as the main threat to its existence and to regional stability. These antagonistic perceptions have taken new dimensions since the early 1990s in response to regional and international developments. During the Cold War Israel was seen as a bulwark against the expansion of communism and the Soviet Union. With the collapse of the latter, the strategic value of Israel came into question. Put differently, with the passing of the bilateral global system some analysts argued that the special relations between Washington and Tel Aviv would disappear.[3] According to this line of thinking, the diminished strategic value of Israel was demonstrated in the Gulf War where its role was intentionally restrained. Furthermore, the argument goes, Israeli leaders were searching for a new menace to revive their country's strategic asset. This 'new enemy' was found in 'Islamic

fundamentalism' represented by the Islamic regime in Tehran.

The close military alliance between Tel Aviv and Ankara since the mid 1990s should be seen as a demonstration of this strategy. The two secular democracies can contain the military and ideological threats from the Islamist Iran or the Arab nationalism of Iraq and Syria. Moreover, the progress in the peace process between Israel and the Palestinians (particularly before Benjamin Netanyahu was elected in 1996) opened the door for economic and diplomatic relations between Israel and some of the Arab Gulf states.[4] This rapprochement came to almost a complete halt since the Likud government came to power but it can be resumed again when the peace process is back on its feet under Barak's government. This Israeli penetration of Iran's backyard is perceived in Tehran as a threat to its security and strategic interests. Similarly, Iran is furious about Israel's growing cooperation with several of its Central Asian neighbours, particularly Azerbaijan and Turkmenistan. On the other side, Tehran has close relations with *Hezbollah* (Party of God) in south Lebanon (Israel's backyard) and for almost two decades has been engaged in a proxy war with the Jewish state.

Against this background it is very hard to see any sign of reducing tension or detente between the Islamic Republic and the Jewish state. The contention of this study, however, is that there will not be lasting and stable peace in the Middle East without reaching some level of understanding between the two regional powers. From the outset, two fundamental propositions need to be emphasized. First, instability in the Persian Gulf and the Arab-Israeli conflict are interconnected. Tension in one region spills over into the other. The two sub-systems cannot be separated. Second, a detente between Tehran and Tel Aviv, if it happens, should not be directed against a third party. There is no need for more axes. Long-term stability in the Middle East should be built on inclusion not exclusion. A lasting peace would involve the Arab states, Turkey, Israel, and Iran.

In order to achieve detente between the last two players, both Tel Aviv and Tehran have to reach an understanding on two issues: the Arab-Israeli peace process and the proliferation of weapons of mass destruction (WMD). In the following, an assessment of the two sides' position on each of these controversial issues is provided but first a brief review of the relations between Iran and Israel is in order.

The Legacy of the Past
The relations between Iranians and Jews have their roots thousands of years back. Interestingly, their interaction with each other has been

mostly positive. An important landmark in this long history occurred in 538 B.C. when Cyrus the Great liberated the Hebrews from the Babylonians. This legacy of ancient past contributed, among other factors, to shaping the relations between Iran and Israel since the establishment of the latter in 1948. For three decades the two sides shared economic and strategic interests and worked side by side to achieve their respective goals.

The overthrow of the Pahlavi regime in 1979, however, turned this relation on its head and since then the two countries have seen each other as adversaries. An analysis of the evolution of Iranian-Israeli relations since 1948 should take into considerations several variables. These include the perception of the leadership, economic and strategic considerations, the rise and fall of Arab radicalism, the Jewish minority (*Aliyah*) in Iran and Iraq, the Palestinian question, and relations with the United States. It is important to point out from the outset that these factors are interrelated, some of them have changed and others are constant.

First, in 1961 Muhammad Reza Shah stated, 'Iran's relations with Israel are like true love that exists between two people outside of wedlock.'[5] This warm perception can be seen as the extreme opposite to that of the Islamic regime. Ayatollah Khomeini accused the Shah of allowing Israel an open hand in Iran and proclaimed the struggle against Israel and Zionism to be one of the major principles of the revolution.

Second, in line with the Pahlavi regime's perception of Israel, economic and military cooperation between the two countries had flourished for most of the Shah's reign. This cooperation was based on profound Iranian admiration of Israeli technological advances particularly in agriculture and water resources as well as military technology. On the other side, Israel badly needed oil supplies from Iran. Thus, many Iranian officers received part of their military training in Israel and the two countries worked together on several economic schemes. Particularly important was the Shah's willingness to meet Israel's oil needs. Unlike Arab oil producing countries, Iran refused to use petroleum as a political weapon and considered it a purely economic transaction. Accordingly, when the Soviet Union terminated oil shipments to Israel in 1957 Iran became a major supplier.[6] Furthermore, in the aftermath of the 1973 Arab-Israeli War the Shah refused to participate in the embargo and continued selling oil at normal price to Israel.

Third, this military and economic cooperation was reinforced by shared strategic considerations. Shortly after Israel was created Prime

Minister Ben-Gurion articulated a strategy known as 'Peripheral Alliance' in order to break the wall of isolation that surrounded it. The proposed alliance included Sunni Muslim but non-Arab Turkey, Shi'a Iran, primarily Christian Ethiopia as well as the Christians of Lebanon, the Kurds in Iraq, and the non-Muslim population of Sudan.[7] Additionally, most of these parties were deeply concerned about the Soviet Union's aspirations to penetrate the region.[8] In his memoirs, the Shah wrote that 'I have lived as neighbour to the masters of the Kremlin my whole adult life. In forty years I had never seen any wavering of Russia's political objective: a relentless striving toward world domination'.[9]

Thus, a principal factor underlying the Iranian policy was the perceived political and strategic utility of Israel in the context of Iran's primary objective of forestalling the advance of Soviet power and influence and the spread of communism in the Middle East.[10] The good relations both Israel and Iran had with the other superpower, the United States, brought them even closer. Indeed, some Iranian leaders believed that warm relations with the Jewish state would protect and promote their interests in Washington.[11]

Fourth, this Iranian/Israeli perception of relations with the two superpowers during the Cold War cannot be separated from the stand they adopted toward the regional or Arab Cold War. This undeclared confrontation between the 'radical' and 'conservative' camps within the Arab World (mostly during the 1950s and 1960s) ironically contributed to the consolidation of cooperation between Tehran and Tel Aviv. Nationalist and leftist leaders in Cairo and Baghdad were seen as a threat to both Israel and the Pahlavi regime with their close association with the West in general and the United States in particular. Playing the 'Kurdish card' can be seen as a response to this threat. For several years both Iran and Israel provided military aid and training to the Iraqi Kurds. The purpose was to keep the government in Baghdad busy fighting the Kurds in the north.

It is important to point out that the configuration of Iran-Arab relations changed during the 1970s. The death of President Nasser and his replacement by Sadat on one side and Iraq's improved relations with France convinced the Shah that there was a sense of moderation in the Arab World and consequently he signed an agreement with Saddam Hussein and stopped supporting the Iraqi Kurds. It is important to emphasize that this detente in Iran-Arab relations was not at the expense of Israel. The Shah managed to maintain the solid rapport with Israel. This understanding was further shaped by two developments: the fate of the Jewish minority in Iraq and Iran (*Aliyah*) and developments

in the Arab-Israeli conflict.

Fifth, shortly after the creation of Israel in 1948 Iran was used as a transit point to relocate the Iraqi Jews into Israel.[12] In contrast, not many Iranian Jews felt the need to leave their country. This can be explained by the relative freedom they enjoyed in comparison with Jewish communities in other Arab countries. It is worth mentioning that after the revolution Khomeini guaranteed that Iranian Jews could live and worship in Iran in a much better manner than under the Shah.[13] This good manner was not affected by the evolution of Tehran's position toward the Arab-Israeli conflict.

Sixth, the Iranian stand on the dispute between Arab states and Israel was shaped by two contradictory forces: the public's sentiment against the Jewish state on one side and the elite's eagerness to forge an alliance with the same state. Accordingly, Iran voted against Israel's entry into the United Nations but did not participate in any military confrontation against it. Another illustration of this hesitancy is the fact that unlike Turkey (the other non-Arab Muslim country in the Middle East), which granted Israel a *de jure* recognition, Iran gave it a *de facto* one. Furthermore, the Pahlavi regime's attitude on the question of Jerusalem had been quite consistent—calling for an Islamic control over the city and rejecting the Israeli claims. Additionally, the Shah supported the UN resolution 242 which called for an Israeli withdrawal from Arab land occupied during the 1967 war. This war transformed Israel, in Iran's eyes, from a victim of Arab aggression to an occupier force and narrowed the gap between how the regime and the public in Tehran viewed Israel.

The dramatic change, however, came with the revolution in 1979. The new rulers in Tehran perceived Israel in a completely different way than their predecessors. Anti-Zionism is a central component of the ideological orientation of the Islamic Republic. Not surprisingly, Yasser Arafat was the first foreign dignitary to visit Iran after the revolution and a Palestinian embassy replaced the Israeli diplomatic mission in Tehran.

It is worth mentioning that the Islamic Regime's fiery rhetoric against Israel did not stop collaboration between the two states during the Iran-Iraq war (1980-88). This war was seen as a blessing to Israel since it weakened two of its enemies. Tel Aviv's role in selling arms to Iran (the so-called Iran-Contra Affairs), can be explained by financial incentives as well as its desire to keep channels open to moderates in the Khomeini regime. It is hard to make any assessment of the impact of this affairs on the long-term Iranian-Israeli relations.

This analysis of the forces which shaped the relations between the

two Middle Eastern powers suggests that beyond the rhetoric on the
surface there are demographic, historical, economic, and strategic
dynamics pointing to different direction. As in the past, these dynamics
can bring the two states together or bring them apart. At the turn of the
century tremendous efforts need to be invested to reduce tension. More
urgently, Iran and Israel need to overcome two substantial obstacles:
their stand on the Arab-Israeli conflict and the proliferation of weapons
of mass destruction (WMD).

The Arab-Israeli Conflict

One of the most drastic changes in Iran's foreign policy after the
revolution has been its relations (or lack of) with Israel.

From the very beginning the leaders of the Islamic regime have
considered the mere presence of the Jewish state as illegitimate. Not
surprisingly, since 1979 Tehran has been one of few Middle Eastern
states to oppose the evolving peace process between Israel and its Arab
neighbours. The nature and magnitude of this opposition, it is argued,
has been exaggerated. A close examination of the Iranian stand
suggests that the Arab-Israeli conflict is intertwined with several central
issues for the Islamic regime.

First, rejecting the Israeli control over Muslim holy sites is
fundamental for the legitimacy of the regime in Tehran. Second,
resisting the Israeli occupation of southern Lebanon (where the
majority are Shi'as) is related to the historical relations between these
Lebanese Shi'as and Iran. Third, so far Tehran has not been included
in the peace process. Put differently, peace between the Arabs and the
Israelis might isolate Iran and threaten its economic and strategic
interests. Finally, given the fact that the peace process is sponsored by
the United States which is perceived as a hostile power by Iran, its
success would further strengthen Washington's penetration of the
Middle East and weaken Tehran's efforts to get foreign powers (i.e. the
United States) out of the region.

Taking all these dynamics into consideration, one can argue that
the Iranian opposition to the peace process is based more on ideology
and less on pragmatic (i.e. strategic and economic) considerations.
More accurately, Tehran's worry of being isolated and its concern over
the increase of American 'hegemony' in the region can be addressed.
A genuine peace should include all parties in the Middle East.
Furthermore, two decades after the revolution, ideology is taking a
back seat in determining Tehran's priorities and shaping its policies. In
line with this perception Iranian President Muhammad Khatami told
Palestinian leader Yasser Arafat 'Whatever the Palestinians can agree

to with Israel we can live with.'[14] Finally, it is important to remember that even if Iran tries to disrupt the peace process (which it strongly denies), its options are very limited, consisting mainly in support to Islamist organizations in the West Bank and Gaza and close association with *Hizbollah* (Party of God) in southern Lebanon.

Several policy-makers in both Tel Aviv and Washington have frequently accused Tehran of supporting terrorist attacks against Israel. The two organizations often alleged to carry out these attacks are the Islamic Resistance Movement (*Hamas*) and Islamic *Jihad*. Any attempt to assess the Iranian involvement should consider the following points.

First, Islamic radicalism is not the result of a conspiracy directed by a foreign power. Rather, the mere existence and any popularity these two organizations (Hamas and Jihad) have can be attributed to Palestinian grievances against the Israeli occupation and the corruption of the Palestinian Authority as well as its failure to gain any meaningful concession from the Israeli government. Second, initially Hamas was fostered by Israel as a counter to the Palestine Liberation Organization (PLO).[15] Additionally, it receives financial and political support from different sources including Saudi Arabia and other Gulf states as well as Muslims residing in Europe and the United States. Finally, it is important to remember that both *Hamas* and *Jihad* are Sunni. They lack the historical and religious ties of the Lebanese Hizbollah to Iran.

Hizbollah was formed in 1982 with Iranian help during Israel's invasion of Lebanon and began as a radical offshot of Amal, a Shi'a Muslim movement.[16] The creation of Hizbollah and the consolidation of Iranian political and military presence in Lebanon were main achievements of Ali Akbar Mohtashemi, then Iranian ambassador to Syria. Since then, the party has gained legitimacy as a resistance movement against the Israeli occupation of a 'security zone' set up in 1985. Thus, when Lebanese militia signed the Taif Agreement in 1989 and agreed to lay down their arms, Hizbollah was excepted in order to keep the fight against the Israeli occupation. Meanwhile, unlike the case with *Hamas* and *Jihad*, the Iranians do acknowledge providing assistance to *Hizbollah*, albeit merely a humanitarian one.[17]

Two important conclusions can be drawn from the on-going confrontation in the south Lebanon between Hizbollah and Israel. First, Hizbollah's military campaign to expel the Israelis out of the 'security zone' is not of the nature of an ideological crusade to destroy the Jewish state. The party does not have the stomach or the means to launch such a campaign. Instead, it has a specific and limited goal, which is to liberate south Lebanon from a foreign occupation. The fact

that Hizbollah's attacks have been mostly carried out within the 'security zone' and not inside Israel underscores this conclusion. Second, since the establishment of this zone, more than 900 Israelis have been killed in south Lebanon. This rising number of casualties has convincing a large segment of the Israeli public that 'a war against a guerrilla army in a foreign country cannot be won.'[18] No wonder, the idea of a unilateral Israeli withdrawal from south Lebanon has been seriously considered at least since 1998. [This actually happened in May 2000, *the Editor*].

This withdrawal from the 'security zone' can put an end to this proxy war between Iran and Israel in south Lebanon. Other steps which might lead to similar conclusions include a peace agreement between Tel Aviv and Damascus, the evolution of the Palestinian autonomy into statehood, and a breakthrough in the Arab-Israeli peace process. Will any of these scenarios ever materialize? There is a great deal of uncertainty in any attempt to answer this question. The same can be said regarding the proliferation of non-conventional weapons.

Weapons of Mass Destruction

In addition to the proxy war between Iran and Israel in south Lebanon, the two countries perceive each other as a military threat, particularly with respect to non-conventional weapons.

Unlike Iran, Israel is not a signatory of the Non-Proliferation Treaty (NPT) and is universally believed to have nuclear weapons. Furthermore, Iran is concerned about Israel's strategic reach which includes long-range aircraft and ballistic missiles.[19] In response, the Iranian leaders believe that they have the right to defend themselves.[20] On the other side, Israeli leaders are convinced that given the country's natural and human resources and its declared hostility toward the Jewish state, Iran has the potential to bring about major strategic changes in the Middle East. Accordingly, Tel Aviv has taken the lead since the early 1990s in sounding the alarm over Tehran's growing military capability.

In the closing years of the twentieth century these concerns and threats have intensified. Two developments can explain this intensity. First, the acquisition and development of different weapon systems. In July 1998, Iran flight-tested its Shehab-3 medium-range ballistic missile which is designed to have a maximum range of 1,300 kilometres.[21] This range means that Shehab-3 is capable of reaching targets in Israel. In response, the Israeli cabinet approved the formation of a National Security Council which will focus on the threat from non-conventional weapons and ballistic missiles.[22] In addition, the production of the

joint US-Israeli *Homa* (formerly Arrow) for ballistic missile defense was accelerated.[23] Equally important, Israel acquired two weapon systems which have substantially increased its striking power. These are F-15I long-range strike aircraft which are considered among the most advanced fighters in the world and, according to some observers, have the capability to launch a pre-emptive attack on Iran's nuclear facilities.[24] The recently delivered three German-built Dolphin Class diesel-electric submarines could give Israel a second-strike nuclear option, using cruise missiles fired from the sea.[25]

The second important reason for the deepening sense of threat between Iran and Israel is the latter's growing military cooperation with another major Middle Eastern state—Turkey. It was the first Islamic country to formally recognize Israel, and since then the two states have enjoyed good relations. Still, the signing of several cooperation agreements since 1996 has given Israel significant strategic advantages. According to these agreements Israeli warplanes are allowed to use Turkish training ranges which is important for a small country that relies heavily on its air power but has limited training space. More important, Israel-Turkey cooperation brought the former's jets closer to the Iranian borders.[26] These joint air and naval exercises have significant impact on the military balance of power in the Middle East in general and between Iran and Israel in particular.

Three characteristics of Tehran's efforts to acquire and develop WMD can be identified. First, there is a great deal of ambiguity and uncertainty regarding these efforts. While the Iranian government has made no secret of its plans to build up its defense industrial capability, it has always denied any interest in non-conventional weapons. At the same time, American and Israeli sources claim the opposite. A recent report by the CIA states that 'Iran remains one of the most active countries in the world seeking to acquire WMD technology.'[27]

In order to confirm its denial and to avoid giving a pretext for preventive strike on its nuclear facilities Tehran has pursued a conscious policy of opening its facilities for inspection by delegations from the International Atomic Energy Agency (IAEA).[28] Second, like other states, Iran has sought foreign cooperation to develop its non-conventional capabilities. Ironically, Iran's nuclear program began with the assistance of the United States. Washington signed a civil nuclear program agreement with Iran in 1957 as part of their Atoms for Peace Program. During the 1960s, America sold hot cells and five megawatt research reactor to Iran.[29] It is worth mentioning that during this time Iran signed the NPT and lent its support to a call to make the Middle East a zone free of WMD (weapons of mass destruction).[30]

All nuclear cooperation between Washington and Tehran, however, came to a halt when the Shah was deposed in 1979. Indeed, this cooperation was replaced with constant efforts by the United States to undermine the Islamic Republic's efforts to acquire non-conventional technology. Thus, under American pressure, Germany, France, Brazil, and India (among others) have suspended any nuclear cooperation with Iran.[31]

Other countries, however, (mainly Russia and China), have resisted this mounting American pressure. Chinese leaders view Washington's policy of containing Tehran as a unilateral initiative designed to ensure its predominance in the Gulf which can endanger Beijing's long-term geo-strategic interests (i.e. growing dependence on oil supplies from the Gulf region). Consequently, China has cooperated with Iran in many areas including developing the latter's defense capabilities. Chinese officials have admitted contributing to Iran's nuclear energy program, but have denied supplying fissionable material or other weapons-related technologies.[32] Given the strong American opposition, this nuclear cooperation between China and Iran has been stalled since 1997.[33]

Washington, however, has not been as successful in terminating Moscow's nuclear cooperation with Tehran. A milestone in this cooperation was the agreement signed in March 1990 by the Iranian Finance Minister and the Soviet Minister for Railways for the completion of the Bushehr plant.[34] More recently (November 1998) the Russian Foreign Ministry said the first bloc of the light-water reactor in Bushehr will be completed in May 2003 and agreed to consider an Iranian proposal that Moscow help build three more nuclear reactors.[35] This close cooperation between Moscow and Tehran should not be taken for granted.[36]

Any assessment of future joint Russian-Iranian nuclear ventures should take into consideration at least three constraints: Although the Russian threat to Iran had significantly diminished with the dissolution of the Soviet Union the Iranians are not ruling out that it can re-emerge. On the other side, considering the fact that the two countries are close neighbours, it is doubtful that a nuclear Iran would be in line with Russia's strategic and security interests.[37] Put differently, it is uncertain that Moscow would like to see a new nuclear power next to its borders. In addition to the American pressure to terminate nuclear cooperation between Russia and Iran, the Israelis have also sought to achieve the same goal by involving Russia's under-funded scientists in joint research projects so they will not be tempted to make money by working for Iran.[38]

Thus, it can be argued that there are limits on how far the Russian-Iranian cooperation can go. Still, since Iran has been subject to heavy American scrutiny for long time, it has gained a significant experience with regard to buying the materials it needs secretly from a variety of sources. In addition, the indigenous military industry has substantially improved.

The third characteristic of Iran's efforts to develop its non-conventional capability is the fact that it has developed more in response to changes in the Persian Gulf and less to those in the wider Middle East. Bluntly, Iran is more concerned about its immediate neighbours (Iraq and the Arab monarchies) than Israel. For example, the Islamic Republic has a territorial dispute with the United Arab Emirates (UAE) over three islands in the Gulf.[39] At the end of the 1990s, the UAE ordered thirty new Mirage 2000-9 from France, eighteen Hawk 200 single-seat combat aircraft from the United Kingdom, and eighty F-16 fighters from the United States.[40] Admittedly, it is hard to imagine a full-scale war between Iran and the UAE, but certainly the stockpiling of all these advanced weapons is of great concern for Tehran.[41]

More important for the Iranian national security is the unsettled situation in Iraq. It is to be remembered that the two countries (Iran and Iraq) fought each other in the 1980s partly over the borders in Shat al-Arab (or, as the Iranians call it, Arvand Rud). Indeed, it can be argued that the Islamic regime's interest in developing non-conventional capability can be explained, almost exclusively, by the lessons it learned during this war. Tehran's inability to respond in kind to Baghdad's missiles and chemical attacks was an essential incentive to develop such weapons during and after the war.[42] Moreover, after the Gulf War Iran, like other countries, seems to have been completely shocked to discover how close Iraq had come to obtaining nuclear weapons.[43]

This Iranian perception of non-conventional threats from Iraq is not likely to recede any time soon at least for two reasons. First, in spite of the United Nations' efforts to destroy Iraq's WMD, the know-how cannot be eliminated. Iraqi scientists know how to make these weapons and this knowledge cannot be taken away from them.[44] Second, regardless of who is in power in Baghdad, Iraq has been dissatisfied with the status quo for most of its modern history. As one scholar put it, 'Iraq is not proliferating simply because its current regime is radical and extreme; it is proliferating because it has good and strategic reasons to do so.'[45]

Ironically, Iran's concerns about Iraq's potential non-conventional

capabilities are shared by Israel. Although Israel and Iraq do not share borders, they have perceived each other as a threat. Since the overthrow of the monarchy in 1958, Israel has viewed the regimes in Baghdad as radical and dangerous. Iraq's continuous opposition to the peace process, and its participation in the Arab-Israeli wars confirmed Israel's perception. Accordingly, Iraq's early efforts to develop a nuclear infrastructure in the mid 1970s were seen with alarm and suspicion in Israel. Without any hesitation, the Israeli government destroyed the Iraqi nuclear facilities in Osiraq in June 1981 before they become operational. This attack was consistent with the Israeli policy of not tolerating nuclear weapons at the hands of a hostile power. The renewed Iraqi threat against Israel in 1990 was silenced by the Gulf War and the substantial destruction of Iraq's WMD. Thus the Gulf War was seen in Israel as a blessing in the sense that it neutralized the Iraqi threat and ensured the nuclear monopoly Israel enjoys in the Middle East.

Since about 1970 it has been commonly assumed that Israel has been a nuclear power. On the eve of the Six-Day War Israel already had a rudimentary, but operational, nuclear weapons which made it the sixth nuclear power in the world and the first, and so far only, one in the Middle East.[46] Given the country's small population and limited strategic depth in comparison with its perceived enemies (both Arabs and Iranians), the nuclear option served as a deterrent. For almost three decades, however, Tel Aviv has neither confirmed nor denied its nuclear status, preferring a general policy of ambiguity. This opacity kept Israel's enemies guessing and prevented the international community from criticizing it. The proliferation of chemical and biological weapons and ballistic missiles in the Middle East prompted a change in Israel's nuclear policy. In July 1998 former Israeli Prime Minister Shimon Peres for the first time publicly admitted that Israel possessed nuclear capabilities.[47]

Another important measure to counter the perceived Iranian threat was the signing of a strategic cooperation agreement by President Clinton and Prime Minister Netanyahu in October 1998.[48] Specifically, the agreement states, 'The United States government would view with particular gravity direct threats to Israel's security arising from the regional deployment of ballistic missiles of intermediate range or greater.'[49] For the foreseeable future, it is expected that Tel Aviv will strive to maintain its nuclear monopoly and to undermine Tehran's efforts to develop non-conventional capabilities.[50]

In closing, four conclusions can be drawn from this discussion of Israeli and Iranian efforts to develop their non-conventional

capabilities. First, Tehran's ambition to acquire nuclear technology is not incited by the ideology of its political system. Originally the program started under the Shah. Given the instability in the Gulf region and the nuclear race between India and Pakistan, it is almost certain that any political regime in Tehran will seek non-conventional capabilities. Second, the American and Israeli efforts to ban the transfer of technology to Iran are likely to slow down, but unlikely to completely prevent Tehran from acquiring and developing different forms of WMD. Such a development, when it happens, will add a new dimension of uncertainty into the security equation in the Middle East.

Third, Israel's preoccupation with security is unlikely to diminish anytime soon, but it is psychological more than it is physical.[51] Iran neither have the motives nor the means to attack Israel. The latter is more advanced in both conventional and non-conventional weapons and the United States is strongly committed to the defense of Israel. Equally important, Iran's hostility toward Israel is driven by ideological not national security considerations.[52] Finally, the question of WMD proliferation in the Middle East and elsewhere is better addressed by political means not a military one. The experience in other countries suggests that these non-conventional weapons are more likely to be eliminated by agreement and cooperation between the parties than by any other way.

Conclusion: Prospects for the Future

The main thesis of this paper is that a stable peace in the Middle East should be based on the inclusion of all the major players in the region.

There is no serious threat to the basic foundations of either the Islamic Republic or the Jewish state. Both of them are here to stay. They have to find out ways to accept and live with each other. Both of them, as well as other states, have to be included in any regional security system. This will not happen overnight, but the first step has to be taken. This study meant to shed light on some of central issues which separate Tehran and Tel Aviv. Its main conclusion is that a detente is possible. It will take a long time and strong leadership on the two sides, but it can be done.

An important contribution toward this end would be an American-Iranian dialogue. A recent publication by Jaffee Center for Strategic Studies at Tel Aviv University supports this approach.[53] Such a dialogue would strengthen the moderates within the religious/political establishment in Tehran. It would accelerate the lifting of American economic sanctions against Iran. A prosperous economy in Iran would enhance its chances to be fully integrated in the regional and

international systems. One can argue, a poor Iran would pursue an aggressive foreign policy while a prosper one would seek peace and cooperation with its neighbours. An Iranian-Israeli peaceful co-existence can be achieved. The sooner the better.

Notes

1. Hudson, Michael C.: 'To Play The Hegemon: Fifty Years Of US Policy Toward The Middle East,' *Middle East Journal*, vol. 50, no. 3 (Summer 1996), p. 334.

2. The World Bank: *World Development Report* (New York: Oxford University Press, 1998), Table 1, pp. 190-191.

3. For example see Evron, Yair: 'The Invasion Of Kuwait And The Gulf War: Dilemmas Facing The Israeli-Iraqi-US Relationship,' in David W. Lesch (ed.): *The Middle East and the United States: A Historical and Political Reassessment* (Boulder, CO: Westview Press, 1996), p. 317; and McGovern, George: 'The Future Role of the US in the Middle East,' *Middle East Policy*, vol. 1, no. 3 (1992), p. 4.

4. For a thorough analysis see Abadi, Jacob: 'Israel's Relations with Oman and the Persian Gulf States,' *Journal of South Asian and Middle Eastern Studies*, vol. 20, no. 1 (Fall 1996), pp. 46-73.

5. Cited in Weinbaum, M.G.: 'Iran and Israel: The Discrete Entente,' *Orbis*, vol. 18, no. 1 (Winter 1975), p. 1070.

6. For a discussion of Israel's oil needs and policies see Longrigg, Stephen Hemsley: *Oil in the Middle East* (New York: Oxford University Press, 1968), particularly pp. 250-253 & 330-333.

7. Yaniv, Avner: 'Israel Faces Iraq: The Politics of Confrontation,' in Amatzia Baram & Barry Rubin (eds.): *Iraq's Road To War* (New York: St. Martin's Press, 1993), p. 239.

8. For a thorough analysis of Iranian-Soviet relations see Sicker, Martin: *The Bear and the Lion* (New York: Praeger, 1988).

9. Pahlavi, Muhammad Reza: *Answer to History* (New York: Stein and Day, 1980), pp. 12-13.

10. Ramazani, R.K.: 'Iran and the Arab-Israeli Conflict,' *Middle East Journal*, vol. 32, no. 4 (Fall 1978), p. 417.

11. Sobhani, Sohrab: *The Pragmatic Entente* (New York: Praeger, 1989), p. 6.

12. Bialer, Uri: 'The Iranian Connection in Israel's Foreign Policy, 1948-1951', *The Middle East Journal*, vol. 39, no. 2 (Spring 1985), p. 295.

13. Souresrafil, Behrouz: *Khomeini and Israel* (London: I. Researchers Inc, 1988), p. 46.

14. 'Iran', *Middle East Economic Digest*, vol. 42, no. 7 (13 February, 1998), p. 21.

15. Ehteshami, Anoushiravan & Raymond A. Hinnebusch: *Syria and Iran: Middle Powers in a Penetrated Regional System* (London: Routledge, 1997), p. 190.

16. For more information on the party see its web site at http://www.Hizbollah.com.

17. In September 1998 President Khatami addressed the United Nations General Assembly and acknowledged non-military aid to 'groups that make efforts and struggle to restore their rights and fight the occupation of their land.' See Gellman, Barton: 'Rushdie Case Termed Finished,' *Washington Post* (23 September 1998), p. A21.

18. Sontag, Deborah: 'Withdrawing from Lebanon Becomes Hot Issue in Israeli Election,' *New York Times* (6 March 1999).

19. Kemp, Geoffrey: *America and Iran: Road Maps and Realism* (Washington, DC: The Nixon Center, 1998), p. 49.

20. For example, President Khatami stated, 'We have over and over again expressed our concern that Israel has become a center for nuclear weapons and for weapons of mass destruction. We too have the right to defend ourselves and make efforts in that respect'. See Gellman, Barton: 'Rushdie Case Termed Finished,' *Washington Post* (23 September, 1998), p. A21.

21. The International Institute for Strategic Studies: *The Military Balance 1998/99* (London: Oxford University Press, 1998), p. 116.

22. 'Israel Forms National Security Council,' *BBC* (7 March, 1999).

23. 'Israelis Start Missile Production,' *Associated Press* (29 November, 1998).

24. Walker, Christopher: 'New Jets Enable Israelis to Hit Iran,' *Times* (25 June, 1998).

25. 'Israel Buys New Subs,' *BBC* (3 July, 1998).

26. Both Israel and Turkey prefer to call their joint plans 'cooperation' not 'alliance.'

27. 'Unclassified Report to Congress on the Acquisition of Technology Relating to Weapons of Mass Destruction and Advanced Conventional Munitions' (Washington: CIA, January 1999).

28. Arnett, Eric (ed.): *Military Capacity and the Risk of War* (New York: Oxford University Press, 1997), p. 5.

29. Simon, Jacqueline: 'United States Non-Proliferation Policy and Iran: Constraints and Opportunities,' *Contemporary Security Policy*, vol. 17, no. 3 (December 1996), p. 371.

30. Hashim, Ahmed: *The Crisis of the Iranian State* (New York: Oxford University Press, 1995), p. 61.

31. Power, Paul F.: 'Middle East Nuclear Issues in Global Perspective,' *Middle East Policy*, vol. 4, nos. 1-2 (September 1995), p. 199.

32. Calabrese, John: 'China and the Persian Gulf: Energy And Security,' *Middle East Journal*, vol. 52, no. 3 (Summer 1998), p. 364.

33. During the US-China October 1997 Summit, China pledged not to engage in any new nuclear cooperation with Iran.

34. Bushehr is the location of two partially-constructed German-built Siemens 1300 megawatt electric power reactors that were more than half completed in 1979 at the time of the Islamic revolution. For more details see

Gerardi, Greg J. & Maryam Aharinejad: 'An Assessment of Iran's Nuclear Facilities,' *The NonproliferationReview*, vol. 2, no. 3 (Spring-Summer 1995), p. 208.

35. 'Russia Says Iran Nuclear Reactor Ready by 2003,' *Reuters* (26 November, 1998).

36. For a recent examination of the Russian-Iranian relations see Gusher, A.: 'On Russian-Iranian Relations,' *International Affairs*, vol. 43, no. 2 (October 1997), pp. 38-44; Vishniakov, V.: 'Russian-Iranian Relations and Regional Stability,' *ibid.*, vol. 45, no. 1 (March 1999), pp. 143-153.

37. For more details on Iran's nuclear capabilities see Koch, Andrew & Jeanette Wolf: 'Iran's Nuclear Facilities: A Profile' (Monterey, CA: Center for Nonproliferation Studies, 1998); Albright, David: 'An Iranian Bomb?' *Bulletin of the Atomic Scientists*, vol. 51, no. 4 (July/August 1995), pp. 21-26.

38. 'Sharansky Discusses Blocking Russian Weapons Leaks to Iran,' *Associated Press* (23 February, 1999).

39. For a thorough analysis of this dispute see Amirahmadi, Hooshang: *Small Islands, Big Politics: The Tunbs and Abu Musa in the Persian Gulf* (New York: St. Martin's Press, 1996).

40. The International Institute for Strategic Studies: *op. cit.* (note #), p. 118.

41. For a discussion of how the UAE perceives Iran see Al-Suwadi, Jamal S.: 'Gulf Security and the Iranian Challenge,' *SecurityDialogue*, vol. 27, no. 3 (September 1996), pp. 277-294. See also his chapter in the present volume.

42. For a detailed discussion see Goodarzi, Jubin: 'Missile Proliferation in the Middle East: The Case of Iran,' *Middle East International*, no. 583 (18 September, 1998), pp. 18-20.

43. Feldman, Shai: 'Middle East Nuclear Stability: The State of the Region and the State of the Debate,' *Journal of International Affairs*, vol. 49, no. 1 (Summer 1995), p. 208.

44. For a detailed review of Iraq's nuclear program see Hashim, Ahmed: 'Iraq: Profile of a Nuclear Addict,' *The Brown Journal of World Affairs*, vol. 4, no. 1 (Winter/Spring 1997), pp. 103-126; and Albright, David & Khidhir Hamza: 'Iraq's Reconstitution of its Nuclear Weapons Program,' *Arms Control Today*, vol. 28, no. 7 (October 1998), pp. 9-15.

45. Cordesman, Anthony H.: 'The Changing Military Balance in the Gulf,' *Middle East Policy*, vol. 6, no. 1 (June 1998), p. 33.

46. Cohen, Avner: *Israel and the Bomb* (New York: Columbia University Press, 1998), p. 1.

47. Center for Nonproliferation Studies: *Israel's Nuclear Posture Review* (Monterey, CA: Center for Nonproliferation Studies, 1999).

48. 'US to Protect Israel against Ballistic Missiles Attack,' *Middle East Monitor*, vol. 28, no. 10 (October 1998), p. 77.

49. For an analysis of this agreement see Feldman, Shai: 'Israel and the Cut-off Treaty,' *Strategic Assessment*, vol. 1, no. 4 (January 1999).

50. For a comprehensive analysis and documentation of nuclear capabilities in Israel and Iran as well as other Middle Eastern states see Office of the Secretary of Defense: *Proliferation: Threat and Response* (Washington DC: GPO, November 1997); Jones, Rodney W., Mark G. McDonough, Toby F. Dalton & Gregory D. Koblentz: *Tracking Nuclear Proliferation: A Guide in Maps and Charts* (Washington, DC: Carnegie Endowment for International Peace, 1998).

51. Neumann, Robert G.: 'Conventional Arms Exports and Stability in the Middle East,' *Journal of International Affairs*, vol. 49, no. 1 (Summer 1995), p. 193.

52. For a detailed discussion of this argument see Chubin, Shahram: *Iran's National Security Policy: Intentions, Capabilities and Impact* (Washington, DC: The Carnegie Endowment for International Peace, 1994).

53. Kam, Ephraim: 'The Iranian Threat: Cause for Concern, Not Alarm,' *Strategic Studies*, vol. 1, no. 3 (October 1998).

7 THE NEVER-ENDING IRAQI CRISIS

Dual Containment and the 'New World Order'

Bjørn Møller

The 'Iraqi Crisis' has been one of the most enduring features of the post-Cold War era. It began in August 1990 with the Iraqi invasion of Kuwait and has remained unresolved ever since, albeit of fluctuating intensity. In the autumn of 1997 the crisis intensified gradually, culminating in December 1998 in a new war code-named 'Operation Desert Fox'. It has been followed by around twice-weekly bombardments of military targets in Iraq by the United States and Great Britain until the time of writing (December 2000).

In the following these events shall be analyzed from a legal, strategic and political angle,[1] followed by a very tentative analysis of the accompanying discourse.

Legal Analysis

There is little doubt that Iraq has been guilty of violating the 1991 cease-fire agreement in general and of the famous 'mother of all resolutions', the UN Security Council Resolution (UNSCR) 687 of 3 April 1991. In the latter the extent and modalities of the disarmament of the defeated aggressor were detailed with, among others, the following provisions:[2]

> The Security Council ... (8) *Decides* that Iraq shall unconditionally accept the destruction, removal, or rendering harmless, under international supervision, of: a) all chemical and biological weapons and all stocks of agents and all related subsystems and components and all research, development, support and manufacturing facilities; b) all ballistic missiles with a range greater than 150 kilometres...

The main issue of controversy has, paradoxically, not so much been Iraq's actual holdings of the proscribed weapons as the international supervision of their destruction. Iraq has on several occasions placed obstacles in the way of, and eventually even completely refused access to, the UN's appointed representatives, i.e. the inspectors of UNSCOM

(United Nations Special Commission), which in 1999 was replaced by the UN Monitoring, Verification and Inspection Commission (UNMOVIC).[3]

Threats and Use of Force
In early 1998, the United States began threatening, as well as materially planning for, a military campaign against Iraq in response to this Iraqi obstruction. After a year's Iraqi provocations and US threats, the crisis was escalated as the US and the UK launched Operation Desert Fox, subsequent to which Iraq demanded the total and irreversible withdrawal of UNSCOM. Even though it does not legally justify Iraq's behaviour, it was later revealed that Iraq's allegations were (at least partly) correct as UNSCOM had indeed allowed itself to be abused as a cover for espionage.[4] In retrospect this might surely be accepted as a significant mitigating circumstance in favour of Iraq, especially in view of the likelihood that some information gathered by these illicit means was used by the US (and perhaps the UK) for the subsequent strikes against Iraq.

The Iraqi violations of resolution 687 and others notwithstanding, both the US and British threats and their subsequent implementation represented clear breaches of international law, *in casu* nothing less than the UN Charter. This states unequivocally that not merely the actual use of force, but also the mere threat thereof is illegal, regardless of the underlying intentions. The only institution with the right to use, or mandate the use of force is the UN Security Council, as clearly stated in the Charter.[5]

> **Article 4(2):** All Members shall refrain in their international relations from the threat or use of force against the territorial integrity or political independence of any state, or in any other manner inconsistent with the Purposes of the United Nations.
> **Article 24(1):** In order to ensure prompt and effective action by the United Nations, its Members confer on the Security Council primary responsibility for the maintenance of international peace and security, and agree that in carrying out its duties under this responsibility the Security Council acts on their behalf.

The advocates of military intervention (the United States, followed by the UK and various other countries, including small and otherwise peaceful and law-abiding states such as Denmark) have argued that prior Security Council resolutions entailed an 'implicit authorization' to use force, referring primarily to UNSCR 678 (29 November 1990),

in which the Security Council authorized 'member States co-operating with the Government of Kuwait (...) to use all necessary means to uphold and implement Security Council resolution 660 and all subsequent relevant resolutions and to restore international peace and security in the area'.

This reading of the resolution, however, does not seem tenable, above all because it clearly referred to a previous resolution (UNSCR 660 of 2 August 1990), which had nothing to do with the disarmament of Iraq, but only with a condition that had already been met, namely the restoration of the sovereignty and territorial integrity of Kuwait. Even though several subsequent resolutions condemned Iraq for non-compliance, none of them contained anything that could be construed as an authorization to use force. Moreover, three of the permanent members of the Security Council (France, Russia and China) made it very clear that they would veto any new resolution to authorize the use of force.[6]

With the explicit US and British threats against Iraq the world was thus in February 1998 heading towards a clear breach of international law perpetrated by two of the Security Council's five permanent members. This threatened to seriously undermine the UN's authority, as there would be very little the rest of the UN could do, if only because the US and UK would be able to veto any condemnation in the Security Council, to say nothing of actual reprisals.

Fortunately, however, UN Secretary General Kofi Annan managed to 'snatch victory from the claws of defeat'. His negotiations in Baghdad produced a Memorandum of Understanding, dated 23 February 1998, between Iraq and the UN, in which Iraq pledged to 'cooperate fully with UNSCOM and the International Atomic Energy Agency (IAEA)', in return for 'the commitment of all Member States to respect the sovereignty and territorial integrity of Iraq'. Concretely, Iraq promised 'to accord to UNSCOM and IAEA immediate, unconditional and unrestricted access'. In return the UN promised to 'respect the legitimate concerns of Iraq relating to national security, sovereignty and dignity'. This was to be ensured by having the controversial presidential sites inspected by a special group headed by a Commissioner appointed by the Secretary-General. The UN further promised to bring the matter of a lifting of sanctions 'to the full attention of the members of the Security Council'.

After some haggling in the Security Council, with the United States and Britain pushing for a resolution that would make the use of force an almost automatic response to Iraqi non-compliance, a compromise resolution (UNSCR 1154) was passed on 2 March 1998, which

warned that Iraqi violations would have 'the severest consequences for Iraq'. However, the resolution clearly left the decision of how to respond to the Security Council. Even if it had not done so, there can be no doubt that the Security Council is the supreme authority on the interpretation of its own resolutions, which cannot even be overruled by the ICJ (International Court of Justice), much less by individual states, however powerful.[7]

When the US and the UK in December 1998 thus used the report by UNSCOM chairman Richard Butler as the pretext for launching Operation Desert Fox, it was, legally speaking, a war of aggression undertaken by two of the permanent members of the Security Council against another UN member state. Not only did the aggressors have no explicit mandate, but the three other permanent members had made it abundantly clear that they were opposed to the use of force. The United States and the UK even had the audacity to launch the strikes while the Council was in session and in the midst of its deliberations on the matter. This did not go down well at all with the other members. In Russian President Yeltsin's words:

> By carrying out unprovoked military action, the USA and Britain have crudely violated the UN Charter and the universally-accepted principles of international law as well as the norms and rules governing the responsible conduct of states in the international arena.[8]

Operation Desert Fox was called off on 19 December 1998, but has since been followed by two other, almost equally serious, breaches of international law on the part of the United States and Great Britain, related to the so-called 'No-Fly Zones' and the 'Iraq Liberation Act'.

The 'No-Fly Zones'
The post-war period has seen regular attacks (about twice a week) against Iraqi air defence systems in the so-called 'No-Fly Zones' in northern and southern Iraq, covering about two thirds of the country. These zones have no U.N. mandate and thus represent a clear infringement of Iraq's sovereignty and territorial integrity. Their prohibition against Iraqi military as well as civilian flights as well as the daily patrolling by US, British and (until 1996) French military aircraft clearly imply that the zones have been withdrawn from Iraq's sovereign domain, hence that its territorial integrity has been violated.

This view is, needless to say, not uncontested. In a U.S. Department of Defense News Briefing (26 January 1999), it was claimed that 'The zones, created after the Gulf War, were mandated by

U.N. Security Council Resolutions 678, 687, and 688 to deter Iraq's use of aircraft against its people and its neighbours.'

In fact, however, none of the quoted resolutions mention the zones at all. The first two are clearly irrelevant, namely UNSCR 678 (29 November 1990) authorizing the use of force to evict Iraq from Kuwait, and UNSCR 687 mandating Iraq's partial disarmament, yet without any authorization to use force. The only relevant resolution is UNSCR 688 which condemned 'the repression of the Iraqi civilian population in many parts of Iraq, including most recently in Kurdish populated areas'. It demanded 'that Iraq, as a contribution to remove the threat to international peace and security in the region, immediately end this repression', and further insisted 'that Iraq allow immediate access by international humanitarian organizations'. Not only was there no mention of no-fly zones, but the resolution explicitly reaffirmed 'the commitment of all Member States to the sovereignty, territorial integrity and political independence of Iraq'.

This lack of legality notwithstanding, the no-fly zones have gradually come to be seen as 'normal', more about which below.

The Iraq Liberation Act
The Clinton Administration in 1999 began (to its credit, somewhat reluctantly and certainly without any enthusiasm) to implement the *Iraq Liberation Act* which had been passed by the US Congress on 5 October 1998. According to this act 'It should be the policy of the United States to support efforts to remove the regime headed by Saddam Hussein from power in Iraq and to promote the emergence of a democratic government to replace that regime.' In addition to support for propaganda and humanitarian assistance, the act explicitly referred to military assistance, i.e. the provision to insurgents against the regime of 'defense articles' (i.e. weapons) and military education as well as training, all to an amount not exceeding 97 million dollars.[9]

Whatever one may think of the Iraqi regime and hope that it will one day be replaced by a democracy, for one state to thus explicitly proclaim its intention to remove another state's government by military means (among others) constitutes a clear violation of the UN Charter, as well as of several UN Security Council resolutions, all of which have pledged respect for Iraq's sovereignty. The Iraq Liberation Act was, furthermore, a violation of the UN General Assembly's *Declaration on the Inadmissibility of Intervention in the Domestic Affairs of States and the Protection of Their Independence and Sovereignty*, which was adopted in 1965 with only one abstention (the UK, but *not* the United States), and in which it was stated:

No state has the right to intervene, directly or indirectly, for any reason whatever, in the internal or external affairs of any other state. Consequently, armed intervention and all other forms of interference or attempted threats against the personality of the State or against its political, economic and cultural elements are condemned.[10]

The United States has thus been in clear breach of international law in several respects during the protracted Iraqi crisis.

Strategic Analysis

The protracted Iraqi crisis has thus seen some very 'creative' attempts at reinterpretation of international law, as well as quite explicit breaches of it. However, all of this might (perhaps) have been justified, if the prevailing assessment of the severity of the problem had been true, in which case a 'bending' or breach of the rules might have been warranted.[11] Unfortunately, on closer analysis this does not seem to be the case.

The Problem of Weapons of Mass Destruction

The core of the problem in 1998 was Iraq's refusal of access for UNSCOM to the presidential sites and various other locations, where it was believed it might conceal either actual weapons of mass destruction or production facilities for WMDs, i.e. for either chemical or biological weapons, or both. This raises the question whether the implicit danger was serious enough to warrant a breach of international law.

Chemical weapons, to be sure, have some very unappealing features. However, except for highly unlikely scenarios (such as very accurate strikes against dense congregations of unprotected victims) the damage they can produce is fairly modest. In other words, quite large quantities are required for chemical weapons to really deserve the label 'weapons of *mass* destruction', and it would be hard for Iraq to conceal such quantities, and even harder to deliver them to the envisaged target. Ballistic missiles generally have too limited throw-weights to be suitable for such missions, while aircraft are better, but less sure to be able to penetrate the air defence array of the target. Finally, a wide range of protective measures are available, which are cumbersome but quite effective.

Biological weapons are, in principle at least, genuine weapons of mass destruction,[12] as some of them can cause infections of pandemic proportions. Moreover, the small quantities required makes it easy to conceal them—the more so, the less stringent the safety precautions

taken by the possessor. There are, however, several drawback to any use of biological weapons:

Their impact is very difficult to control, hence their use may also affect the country using them, including its (invading or occupying) armed forces. The collateral damage would also be considerable, and those segments of the population which might have been singled out as supporters of the aggressor would not be immune. For instance, an Iraqi biological weapons attack against Israel would inevitably have a large toll of Palestinian casualties besides the intended (Jewish) victims.

Certain agents, furthermore, have too long incubation times to make them suitable for supporting a surprise attack, and others may be difficult to deliver, for instance, by means of ballistic missiles, as the micro-organisms would be killed either during the boost or impact phase. Finally, while vaccines are available that may protect the troops using them against some agents, mass inoculations would surely be detected, which would alert the envisaged target country, to which the same vaccines would be available.[13] There have been speculations about genetic engineering to overcome some of these problems,[14] but this would surely require a level of sophistication beyond that available to a country such as Iraq—and even more so as long as it remained under the close and intrusive supervision of UNSCOM.

Even if Iraq should succeed in producing significant stockpiles of chemical and/or biological weapons, it is hard to fathom what would be their possible utility, even in the hands of a ruthless dictator like Saddam Hussein. A few possibilities immediately spring to mind, but none of them (with the possible exception of no. 1) seem to make much sense:

1. As a 'defensive deterrent', intended to protect Iraq against an attack with unlimited objectives that would pose an 'existential' threat to the country or regime. This would, however, not be relevant in the absence of such a threat.
2. As an 'offensive deterrent', under the protection of which Iraq might launch a conventional attack, taking advantage of its possession of WMD to neutralize the deterrent effects of WMD in the hands of the victim of aggression or its allies. This would, however, only really matter against conventionally inferior opponents, while Iraq would undoubtedly be up against a crushing conventional superiority in the event of a renewed attack against Kuwait or other neighbours.
3. As a means of 'offensive compellence', where Iraq would use the

threat of strikes with WMD (i.e. attempt 'WMD blackmail') to compel another state to make concessions. The entire case for such blackmail is, however, extremely vague and could probably safely be dismissed as a figment of the imagination. In any case such blackmail would make no sense vis-à-vis countries aligned with a nuclear-armed superpower who might 'call the blackmailer's bluff'.[15]

4. As a political 'bargaining chip', which Saddam might 'cash in' for concessions such as a complete lifting of sanctions—perhaps in analogy with what may have been the North Korean strategy underlying its threat to withdraw from the Non-Proliferation Treaty (NPT).[16] However, as such a lifting of sanctions is preconditioned on Iraqi compliance with UNSCR 687, an initially clandestine development would seem to defeat its purpose: As long as it would remain hidden, it would have no bargaining utility, whereas a revelation would automatically be labelled as non-compliance, thereby militating strongly against any lifting of sanctions.

While all of the above might make some strategic sense, the purpose most often alluded to would not, namely terror bombardments of neighbouring countries. The stigma that is attached to biological weapons would deprive the country using them of all (or at least most) international support.[17] It might further help lifting the taboo against nuclear first-use, implying that an Iraqi biological attack could provoke nuclear retaliation—as has been intimated by both Israel and the United States.[18] The deterrence strategy on which the national security of both the United States and NATO was premised throughout the Cold War could surely work against a foe such as Iraq which is, after all, much less of a threat than the mighty Soviet Union,

While it would surely be cynical to trivialize B and C weapons, they cannot really compare with the *actual* nuclear weapons that are deployed by, *inter alia*, the United States, the UK and Israel,[19] but which have been almost completely forgotten in the uproar over *potential*, and in any case primitive, Iraqi WMD. Moreover, to the extent that B and C weapons are regarded as a serious danger, the most promising approach to solving the problem would arguably be negotiations on the establishment of a zone free of WMD covering the entire Middle East/Persian Gulf region.[20] This would surely have been preferable to an attack in breach of international law such as Operation Desert Fox.

Operation Desert Fox: War Aims

Operation Desert Fox involved more than 30,000 U.S. troops in the Persian Gulf and 10,000 more from outside Central Command; more than 600 sorties; and more than forty ships performing both support and strike functions, e.g. by launching more than 300 cruise missiles.[21]

Its objectives were never made entirely clear, but the following were mentioned by President Clinton in his announcement of the operation: 'They are designed to degrade Saddam's capacity to develop and deliver weapons of mass destruction, and to degrade his ability to threaten his neighbours'. When calling off the campaign four days later, the US President declared that 'We have inflicted significant damage on Saddam's weapons of mass destruction programmes, on the command structures that direct and protect that capability, and on his military and security infrastructure'.[22] The terms used to describe both the aims and achievements were thus quite vague, and it was never specified to which extent Iraqi capacities should be degraded, making it impossible to evaluate the operation as a success or failure.

In his testimony to the Senate Armed Forces Committee, 28 January 1999, General Anthony C. Zinni, who had directed Desert Fox operations, provided a summary of the tactical and operational achievements of the campaign, yet without explicitation of the strategic and political effects thereof:

> Primary targets struck during Operation Desert Fox were installations associated with development of WMD, units providing security to IKMD programs, and Iraq's national command and control network. Additional targets included selected Republican Guard facilities, airfields, and the Basra oil refinery that was involved in production of illegal gas and oil exports. Iraq's integrated air defenses and surface-to-air missiles (SAM) sites were also heavily struck in order to ensure the safety of coalition aircraft. Due to the destruction of key facilities and specialized equipment, we assess that Iraq's ballistic missile program has been set back one to two years. Several of Iraq's most sensitive security units suffered attrition and the Iraqi command and control network was disrupted, with some degradation remaining today. Regarding the success of Operation DESERT FOX, over 80 percent of the designated targets were hit and damaged. Additionally, every security unit attacked suffered damage. Iraqi claims of civilian casualties and collateral damage remain unsubstantiated. Finally, these successes were realized with no casualties to our coalition forces.

There thus seem to have been, at least, three different objectives: (1)

destroying Iraq's WMD; (2) hampering Iraq's production of WMD; and (3) compelling Saddam Hussein to comply with the UN's requests. In addition to these, there apparently was a fourth objective, which was less clearly spelled out, namely (4) removing, or at least politically weakening, Saddam Hussein.

The Chosen Strategy
Laudable though (some of) these goals may have been, neither did Operation Desert Fox appear to have achieved any of them, nor was this really to be expected, judging from previous experience.

A destruction of the (presumed) Iraqi stocks of biological and/or chemical weapons would be virtually impossible, even by means of the high-precision concrete-penetrating missiles shown in the media, as surgical strikes presuppose the availability of accurate and reliable target coordinates. While such coordinates would be available for possible production sites for nuclear weapons (as demonstrated by the 1981 Israeli attack against the Osiraq nuclear reactor)[23], production sites for B and C weapons could be much more dispersed and easily moved about. In fact, this was exactly what the US accused Saddam of doing, i.e. delaying access for the inspection teams and in the meantime moving the proscribed materials to other locations.

Even in the hypothetical event that the attacks should actually succeed in destroying all existing stocks and production facilities, there could never be any complete certainty thereof. Striking at the presumed locations might be partly successful, but would have to be followed up with renewed strikes *ad infinitum*. This would be a form of gradual attrition and would surely do something to hamper and postpone any Iraqi access to WMD, but there would also be drawbacks.

First of all, a collateral damage would be inevitable, and Saddam might even deliberately magnify it by locating production sites in densely populated areas (viz his usage of hostages during the Kuwait crisis). Secondly, the costs to the United States would be substantial, especially as such an open-ended campaign could probably not count on Arab or Turkish support indefinitely. The 1998 war thus saw Iraqi threats against Saudi Arabia and Kuwait that they would have to 'bear the consequences of providing bases for aggression against Iraq', as well as negotiations with Turkey. Even though the latter have not, so far, produced the intended result, in due course they may well do so.[24] Eventually, the strikes might thus have to be launched from aircraft carriers on station in the Gulf, which are extremely costly.

It was, of course, conceivable that one or several series of air strikes against important targets in Iraq might have compelled Iraq into

submission. However, this did not happen, but Saddam remained recalcitrant in the face of attacks that were massive but not fatal. It did not appear that the United States had any *strategy* to guide its air strike *tactics*, as such a strategy would have to include plans for several rounds of moves and counter-moves. The following options were open:

To simply continue the strikes—but for how long? To discontinue them after a 'decent interval', yet without having accomplished what they had been intended to achieve—with a US loss of face as the inevitable result. To gradually escalate them until the goal was reached. However, should this escalation be undertaken in quantitative or qualitative terms—i.e. by simply increasing the intensity of the strikes, or by proceeding to more important targets or using more destructive means of attack, perhaps even WMD?[25]

A similar strategy of gradual escalation was attempted by both the Kennedy, Johnson and Nixon administrations during the Vietnam War, but to absolutely no avail. Eventually the United States had to withdraw and accept defeat, leaving behind it a trail of destruction of both Vietnamese society and environment.[26] This was surely not a strategy for emulation, but the US nevertheless seemed to have settled for a similar strategy of gradual attrition against Iraq—just as they did in the war against Yugoslavia in the spring of 1999.[27]

As far as the (less clearly articulated) fourth possible war aim of deposing Saddam is concerned, this might have been possible, either by means of successful 'surgical' strikes against his presumed whereabout (the Presidential palaces, for instance) or by marching all the way to Baghdad. Indeed, several observers have argued that it was a mistake not to have proceeded to the Iraqi capital in 1991. However, better late than never![28]

First of all, however, there were surely more effective ways of doing this than by means of air bombardments or AirLand Battle-type operations, e.g. by means of special forces or agents 'with a licence to kill', which would have had the advantage of being more 'discrete'. Even though such an assassination of Saddam, or an instigated coup against him, would have been unlawful, such activities would at least have been deniable. At worst, the US President might have been compelled to dismiss a few high-ranking officials, but he would not automatically have been officially implicated in a breach of international law, hence would have created no unfortunate precedents. It might still have been immoral, but would surely have been more prudent.

Secondly, an attack 'to get Saddam' would have constituted an even more blatant violation of international law than an attack to

ensure compliance with UN resolutions.[29] Thirdly, such an operation would have presupposed that there was somebody ready to take the place of Saddam Hussein, most likely a group of rebellious officers. Their prospects of being accepted as legitimate by the Iraqi population would, however, have been jeopardized by their being seen (correctly) as the agents of foreign powers. Were they to be regarded as illegitimate by (all or large parts of) the population, continuing discord and turmoil would have been the most likely consequence.

It was thus very difficult to make any strategic sense of the campaign. When viewed in the wider context of the Iraq Liberation Act it also appeared politically ill-advised.

Political Analysis

Even if it had been successful according to the above criteria, the December 1998 attack and its follow-up are likely to have severe negative repercussions, both regionally and globally.

First of all, any attack without UN Security Council authorization is a clear violation of the Kellogg-Briand Pact of 1928 as well as of the UN Charter and other elements of international law. International law explicitly proscribes war, not through a ban on specific types of war but in the form of a general prohibition with certain explicit exceptions. Only wars of self-defence and of collective security are permitted, and in both cases the legality is conditional upon Security Council approval, either *ex ante* or *ex post*.[30]

That war has thus been outlawed must be acknowledged as one of the most significant advances in the progressive civilizing of international relations. Just compare the present situation to that of the 19th century when war was a matter of expediency. If the prospects of success were good enough, it was regarded as perfectly legitimate (perhaps even imperative) to go to war for such political goals as territorial expansion. A violation of these rules thus contributes to making war, once again, a legitimate means to political ends, and the more so as Operation Desert Fox could not even be condemned by the United Nations (if only because of predictable US and British vetoes), whereby a most unfortunate precedent has been set. What should prevent other states from using war as a means to their political ends in the future, if only they possess the requisite military strength?

Secondly, by 1998 the assembled anti-Iraqi coalition had crumbled significantly in comparison with that of 1990/91. No serious attempts had been made at enlisting regional support prior to Operation Desert Fox, and there had been no discernible interest in creating a regional coalition which might, in due course, have come to constitute a

regional collective security system *in embryo*. Instead, the US-British 'coalition' must have looked very much like a real-life manifestation of a (Huntingtonian) war of 'the West against the rest'[31], yet with the unfortunate twist that 'the West' was now cast in the role of the aggressor. In all fairness, however, it should be mentioned that the very same Samuel Huntington who coined the term has warned against such 'bullying'.[32]

The immediate response to Operation Desert Fox were large protest rallies in several Arab countries. The longer-term effect may be a swell of anti-western sentiments in the Arab and Muslim world (including Turkey),[33] which could produce a growth of radical islamist parties and groupings. As several of the regimes in the region have a fragile basis, it is quite conceivable that some of them (Saudi Arabia, for instance) could be overturned in favour of radical islamist rule—or, even worse, be replaced by stateless chaos.[34] One could also envisage endangered regimes adopting more oppressive means of government (or military rule) as a safeguard against democratic victories for the radicals (as happened in Algeria in 1992). A renaissance for pan-Arabist or pan-Islamist policies would also seem a possibility, even though the plethora of rivalries would probably prevent this from proceeding far beyond rhetoric to actual politics.[35]

A worst-case scenario would involve a virtual dissolution of Iraq, for instance as a result of the aforementioned political instability caused by a future 'Western' (or U.S.) attack aimed at dethroning Saddam, which might escalate to civil war. The Shi'ites in the southern parts of Iraq might secede, perhaps with a view to merging with Iran; and the Kurds in northern Iraq might secede in order to create an independent Kurdistan. This would put further pressure on the other states hosting Kurdish minorities, i.e. Syria, Iran and Turkey.[36] Both eventualities would place severe strains on the already extremely delicate balance of power in the Persian Gulf region, especially if combined with political instability in Saudi Arabia.

Discourse Analysis
None of the above political or military strategies thus seem politically prudent, and they might thus be dismissed as simply the most recent in a long chain of counter-productive U.S. strategies for the Persian Gulf (as described in the introductory chapter by the present author).

The 'New World Order' Discourse
An alternative explanation may be that the US behaviour vis-à-vis Iraq has had little to do with Iraq as such, but has been intended for the

'global audience'. Perhaps the US is trying to create a new set of rules for the 'unipolar moment', i.e. for the (probably ephemeral) *'Pax Americana'* that the world is now experiencing.[37] Judging by recent events one might fear that these rules may be reminiscent of those advocated by the Athenians in the famous Melian Dialogue recorded by Thucydides: 'The strong do what they have the power to do and the weak accept what they have to accept'.[38]

Ironically, however, from beginning to end the handling of the Iraqi crisis has been embedded in a discourse on 'the New World Order',[39] the connotations of which are not those of power politics or superpower domination, but rather the exact opposite thereof. In his message to a joint session of the US Congress, 11 September 1990 (i.e. during the 'Desert Shield' phase of the Gulf conflict), President George Bush thus described the 'new world order' as '... a new era, free from the threat of terror, stronger in the pursuit of justice, and more secure in the quest for peace. An era in which the nations of the world, East and West, North and South, can prosper and live in harmony.'[40]

This vision was further elaborated in a similar presidential statement to Congress after the victorious Operation Desert Storm, 6 March 1991, in which the president associated the emerging new world order with 'the new principles of justice and fair play', credited it with the ability to 'protect the weak against the strong', and predicted that this would be '... a world where the United Nations, freed from the Cold War stalemate, is poised to fulfil the historic vision of its founders. A world in which freedom and respect for human rights find a home among all nations.'[41]

The Clinton Administration couched its policies in similar terms. In the White House document of October 1998 *A National Security Strategy for a New Century*, it was thus stated that

> As we approach the beginning of the 21st century, the United States remains the world's most powerful force for peace, prosperity and the universal values of democracy and freedom (....) At this moment in history, the United States is called upon to lead—to organize the forces of freedom and progress; to channel the unruly energies of the global economy into positive avenues; and to advance our prosperity, reinforce our democratic ideals and values, and enhance our security.[42]

Few would disagree with such lofty goals: freedom, justice, peace, human rights, rule of law, etc. In fact the vision is couched in terms that command consent. Even though one may disagree on what the terms imply, one cannot be against 'justice' or 'freedom'. However, as

argued above, the reality underlying this discourse is almost the exact opposite, namely breaches of international law, an undermining of the authority of the United Nations, and a general militarization of international relations.

Discursive Anomalies

The above conclusion takes us into the somewhat nebulous realm of 'discourse analysis'. However, even though it is somewhat inspired by the writings of David Campbell and others, the following does not pretend to be a 'genuine' analysis of the discourse accompanying the action of the Iraq crisis.[43] The ambition is simply to highlight some paradoxical features of the language used about the crisis, both by politicians and the media. Some of them can be explained with reference to the findings of what one might call 'the social psychology of conflict'.

The quest for avoidance of 'cognitive dissonance' was already highlighted in the 1950s by Leon Festinger,[44] according to whom individuals seek world views without contradictions, i.e. cognitive consonance. If Saddam is 'bad' such consonance demands that all his actions are also seen as objectionable; and if the United States is 'good', then so its actions must be. No need for further analysis.

Another cognitive pattern is the proclivity for developing stereotyped, or even demonized, 'enemy images' of one's opponent which tend to become nearly irrefutable.[45] As Saddam is unquestionably a gross violator of human rights,[46] all his foreign policy initiatives are automatically assumed to bear the same demonic traits. Once again: no need for concrete analysis, and if somebody should question the assumptions they can conveniently be dismissed as defenders of 'evil personified'.

The well-documented phenomenon of 'group think' was long ago described by Irving Janis[47] as a mechanism that ensures conformity, thereby narrowing the span of options available to decision-makers in a complex decision-making situation. Dissent is depicted as illoyal behaviour, a pattern that apparently also holds true for alliance politics, especially in NATO, where member states have shown a similar propensity for groupthink.

The propensity for what one might call 'action-reaction inversion' also plays a role, where an actor views his own behaviour as forced reactions to what the other side does as a matter of choice. *Alter* is thus seen as proactive, i.e. on the offensive, while *Ego* is merely reacting defensively.[48] In real life, of course, this is nearly always a chicken-and-egg situation.

A final cognitive pattern of relevance for Iraq is widespread use of images,[49] myths and spurious historical analogies, which 'in a split-second conjure up in the minds of audiences and readers certain associations, which the writer or orator wants to evoke', and which (...) pretending that there is a law of historical repetition, serves as pseudo-rationalisation, furnishing bogus scientific evidence for a decidedly unscientific argument'.[50]

Others features of US behaviour towards Iraq might be explained by economic theory, e.g. with reference to the need of the (American and, to a lesser extent, British) 'military industrial complex' (MIC) for an enemy to replace the USSR. Even though defence planning can, in principle, proceed without an enemy, it is much easier with one.[51] Had a Saddam Hussein not existed in real life, it would thus have been in the Pentagon's interest to create one. By combining despotic features and an alien culture (Islam) with 'the right size', the Iraqi leader represented 'the ideal enemy'.

The social-psychological and the economic explanations are, of course, not mutually exclusive. It is entirely conceivable that the MIC pursues its vested interest by capitalizing on familiar cognitive patters such as the above, *inter alia* by means of a manipulation of the mass media.[52] However, it is also possible that (at least parts of) the intelligence services and other employees of the MIC have themselves fallen prey to these patters, hence have come to believe in enemy images of their own creation.

The War of Words against Iraq

Regardless of their explanation, the following are some of the anomalous features of the 'discourse' on Iraq which have been intertwined with the above on the 'New World Order':

Especially prominent has been the comparison of Saddam Hussein with Hitler, and the accompanying 'Munich analogy'.[53] The logic is that, just as it proved fatal to have placated and appeased Hitler and believed in his peaceful rhetoric, it would be naive and dangerous to compromise with his modern counterpart—as allegedly proposed by, among others, the Russians, the French and the United Nations with their preparedness to 'go the extra mile' diplomatically. However, their unappealing personal characteristics notwithstanding, there are more differences than similarities between Hitler and Saddam Hussein. The former was the leader of a European great power on the rise and with obvious aggressive ambitions, while the latter is the leader of a minor power which has already been quite decisively defeated.

Another pervasive feature was the talk about 'punishing Iraq',

which alludes to an analogy with criminal justice or even pedagogy. However, while it is arguably fair to punish a felon or a disobedient child, it is quite something else to 'punish' a country by means of sanctions which only tangentially punish the real culprit(s), i.e. Saddam Hussein and his immediate entourage, but which cause immense suffering among the civilian population, including Iraqi infants who are surely innocent of any invasion of Kuwait, if only because they were not born at the time (*vide infra*).

The conflict was almost consistently personified as implied by the frequent use of 'Saddam' as a short-hand for Iraq, as in the above quote or the frequently heard phrase to 'Get Saddam'. This facilitates the use of enemy images, as it is inherently more credible that a person is 'evil' than that an entire nation should be so. The exact opposite happens for the other side, where terms such as the 'World Community' or at least 'the West' are often used for what is in reality merely a couple of countries (the United States and the UK) acting on their own behalf. Sometimes completely abstract expressions are used which obscure who did what, hence avoid the obvious questions 'with what right?' or 'on whose authority?'. This has, for instance, been the case of the aforementioned no-fly zones in northern and southern Iraq. While they were, in reality, established by the US, UK and France (that later withdrew its support) without any UN mandate, the favourite terms seem to have become that they 'have been established', with the even more absurd corollary that they 'were expanded' in 1996—as if they could grow organically.[54]

To the extent that it has to be acknowledged that the 'world community' is not unanimous, opposition to the action is often dismissed with reference to (presumably sordid) 'special interests'. While it is probably true that neither Russia nor France have been completely unselfish, the same could surely be said of the US and the UK. It would thus be more fair to either compare what the two sides actually do or say for the intrinsic merits thereof, or to compare their respective 'hidden agendas'. To take merely one of the opposing sides' words or actions at face value, however, is obviously biased. Opposition (by Russia, France or others) is, furthermore, often labelled 'obstruction', while a better explanation might be that they simply disagree with the US and/or Britain on the right course of action. It becomes even more absurd when it is a minority of two who dismiss the dissent of the majority as 'obstruction'.

The very term (dual) 'containment' with the implied analogy with the East-West conflict is also profoundly misleading (*vide infra*). Finally, the depiction of the US (and British) armed forces as 'heroic'

is undoubtedly welcomed by the American public, but devalues the meaning of the term. The risks involved with launching cruise missiles against another country in order to neutralize its air defence and subsequently conduct air raids against it are minimal—and to do so is thus hardly 'heroic' in the usual sense of the word. This lack of any need for heroism might also, according to some analysis, even make the label 'war' inappropriate, which may presuppose as least some duel features, while 'slaughter' may be a more suitable term for what has been happening.[55]

Offence-Defence Inversion

A particularly perverse feature of this discourse about Iraq has been the complete inversion of the distinction between offence and defence. 'Defence' is usually (on the grand strategic level) held to be synonymous with defending one's own territory, territorial waters and airspace against invaders or intruders, and (on the lower levels) with 'parrying and awaiting a blow' (Clausewitz), while 'offence' usually refers to striking a blow against the defender or even invading.[56] With regard to Iraq, the roles have been inverted, so that Iraq is depicted as 'offensive' or 'provocative' when it seeks to defend its own airspace against enemy aircraft, while it is portrayed as 'defensive' for the US Air Force to strike against ground-based Iraqi air defences—and even to do so pre-emptively, i.e. as soon as they turn on their radars, or even just because of their being there, i.e. on Iraqi soil.

According to the military commander of the U.S. Central Command (USCENTCOM), Marine General Anthony Zinni, 'Iraq's entire air defense system is a threat to us', referring mainly to the surface-to-air missiles (SAMs), which are only operational in Iraq's own airspace. Indeed, on the same occasion, the general complained about early-warning systems as well as optical guidance systems being used 'obviously to prevent turning on radars which would make targeting for us much easier'. By implications, for Iraq to even receive early warning of US strikes would be 'offensive' and 'threatening'. 'We responded within our rules of engagement by defending ourselves and attacking Iraq's air defense system, including its radars, communications facilities and surface-to-air missile (SAM) batteries'.[57]

War and Sanctions as Normality

An almost 'normal situation' has been created by means of the above-mentioned practice and discourse, aided and abetted by subservient news media. It is characterized by twice-weekly small-scale air attacks against Iraqi military targets which inevitably produce accidental hits

on civilian targets (such as Basra, 25 January 1999). Such 'incidents' are habitually 'regretted', but trivialized.[58]

In this way, both the media and possible opponents gradually lose interest. Even though it would be justified, it is obviously impossible to bring the matter up in the UN Security Council each time—and especially not considering the fact that any motion to condemn would meet with a US and/or British veto. The United States may even hope to thereby create some perverted kind of 'customary international law'. If something goes virtually unopposed and uncontested for long enough, it may be possible (especially if one is a superpower) to claim that a new set of rules has emerged that justify it *ex post facto*. This was how the no-fly zones achieved the status they possess today, in the eyes of many observers at least. Both the media and most politicians have long ago forgotten about their actual origins, and some have even come to believe that the zones were mandated by a Security Council resolution in the first place.

Even though there are no signs that this low-intensity war of attrition against Iraq has any effect, it continues—apparently because of a curious logical twist of the argument. The question being asked is not whether the two Western powers should continue doing something that does not achieve its intended results and constitutes a standing violation of international law, but whether 'Saddam' has done anything to deserve a discontinuation of the bombardments. War has thus become the normal situation requiring no explanation, whereas peace has become the anomaly calling for a special reason.

The same curious 'logic' seems to apply to the sanctions regime which was originally imposed on Iraq in 1990 and 1991, i.e. during and in the immediate aftermath of its invasion of Kuwait, and which remained in effect by the time of writing (December 2000). There is absolutely no evidence that this sanctions regime has had any success in influencing Iraqi behaviour, just as the evidence for sanctions ever working is highly questionable.[59] The sanctions also raise serious ethical questions. When President Clinton in his speech announcing Operation Desert Fox thus claimed that 'Sanctions have cost Saddam more than $120 billion', it may have appeared fair and just. However, in actual fact it is, of course, not Saddam but Iraq that must bear the costs. Moreover, the more dictatorial Iraq is portrayed as being, the more obvious the injustice becomes which is inherent in such a punishment scheme. The estimated one million malnourished children in Iraq of the year 2000 were certainly innocent of the invasion of Kuwait in 1990, but they are among the main victims of the sanctions (even though the regime is certainly also to blame for their dismal

fate).[60]

The question being asked, however, is usually not whether to uphold a sanctions regime that does not work as intended, and which has severe (bordering on genocidal) consequences, but whether Saddam has done anything to deserve the 'reward' that a lifting of sanctions would amount to. In principle the sanctions can thus continue indefinitely, also because of the special rules of decision-making pertaining to them.

Contrary to the war of attrition, the sanctions do have a mandate from the UN Security Council, making them lawful. However, rather than mandating sanctions of a finite duration against Iraq, which might have been renewed (e.g. on a annual basis) if still deemed warranted, the Security Council imposed sanction of indefinite duration. Hence they can only be lifted (or even relaxed) by a new decision in the Security Council, which the United States could simply veto.

Rogueness and Dual Containment

A central part of the above discourse has been played by the notion of 'rogue states' which has been combined with that of 'containment' in the sense that the US strategy is allegedly about 'containing the rogues', *in casu* Iraq as well as Iran. Closer inspection, however, reveals this strategy as deeply flawed and the discourse about it to be deceptive, as both 'rogueness' and 'containment' are used in a highly questionable manner.

The containment strategy proposed in the late 1940s by George Kennan and others vis-à-vis the Soviet Union and its allies was basically a defensive political strategy. It was based on the assumption (right or wrong) that the USSR was fundamentally expansionist, but rational. Hence, not only did the USSR require containment, it was also basically containable. The means to do so were (nuclear and other forms of) deterrence, defensive alliances and other forms of support to friendly states (or states hostile to the USSR). The more sophisticated versions of the strategy, including that of Kennan himself, placed the main emphasis on political and economic means. The rationale for this was that communist expansion was more likely to be political than military, hence that political and social stabilization would work in the West's favour, as it would deprive communism of popular support.[61]

During the Cold War, containment was surely taken too far on occasions, for instance when excessive emphasis was placed on factors such a 'reputation', which entailed a need for exhibiting 'toughness', even in non-vital questions;[62] or when it concentrated on weakening the East rather than on strengthening the West; or when the political

aspects of containment came close to jeopardizing, rather than securing, freedom and democracy.[63] Surely there were also occasional problems with drawing the line between the containment and a 'roll back' of communism, for instance during the Korean War or under the Reagan Administration.[64] On balance, however, containment was largely defensive. The Cold War, moreover, saw plenty of 'cooperation among adversaries', including persistent (and successful) efforts to avoid any direct armed confrontation, an extensive use of arms control, confidence-building measures and summit meetings.[65]

Not so in the Persian Gulf region, where the US policy of 'dual containment' of the two alleged rogues, Iran and Iraq, has exhibited virtually no such cooperative features, has not been based on any appreciation of the other side's legitimate security interests, and where nearly no serious dialogue or negotiations have been attempted. Moreover, with regard to both the Persian Gulf 'rogues' US policy has exhibited unmistakable, if not persistent, elements of 'roll back' ambitions,[66] as in the aforementioned US 'Iraq Liberation Act of 1998'.

Moreover, the very notion of 'rogueness' appears deeply flawed as well as biased. If one were to compare US with Iranian and Iraqi behaviour according to the US definition one would find the United States to be much 'roguer' than both Iran and Iraq. With one third of the world's military expenditures for a mere five percent of its population the United States obviously has defence expenditures vastly in excess of its defence needs.[67] It possesses huge quantities of weapons of mass destruction, and has shown the willingness to also use them (against Hiroshima and Nagasaki in 1945). It has on several occasions launched illegal attacks against other states, and it has supported a wide array of (what others would call) terrorists—all of which is amply documented in open sources.[68]

Another surprising conclusion is that the alleged rogues have behaved most 'roguely' precisely when they enjoyed US support, i.e. that the US appears to have (inadvertently, one must assume) invited rogueness rather than deterring or even containing it. All of the Iranian instances of aggression and intervention thus occurred under the auspices of the 'Nixon Doctrine' that assigned the role of 'maintaining order' in the region to Iran of the Shah.

For all its flaws, however, the 'rogueness discourse' serves an important purpose for the United States. By depicting certain states as lawless, it also places them in the position of not having (or at least deserving) the protection of the law. Hence, against them 'anything goes'.

Conclusion

We have thus seen that the US and British behaviour vis-à-vis Iraq is questionable in several respects. It is unlawful, militarily unsuccessful and probably counter-productive, both with regard to its immediate and regional repercussions and in terms of long-term and global implications. This conclusion is supported by the following chapters by Anthony McDermott and Jalil Roshandel, whereas the chapter by Birthe Hansen looks somewhat more favourably at US policies.

Notes

1. These parts are an expanded and updated version of the appendix to Møller, Bjørn: 'Resolving the Security Dilemma in the Persian Gulf. With a postscript on the 1997/98 Iraqi Crisis', *Working Papers*, no. 8/1998 (Copenhagen: Copenhagen Peace Research Institute, 1998).

2. Molander, Johan: 'The United Nations and the Elimination of Iraq's Weapons of Mass Destruction: The Implementation of a Cease-Fire Condition', in Fred Tanner (ed.): *From Versailles to Baghdad: Post-War Armament Control of Defeated States* (Geneva: UNIDIR, 1992), pp. 137-158; Sur, Serge (ed.): *Disarmament and Arms Limitation Obligations. Problems of Compliance and Enforcement* (Aldershot: Dartmouth, 1994), pp. 63-80; Weller, M. (ed.): *Iraq and Kuwait: The Hostilities and their Aftermath.* Cambridge International Documents, vol. 3 (Cambridge: Grotius Publications, 1993), pp. 8-12, 494-536.

3. For a personal account by the chief UNSCOM inspector see Ritter, Scott: *Endgame. Solving the Iraq Problem—Once and for All* (New York: Simon & Schuster, 1999).

4. Lippman, Thomas W. & Barton Gellman: 'U.S. Says It Collected Iraq Intelligence Via UNSCOM', *Washington Post* (8 January 1999).

5. For an otherwise quite 'permissive' (Israeli) interpretation of the Charter to the same effect see Dinstein, Yoram: *War, Aggression and Self-Defence*. Second Edition (Cambridge: Grotius Publications, 1994), pp. 83-97.

6. For an elaborate analysis of all the resolutions see White, Nigel: 'The Legality of the Threat of Force against Iraq', *Security Dialogue*, vol. 30, no. 1 (March 1999), pp. 75-86.

7. Sohn, Louis B.: 'The UN System as Authoritative Interpreter of Its Law', in Oscar Schachter & Christopher C. Joyner (eds.): *United Nations Legal Order*, Vols. 1-2 (American Society for International Law and Cambridge: Grotius Publications, 1995), vol. 1, pp. 169-230.

8. *CNN* (17 December 1998).

9. *Public Law 105-338*, 105th Congress, sections 3 and 4.a.2.

10. Murphy, John F.: 'Force and Arms', in Schachter & Joyner: *op. cit.* (note 7), pp. 247-317, especially pp. 251-265 and 277-292 (quotation from p. 248).

11. See, e.g., the chapter on 'Supreme Emergency' in Walzer, Michael: *Just and Unjust Wars. A Moral Argument with Historical Illustrations* (New York: Basic Books, 1977), pp. 251-268.

12. On biological weapons and warfare see, for instance, Dando, Malcolm: *Biological Warfare in the 21st Century* (London: Brassey's, 1994); Lederberg, Joshua (ed.): *Biological Weapons. Limiting the Threat* (Cambridge, MA: MIT Press, 1999).

13. Geissler, Erhard & John P. Woodall (eds.): *Control of Dual-Threat Agents: The Vaccines for Peace Programme*. SIPRI Chemical and Biological Warfare Studies, no. 15 (Oxford: Oxford University Press, 1994).

14. Geissler, Erhard: 'Implications of Genetic Engineering for Chemical and Biological Warfare', *SIPRI Yearbook 1984*, pp. 421-454.

15. On compellence, see Schelling, Thomas C.: *The Strategy of Conflict* (Cambridge, MA: Harvard University Press, 1960), pp. 195-199; idem: *Arms and Influence* (New Haven: Yale University Press, 1966), pp. 69-91. On blackmail see Betts, Richard K.: *Nuclear Blackmail and Nuclear Balance* (Washington DC: The Brookings Institution, 1987).

16. Mazarr, Michael J.: *North Korea and the Bomb. A Case Study in Nonproliferation* (New York: St. Martin's Press, 1994); Sigal, Leon V.: *Disarming Strangers. Nuclear Diplomacy with North Korea* (Princeton, NJ: Princeton University Press, 1998); Reiss, Mitchell: *Bridled Ambitions. Why Countries Constrain Their Nuclear Capabilities* (Washington, DC: Woodrow Wilson Center Press, 1995), pp. 231-319; Kihl, Young Whan: 'Confrontation or Compromise? Lessons from the 1994 Crisis', in idem & Peter Hayes (eds.): *Peace and Security in Northeast Asia. The Nuclear Issue and the Korean Peninsula* (Armonk, NY: M.E. Sharpe, 1997), pp. 181-204.

17. Price, Richard M.: *The Chemical Weapons Taboo* (Ithaca: Cornell University Press, 1997).

18. Proponents of such a strategy include Betts, Richard K.: 'The New Threat of Weapons of Mass Destruction', *Foreign Affairs*, vol. 77, no. 1 (Jan-Feb. 1998), pp. 26-41; Gompert, David, Kenneth Watman & Dean Wilkening: 'Nuclear First Use Revisited', *Survival*, vol. 37, no. 3 (Autumn 1995), pp. 27-44. For an argument against this see Sagan, Scott D.: 'The Commitment Trap: Why the United States Should Not Use Nuclear Threats to Deter Biological and Chemical Weapons Attacks', *International Security*, vol. 24, no. 4 (Spring 2000), pp. 85-115.

19. On Israel's nuclear weapons see Evron, Yair: *Israel's Nuclear Dilemma* (London: Routledge, 1994); Shahak, Israel: *Open Secrets. Israeli Foreign and Nuclear Policies* (London: Pluto Press, 1997); Cohen, Avner: *Israel and the Bomb* (New York: Columbia University Press, 1998).

20. See, for instance, Prawitz, Jan & Jim Leonard: *A Zone Free of Weapons of Mass Destruction in the Middle East* (Geneva: UNIDIR, 1996).

21. Press briefing by Army Gen. Hugh Shelton, *American Forces Press Service* (6 January 1999).

22. Both quotations are from the CNN's homepage.

23. Schneider, Barry R.: *Future War and Counterproliferation. U.S. Military Responses to NBC Proliferation Threats* (Westport, CT: Praeger, 1999), pp. 151-153.

24. 'Turkey Reportedly Criticizes some U.S. Strikes in Iraq', *CNN Interactive* (29 January 1999); 'US Warns Iraq against Attacks', *BBC Online Network* (16 February 1999).

25. The most systematic analysis of this is the herostratically famous 44-rung 'escalation ladder', developed by Kahn, Herman: *On Escalation. Metaphors and Scenarios* (London: Pall Mall Press, 1965), pp. 50-51, 194-195.

26. Gibson, James William: *The Perfect War. The War We Couldn't Lose and How We Did.* (New York: Vintage Books, 1988); Clodfelter, Mark: *The Limits of Air Power. The American Bombing of North Vietnam* (New York: The Free Press, 1989); Pape, Robert A.: *Bombing to Win: Air Power and Coercion in War* (Ithaca: Cornell University Press, 1996).

27. Daalder, Ivo H. & Michael E. O'Hanlon: *Winning Ugly. NATO's War to Save Kosovo* (Washington, DC: Brookings Institution Press, 2000), pp. 101-136 *& passim*; Byman, Daniel A. & Matthew C. Waxman: 'Kosovo and the Great Air Power Debate', *International Security*, vol. 24, no. 4 (Spring 2000), pp. 5-38.

28. Dowdy, William L. & Barry R. Schneider: 'On to Baghdad? Or Stop at Kuwait? A Gulf War Question Revisited', *Defense Analysis*, vol. 13, no. 3 (December 1997), pp. 319-327.

29. It would, for instance, constitute a breach of the above-mentioned *Declaration of the Inadmissibility of Intervention.* See Murphy: *loc. cit.* (note 10), pp. 248.

30. Baratta, Joseph Preston: 'The Kellogg-Briand Pact and the Outlawry of War', in Richard Dean Burns (ed.): *Encyclopedia of Arms Control and Disarmament*, vols. I-III (New York: Charles Scribner's Sons, 1993), vol. II, pp. 695-705.

31. Huntington, Samuel: 'The Clash of Civilizations', *Foreign Affairs*, vol. 72, no. 3 (Summer 1993), pp. 22-49; idem: *The Clash of Civilizations and the Remaking of World Order* (New York: Simon & Schuster, 1996), especially pp. 328-331. On Middle Eastern perceptions of the West see Fuller, Graham E. & Ian O. Lessler: *A Sense of Siege. The Geopolitics of Islam and the West* (Boulder, CO: Westview, 1995), pp. 27-46.

32. Huntington, Samuel P.: 'The Lonely Superpower', *Foreign Affairs*, vol. 78, no. 2 (March-April 1999), pp. 35-49.

33. 'Arab Deputies Condemn Air Strikes', *BBC Online Network* (27 December 1998); 'Arab League, Egypt Stress Iraq's Territorial Unity', *CNN Interactive* (26 January 1999).

34. On the fragility of the 'social contract' in the GCC countries see Gary G. Sick: 'The Coming Crisis in the Persian Gulf', in idem & Lawrence Potter (eds.): *The Persian Gulf at the Millennium. Essays in Politics, Economy, Security, and Religion* (New York: St. Martin's Press, 1997), pp. 11-30; Mottahedeh, Roy P. & Mamoun Fandy: 'The Islamic Movement: The Case for

Democratic Inclusion', *ibid.*, 297-318; Long, David: 'Revolutionary Islamism and Gulf Security in the Twenty-first Century', in idem & Christian Koch (eds.): *Gulf Security in the Twenty-First Century* (Abu Dhabi: Emirates Center for Strategic Studies and Research, 1997), pp. 121-132.

35. A good analysis of the rise and fall of pan-Arabism is Sela, Avraham: *The Decline of the Arab-Israeli Conflict: Middle East Politics and the Quest for Regional Order* (Albany, NY: State University of New York Press, 1997). See also Barnett, Michael N.: *Dialogues in Arab Politics: Negotiations in Regional Order* (New York: Columbia University Press, 1998).

36. See, for instance, Entessar, Nader: *Kurdish Ethnonationalism* (Boulder, CO: Lynne Rienner, 1992).

37. On unipolarity see Layne, Christopher: 'The Unipolar Illusion: Why New Great Powers Will Rise', *International Security*, vol. 17, no. 4 (Spring 1993), pp. 5-51; Mastanduno, Michael: 'Preserving the Unipolar Moment. Realist Theories and U.S. Grand Strategy after the Cold War', *ibid.*, vol. 21, no. 4 (Spring 1997), pp. 49-88; Kupchan, Charles A.: 'After Pax Americana. Benign Power, Regional Integration, and the Sources of Stable Multipolarity', *ibid.*, vol. 23, no. 2 (Fall 1998), pp. 40-79. For a more optimistic assessment see Kapstein, Ethan B. & Michael Mastanduno (eds.): *Unipolar Politics. Realism and State Strategies after the Cold War* (New York: Columbia University Press, 1999).

38. Thucydides: *The Peloponnesian War* (Harmondsworth: Penguin, 1972), p. 402.

39. On world order discourses see Williams, Andrew: *Failed Imagination? New World Orders of the Twentieth Century* (Manchester: Manchester University Press, 1998); Knutsen, Torbjørn L.: *The Rise and Fall of World Orders* (Manchester: Manchester University Press, 1999).

40. Quoted from *Keesing's Contemporary Archives*, vol. 36, art. 37694A.

41. Quoted from Weller: *op. cit.* (note 2), pp. 281-283.

42. http://www.whitehouse.gov/WH/EOP/NSC/html/documents/nssr.pdf.

43. Campbell, David: *Politics Without Principle. Sovereignty, Ethics, and the Narratives of the Gulf War* (Boulder, CO: Lynne Rienner, 1994). Comparable analyses of the war against Iraq include Baudrillard, Jean: *The Gulf War Did Not Take Place* (Bloomington: Indiana University Press, 1995); Norris, Christopher: *Uncritical Theory. Postmodernism, Intellectuals, and the Gulf War* (Amherst: University of Massachusetts Press, 1992); Der Derian, James: *Antidiplomacy. Spies, Terror, Speed and War* (Oxford: Polity Press, 1992), pp. 173-202. On discourse analysis see also Campbell, David: *Writing Security. United States Foreign Policy and the Politics of Identity*. Revised Edition (Manchester: Manchester University Press, 1998), *passim*; George, Jim: *Discourses of Global Politics: A Critical (Re)Introduction to International Relations* (Boulder, CO: Lynne Rienner, 1994), pp. 29-34; Jabri, Vivienne: *Discourses on Violence: Conflict Analysis Reconsidered* (Manchester: Manchester University Press, 1996); Wæver, Ole: *Concepts of Security*

(Copenhagen: Institute of Political Science, University of Copenhagen, 1997), pp. 1-25 & *passim*. An interesting application of discourse analysis to Iraq is Bengio, Ofra: *Saddam's Word. The PoliticalDiscoursein Iraq* (Oxford: Oxford University Press, 1998). For an analysis of the discourse of Pan-Arabism see Barnett: *op. cit.* (note 36).

44. Festinger, Leon: *A Theory of Cognitive Dissonance* (Stanford: Stanford University Press, 1957); Jervis, Robert: *Perceptionand Misperception in InternationalPolitics* (Princeton, NJ: Princeton University Press, 1976), pp. 117-202, 382-406; Lebow, Richard Ned: *Between Peace and War. The Nature of International Crisis* (Baltimore: John Hopkins University Press, 1981), pp. 101-147.

45. Fiebig-von-Hase, Ragnhild: 'Introduction', in ida & Ursula Lehmkuhl (eds.): *Enemy Images in American History* (Oxford: Berghahn Books, 1997), pp. 1-40; Spillmann, Kurt R. & Kati Spillmann: 'Some Sociobiological and Psychological Aspects of "Images of the Enemy"', *ibid.*, pp. 43-64; Beck, Ulrich: 'The Sociological Anatomy of Enemy Images: The Military and Democracy after the End of the Cold War', *ibid.* 65-87; Shimko, Keith L.: *Images and Arms Control. Perceptions of the Soviet Union in the Reagan Administration*(Ann Arbor: University of Michigan Press, 1991), pp. 11-41; Fischer, Ronald J.: *The Social Psychology of Intergroup and International Conflict Resolution*(New York: Springer Verlag, 1990), pp. 39-57. See also Hermann, Richard K. & Michael P. Fischerkeller: 'Beyond the Enemy Image and Spriral Model: Cognitive-Strategic Research after the Cold War', *International Organization*, vol. 49, no. 3 (Summer 1995), pp. 415-450; Rojo, Luisa Martin: 'Division and Rejection: From the Personification of the Gulf Conflict to the Demonization of Saddam Hussein', *Discourseand Society*, vol. 6, no. 1 (January 1995), pp. 49-80.

46. See, for instance, Makiya, Kanan: *Republic of Fear. The Politics of Modern Iraq* (Berkeley, CA: University of California Press, 1998).

47. Janis, Irving: *Victims of Groupthink* (Boston: Houghton Mifflin, 1972); Fischer: *op. cit.* (note 46), pp. 68-74.

48. Jervis: *op. cit.* (note 45), pp. 32-57, 343-355.

49. Glad, Betty & Charles S. Taber: 'Images, Learning, and the Decision to Use Force: The Domino Theory of the United States', in Betty Glad (ed.): *Psychological Dimensions of War* (London: Sage, 1990), pp. 56-81.

50. Heuser, Beatrice & Cyril Buffet: 'Conclusions. Historical Myths and the Denial of Change', in Cyril Buffet & Beatrice Heuser (eds.): *Haunted by History. Myths in International Relations*(Oxford: Berghan Books, 1998), pp. 259-274, quotations from 265-266, 272.

51. Klare, Michael: *Rogue States and Nuclear Outlaws. America's Search for a New Foreign Policy*(New York: Hill and Wang, 1995). See also Goldman, Emily O.: 'Thinking About Strategy Absent the Enemy', *Security Studies*, vol. 4, no. 1 (Autumn 1994), pp. 40-85. For an attempt at planning without a stipulated enemy see Davis, Paul: 'Planning Under Uncertainty Then and Now: Paradigms Lost and Paradigms Emerging', in idem (ed.): *New*

Challenges for Defense Planning. Rethinking How Much is Enough (Santa Monica, CA: RAND, 1994), pp. 15-58; Khalilzad, Zalmay M. & David A. Ochmanek (eds.): *Strategy and Defense Planning for the 21st Century* (Santa Monica, CA: Rand, 1997). On the MIC see Pursell, Carroll W. Jr. (ed.): *The Military Industrial Complex* (New York: Harper & Row, 1972); Barnett, Richard: *The Economy of Death. A Hard Look at the Defense Budget, the Military Industrial Complex, and What You Can Do About Them* (New York: Atheneum, 1970); Senghaas, Dieter: *Rüstung und Militarismus* (Frankfurt, Suhrkamp Verlag, 1972). For a critique see Sarkesian, Sam C. (ed.): *The Military-Industrial Complex. A Reassessment* (Beverly Hills: Sage, 1972).

52. Taylor, Philip M.: *War and the Media. Propaganda and Persuasion in the Gulf War.* 2nd edition (Manchester: Manchester University Press, 1998); Hayward, Malcolm: 'The Making of the New World Order: The Role of the Media', in Tareq Y. Ismael & Jacqueline S. Ismael (eds.): *The Gulf War and the New World Order: International Relations in the Middle East* (Gainesville: University Press of Florida, 1994), pp. 224-242; Parasitil, Andrew T.: 'Defeating the Vietnam Syndrome: The Military, the Media, and the Gulf War', *ibid.*, pp. 242-262; Manheim, Jarol B.: 'The War of Images: Strategic Communication in the Gulf Conflict', in Stanley A. Renshon (ed.): *The Political Psychology of the Gulf War. Leaders, Publics, and the Process of Conflict* (Pittsburgh: University of Pittsburgh Press, 1993), pp. 155-171; Mueller, John: 'American Public Opinion and the Gulf War', *ibid.*, pp. 199-226.

53. Chuter, David: 'Munich, or the Blood of Others', in Buffett & Heuser (eds.): *op. cit.* (note 51), pp. 65-79.

54. An example is the testimony of Under Secretary of Defense for Policy Walter B. Slocombe, speaking before the Senate Armed Services Committee January 29. He used the expression 'the sanctions, the no-fly zones in the north and south, and the no-reinforcement zone in the south—which *were placed* upon Iraq pursuant to resolutions of the Security Council'. In actual fact only the sanctions were mandated by the UN.

55. Baudrillard: *op. cit.* (note 44), p. 26. See also Gelven, Michael: *War and Existence. A Philosophical Inquiry* (University Park, Pennsylvania: Penn State Press, 1994), pp. 116-124. On the lack of heroism see Luttwak, Edward N.: 'A Post-Heroic Military Policy', *Foreign Affairs*, vol. 75, no. 4 (July-August 1996), pp. 33-44; Gentry, John A.: 'Military Force in an Age of National Cowardice', *The Washington Quarterly*, vol. 21, no. 4 (Autumn 1998), pp. 179-191.

56. Clausewitz, Carl von: *On War*, edited and translated by Michael Howard and Peter Paret (Princeton, NJ: Princeton University Press, 1984), p. 357 (Book VI.1.1.). See also Gat, Azar: 'Clausewitz on Defence and Attack', *Journal of Strategic Studies*, vol. 11, no. 1 (1988), pp. 20-26.

57. *USIA Security Affairs* (25 January 1999).

58. *American Forces Press Service* (26 January 1999) confirmed that 'A U.S. missile fired at an Iraqi radar site Jan. 25 went astray and exploded in a residential neighbourhood near the city of Basra in southern Iraq', justifying it with the explanation that 'At the time, U.S. forces were responding to provocative attacks against coalition aircraft by targeting elements of Saddam Hussein's air defense system'. Pentagon spokesman Ken Bacon added that 'Coalition forces take every step possible to avoid targeting civilians or creating collateral damage. ... We are not attacking the people of Iraq. We have no animus against them whatsoever. In fact, we have a lot of sympathy for the people of Iraq. But we are attacking a large air defense system being used in an attempt to defeat the policing of the no-fly zones.'

59. Major studies include Hufbauer, Gary Clyde, Jeffrey J. Schott & Kimberly Ann Elliott: *Economic Sanctions Reconsidered. History and Current Policy*, 2nd edition, vols. 1-2 (Washington, DC: Institute for International Economics, 1990); Cortright, David (ed.): *The Price of Peace. Incentives and International Conflict Prevention* (Lanham, Maryland: Rowman & Littlefield, 1997); idem & George A. Lopez (eds.): *Economic Sanctions. Panacea or Peacebuilding in a Post-Cold War World?* (Boulder, CO: Westview, 1995); Preeg, Ernest H.: *Feeling Good or Doing Good with Sanctions. Unilateral Economic Sanctions and the U.S. National Interest* (Washington, DC: CSIS Press, 1999); Simons, Geoff: *Imposing Economic Sanctions. Legal Remedy or Genocidal Tool?* (London: Pluto Press, 1999). See also Mansfield, Edward D.: 'International Institutions and Economic Sanctions', *World Politics*, vol. 47, no. 4 (July 1995), pp. 575-605; Mueller, John & Karl Mueller: 'Sanctions of Mass Destruction', *Foreign Affairs*, vol. 78, no. 3 (May-June 1999), pp. 43-53; Boudreau, Donald G.: 'Economic Sanctions and Military Force in the Twenty-First Century', *European Security*, vol. 6, no. 2 (Summer 1997), pp. 28-46; Pape, Robert A.: 'Why Economic Sanctions Do Not Work', *International Security*, vol. 22, no. 2 (Fall 1997), pp. 90-136; idem: 'Why Economic Sanctions *Still* Do Not Work', *ibid.*, vol. 23, no. 1 (Summer 1998), pp. 66-77; Elliott, Kimberly Ann: 'The Sanctions Glass: Half Full or Completely Empty', *ibid.*, pp. 50-65; Baldwin, David A.: 'The Sanctions Debate and the Logic of Choice', *ibid.*, vol. 24, no. 3 (Winter 1999/2000), pp. 80-107; Rogers, Elizabeth S.: 'Using Economic Sanctions to Control Regional Conflicts', *Security Studies*, vol. 5, no. 4 (Summer 1996), pp. 43-72; Kirshner, Jonathan: 'The Microfoundations of Economic Sanctions', *ibid.*, vol. 6, no. 3 (Spring 1997), pp. 32-64; Lavin, Franklin L.: 'Asphyxiation or Oxygen? The Sanctions Dilemma', *Foreign Policy*, vol. 104 (Fall 1996), pp. 139-153; Weiss, Thomas G.: 'Sanctions as a Foreign Policy Tool: Weighing Humanitarian Impulses', *Journal of Peace Research*, vol. 36, no. 5 (September 1999), pp. 499-510.

60. 'Situation Analysis of Children and Women in Iraq', *UNICEF Report*, 30 April 1998, extracts available at http://leb.net/iac/UNICEF1998.html. For additional documentation see Graham-Brown, Sarah: *Sanctioning Saddam. The Politics of Intervention in Iraq* (London: I.B. Tauris, 1999); Arnove, Anthony (ed.): *Iraq under Siege. The Deadly Impact of Sanctions and War*

(London: Pluto Press, 2000).

61. Gaddis, John Lewis: *Strategies of Containment. A Critical Appraisal of Postwar American National Security Policy* (New York: Oxford University Press, 1982), *passim*; Kennan, George F.: 'Reflexions on Containment', in Terry L. Deibel & John Lewis Gaddis (eds.): *Containing the Soviet Union. A Critique of US Policy* (London: Pergamon-Brassey's, 1987), pp. 15-19; idem: 'Containment Then and Now', *Foreign Affairs*, vol. 66, no. 2 (Spring 1987), pp. 885-890; Mayers, David: 'Containment and the Primacy of Diplomacy: George Kennan's Views, 1947-1948', *International Security*, vol. 11, no. 1 (Summer 1986), pp. 124-162.

62. On the general logic see George, Alexander L.: 'Superpower Interests in Third Areas', in Roy Allison & Phil Williams (eds.): *Superpower Competition and Crisis Prevention in the Third World* (Cambridge: Cambridge University Press, 1990), pp. 107-120. For a critique see Hopf, Ted: *Peripheral Visions. Deterrence Theory and American Foreign Policy in the Third World, 1965-1990* (Ann Arbor: University of Michigan Press, 1994).

63. Corke, Sarah-Jane: 'Bridging the Gap: Containment, Covert Action and the Search for the Missing Link in American Cold War Policy, 1948-1953', *The Journal of Strategic Studies*, vol. 20, no. 4 (December 1997), pp. 45-65.

64. On the Korean War (where the 38th parallel and the Yalu River signified the dividing between containment and roll-back, in the strict and more 'liberal' sense, respectively) see Whelan, Richard: *Drawing the Line. The Korean War, 1950-1953* (Boston: Little, Brown & Co., 1990), pp. 217-240; Gaddis: *op. cit.* (note 61), pp. 89-126. On the Reagan Administration see Posen, Barry R. & Stephen Van Evera: 'Defense Policy and the Reagan Administration: Departure from Containment', *International Security*, vol. 8, no. 1 (Summer 1983), pp. 3-45.

65. See, for instance, Lynch, Allen: *The Cold War is Over—Again* (Boulder, CO: Westview, 1992); George, Alexander L., Philip J. Farley & Alexander Dallin (eds.): *U.S.—Soviet Security Cooperation. Achievements, Failures, Lessons* (New York: Oxford University Press, 1988), *passim*; Kanet, Roger E. & Edward A. Kolodziej (eds.): *The Cold War as Competition. Superpower Cooperation in Regional Conflict Management* (Baltimore: John Hopkins University Press, 1991), *passim*. For a theoretical perspective see Milner, Helen: 'Review Article: International Theories of Cooperation Among Nations: Strengths and Weaknesses', *World Politics*, vol. 44, no. 3 (April 1992), pp. 466-496; Miller, Benjamin: *When Opponents Cooperate. Great Power Conflicts and Collaboration in World Politics* (Ann Arbor: University of Michigan Press, 1995).

66. Byman, Daniel, Kenneth Pollack & Gideon Rose: 'The Rollback Fantasy', *Foreign Affairs*, vol. 78, no. 1 (Jan-Feb. 1999), pp. 24-41.

67. Figures from *World Military Expenditures and Arms Transfers 1998* (Washington, DC: U.S. Department of State, Bureau of Verification and Compliance, 2000), pp. 61, 109.

8 INTERVENTION, SOVEREIGNTY AND IRAQ

Absorbing and Deflecting the Blows

Anthony McDermott

Introduction

Historically, the Middle East can lay claim to the title of having been the target of more interventions and outside attentions than any other region. Internally, the region has not been at one with itself. Countries have invaded neighbours and interfered in each other's internal affairs. A variety of features and interests—ranging from religion and race to geography and natural resources—have all left their mark on the area broadly and loosely defined as the Middle East and made it attractive to outsiders. A comprehensive identification of local modern attitudes towards intervention (whether on the level of governments, popular opinion, traditional attitudes or groupings of a nongovernmental origin) becomes something of an adventure. It is also, in the course of a single chapter, an unattainable task, if the objective is to be all embracing.

This chapter examines one singular case that raises the issue of intervention: Iraq during the crisis between November 1997 and February 1998 over UNSCOM, the UN's special commission with the job of stripping Iraq of its weapons of mass destruction. In the period under study, direct military intervention of the order of magnitude seen at the end of 1998 did not take place, although other pressures were brought to bear from the outside. Iraq's sovereignty had for some years already been breached and interventions effected to the extent that no-fly zones were being enforced in the northern and southern parts of the country. Economic sanctions had been in operation.

That new, direct intervention did not occur at the turn of the 1997/98 year nevertheless aroused reactions which shed light on local attitudes towards intervention and which continue to hold true. They also sustained Iraq and Saddam Hussein, the president, through the US and UK air raids of December 1998.

Iraq is firmly part of the Middle East, predominantly Arab and Muslim, and run by an undemocratic military-dominated government, personified by Saddam Hussein, a dictator almost *nonpareil*. Its

geographical position at the head of the Gulf brings regional special security implications connected with the stability of the regime. This chapter does not address in detail those aspects, which have been examined elsewhere.[1]

The Importance of the Middle East

Under this rubric, this excursion sets out to avoid some of the familiar paths regarding why outside states or organisations find the Middle East worth trying to get into, stay in or just pass through. In the last half-century, four factors in particular have had a deep influence on the nature of regional intervention: the creation of Israel, the presence of the United States, the Cold War and its aftermath, and Arab nationalism. George Lenczowski, in his review of US relations with the Middle East during the presidencies from Truman to Reagan, wrote that

> Eisenhower realised that this was the arena of great confrontations of the mid-twentieth century: Communist imperialism vs. Western democracy, emerging nations of Afro-Asia vs. old colonialism, and Arab vs. Israeli nationalism. He viewed these confrontations as 'a constant test to the United States will, principle, patience, and resolve.'[2]

For the US, the focus of its concern in the past was on the Soviet challenge, the role of oil and the Arab–Israeli feud. All three issues might have provoked direct US military intervention. Since the end of the last decade, the Soviet challenge in Cold War terms has disappeared. Other, different interventional targets—mainly in connection with Iraq (and here the Kurds are included)—have emerged. There has always been a deeply political and global dimension to outside interests and interference.

This factor has tended to colour even ostensibly local disputes. Israel, which has frequently resorted to military intervention, still has outstanding political, territorial, refugee and economic disputes with all its neighbours, except perhaps Egypt. Iraq has territorial and religious disputes and contests over resources with Syria, Kuwait, Iran and Turkey. Iran, after Israel and Turkey the most influential non-Arab state in the area, has territorial disputes in the Gulf and has long been seen as a threat to regional stability through its support of religious Shi'ite fundamentalism. In a broader definition of the Middle East, border and territorial disputes persist as far apart as the Arabian Peninsula and the Maghreb. The brutal disputes of the Algerian (and Turkish) governments with their religious and ethnic minority opponents are a constant focus of outside attention, prompting questions

of intervention.

At stake is the issue of when there is a confluence or conflict of interests. It has to be decided whether any intervention has come about with the dominant motivation of economic, humanitarian or social benefits. Or are they all just motivated by political, external self-interest? Above all, can intervention be effective?

An almost cursory list later should provide sufficient evidence of the reasons why states and organisations have chosen countries of the Middle East as their targets. A random selection of the varieties of cases where Arab countries have been involved in intervention of one sort or another makes clear the difficulties of where any analysis can or should begin. They may give some answers to the questions of the nature of intervention in this region. The Suez campaign of 1956, involving Britain, France and Israel, can still today stir memories of old-fashioned imperialist and colonialist invasion for the re-establishment, in part, of political rights and economic interests of an empire lost. The Algerian war of independence against France, 1954–62, was both a brutal reminder of this and the forerunner of this decade's internal civil wars there.

A decade or so later, the UN-backed allied victory over Iraq (and this involved some Arab states) in the Gulf War of 1990–91 after the Iraqi invasion and conquest of Kuwait in August 1990 was reckoned to have been a successful intervention, judged against some limited and short-term objectives. The violation of sovereignty (and of Arab solidarity) was punished and the *status quo ante* affecting Kuwait restored. It might well turn out to have been one of the last set piece, traditional wars fought in this century.

Linked to this war, the humanitarian intervention on behalf of the Kurds in 1991 in northern Iraq through Operation Provide Comfort is believed by some to have been a rare success, if only in the short term.[3] Elsewhere, the sovereignty of Lebanon has been violated most conspicuously by Israeli invasions twice since the 1980s, and parts of that country remain under Israeli and Syrian tutelage today. The Israeli–Palestinian relationship over the years of competing nationalisms to establish a state resists any easy analysis about intervention, its causes and its interpretations.

All of these had some influence on the understanding of the nature of intervention. As we have seen, intervention itself is no new operation or activity. It has taken many forms in the Middle East and has been largely inspired neither by altruism nor humanitarian motives. The Bible, Crusaders and Ottomans have provided only a few of the accounts of intrusions and incursions. These traditions were carried in

later centuries mainly by British and French colonialists and imperialists and latterly by the Zionists and the US. The Cold War was played out here, too.[4]

Globalization has reinforced and made more pressing the vast, varied and interlinked interests at stake, which need not necessarily be connected to military intervention: oil and gas, downstream industrial activities, pipelines, water supplies and the environment; shipping lanes, canals and roads; banking and finance, debts, investment and trade; internal political behaviour, democracy and human rights; and geographical strategic positions, arms, both conventional and unconventional, regional political dominance and security.

Globalization has also notably undermined the state's control over its own resources. But this was not a new phenomenon, as foreign companies and governments had already exploited these resources. Any one of these listed factors alone could justify some of the reasons for intervention on one level. At the same time, the writing of Western guides to sovereignty and intervention has long stopped being a mere cottage industry; it has become an established way of life. This chapter attempts to provide one contemporary experience to complement those analyses.

The choice of Iraq as an example of a victim of intervention may at first seem wayward, since at the time under study no intrusive international intervention actually took place, although in Iraq's case the US, supported by some allies, appeared on the brink of doing so.[5] Iraq is not geographically on the front-line of what used to be known broadly as the Arab–Israeli conflict. Arab nationalism and, by inference, sovereignty shows itself in a particular forms. In Iraq's case, nationalism is outward looking, calling for support from fellow Arabs. Iraq has tried to broaden its cause to involve pan-Arab and international issues. In this the use of the Arabic language has been crucial to Saddam's ability to stay in power and gather regional support.

Although intervention and direct intrusion from outside did *not* take place on a new scale, the threat and discussion of it, whether in Europe or the UN, were sufficient to trigger revealing and informative reactions in Iraq. To a certain extent, this local reaction, backed by some limited echoes in the rest of the Arab world helped prevent intervention. Saddam was able to exploit to some degree the frustration sensed by the lack of progress in negotiations between Israel and the Palestinians and what the Arabs saw as Washington's lack of evenhandness in the peace process.

The particular case of Iraq neither confounds nor confirms

comprehensive or established theories of intervention and sovereignty. The aim of this chapter is to provide through analytical narrative a view of how complex and varied the region of the Middle East is, even if one of its components is deliberately selected as a singular example. The emphasis and focus is on local Arab reactions and interpretations. Some non-Arab examples and attitudes—such as through Israel, Iran and Turkey—appear and provide regional points of comparison and allusions to alternative perspectives to concepts of nationalism, secularism and sovereignty. In particular, these three countries stand as reminders that the Arabs do not have a complete hold on nationalism in the region. After the Shah's departure in January 1979 and until the eight-year war with Iraq, Iran became something of a passing hero in the Arab world by undermining US credibility in the whole region. Some Arab nationalist quarters appeared to be favourably impressed and pleased by the Islamic revivalism that the revolution was said to inaugurate.[6]

Though the dependence here is largely on secondary sources, it should also become clear how the internal and external constituencies to these crises have reacted and interacted. It would be hard to deduce that any conclusions drawn from the case under study could have immediate general lessons for application elsewhere, except in the broadest sense and as a guide to what defiant leadership can achieve as with President Milosevic in Yugoslavia. Saddam's defiance could have implications for security in the Gulf region.

The situation of nexus and tension between intervention and sovereignty (and this is based on the assumption that the two involve each other) has found its way into the Arabic language. This in turn reveals a gap in understanding between East and West of these concepts. In addition, language is, in the Iraqi case, an important factor. Arabic is both one regional political and cultural unifying element and a contentious issue both within predominantly Arab countries and for non-Arab countries, as the notions of Pan-Arabism and nationalism revolve around it. Native academic speakers and writers have absorbed concepts of sovereignty and often invented political and scientific terms in Arabic which can distract attention away from the way local inhabitants express their views on such issues and react. Outsiders, mainly from the West, betray traces of surprise that local rulers and states do not share some of these largely Western concepts and interpretations. Language is only part of the problem.

The UN's role in the area has lasted longer than in any other part of the world, going back to involvement in Palestine in 1947 and, for example, the establishment of Mixed Armistice Commissions between

Israel and Egypt, Jordan, Lebanon and Syria.[7] The UN has been called upon to engage in political mediation, conflict resolution, peacekeeping, the monitoring of human rights violations and humanitarian relief activities. The acronyms give most of the picture: UNSCOP (for Palestine), UNTSO (Middle East observers), UNEF I & II (Egypt/Israel), UNOGIL (Lebanon), UNYOM (Yemen), UNDOF (Israel/Syria), UNIFIL (south Lebanon), UNIIMOG (Iran/Iraq), MINURSO (Western Sahara), UNIKOM (Iraq/Kuwait), and UNRWA and UNHCR (development and refugees).[8]

All involved a measure of some form of intervention, sponsored by the UN, and all trespassed on sovereignty to varying degrees. They were there to cover and prevent the full gamut of human behaviour in wars and afterwards. The UN, through these different operations and debates and votes in the General Assembly, may well have worked broadly to the benefit of the Arab states in resolutions, and in action more particularly in its humanitarian services than through its political policies.[9] (There are some notable exceptions. Iraq might not share that view, given the Security Council resolutions imposing economic sanctions). Nevertheless, the Arabs have viewed the UN with considerable suspicion, particularly in the UN Security Council.[10]

For example, although the states of the Middle Eastern region may be members of the UN—the world's largest intergovernmental organisation and deeply involved in the Middle East from the beginning of its existence—and may, to varying degrees, also value the activities of nongovernmental organisations (NGOs), countries differ greatly in their ideas of what NGOs may be doing or think they are entitled to do on their own territory. They are seen in some Arab countries as an affront to the authority of the local governments. There is a clash here of conceptual approaches to common problems and interpretations. One organisation's humanitarian contribution and intervention may be seen as another state's intrusion or violation. This often applies to the UN and NGOs alike.[11] Contrary and sometimes undemocratic (in a Western sense) as some of these ideas might seem, they deserve a hearing and, ultimately, have to be taken account of in any form of intervention.

Where and What Is the Middle East?

If left to his own devices, this writer would settle for the term The Levant, for it has a convenient romanticism which ignores grimmer realities of Arabia, once known as *deserta*.[12] Geographically, it should be remembered, what the West calls the Middle East is for others, from the different perspective of the Far East, sometimes West Asia. The

UN, for example, has no separate regionally classified grouping for the Middle East, although Arab voting as a bloc in the General Assembly is, unsurprisingly and generally, united.[13]

Seen from another geographical aspect and as a different approach to resolving the Arab–Israeli conflict as a whole, under the influence of the European Union and its interests, and the round of Middle East peace negotiations started by the Madrid conference of November 1991, there were deliberate efforts to put perceptions of the area in a broader and more Mediterranean context.

The membership of regional organisations does not provide a complete guide. Although political developments affecting Sudan, Djibouti, Mauritania and Somalia are often put in an African context, these states have all been members of the Arab League for more than a decade. The Organisation of the Islamic Conference embraces a large clutch of nations outside 'The Middle East'. The dissolution of the Soviet Union extended one notion of the Middle East northwards towards the Muslim regions of the Caucasus (and renewed Russia's interest in disputes of the Arab–Israeli region). Its strategic position and copious oil and gas reserves have provided other solid material reasons for making it a focus of international attention. This 'Greater Middle East' is defined elsewhere in this volume, in the chapter by Gulshan Dietl. Geoffrey Kemp and Robert Harkavy have made a determined and detailed attempt to define the region and its importance. Looking ahead, they write expansively:

> We will be emphasising again and again the point that the Middle East (including the Caspian Basin region) has now assumed the role of the strategic high ground, a key strategic prize in the emerging global system at the juncture between the twentieth and twenty-first centuries.[14]

All point to the same conclusion: that the region of the Middle East, however it is defined in detail, will remain the focus of outside attention. Iraq is only one shard of the broader regional pottery—but a vital one in the Gulf.

The region is, furthermore, not ethnically uniform. The Kurds and Berbers are only two of the most easily identifiable of the area's many ethnic groups, which further complicate its definition. Under the broader heading of stateless peoples and minorities come the traditional numerical minorities such as the Christian, Jewish, Zoroastrian, Alawi, Druze and Baha'i communities, and majority populations which are powerless (Iraqi Shi'a and Syrian Sunnis) as well as minorities in power such as the Alawis in Syria and the Maronites in pre-civil war

Lebanon. There are the stateless peoples, such as the Kurds and the Palestinians in the West Bank and Gaza Strip. Israel's minority position, as a non-Arab state in a predominantly Arab Middle East, is of a special order.[15] Relevant here is the fact that the presence of these minorities have not only made more complicated the definition of the Middle East but also created tensions which have attracted outside attention and, often, military intervention on whatever pretext. Schultze et al. have observed that:

> The changing relationship between minorities, diasporas and majorities is bound up with the changing nature of the nation-state in the Middle East. The practices and cultures of nationalism that have dominated the Middle East over the last half century, based on the relative certainties of the anti-colonial struggle, and the inevitable victory of rational bureaucratic modernism, have collapsed. In place of the cold war structures which have defined and contained the experience of nationalism in the Middle East, 'structural adjustment', the emergence of new transnational blocs, anti-state Islamism, and political exclusion from 'fortress Europe' have rendered the whole idea of the nation-state problematic.[16]

These changed and changing circumstances raise questions about the sorts of entities a government plays host in or defends when intervention, sought or unsought, civilian or military, occurs.

Arab nationalism, as has been noted, has never been the exclusive preserve of Muslims, drawn on one single source of inspiration or adopted a uniform pattern. Single-party regimes emerged, almost entirely as a result of military action and patriotism, and the states linked to them were, with the difficult exception of the disputed territory of Israel/Palestine,[17] concentrated on areas drawn by colonial boundaries.[18] Royal family rule on the Arabian Peninsula and in Jordan and Morocco provides a pattern which runs against the trend elsewhere in the region. Borders and national sovereignty were disregarded when it came to trying to influence an Arab neighbour, and over the years this has taken the form of direct military intervention, assassinations, kidnappings, bombings, sabotage, newspaper and radio campaigns, and support for the political opponents of rival regimes.[19] Arab regimes have become, over the years, more durable with more state nationalism than region-wide Arab or even religious solidarity.[20] This would seem to be the case still today, with Egypt remaining the critical and central Arab state in the region. All this has taken place against the background, in this century, of the impact of modernisation

on national consciousness and the social, educational and political spheres of daily life.[21]

Illustration by Non-Intervention: Iraq's Stubbornness

Iraq is an authoritarian state ruled by a small, violent, ruthless Sunni minority faction. It has no modern tradition of legitimate representative government or of providing representation that reflects the ethnic and sectarian differences within its population. Iraq's politics are in general highly nationalistic and violent in character.[22]

The regime, normally equated with the rule of Saddam Hussein and complemented by an extreme example of the cult of personality, survived Iraq's defeat in the Gulf War and several years of post-war sanctions. Saddam has become isolated from many of his traditional supporters, but still he and his immediate coterie continue to rule through brutality, coercion, and military and political diversions and a regional paranoia of being encircled by hostile states on the Arabian Peninsula, and its neighbours Jordan, Syria, Iran and Turkey. Through continuous repression, the regime has managed to suppress almost all active dissent.[23] As one measure of the brutality of Saddam's regime, *The Observer* compiled a Human Rights Index of the world's states in which Iraq came eighth (and, among other Arab countries, Algeria came first, Libya fifth and Syria seventh).[24]

A description of Iraq's power structures is essential to understand Saddam's survival after eight years of war with Iran and the conflict with the international community during and after the Gulf War, and in 1997–98. It helps to explain why Saddam may survive several more years of UN sanctions and why it is so difficult to change the fundamental character of Iraq's regime.[25]

Saddam exerts control over a number of strong instruments of state power. At the centre lies the internal security structure with numerous agencies directly accountable to the president.[26] It could number up to 100,000 men and includes massive civil police forces, ruthless intelligence services and such paramilitary forces as the Republican Guard, the quite separate and vital Special Republican Guard[27] and Saddam's own bodyguards and elite security forces. In addition, these instruments include the Revolutionary Command Council (RCC), the Ba'ath party, the armed forces and important Sunni tribes. He depends, too, on a network of nepotism and personal patronage, surrounding himself with a closely controlled group of relatives and friends. These instruments help to preserve the regime and make it difficult for any rival other than another Sunni authoritarian elite to come to power.[28]

One key institution of the state is the Ba'ath party. Over the years, it has shifted from being a pan-Arab socialist party to an extension of the Iraqi ruling elite. Now, it functions basically as an arm of the regime in the administration of its policy.[29] Saddam made the Ba'ath party into a cover for Iraqi nationalism at the expense of pan-Arab nationalism. As part of an effort to unite Iraqis of all ethnic and sectarian backgrounds, he developed the idea and practice of a Mesopotamian and Iraqi identity that was both Arab and non-Arab, and Islamic and non-Islamic. He accelerated this trend during the 1980–88 Iran–Iraq war when he accused the Arab world of failing to support Iraq in the struggle against a 'hated' Persian enemy.[30] But since then, and notably during the 1997–98 crisis, he has reverted to invoking images of pan-Arab nationalism and its role in confronting the West, personified by the US and Israel. In these different approaches, the use of Arabic in official communiqués and rhetoric has been vital.[31] Saddam has made a fine art of using and controlling political discourse as one means of gathering and sustaining support in a country under perpetual domestic and external pressure.[32]

The armed forces are the largest instruments of government power and, at the top, highly politicised. They have also a long history of playing a violent role in Iraqi politics and have fought repeated civil wars against Iraq's Kurds and Shi'ites.[33]

One striking feature of the Iraqi method of rule, especially emphasised in the years after the Gulf War, is the increasing dependence on tribalism. Tribalism is a patriarchal, pyramidal structure of loyalty.[34] Within a tribal community, the loyalty follows the leader who emerges from within the community. The patrimonial leader's position is based on his ability to distribute tangible and concrete material rewards, on his control of instruments of the State and on a variety of personality characteristics such as charisma and ruthlessness that enable such a leader to maintain authority.[35]

The extraordinary feature of the period under review is the extent to which effective centres of opposition to Saddam's rule did not emerge. There was no apparent connection made (or allowed to be made publicly) between Iraq's plight and the strategies and policies of its ruler over the years.[36] The Iraqi media portrayed the people, not Saddam, as the target of the West's policies. Saddam's role was to defend the wider Arab cause in a context detached from the real causes and consequences of the conflict and crisis. Hostility was directed towards the US, Kuwait and Saudi Arabia—rather than the regime. Nevertheless, the centre feels a growing bitterness towards Saddam and the regime because of the steady erosion of Iraq's wealth and power.[37]

By some, he is now regarded as the man who reduced one of the Arab world's most prosperous and important countries to the status of an international pariah.[38] Ahmad S. Hashim described Saddam's policies as having transformed Iraq from a regional superpower to a regional 'superpauper'.[39]

Iraq, especially through the Ba'athist Arab socialist movement, has always yearned to be the leader of pan-Arabism. In modern decades, it has vied with Egypt (under Nasser) and Syria (another Ba'athist state) for this role. As a result, Iraq perversely almost wanted to bring about intervention, first because its sovereignty had already been battered by the Gulf War, no-fly zones, UN Security Council Resolution 687 of 3 April 1991,[40] the Kurds and Turks in the north, and constant wariness about Iran, and second because it wanted a say in the Arab–Israeli conflict (a point it made through its Scud missile attacks on Israel during the Gulf War).

In seeing for himself a role as the vanguard of Arabism, Saddam invokes the historical battle of Qadisiya of AD 636, where the Arabs defeated the Persian Sasanid dynasty, and Muslim resistance to the Christian Crusaders. His name is linked to some of the greatest leaders in Iraq's history, such as Hammurabi, Harun al-Rashid and Nebuchadnezzar.[41] On the eve of the invasion of Kuwait, Saddam spoke of the Arab nation's unique opportunity to regain, through the efforts of Baghdad, its former place of global centrality.[42]

Nowhere is his obsessive personality cult more patently demonstrated than through the monumental architecture and heroic statues erected in and around Baghdad. One writer, commenting on 'the scale and single-mindedness of his building campaign' observed: 'More and more are being planned all the time. Some refer directly to the past, others vaguely to what might be; most do both, invoking a proud national history as a model for an even more glorious future.'[43]

Saddam enjoys the role of facing down the US and the West. Although a ruthless tyrant at home, he skilfully uses the populist political tools of his position, showing off the human effects of economic sanctions (another form of UN intervention!), knowing that in the long run sanctions will be ended. The use of language, as Ofra Bengio shows, has been crucial. In an article marking the first anniversary of the Gulf War and personifying the regime, *al-Qadisiyya* wrote: 'We have Saddam Hussein and they have their democracy'.[44]

The Crisis of 1997–98

The crisis between the autumn of 1997 and February 1998 arose over the UN's rights of inspection for weapons of mass destruction through

the UN Special Commission (UNSCOM). It had been long in the making and had wide international implications. This was because the UN, including in particular the five permanent members of the Security Council, was involved, and simultaneously a massive military build-up, led by the US and supported mainly by Britain, was developing in the Gulf region. At one stage, it looked as if a large-scale attack was inevitable.

In propaganda terms, Iraq played heavily on the humanitarian effect of UN sanctions. In reality, the sanctions had brought suffering. In May 1996, a $2 billion Oil-for-Food deal was struck with the UN, of which $1.32 billion would be used for humanitarian items. UN agencies and programmes reported that malnourishment was rife, previously controlled diseases had returned and infant mortality for children under five had increased sixfold between 1990 and 1995.[45]

Iraq tried to broaden the crisis, as it had during the Gulf War years earlier, to embrace wider Arab–Israeli issues. Although the self-proclaimed 'sword of the Arabs' had suffered a massive defeat in the Gulf War, in which some Arab countries participated in the US-led alliance, there seemed to be little difficulty in manufacturing nationalist support for Saddam for international media consumption. Perhaps, too, he calculated that 'his grip on domestic power seemed to be stronger than it had been for a number of year'.[46] Because it was clear that Iraq's sovereignty *was* indefensible, its violation, or potential violation, was accepted and the appeal made broader towards the Arabs as a whole. And there he knew he had some fertile ground, because it was apparent that, while a majority of Arab politicians might have been happy to see Saddam go, they were unable to say so publicly and, in any case, felt disillusioned with the role of the US in the troubled Israeli–Palestinian peace negotiations. In addition, Iraq tried to harness Islam as an additional support while not facing a direct Islamist threat.

There could be observed at the time the glimmerings of old reactions in the Arab world. For many, US policies (backed by Britain) were interpreted as efforts to humiliate the Arabs and violate their sovereignty rather than a genuine attempt to make the world a safer place. In one additional sense, the earlier humanitarian intervention in 1991 to help the Kurds in northern Iraq, combined with Western abhorrence of the regime, made the idea of military intervention at the turn of the year more acceptable to the world outside, although important questions were raised about the legality of it in international and UN terms. But it did not come about, for the time being.

The crisis was settled by Kofi Annan's mission and the signing in Baghdad on 23 February of a Memorandum of Understanding

between the UN and Iraq. The agreement was endorsed by the Security Council on 2 March 1998 in Resolution 1159. In Annan's view, the military threat had been crucial: 'Diplomacy can be effective, but it helps to have a military presence in the region. You can do a lot with diplomacy, but with diplomacy backed up by force you can get a lot more done.'[47]

In New York, he implicitly endorsed the tough line taken by the US and Britain by describing their leaders as 'perfect UN peace-keepers', who worked on the principle that 'the best way to use force is to show it, in order not to use it'.[48] The crisis was headed off, but the underlying problems were now seen in a different light and remained unsolved. Until the bombings by the US and Britain in December 1998, Iraq's sovereignty remained as unviolated as before by direct, heavy military intervention.

Whose Sovereignty and for Whom? Interests, Intervention or Intercourse?

What of modern-day intervention? On 26 June 1998, UN Secretary-General Kofi Annan put forward some provocative views on how he saw both the UN's role and the nature of sovereignty.[49] In his broad review, he observed:

> The Charter of the United Nations gives great responsibilities to great Powers, in their capacity as permanent members of the Security Council. But as a safeguard against abuse of those powers, Article 2.7 ... protects national sovereignty even from intervention by the United Nations itself.

He raised a central dilemma in reminding his audience that this article forbade the UN to intervene 'in matters which are essentially within the domestic jurisdiction of any State.' But then came some qualifications. 'Even national sovereignty', he said, 'can be set aside if it stands in the way of the Security Council's overriding duty to preserve international peace and security.' And this distinction became blurred. He went on:

> The Charter protects the sovereignty of peoples. It was never meant *as a licence for governments to trample on human rights and human dignity. Sovereignty implies responsibility, not just power.* [Emphasis added] (...) State frontiers should no longer be seen as a watertight protection for war criminals or mass murderers. The fact that a conflict is 'internal' does not give the parties any right to disregard the most basic rules of human conduct. Besides, most 'internal' conflicts do not stay internal for very long. They soon 'spill over' into neighbouring countries.

Annan made a reference to his mission in Iraq the previous February to defuse the tension over the UNSCOM mission, which 'had brought us to the brink of a new war in the Gulf'. It was a success for intervention in non-military ways, and he said again: 'It underscored ...that if diplomacy is to succeed, it must be backed both by force and by fairness.'

Annan was talking specifically about the UN's position on intervention and sovereignty. But it is clear that unavoidably linked with the notion of intervention come other concepts such as sovereignty, state power, failed states, religious authority and nationalism.

It is a truism, for example, that Arab nationalism, perhaps particularly today, carries some faint echoes of a Nasserite approach which, more tinged with Islam now than then, transcends the sovereignty of individual states. It is a line Saddam Hussein has taken up. The stridency of Nasser's pan-Arab call, which led at one stage to the creation of the United Arab Republic, comprising Egypt and Syria (and briefly Yemen), disappeared long ago. Nevertheless, the Arab nationalism of today makes intervention, whether for military, political or humanitarian reasons, more complicated to carry out and equally difficult to be accepted by host governments, since it comes mainly from the West.

This particular, modern form of regional nationalism has tended to be seen in the Arab world in the context of the Arab–Israeli conflict, personified by the Palestinians and, in the broadest senses, as one more experiment in Western economic and political plotting against the Arabs and Islam. The crisis over the UN inspection team's right of access in search of Iraqi weapons of mass destruction carried the issue of intervention to new levels, as the military events of December 1998 showed. It was a curious crisis in terms of intervention and sovereignty in that it had its origins in the Iraqi invasion of Kuwait and the subsequent Gulf War. Seven years earlier, it had almost seemed a satisfying cut-and-dried case of almost universal support for an ultimately UN-sponsored alliance forcing a predatory state, easily personalised into its hate figure of a dictator, Saddam, to disgorge Kuwait, the fruit of its conquest.

It did not work out that way, partly because Saddam remained resilient and steadfast in the face of domestic revolts. Backed by a formidable and ruthless domestic security system, Saddam has been able to ignore the infringements of Iraq's sovereignty carried out with international backing in the form of no-fly zones, the humanitarian intervention of Operation Provide Comfort for the Kurds in the north

and severe economic sanctions. The checklist of conditions which should have presaged his overthrow and replacement has long been proved useless.

In this process, Saddam has been successful in moving his points of reference for sovereignty from a local, national level to one embracing broader Arab interests. These include a pro-Palestinian settlement of the conflict with Israel, confronting the US and, when and if Iraq's oil production is allowed to return to full levels, having a significant effect on oil prices. In the earlier part of this decade, it had been possible to ignore his pretensions towards making a local deal dependent on a settlement of the Israeli–Palestinian issue. The economic sanctions imposed became more of a humanitarian issue affecting Iraq's people and, in particular, its children than a political lever, with the backing of the UN Security Council's Resolution 687 of 3 April 1991, to force Saddam to get rid of his weapons of mass destruction and the means of making and delivering them.

Between November 1997 and February 1998, there was the growing possibility of military intervention by the US and Britain. This alienated, or at least discomforted, many of their Arab allies, who might well privately have welcomed an intervention resulting in the fall of Saddam. It became linked with ideas and feelings of Arab nationalism, which find a more natural outlet over the Arab–Israeli crisis—these days seen much more in the context of the Palestinians. In this sense, the issue of intervention has again become blurred by regional nationalistic passions, which broaden the concept of sovereignty beyond the borders of a single state.

Added to the change in political circumstances over the decade, there were also conceptual misunderstandings between the West and the Middle East and a basic linguistic gap, seen in such Arabic terms as *umma, sulta, wataniya* and *siyada,* whose translation alone poses problems of comprehension, even before their emotive or analytical usage in the press, in broadcasts or by politicians (see below).

Local Views, Fears and Interpretations

Several authors have attempted to put Middle Eastern attitudes towards statehood and sovereignty and intervention into some perspective. Ideas about the state, or the nation-state, came often from Western historical experience and have been frequently defined within those terms.[50] This cultural and definitional clash is summed up inadvertently and somewhat improbably by Michael Barnett:

Since the beginning of the Arab states system state and nonstate actors

have engaged in an active and occasionally violent dialogue over how regional life should be organised in general and how the Arab states should manage the legacy of Westphalia and the demands of Arab nationalism in particular.... Such a debate highlights how Westphalia and the norms of international society conflicted with (and shaped) the existing (and emerging) regional society.[51]

For the Arabs, this also produced some clashes between local and regional loyalties, making their states more vulnerable to the attentions of outsiders. Whether Westphalian concepts of sovereignty became a popular topic of debate remains a doubtful idea.[52]

Further complexities arise because definitions can change to become complicated emotional expressions. The Arabic word *umma* has moved from meaning the whole Islamic religious community to meaning the Arab nation in general, and just part of it, for example Egypt or Syria.[53] The translations of the key, identifiable words can only be *approximate* and limited: for example, *umma* as 'community of believers; nation'; *sulta* 'sovereign power'; *siyada* 'sovereign rule'; *wataniya* 'nationalism', with the emphasis on the land/territory; *qaumiya* 'nationalism', with the emphasis on the people; *daula* 'state'; and *qutriya* 'regionalism'.

The problem with some of these words is that they are translations of Western political and academic terms, thereby blurring local perceptions of political and geographical entities on the receiving end of intervention. For example, as early as the 1930s and 1940s, the Muslim Brethren in Egypt tried to argue against acceptance of the European interpretations of such words as *wataniya,* in the sense of 'patriotism', and *qaumiya*. Hassan al-Banna, their founder, argued that the words should be given meanings in keeping with the spirit of Islam.[54] The use of language as a means of preserving a government in power has never been clearer than in Iraq, as personified by Saddam's repressive rule of thirty years.

Some years earlier, President Kennedy had attached great importance to US relations with Egypt. Lenczowksi summarises the problems of his administration in dealing with a region which was extremely sensitive to the specific form of political intervention embodied in developing diplomatic relations:

> The first, and fundamental, question Kennedy had to deal with was to define his attitude toward Arab nationalism in its current phase. The nationalism professed by the new Arab leaders (especially those in Egypt and Syria) had two dimensions deserving America's attention: it reflected

a revolt of the middle and lower classes against the privileged and tradition-bound ruling groups, and it was Pan-Arab in character. In the early stages of their struggle for freedom from Western imperial control, individual Arab countries had developed local nationalisms—Egyptian, Syrian, Iraqi, etc.—but once their independence was achieved, a new Pan-Arab nationalism began to emerge. This new movement even coined a special political vocabulary to account for the difference: the old local nationalism was to be known as *wataniyah* (patriotism) from the word *watan*, meaning a homeland or fatherland. The new Pan-Arab version acquired the name of *qaumiyah* (nationalism) from the word *qaum*, meaning a nation. Whereas, in the early, pre-Nasser, era *wataniyah* was perceived as a virtue, during the Nasser period it began to be seen as a parochial obstacle to all-Arab unity. Consequently, it was replaced by a new expression *iqlimiyah* (regionalism), with a negative connotation in terms of the pan-Arab ideal, because the 'region' (that is, a country) was being contrasted to the entire 'nation' (extending from the borders of Iran to the Atlantic) which was to hold primacy in Arab loyalties.[55]

Since that era, the swing has been back to different, local Arab nationalisms with a stronger and more assertive Islamic overtone. The reactions to contacts with states, organisations and ideas from outside are nevertheless liable to a friendly or hostile interpretation on several different levels. In many ways, one of the most persistent stems from what has been identified as the 'mental invasion' of Westernization, setting up an emotional reaction to the impact of the West.[56]

Some Conclusions

From the example of Iraq and against the broader background of the Middle East as defined earlier, it should be possible to draw some general conclusions about, and create some loose categories for, the special nature of intervention and its reception.

Non-intervention after the serious threat of intervention can be as instructive as intervention itself because of the reactions it provokes. The focus must be to attempt to classify these reactions. Many will be, to Western ears, strangely irrelevant—hence the importance of language with the concepts that lie behind it. In Iraq, it seems to outsiders inconceivable that connections are not made to the miserable state of the country and the leader—Saddam Hussein—who, moved by personal ambition and misconceived nationalism, has led Iraq into two disastrous wars in two decades. There is, indeed, a sense that while Iraqis may, like others, make eloquent pleas for peace, in practice since 1980 they have had almost unbroken years of war and domestic brutality. What is shifting marginally is the possibility that Iraq will

make some sort of a comeback of acceptability into the Arab fold, but few governments trust Saddam.

The above case, in the context of the Middle East, leaves some broad, unsatisfactory and even contradictory conclusions:

The patterns of intervention over the years have been extremely varied and for equally varied motives. Few interventions have been welcomed (except possibly in some cases involving refugees; the Gulf War is an exception, *and* it involved non-Muslim intervention). The majority of interventions have been for highly political and dissimilar motives—and have been interpreted in the region as such. The possibility of democracy being restored through the overthrow of Saddam is invoked, but without conviction. As far as can be discerned, the local reactions are related, mainly in emotional terms, to concepts of intervention, sovereignty and democracy which do not necessarily fit easily into the patterns that Western analyses ascribe to them. The notion of nationalism and its various forms cause further problems in defining reactions to intervention, even on humanitarian grounds. Nationalism is a strong part of the reaction to intervention. It is not always possible to make a cost–benefit analysis of intervention in political, social or humanitarian categories, for either the intervenor or the intervenee. There has been a significant watershed in the UN's roles in Iraq (Annan's diplomacy backed by military strength).

A highly repressive regime may deter direct intervention, in part for fear of the unpredictable nature of the government that might follow its overthrow.[57] Violations of human rights are given comparatively restrained and limited attention by the outside world. There might even be a case for saying that Iraq, through Saddam Hussein's intransigence, qualified, *at that time*, as a rare anomaly and example of a state that has claimed and exercised the right to non-intervention, or at least only comparatively limited intervention. In any case it was not amenable or not easily amenable to direct and sustained outside intervention.

The events of December 1998 and the NATO bombing of Yugoslavia in 1999 would appear paradoxically to confirm this because of the limited, immediate success that violent intervention produced.[58] Iraq's political behaviour, both domestically and internationally, could be, at best and at a reasonable cost to those intervening, only contained. That conclusion would in effect lend support to other governments whose wayward approaches towards human rights and civil liberties might justify their belief, not usually made explicit officially, that they had earned the right to non-intervention. This would be an uncomfortable and, ultimately, untenable conclusion, but one which

Notes

1. Notably by Møller, Bjørn: 'Resolving the Security Dilemma in the Persian Gulf—With a Postscript on the 1997/98 Iraqi Crisis', *Working Paper*, no. 8/1998 (Copenhagen: Copenhagen Peace Research Institute, COPRI, 1998), p. 70 (including March postscript pp. i-xi). See also chapters I and VIII in this volume.

2. Lenczowski, George: *American Presidents and the Middle East* (Durham, NC: Duke University Press, 1990), p. 46.

3. Weiss, Thomas G.: *Military–Civilian Interactions: Intervening in Humanitarian Crises* (Lanham, MD: Rowman & Littlefield, 1999). See also Ramsbotham, Oliver P.: 'Islam, Christianity, and Forcible Humanitarian Intervention', *Ethics & International Affairs*, vol. 12 (1998), pp. 81–102. In an interesting examination of the different approaches, Ramsbotham concludes that there may be a surprising measure of agreement among Muslims and Christians.

4. For a comprehensive, if now dated, account, see Morris, Mary E.: *The Persistence of External Interest in the Middle East* (Santa Monica, CA: Rand, 1993).

5. To the extent that the UN General Assembly adopted a resolution urging member-states 'to observe the Olympic Truce during the XVIII Olympic Winter Games', to take place in Nagano, Japan, 7–22 February 1998! See Doc. A/RES/52/21m (8 December 1997).

6. Rejwan, Nissim: *Arabs Face the Modern World: Religious, Cultural, and Political Responses to the West* (Gainesville, FL: University Press of Florida, 1998), p. 86.

7. Saikal, Amin: 'The Role of the United Nations in the Middle East', in Tom Woodhouse, Robert Bruce & Malcolm Dando (eds.): *Peacekeeping and Peacemaking: Towards Effective Intervention in Post–Cold War Conflicts* (Basingstoke: Macmillan, 1998), pp. 133–144; McDermott, Anthony: 'The Arab–Israeli Mixed Armistice Commissions of Yore: Relevant Today?', *Geopolitics and International Boundaries*, vol. 1, no. 1 (Summer 1996), pp. 93–114.

8. To these should be added the unsuccessful non-UN Multinational Force in Beirut in 1982–84 and the effective Multinational Force and Observers monitoring, since the April 1982 Egypt–Israel peace treaty, Sinai.

9. Laugen, Torunn in 'The World Bank and the UN in the Occupied Territories', *Security Dialogue,* vol. 29, no. 1 (March 1998), pp. 63–77, describes how more than $2.2 billion in humanitarian relief and development aid has been committed to the West Bank and the Gaza Strip, in particular by the World Bank, UNRWA and UNDP. Their efforts have been hampered by local and regional political instability and the weak administrative structures of the Palestinian Authority.

10. For an interesting perspective, see Lia, Brynjar: 'Islamic Perceptions of the United Nations and Its Peacekeeping Missions: Some Preliminary Findings', *International Peacekeeping*, vol. 5, no. 2 (Summer 1998), pp.

38–63.

11. Saikal: *loc. cit.* (note 7).

12. As in Doughty, C. M.: *Travels in Arabia Deserta* (Cambridge: Cambridge University Press, 1888).

13. Marín-Bosch, Miguel: *Votes in the UN General Assembly* (The Hague: Kluwer Law International, 1998); the table on p. 120 illustrates this consistently high level of Arab coincidence voting.

14. Kemp, Geoffrey & Robert E. Harkavy: *Strategic Geography and the Changing Middle East* (Washington, DC: Brookings Institution Press, 1997), pp. 7–8. On p. 14, there are two maps. One shows the US State Department's 'bureaucratic parameters for the Near East' as stretching from Morocco (excluding Sudan) across to and including the Arabian Peninsula and Iran (not Turkey). The Pentagon divides the area another way. US Central Command (CENTCOM) has responsibility for military operations in a region that includes Egypt, Sudan, Ethiopia, Djibouti, Kenya, Somalia, Jordan, Saudi Arabia, Iraq, Iran, the states of the Gulf Cooperation Council, Afghanistan and Pakistan. Turkey, Israel and Syria remain the responsibility of the European Command (EUCOM).

15. Schultze, Kirsten E., Martin Stokes & Colin Campbell (eds.): *Nationalism, Minorities and Diasporas: Identities and Rights in the Middle East* (London: Tauris Academic Studies, 1996), p. 1.

16. *Ibid.* See the editors' chapter, p. 11.

17. For a discussion of the Palestinians' stateless nationalism, see Sayigh, Yezid: *Armed Struggle and the Search for State: The Palestinian National Movement, 1949–1993* (Oxford: Clarendon Press, 1997).

18. Lustick, Ian S.: *Unsettled States, Disputed Lands: Britain and Ireland, France and Algeria, Israel and the West Bank/Gaza* (Ithaca, NY: Cornell University Press, 1993).

19. Owen, Roger: *State, Power & Politics in the Making of the Middle East* (London: Routledge, 1997), pp. 94–95.

20. *Ibid.*, p. 286.

21. Hisham Sharabi explores this in *Neopatriarchy: A Theory of Distorted Change in Arab Society* (Oxford: Oxford University Press, 1988). Interestingly, in *Theory, Politics and the Arab World: Critical Responses* (New York: Routledge, 1990), which Sharabi edited, some of these issues are taken up but in the context of mainstream academic scholarship on the Arab world and the Middle East. Rejwan (see note 6), in the debate about Westernization's accommodation and integration, places Sharabi among those with 'emotional rejection' (p. 138). On Sharabi in detail, see pp. 151–159.

22. Cordesman, Anthony H. & Ahmed S. Hashim: *Iraq: Sanctions and Beyond* (Boulder, CO: Westview, 1997), p. 4.

23. *Ibid.*, p. 8.

24. *The Observer* (28 June 1998), pp. 11–13. The panel included four Nobel Peace Prize laureates. It was arrived at by multiplying abuses of human rights over thirteen categories by a country's Human Development Index as

defined by the UNDP.

25. *Ibid.*, p. 11.

26. Boyne, Sean: 'Inside Iraq's Security Network, Part One', *Jane's Intelligence Review*, vol. 9. no. 7 (1997), pp. 312-14.

27. Sean Boyne provides extensive details of its numbers, deployment and responsibilities in 'Saddam's Shield: the Role of the Special Republican Guard', *Jane's Intelligence Review*, vol. 11, no. 1 (1999), pp. 29-32.

28. Cordesman & Hashim: *op. cit.* (note 22), p. 36.

29. Marr, Phebe: 'Iraq after the Gulf War: The Fallen Idol', in Robert Owen Freedman (ed.): *The Middle East and the Peace Process: Impact of the Oslo Accords* (Gainesville, FL: University Press of Florida, 1998), p. 230.

30. *Ibid.*, pp. 37–38.

31. Bengio, Ofra: *Saddam's Word: Political Discourse in Iraq* (New York: Oxford University Press, 1998), provides a detailed and extended illustration and explanation of the political role of the Arabic language in Ba'athist Iraq.

32. Indeed, in 1988, *Qamus Saddam Husayn al-Siyasi* [The Political Dictionary of Saddam Hussein] was published, containing some 500 entries of his favourite words, expressions and 'memorable quotes'. See Bengio: *op. cit.* (note 31), p. 78.

33. Marr: *loc. cit.* (note 29), pp. 48–49.

34. Dawisha, Adeed: 'Iraqi Politics: The Past and Present as Context for the Future', in John Calabrese (ed.): *The Future of Iraq* (Washington, DC: Middle East Institute, 1997), p. 12.

35. Cordesman & Hashim: *op. cit.* (note 22), p. 19.

36. Saad Eddin Ibrahim wrote: 'The truth of the matter is that Saddam Hussein is an indisputable Evil. In his 30 years of tyrannical rule, he has ordered, caused, or carried out with his bare hands the killing of about two million people, 99% of whom are Arabs and Muslims, not Americans or Israelis. His wrath is primarily directed at his own people and immediate neighbors, not against those who are thousands of miles away.' See idem: 'For Iraq, Not for Saddam Hussein: Evil and Super-Evil in the Middle East', *Civil Society* (Cairo), March 1998, p. 3. Khalid Salih describes more fully the abysmal state of civil liberties in 'Might vs Right: Human Rights in Iraq', *Civil Society* (December 1998), pp. 4-6.

37. Cordesman & Hashim: *op. cit.* (note 22), pp. 14–15.

38. Dawisha: *op. cit.* (note 34), p. 12.

39. Hashim, Ahmad S.: 'Iraq's Regional Policies in the 1990s: From Regional Superpower to ''Superpauper''', in Calabrese (ed.): *op. cit.* (note 34), p. 91.

40. Bjørn Møller described 687's terms as 'the most intrusive and rigid constraints ever imposed on a sovereign state since those imposed on the vanquished after WWII'. See idem: *op. cit.* (note 1), pp. 15, where he summarises the conditions. See also related notes 78 and 79 on p. 51.

41. Dawisha: *op. cit.* (note 34), p. 13, drawing on Karsh, Efraim & Inari Rautsi: *Saddam Hussein: A Political Biography* (New York: The Free Press, 1991), p. 124.

42. Bengio: *op. cit.* (note 31), p. 37.

43. *The Ecomonist* (6 March 1999), pp. 85-86.

44. Bengio: *op. cit.* (note 31), p. 69.

45. Adebajo, Adekeye: 'Saddam's Bazaar', *The World Today*, vol. 54, no. 3 (March 1998), p. 62.

46. The International Institute for Strategic Studies: *Strategic Survey 1997/98* (Oxford: Oxford University Press, 1998), pp. 153–154.

47. Annan's press conference on 24 February 1998, *UN Chronicle*, no. 1, 1998, p. 71.

48. *Ibid.*, p. 5.

49. The thirty-fifth annual Ditchley Foundation Lecture, Doc. SG/SM/6613/Rev.1, 26 June 1998. An edited version of this speech appeared in the *International Herald Tribune*, 27–28 June 1998.

50. See Owen: *op. cit.* (note 19), pp. 1–7, where he discusses in this context the relationship between state and society. He draws, in part, on Zubaida, Sami: *Islam, the People and the State* (London: Routledge, 1989).

51. Michael N. Barnett, 'Sovereignty, Nationalism, and Regional Order in the Arab States System', *International Organization*, vol. 49, no. 3 (Summer 1995), pp. 479–510. On p. 508 the author analyses comprehensively and usefully the interaction between these elements, in particular that of the sovereign state and pan-Arabism (pp. 494–495). Elsewhere Barnett, in *Dialogues in Arab Politics. Negotiations in Regional Order* (New York: Columbia University Press, 1998), relates admirably through 'a narrative of Arab politics' (*passim*) the changing nature of Arab politics and nationalism since the 1920s until the years following the turning point of the Gulf War (after which 'any notions of Arab collective security lay in ruins', p. 228.) The interplay between Arabism and sovereignty is again an important recurrent theme. Vatikiotis, P. J.: *The Middle East from the End of Empire to the End of the Cold War* (London: Routledge, 1997) provides an invaluable account of regional developments, drawing extensively on Arabic sources. It provides, for example, an insightful analysis of Arab perceptions of the 1973 Arab–Israeli war (through the Egyptian and Lebanese press) and the 1990–91 Gulf crisis and war.

52. In the same sort of vein as a Western perspective, Musallam Ali Musallam wrote: 'The three principal causes of conflict outlined in the work of Thomas Hobbes—competition, self-defence (or the perception thereof), and glory—seem to underlie all the international and local political strategies of Saddam Hussein.' See idem: *The Iraqi Invasion of Kuwait: Saddam Hussein, His State and International Power Politics* (London: British Academic Press, 1996), p. 59.

53. Owen: *op. cit.* (note 19), p. 19. Bengio draws attention to the use of the word *umma* for arousing popular political support in Iraq. See *op. cit.* (note 31), pp. 35-36.

54. Rejwan: *op. cit.* (note 6), p. 63.

55. Lenczowski: *op. cit.* (note 2), pp. 75–76. The italics are in the original text.

56. Rejwan: *op. cit.* (note 6), p. 138.

57. Gawdat Bahgat concludes that the next regime in Baghdad, when it comes, is likely to be less ruthless but still not democratic. See idem: 'Iraq After Saddam—What Lies Ahead?', *Journal of Social, Political, and Economic Studies*, vol. 23, no. 1 (Spring 1998), pp. 39–52.

58. Indeed, these air interventions have unsurprisingly forged alliances of victim states. Sir Charles Guthrie, the chief of the UK defence staff, described in *The Guardian* of 1 April 1999, the growth over six months of the relationship between Saddam Hussein and Slobodan Milosevic, the Yugoslav President on military, tactical and technical levels in response to the pressure from the West. He said: 'All this adds up to a close relationship between Saddam and Milosevic; a marriage of convenience, based on the suffering of their peoples.'

9 TOWARDS COOPERATIVE SECURITY IN THE PERSIAN GULF

Jalil Roshandel

The Legacy of Two Wars

During the past two decades, three wars have occurred in the Persian Gulf: The eight-years Iran-Iraq war (1980-1988); the 1990 occupation of Kuwait by Iraq and the international community's response in the form of the second Persian Gulf War (1991); and the seventy-hour bombing campaign against Iraq (17-20 December 1998), followed until the time of writing (end of March 1999) by continuous attacks against the so-called 'no-fly zones'.

No doubt Saddam Hussein was the primary, if not the only, instigator of all three wars. Even though these wars could probably have been avoided if he had not been in power, his absence would not have assured the end of all forms the hostilities in the region. The area is marred with inter-state tensions which are intensified by the involvement of extra-regional forces.

Some might argue that the US involvement in the region with operations 'Desert Shield', 'Desert Storm' and 'Desert Fox' has been a result, rather than a contributing cause, of the wars in the region. However, one could equally plausibly argue the United States has escalated the wars, as when it, during the 1980-88 war, helped Iraq reduce Iran's power.[1] Notwithstanding the assertions by outside powers that their aim has been to enhance security in the region, each of the three wars has produced deteriorating regional security.

The wars have, furthermore, imposed heavy economic burdens on the countries involved. The first war ruined the military might of both Iran and Iraq and set their development back for many years, thereby endangering regional peace and security. The subsequent wars further produced insecurities for Saudi Arabia and Kuwait. Even though Kuwait regained sovereignty over its territory, a profound sense of insecurity persists. Moreover, the inspection regime created in the wake of the 1991 war to control Iraq's WMD (weapons of mass destruction) and related delivery systems did not succeed in providing the wished-for security, and it was ultimately dismantled as an unintended

consequence of the US-UK operation against Iraq in December 1998.

During this third war more than 400 Tomahawk cruise missiles were launched, and over a hundred targets were destroyed. After four nights of intense strikes, President Clinton announced a halt to the bombing, claiming that the strikes had 'significantly' damaged Iraq's military capabilities and its ability to produce WMD, hence that the operation had been a success: 'I'm confident that we have achieved our mission'.[2] This all raises a number of questions such as: What has changed as a result of the bombings? What were the U.S. objectives vis-à-vis Iraq and the region? How effective was the bombing in terms of these objectives? and What are the security implications for the Persian Gulf countries?

These are some of the questions addressed in the following. It is further argued that the strategic importance of the Persian Gulf can still be captured in one word, namely 'Oil'. As the low oil prices are very beneficial to the West, whatever can prolong the current situation will probably be supported by the West. The paper concludes with suggestions for how to promote stability and cooperative security for the region.

Iran-Iraq War 1980-1989
The Iran-Iraq war came in the immediate wake of the 1979 Iranian Revolution which 'shocked the world and set in motion a process that continues to baffle many observers.'[3] Lasting for almost eight years this war exhausted both Iran's and Iraq's military and economic resources as well as undermined regional security as a whole.

Both countries could have embarked on a period of development, as would have been the case for revolutionary Iran, had it not been for the war. The war meant a diversion from Iran's natural path towards prosperity, development, and 'stability through the consolidation of central control and a development program that (could) enhance (its) position and the security of the state.'[4] Instead of the direct and active participation in the international community that would otherwise have occurred, Iran was forced to adopt a more defensive attitude. The resultant isolation continues to mar Iran to the present day, when it still struggles to neutralize the effects of the US-imposed sanctions and containment policy. The isolationist posture is thus a consequence of both the war with Iraq and of US policies.

From a narrow military point of view the war had no winner, even though both parties declared victory. Even though it was the aggressor Iraq escaped with impunity, as the United Nations Security Council imposed no penalties—nor did the United States penalize Iraq

for its use of chemical weapons.

Together with the 1979 Iranian Revolution, the Iran-Iraq war produced significant changes in the Persian Gulf security configuration, bringing about new forms of alignment in the region. The GCC (Gulf Cooperation Council) was created as a result of the war, and the US involvement grew. Hence, when the second Persian Gulf war broke out, the American allies found themselves completely dependent for their security on a permanent American military presence and support.

The Second Persian Gulf War

The 1990 Iraqi invasion and occupation of Kuwait, followed by the international community's response in the form of the Second Persian Gulf War (1991), gave a further shock to the security and economy of the countries in the region. While this war was much shorter than its predecessor, it produced a more direct involvement of various states from inside and beyond the region. It furthermore led directly to the third war.

The US, UK and other industrialized countries together with Japan (in an indirect, supportive role) forged an anti-Iraqi coalition, which even included some Arab states of the region, and waged a devastating war against the country. However, at the end of the war the primary problems remained unsolved. One could thus argue that the Second Persian Gulf War never ended, but that it has reemerged over and over again in different forms, each time depleting the wealth and strength of the Persian Gulf nations. In 1993 Stanley Renshon wrote:

> Because the Gulf War was short, apparently successful, and minimally costly in American lives, newer concerns have engaged our attention. The war has receded from national consciousness yet has also left an unsettled feeling. Saddam Hussein is still in power and threatens to be a source of difficulty in the near future and possibly longer. The movement for an overall Middle East settlement proceeds slowly and will be long and difficult, if it succeeds at all. And the world scarcely seems to be a more secure place in spite of the performance of the anti-Iraq coalition.[5]

It is thus a gross simplification to praise the war as one that put an end to Saddam Hussein's aggressive stance vis-à-vis Iraq's neighbours. Not until confidential files are opened will we be able to realistically assess the process and the outcomes of this war.

Both during and after the war, the US policy was criticized for not giving negotiations a fair chance. According to Herbert Kelman,

'the decision to go to war in January 1991 was flawed because it gave no serious consideration to alternatives short of military action, particularly to the possibilities of negotiating an agreement. (...) The fact remains that negotiations were not tried, and so we cannot say with any degree of certainty that they would *not* have succeeded'[6]

Intrusive Containment, 1991-1998

After the second war, American policy in the Persian Gulf followed an 'intrusive containment' pattern. To this end different instruments were used, underpinned by UN resolutions.

An inspection regime was created for WMD and ballistic missiles with ranges in excess of 150 kilometres, and UNSCOM (United Nations Special Commission) was tasked with inspecting Iraq's WMD facilities. In defiance of UN resolutions, Saddam Hussein obstructed UNSCOM's mission whenever possible, thereby provoking recurrent crises. The most recent of these led directly to the operation 'Desert Fox', which was provoked by USCOM's latest report. This not only denied real progress in terms of disarmament, but also highlighted several impediments to the inspections imposed by the Iraqi authorities. Indeed, the report claimed that Iraq had 'routinely interrupted' the commission's work.

The so-called policy of 'Dual Containment' policy has apparently been intended to maintain a 'balance of weakness' between Iran and Iraq while upholding the embargo against Iraq's oil exports. According to President Clinton these sanctions 'have cost Saddam more than $120 billion.'

Another element in this containment has been the creation of 'no-fly zones' in northern and southern Iraq, the latter demarcated by 33rd parallel and the former by the 36th. The northern zone was established 1991, while that in the south was created in August 1992 and expanded in 1996, in both cases unilaterally by the western powers. The official rationale was to protect the Kurdish population in the north and Shi'ite Muslims in the south. Iraq has always opposed this arrangement, even though it formally accepted the UN Security Council Resolution 688 which indirectly gave birth to the northern zone, yet without any explicit reference to it.

Unfortunately, none of these tools, intended to 'tame' Iraq, have really worked. Iraqi jets have 'violated' the zones whenever they could. Even though both U.S and British pilots have patrolled both zones, all clashes have occurred with the U.S. The first incident took place on 27 December 1992, when a U.S. F-16 shot down an Iraqi MIG-25'[7].

The bombings in December 1998 have been followed by several

clashes between the US and British forces enforcing the no-fly zones and Iraq, which has vowed to challenge them. This has also produced a questioning of the legality of US-UK bombing by many observers and analysts. Do any of the cited UN resolutions actually authorize states to use force or threaten such use? Apparently there is no such authorization. Nigel White thus in a recent article argued, 'To accept the contrary would mean any state could take upon itself the right to use force to enforce a Security Council resolution whenever it perceived that the resolution required enforcement. This is not mere delegation, but would constitute unilateral or multilateral action outside the UN system.'[8]

Perhaps Iraq could have used legal means to have the no-fly zones dismantled, but apparently the Iraqi leadership is more attuned to use military means. However, it has to be acknowledged that the Iraqi response probably reflects a legitimate desire to defend its sovereignty and territorial integrity. As far as the legality of the 'no-fly zones' is concerned, I do not personally find any legal justification for it, but in application, backed by American bombings, they proved efficient.

Even though the zones have been challenged by Iraqi, they have been welcomed by part of the Kurdish factions, especially those shielded by them. Previously, the Iraqi Kurds were subjected to several air attacks by Saddam Hussein's forces; and during the Iran-Iraq war they were the victims of attacks by means of chemical weapons, ethnic cleansing, and forced deportations. Hundreds of thousands of Kurds were forced to cross the nearest border into neighbouring countries, with close to one million in Iran. More than 180,000 civilians were killed during the *Anfal* campaign alone, and over one million left the country again in 1991.

This long history of Iraqi repression has made the Kurdish population support the no-fly zone. According to a recent report on the Developments in Iraq, prepared by the Staff of *Radio Free Europe,* 'the Patriotic Union of Kurdistan (PUK) has called on the international community to extend the northern no-fly zone so as to provide Iraqi Kurdistan with better security'. Among other points the report quotes from the director of the Bureau of International Affairs (BIA) of the PUK: Some forty percent of Kurdistan, he notes, are not now covered by the present no-fly zone. As he argued in a statement released earlier that month such a step 'would provide the Kurdish people a credible international security guarantee against future Iraqi ground assaults.'[9]

While the main objective of Iraq is a normalization of the situation and a regaining of full sovereignty over its territory, the Iraqi Kurds fear Saddam Hussein's hidden objective, they are convinced that

a new wave of ethnic cleansing will start as soon as Saddam regains full control over the zones. Quoting from the director of the BIA the report mentions the danger of military action against the Kurds:

> The Iraqi government's latest assertion that the no-fly zones lack international validity, together with the constant threat posed by Iraq's armed forces, suggests that Baghdad may plan to again step up repression against the Kurds as well as other Iraqis. (...)
> Baghdad has recently denounced international NGOs operating in Iraqi Kurdistan, especially those NGOs which have been engaged in clearing land mines in the countryside. He notes that the Iraqi military which planted these throughout Kurdish territory has refused to provide these NGOs with the necessary maps showing where the mines are located.[10]

From Baghdad's point of view the Kurdish issue is best dealt with during periods of external pressure and crisis. While the international community is involved with Iraq itself, especially with regard to issues such as disarmament, Iraq has better opportunities to suppress the Kurds. As such, Iraq exploits external problems and pressure as an opportunity to conceal internal massacres and cleansing.

Iraqi WMD and UNSCOM

Resolution 687 as well as a number of other resolutions, all accepted by Iraq, place the country in a difficult situation. Iraq had to accept 'the forming of a Special Commission, which shall carry out immediate on-site inspection of Iraq's biological, chemical and missile capabilities, based on Iraq's declaration and the designation of any additional locations by the Special Commission itself...'

Even though UNSCOM was thus created with Iraq's consent, Baghdad has consistently used all available means to hamper its activities, render them more expensive, or force the inspectors to temporarily leave the country. In one of the last UNSCOM reports, numerous examples were given from the period 17 November-2 December 1998. Among the relevant incidents one could mention the following:

> On 23 November 1998, an Iraqi escort helicopter took off and passed over a UN helicopter at low speed and low altitude, not more than ten meters from the ground. The Iraqi helicopter continued to fly over the area only slightly higher, making two full circles above the UN helicopter on the ground.

However, compared to UNSCOM's overall achievements, the above was really a rather trivial incident. It thus seems that UNSCOM, for some reason, had decided to highlight quite insignificant events. The problems mentioned in the subsequent report, covering the week 2-9 December 1998, appeared even more trivial:

> During the first inspection day of UNSCOM 261 (BW 74), on 5 December, the Iraqi representatives made efforts to prevent videotaping and interrupted and sought to direct site personnel's responses. An attempt (in the end unsuccessful) was made to prevent the team photocopying a set of documents.[11]

According to UNSCOM reports, despite all the barriers and until the inspections came to a complete halt (only few days before the bombings), undeclared dual-use pieces of production equipment were found. A BBC report shows UNSCOM to have been more successful than formal statements have suggested in uncovering Iraq's weapons of mass destruction as well as its stock of long-range missiles. This report, based on 'a UN assessment' gave the following picture of UNSCOM's accomplishments with regard to Iraq's capabilities:

> **Nuclear weapons**: Iraq came close to developing a workable nuclear device shortly before the Gulf War, in violation of the Nuclear Non-Proliferation Treaty. However, the IAEA (International Atomic Energy Agency) is optimistic that it has succeeded in shutting down potentially dangerous nuclear weapon projects. Indeed, on January 22, Russia called on the UN to adopt a resolution declaring Iraq free of nuclear weapons. However, this attempt was rebuffed by the UN Security Council.
> **Super gun**: UNSCOM has destroyed a variety of assembled, and non-assembled 'supergun' components. Many of these were imported from the UK.
> **Missiles**: UNSCOM says the following have been destroyed: 48 operational SCUD missiles; 6 missile launchers; 30 special warheads for chemical and biological weapons. Most of the equipment that Iraq has actually admitted to owning has been old and barely working. It is thought that Iraq could still be hiding as many as 16 proscribed missiles. UNSCOM says critical components and missile propellant are unaccounted for.
> **Chemical Weapons**: Iraq is known to have produced mustard gases and a deadly nerve gas called VX. In August 1988, Iraqi forces used both chemical and gas munitions against Kurdish civilians in the area around Halabja in Iraqi Kurdistan.

UNSCOM has also been investigating Iraqi interest in sarin, tabun and

other chemical agents. On 2 November 1997, *The Observer* reported that the UN believed that Iraq was holding secret stocks of the lethal VX liquid nerve agent, and that UNSCOM was on the verge of uncovering it when Saddam Hussein ordered the US members of the team to leave.

According to its own reports UNSCOM had destroyed: 38,537 filled and empty chemical munitions, 480 tons of live chemical weapons agent, more than 3,000 tons of precursor chemicals, several hundred pieces of chemical weapons production equipment and related analytical instruments. It estimated 4,000 tons of precursor chemicals to remain unaccounted for.[12]

Perhaps the most important concern for the UN, as reflected in the report, had been Iraq's production of biological weapons. When UNSCOM started working in Iraq, shortly after the end of the war in 1991, Iraq denied having any biological weapons programme, which UNSCOM verifications proved to be absolutely wrong. In fact UNSCOM learned that Iraq had produced 19,000 litres of botulinum, 8,400 litres of anthrax, and 2,000 litres of aflatoxin and clostridium. In July 1995, Iraq finally admitted to having sought an offensive biological warfare capability. In 1988 alone, it had imported 39 tons of growth material for virulent agents such as anthrax and botulinum, only 22 tons of which could be satisfactorily accounted for in peaceful production. UNSCOM has destroyed much of the growth media, but an estimated seventeen tons remain unaccounted for. UNSCOM further claimed to have destroyed the entire *Al Hakam* biological weapon production factory complex which the Iraqis claimed was used to produce animal feed.[13]

In his statement on 16 December 1999, on the eve of the launching of air strikes against Iraq, British Prime Minister Tony Blair, also provided some important statistics. While claiming that [Saddam Hussein's] 'threat is now, and it is a threat to his neighbours, to his people, and to the security of the world,' he still admitted that, 'Since 1991 the inspectors destroyed or rendered harmless 48 Scud missiles, 49,000 chemical munitions, 690 tones of chemical agents, 3,000 tones of precursor chemicals and the Al Hakam biological weapons factory, destroyed in 1996. However, over 30,000 chemical weapons warheads and 4000 tones of precursor chemicals remain unaccounted for'.[14]

UNSCOM had thus been quite successful in finding and destroying Iraqi WMD sources. Though one may rightly argue that UNSCOM's achievements were less than complete, this does not mean that a bombing campaign would be a better means to peace and security. Hence, the official rationale for the US-UK bombings cannot

be accepted at face value, but we need to look for hidden or unstated objectives.

One could also argue that UNSCOM might have continued its inspections with sufficient rigour if only it had been able to gain the confidence of the Iraqi regime. Perhaps one of the reasons UNSCOM had to discontinue its mission in Iraq was that it had ventured into areas which they were unable to convince Iraq were in accordance with their mission.

Operation Desert Fox
While mentioning 'international supervision', the aforementioned UNSCR 687 gave no authorization to use force, but this was what happened.

The Motives
When the bombings started on 16 December President Clinton was accused by critics of trying to conceal his 'principal objective of self-preservation.'

White House officials, of course, insisted that 'Iraq was solely responsible for the timing' and that the timing had nothing to do with the impeachment of Clinton over the Monica Lewinsky scandal.[15] However, it is now clear that the military action was decided in a highly ambiguous, if not bizarre, domestic situation related to Clinton's personal affairs and his ongoing conflict with the Republicans in Congress. As it happened, in the light of the military strikes against Iraq, the impeachment debate was in fact delayed, but only for a short while, and certain congressmen questioned the timing. House Majority Leader Dick Armey, for instance, released a statement saying that 'people's suspicions that the attack on Iraq was motivated by the president's desire to avoid or distract from the impeachment debate are themselves a powerful argument for impeachment.'[16]

Everything was done to disconnect the two events. British Prime Minister Tony Blair thus referred to UNSCOM's findings as 'a catalogue of obstruction', claiming that they showed that 'Saddam has no intention whatever of keeping to his work. He is a serial breaker of promises'. He further made it clear that the quarrel was not with the Iraqi people, but with Saddam himself 'and the evil regime he represents', concluding that 'we have exhausted all other avenues. We act because we must act.'[17] In actual fact, however, the attacks were aimed at Saddam Hussein's power base rather than at the WMD capabilities that had been scrutinized by UNSCOM.

The *Jerusalem Post* revealed other aspects of the operation, noting

that some of the targets hit during the operation 'were important to Saddam from the point of view of his personal security.' According to Amitzai Baram of the Haifa University, whereas 'the minimum aim is to force Saddam to comply with UN resolutions,' there was another objective that was not publicly stated, namely 'to try to create a situation in which it would be easier for Saddam to be toppled'. In Baram's view the overthrow of Saddam might come about by encouraging a military coup d'état or a major uprising, possibly initiated by Iraqi Shi'ites. Such ambitions might explain the selection of such targets as the Republican Palace in Baghdad. While admitting that substantial damage to Sadam's military infrastructure might 'cause cracks in the regime,' Baram also mentioned having information about no less than three abortive attempts at *coups d'état* in the past three years from within the Republican guard.[18]

The *Jerusalem Post* further mentioned that by sub-delegation of authority Saddam had created 'an effective personal defense.' Hence, according to IDF (Israeli Defence Force) assessment, any American intention to kill Saddam would be problematic.[19] Acknowledging that the U.S. had refrained from admitting to be personally targeting Saddam, the journal concluded that 'the Iraqi leader is aware that this is the long-term American intention, and has prepared for it.'[20]

The Achievements

The extent to which the seventy hours' Operation Desert Fox was effective is difficult to determine. There is no doubt that some military and weapons production facilities were hit. According to U.S. Defense Secretary William S. Cohen the military action was 'substantial' and Saddam's ballistic missile programme was set back by at least a year. However, on the same day, an anonymous senior military commander was quoted by the *New York Times* as agreeing that the attacks had certainly set back Iraq's military, but conceding that it was difficult to quantify this.[21]

In a Pentagon briefing session during the operation it was revealed that more than 400 Tomahawk cruise missiles had been launched, and over a hundred targets destroyed, to which should be added undisclosed numbers of laser-guided bombs and other ordnance. Apparently the poor Muslims of Iraq were only saved by the holy month of Ramadan which gave the American president a good excuse to stop the attacks.

After four nights of intense strikes, President Clinton announced a halt to the bombing, claiming that the American and British missiles and war planes had 'significantly damaged Iraq's military capabilities

and its ability to produce weapons of mass destruction.' He also called the operation a 'success' and claimed that 'I'm confident that we have achieved our mission'.[22]

According to Defense Secretary Cohen, Iraq's 'command and control' systems and networks had been substantially damaged, but he also had to concede that 'Saddam may rebuild, and attempt to rebuild, some of this military infrastructure in the future, just as he has replaced many facilities, including lavish palaces, after Desert Storm, but we have diminished his ability to threaten his neighbours with both conventional and non-conventional weapons.'[23]

The table bellow gives only a preliminary damage assessment of attacks during four nights of attack. Many of the cases appearing as 'under assessment' turned out to be of much lower importance than first assumed.

TABLE 8: TYPES OF SITES TARGETED DURING THE ATTACKS[24]	Total	D/SD	M/LD	UA
Surface-to-Air Missiles (SAM),Integrated Air Defense Systems (IADS)	32	6	8	18
Command and Control Facilities	20	11	6	3
Weapons Security Facilities	18	7	11	0
Weapons Production, Research and Development, Storage Facilities	11	1	9	1
Airfields	5	0	5	1
Economic Targets	1	0	1	0
Legend: D/SD: Destroyed/Severely Damaged,				

On the whole only a minority of targets were destroyed and the only economic target (the oil refinery complex at Basra) was only 'lightly' damaged. Moreover, the attacks left Saddam Hussein in power, perhaps in an even more defiant posture than before and challenging the international community at every possible way.

At the local level, a purge of several high-ranking officers from the Iraqi army took place with a view to strengthen the rule of Saddam. Saddam proclaimed victory over 'enemies of God.' In his taped address to the Iraqi people and members of the armed forces shortly after the halt of the attacks, the Iraqi leader thus claimed that 'You were up to the level that your leadership and your brother and comrade Saddam Hussein had hoped you would be at, so God rewarded you and delighted your hearts with the crown of victory'.[25]

Saddam has on several occasions fired against the American jets

patrolling the Iraqi no-fly zones. He has further refused to allow the United Nations to resume the weapons inspections, accusing UNSCOM teams of having 'collected sensitive electronic intelligence for the Clinton administration designed to topple the government of Saddam Hussein.'[26] Later developments confirmed that this accusation was not baseless, but that at least some members of the team were indeed on such a mission. Finally, he threatened to terminate the UN 'Oil for Food' programme.

A Continuing War of Attrition

Ever since the end of the seventy hours' bombings in December, there have been almost daily raids against the Iraqi air defense system in both the northern and southern no-fly zones. This deserves the label of a war of attrition, even though US sources claim that their activities are 'in response to anti-aircraft fire directed at allied planes and an Iraqi violation of the southern exclusion zone.'[27]

Moreover, soon after Operation Desert Fox, U.S. efforts to encourage an overthrow of the Iraqi President commenced, in accordance with a law passed by the US Congress in October 1998. The United States pledged $97 million in military support to seven Iraqi opposition groups working to depose Saddam Hussein. During the last week of January 1999 Secretary of State Madeleine Albright toured the Middle East to discuss the overthrow of the Iraqi leader, accompanied by Assistant Secretary of State Martin Indyk, known as the designer of 'Dual Containment'. The immediate response of Saddam Hussein was to offer of a $14,000 reward to any Iraqi who shot down an enemy plane. The regime further referred to the opposition groups as 'traitors, agents and aging mules who call themselves opposition.'

Diplomats in Baghdad see few signs that any opposition groups would be able to dethrone Saddam Hussein. According to CNN:

> The main pillars of the Iraqi regime are stable—the ruling Ba'ath party, the armed forces and internal security forces are firmly under the Iraqi president's control. Hussein himself is surrounded by a tightly knit circle of relatives and old comrades. Years of sanctions have weakened Iraq's once-formidable army, but it still outnumbers and can outgun the opposition. Although Baghdad does not have total control over squabbling Kurdish groups in the north or Iranian-backed Shi'ite guerrillas in the south, Iraq officials say the rebels pose no threat.[28]

The external players apparently do not sincerely want to promote peace

and tranquillity in the region, unless this unconditionally serves their interests. Regional players, on the other hand, are handicapped by their lack of sense for strategy, hence remain vulnerable to both external and internal threats.

The International and Arab World Reaction

During the last twenty years in the Middle East, Saddam Hussein inflicted brutal harm on his own people, as well as threatened his neighbours and regional stability. Nevertheless, regardless of how much the people in the region may hate Saddam and dislike his politics, they have generally not been supportive of the US-UK military raids against Iraq.

Many thought that 'the United States should hit at the regime and not the people.'[29] During and after the December attacks anger spread in immigrant Iraqi communities across Europe and emotions erupted around the world, especially among Arabs. The most restrained reactions consisted of short notes in journals, telephone calls to news agencies and e-mail messages to U.S. President Bill Clinton. In most cases, the protesters pretended to represent a global view, hence their messages typically stated that more than 250 million Arab people were deeply saddened and hurt by the way Iraq and its people were treated.

More significant expressions of grievances were anti-British and American demonstrations such as those in Damascus, reported by the *Washington Post*.

> In Damascus, thousands of stone-throwing demonstrators attacked the U.S. Embassy and the British cultural mission. Some demonstrators managed to scale the wall of the embassy compound, where they tore down and burned an American flag. Embassy guards held off the protestors with tear gas before Syrian security forces waded in and dispersed the crowd.[30]

In Palestine, the positive memory of the recent visit by president Clinton was soon overshadowed by anger, and cries of 'Death to America' were heard and U.S and British flags burned on the West Bank, in Hebron, Jenin and the Gaza strip. Palestinian Authority cabinet secretary Ahmed Abdel-Rahman, was quoted by the *Jerusalem Post* as saying:

> Stop unconditionally and without delay. Solve the problem peacefully on the basis of UN resolution. What is going on now is without international legality and should stop immediately. The bombings will have bad

consequences in the Arab world...This military [operation] will not help stability or the peace process.[31]

Besides the U.S and Britain, countries such as Jordan, Egypt, Austria, Denmark and even Bulgaria saw demonstrations against the bombings. On the official level too, both allies and enemies urged Bill Clinton 'to end military operations on Iraq as quickly as possible'.[32] Egyptian Foreign Minister Amr Moussa was quoted as demanding that the assault be discontinued immediately because of 'the extreme damage it is causing to Iraq and its people and the region.'[33] Quoting from Daoud Talhami, a leader of the Democratic Front for the Liberation of Palestine and member of the Palestinian National Council, the journal wrote:

> This action is morally shocking to our people because Israel is not respecting any of the UN resolutions or even the [Wye] accord signed in the presence of the US president. Nothing is done to Israel, while Iraq is bombarded on every occasion. The people are saying this isn't just a strike against Iraq, that is a strike against all Arabs from the Strait [of Gibraltar] to the Persian] Gulf.[34]

The opponents of Saddam Hussein, *Hizb-ut-Tahrir*, by means of their electronic message system in England, protested against the bombings, accusing the US and Britain of having attacked 'the Muslims in Iraq without warning.' Their analysis identified Richard Butler's report 'as a pretext to attack the Muslims in Iraq.'

Hence not even avowed anti-Saddam forces appreciated the attack, even though they mights have construed it as furthering their own cause. On the contrary, the attack was depicted as an attack by *Kuffar* (infidels) against the Muslims of Iraq.

> The military attack that Clinton ordered against the Muslims in Iraq is not because of Iraq's dispute with the inspection team regarding the exposure of some locations. Neither is it to protect the neighbours of Iraq from the threats of Saddam. Nor is it in fear of the chemical and biological weapons as claimed. Rather it is because of the first American objective, which is the strengthening of the American presence in the Gulf and tightening control over it and the attempt to be alone in terms of influence in it.[35]

Arab leaders, like the Arab peoples, regarded the military operation as an instance of the 'jungle law' operating, referring to the lack of international backing. It was very easy to compare Iraq with Israel and

reach conclusions such as: 'If we were to compare Iraq's mistakes to Israel's, we would find that the latter's are much bigger by far, without the U.S. even thinking of once reproaching it for its jungle law.'[36] As a result of these impressions, the United States will find it hard to come up with convincing justifications for this or similar operation in the future, and it may thus have to refer to purely national security and interests criteria.

Even Turkish leaders, including the new Prime Minister, Bülent Ecevit have criticized U.S. policy, finding it increasingly difficult to support the American use of a Turkish air base for the enforcement of the no-fly zone in northern Iraq. He even said, according to a *Washington Post* report, that 'he favors lifting some economic sanctions against Iraq.' On the one hand, the Turkish leaders may appreciate having a weakened Iraq on their southern borders, which will give them a free hand to punish Kurdish rebels every now and then. On the other hand, they clearly do not want the Kurds to receive direct support from United States. Any excessive American intervention in the Kurdish region can cause problems much more severe than the current Iraqi problem. Ankara is in fact concerned that 'US policies towards Turkey's southern neighbor, Iraq, might result in the establishment of an independent Kurdish state in northern Iraq.'[37]

Iran shares some of these concerns and has recently had contacts with Turkish decision-makers. During a visit to Iran by the Turkish National Assembly Speaker, Hikmet Cetin, one of the main issues for discussion was apparently Iraq. According to the Iranian Journal *Ettela'at*, Cetin on his return to Turkey said that the 'Iranian and Turkish officials share similar views on the need to preserve Iraq's territorial integrity.'[38]

Another sign of such a rapprochement between Tehran and Ankara was President Khatami's message to President Demirel, submitted by his special envoy, Deputy Foreign Minister for Asia-Pacific Affairs Mohsen Aminzadeh. According to the International edition of *Ettela'at*, President Demirel expressed his satisfaction with the message, praised Iran's 'constructive role', touched on 'the identical views shared by the two countries on developments in Iraq' and expressed his conviction that 'a continuation of U.S. interference in Iraq will bear no results.' Furthermore, quoting from Aminzadeh the journal reported that 'Tehran and Ankara severely condemn the alien interference in the region specifically in Iraq, demanding an immediate stop of the U.S. strike against the nation'. He further stressed that 'both Turkey and Iran believe in the territorial integrity of Iraq and that the U.S. attack on Iraq will bear no result except the augmentation of pains

and suffering of the Iraqi Muslim people and enchantment of the crisis in the region.'[39] This message came only a few days after the announcement that the United States had pledged military support to the Iraqi opposition.

Moreover, during Operation Desert Fox Iran unequivocally condemned the US-UK raids. In the words of Minister Kharrazi, 'We contacted governments in the region as well as Russia, France and Britain to put an end to the attacks. We made it clear to British officials that the continuation of military actions is not acceptable to Islamic countries and demanded an end to the attacks before the start of the holy month of Ramadan. We are happy that the attacks have ended.'[40]

Even though the Vatican rarely intervenes in international war and peace issues, it did so this time, criticizing the air strikes and claiming that military action did not resolve but aggravate problems, according to the CNN.[41]

Even more importantly, having launched the attack without UN support or authorization, both the US and the UK were criticized by many of the Security Council members. While most were of the opinion that 'Iraq bore the responsibility for the situation because its refusal to cooperate with UN weapons inspection,'[42] not all members shared this view, and there were two major exceptions: Russia and China. The Chinese Ambassador charged the two attackers with having 'violated the UN Charter', and the Russian Ambassador called it a 'gross violation of the rule of law'.[43] France, too, did not appreciate the bombings and expressed its disappointment and regret.

However, the reaction of these countries should probably neither be understood as support for Saddam Hussein, Iraq and the Iraqi people in general, nor for regional peace and stability. Rather, their objections to the U.S-UK operation should be seen in the context of the existing rivalries over the so-called New World Order.

Soon after the bombings a rift appeared among the permanent members of the UN Security Council over sanctions. One of the main arguments have been that sanctions simply do not work, but rather tend to create a sense of national unity in the face of external intrusion, thereby promoting a willingness to suffer. Iraq has therefore been unwilling to accept any American-proposed relaxation of restrictions, claiming that the only satisfactory solution is a complete lifting of sanctions. Softening its position on humanitarian issues, the United States has been prepared to increase the quota under the 'Oil for Food' programme, but this was not acceptable for Iraq. Russia took a more lenient stand, proposing even softer measures which would permit Iraq

virtually full reintegration into the international community.

When the air strikes targeted pipeline communications centres and began to impact on the UN Oil-for-Food program, UN officials expressed deep concern. In fact the U.S. air strike interrupted the flow of oil to Turkey by hitting a pipeline communications tower on the 18th of February. This time they could not deny it, and even the Americans were not eager to accept responsibility for endangering the flow of the cheap oil. This incident illustrates my next point, namely that everything in the Persian Gulf region revolves around oil.

Strategic Importance of the Persian Gulf

The direct relation between 'oil' and 'war' in the Persian Gulf is obvious. On 7 December 1998, only ten days before the US-UK bombings, the Persian Gulf countries agreed to cut oil production and to ask other producers in the Organization of Petroleum Exporting Countries (OPEC) to join them in cuts. They also planned to ask Mexico to join in their efforts at reducing oil production. When in the 1970s a similar decision was taken together with Iran, Libya and other oil states it produced the so-called 'oil shock'. In 1998 the response was Operation Desert Fox which began on 16 December.

In an effort to head off a growing economic crisis, the oil producing countries in the Persian Gulf had discussed reducing oil production. Such decisions are not taken lightly by countries depending for more than 75 percent of their revenues on the export of oil. However, in the Persian Gulf region it manifested one of those rare simultaneous changes of politics and economics. This change will bring both new opportunities and instabilities to this the world's most volatile region. A symbol of this change is the remarkable development of Iranian politics which will shape regional politics and provide a model for all its neighbours.

What provoked the political change was a combination of the permanent threat from the regime of Saddam Hussein to other countries of the region with the U.S. quest for domination by a variety of means, including efforts to antagonize intra-regional relations thereby making them replicate Cold War patterns on a smaller scale. As for the economic aspect of this shift, the main factor is 'oil politics', which is bound to become risky when the players are not familiar with the game.

When the Middle Eastern states embarked on their 'oil game' in the 1970s, no Arab state really anticipated the likely outcomes of such a game. After about three decades of oil politics, today's oil prices are comparable to what they were thirty years ago, and the competition for

oil sales at attractively reduced prices is as strong as ever. This trend is likely to continue despite the very problematic, high-cost and high-risk oil from the Caspian Sea.

Using the 'oil factor' as the independent variable makes it easier to understand why France, Russia and China do not support the U.S. policy towards Iraq, but are considered Iraq's best friends on the UN Security Council. Iraq has huge debts to Russia and France, and these two states as well as China are hoping for favourable future oil deals with Iraq. While countries like Iran, as of April 1999, were doubling their price at local gas pumps in order to cover part of their large budget deficit, the U.S. was transferring oil to bolster prices.[44] The Iranians will buy their own regular unleaded gas at a price almost ninety percent higher than last year, whereas the American consumer can expect to pay eighty cents a gallon, i.e. twenty percent less than last year.

The *Washington Post* reports that the U.S government plans to transfer 28 million barrels of cheap oil from the market into the federal Strategic Petroleum Reserve, a move which oil industry officials believe will bolster U.S. energy security. According to the president of the Washington-based American Petroleum Institute, 'It Makes a great deal of sense to replenish the reserve now when crude oil can be obtained at historically low prices, substantially saving money for American tax payers.'[45]

According to the statement by President Clinton issued only few minutes after the air raids began in the night of 16 December 1998, 'The purpose [of the military raids against Iraq] is to protect the national interest of the United States, and indeed the interests of the people throughout the Middle East and around the world.' However, it strains the imagination to believe that the U.S. should take such steps for entirely unselfish reasons. The primary motives are rather to be found in a complex set of national interests, central among which is oil.

The cheap and accessible oil which is essential for almost all industrialized countries is only to be found in the Persian Gulf. Indeed, approximately two-thirds of the world's proven oil and one-third of its natural gas reserves are controlled by the Persian Gulf states, as shown in Table 9. Furthermore, the best routes from the Caspian Basin to the West pass through the Persian Gulf. If the estimated reserves of the Caspian Basin are added to those of the Persian Gulf, the regional share rises to perhaps seventy percent for oil and over forty percent for natural gas. Hence, the combined Persian Gulf and Caspian Basin energy reserves represent 'the most significant geo-strategic realities of our time'.[46]

TABLE 9: WORLD OIL AND GAS	Oil	Gas
Saudi Arabia	257,800	5,200
Iraq	100,000	3,100
UAE	98,100	5,800
Kuwait	94,000	1,500
Iran	92,900	19,800
Neutral Zone	5,000	n.a.
Oman	4,500	500
Qatar	3,700	6,400
Bahrain	n.a.	500
Persian Gulf (total)	656,000	42,500
Rest of the world	350,800	95,800
World total	1,006,800	138,300
Legend: mb: million barrels, bcm: billion cubic metres		

The need for oil from the Persian Gulf creates a requirement for safe passage through its waters. For many industrialized countries of the West the region is, furthermore, economically very important as an export market for their civilian commodities as well as armaments. These exports also presuppose the secure passage of oil, as oil exports provide the revenue needed to purchase weapons and other goods.

These trade flows would be placed in jeopardy by the domination or occupation of these territories by external powers who would then also control trade. A statement by British PM Tony Blair during the last war against Iraq contained a phrase that deserves more attention than it has received, and which must frighten any oil producing country: 'The whole world knows *we have allowed* Saddam to sell oil to buy as much as *food and medicine* for the Iraqi people *as necessary.*' For countries possessing natural resources, but dependent on trade it must be a frightening prospect to become dependent on the good will of a foreign power for access to the world market. Instability in the Persian Gulf will almost automatically endanger the safe passage of oil and is thus a potential threat to both oil importing and exporting countries, both of which are dependent on it. As a corollary, the defence of 'oil' in the Persian Gulf cannot be a monopolistic task for the Americans.

Conclusion and Recommendations

For the entire period from 1991 to 1998 the Persian Gulf region has hoped for 'light at end of the tunnel' and a brighter future. However, the events of December 1998 proved that Saddam Hussein remained capable of threatening the region. The attack by the British and

American Air Forces merely set back his capabilities for a year or so. It also proved the Clinton administration's policy of 'dual containment' to be a failure.

Hence the need for the Persian Gulf countries themselves to think about their own regional security arrangements. Most preferable would be a cooperative security arrangement in which all interested parties could play a role proportional to their capabilities—a system of security based on the necessity to coexist peacefully with neighbours and to live in peace, based on mutual respect, confidence, and protection.

The American dual containment policy is both confused and confusing. It is incompatible with regional security and stability and has undesired political, social, and economic consequences for the Persian Gulf countries. A good example of how Western, and specially American, scholars see the region is Geoffrey Kemp's recent article 'The Persian Gulf Remains the Strategic Prize', in which the author argues: 'There are three general categories of threat that could disrupt Persian Gulf oil supplies: the overt use of force by regional hegemons armed with WMD; domestic instability and terrorism within the Gulf states themselves; and conflict between regional and outside powers over control and access to the Caspian Basin.'[47]

While this is, of course, correct, Kemp disregards the, at least equally likely, possibility that a world hegemon such as the United States could be seen as a threat with its deployment of aircraft carrier and naval battle groups armed with hundreds of Tomahawk missiles and aircraft, tens of thousands of troops armed with Tornadoes, Jaguars, heavy B-52 bombers, and its a far-flung network of military bases and strong military presence all around the Persian Gulf.[48] To his credit, Geoffrey Kemp highlights the very real dangers stemming from growing economic pressure (illustrated by the declining GDP growth rates in countries like Saudi Arabia and Iran) in combination with a growing population:

> With Saudi Arabia's population growing at 3.5% a year and its gross domestic product (GDP) stagnant, per-capita GDP has fallen from nearly $10,000 in 1990 to $8,000 in 1998. Many young Saudis are unskilled and unemployed. Since revenues are falling because of low prices, Saudi Arabia has to cut back either on defense spending, cradle-to-grave welfare programs or investment in energy modernization.
>
> Iran's GDP growth-rate dropped from 3.4% in 1997 to an expected 2.3% in 1998. If, as expected, the world oil market remains flat for a period of years, Iran's revenues will continue to fall just when it needs to make key investment decisions. Iran's oil-export income accounts for about 40% of government revenues. Tehran claims that it loses $1 billion

for each $1 drop in the barrel price of oil.[49]

The dangers inherent in these developments notwithstanding, international arms deliveries to the region have not abated, showing how suppliers have only little interest in the stability of the region.

Table 10: Arms Deliveries to the Persian Gulf, 1994-97 (US $M)[50]	1994	1995	1996	1997
Iran	417	522	417	800
Iraq	n.a.	n.a.	n.a.	n.a.
Kuwait	864	939	1,081	700
Saudi Arabia	7,769	9,032	9,439	11,001
UAE	428	913	678	626

Obviously in a tight economic situation, the countries involved face the choices between increasing the percentage of their GDP dedicated to defence expenditures or decreasing their arms purchases.

As the situation of the other countries of the region is no better, it becomes apparent that these nations simply need to learn to coexist. Perhaps a non-aggression pact could be a valuable beginning. In the past countries such as Iran have (at least rhetorically) supported the idea, but it needs elaboration and an explicitation of the functional steps required by each country.

A non-aggression pact could probably increase the sense of security in the Persian Gulf, but only if all countries are involved. It should start from small steps; initially involve NGOs rather than direct contacts between high-ranking officials, and take into account the various peace research proposals for regional conflict resolution and preventive diplomacy. Only after such preparatory steps have been taken and eventually produced a final non-aggression pact is any support from the international community to be expected. A defensive restructuring of the armed forces in the region (elaborated in the chapter by Bjørn Møller in the present volume) would be a useful companion to the suggested non-aggression treaty, both of them representing a Common Security approach to regional security.

Notes

1. Klare, Michael T. & Yogesh Chandrani (eds.): *World Security. Challenges for a New Century,* 3rd ed. (New York: St. Martin's Press, 1998), p. 128.

2. Robinson, Eugene: 'U.S. Halts Attacks on Iraq after Four Days', *Washington Post* (20 December, 1998).

3. Bakhtiari, Bahman: 'The Governing Institutions of the Islamic Republic of Iran: The Supreme Leader, The Presidency, and the Majlis', in Jamal S. Al-Suwaidi (ed.): *Iran and the Gulf: A search for Stability* (Abu Dhabi, Emirates Center for Strategic Studies and Research, 1996), pp. 47-69.

4. *Ibid.*, p. 48.

5. Renshon, Stanley A.: 'The Gulf War Revisited: Consequences, Controversies, and Interpretations', in idem (ed.): *The Political Psychology of the Gulf War, Leaders, Publics and the Process of Conflict* (Pittsburgh: University of Pittsburgh Press, 1993), pp. 329-357.

6. Kelman, Herbert C.: 'The Reaction of Mass Publics to the Gulf War', *ibid.*, pp. 251-265.

7. Michael, Gordon: 'U.S. Shoots Down an Iraqi Warplane in No-Flight Zone', *New York Times* (29 December 1992); Wright, Robin: 'U.S. Strikes Back as Iraq Defies ''No-Fly'' Zone', *Los Angeles Times* (31 December 1998); idem: 'U.S. Pilots Fire on Iraq Jets in ''No-Fly'' Zone Confrontation', *ibid.* (6 January 1999).

8. White, Nigel: 'The Legality of the Threat of Force against Iraq', *Security Dialogue*, vol. 30, no. 1 (March 1999), pp. 75-86.

9. 'A Review of Developments in Iraq', *RFE/RL Iraq Report*, vol. 2, no. 2 (15 January 1999).

10. *Ibid.*

11. UNSCOM: *Report on the Activities of the Special Commission during the period, 2-9 December 1998.*

12. 'Special Report: Iraq's Weapons of Mass Destruction', *BBC* (8 November 1998).

13. *Ibid.*

14. 'Blair's Statement on Iraq Strikes: Full Text', *BBC Online Network* (17 December 1998).

15. Gellman, Barton: 'Why Now? U.S. Says Iraq Determined Timing', *Washington Post* (17 December 1998).

16. 'Impeachment Debate Delayed', *CNN Online* (16 December 1998).

17. Tony Blair's statement, 'We Had No Other Choice', was published in *The Times*, electronic version (17 December 1998).

18. Rudge, David: 'Air Strikes Has 50-50 Chance of Success', *The Jerusalem Post*, Internet edition (18 December 1998).

19. O'Sulivan, Arieh: 'Security Sources: Saddam Starting to Crack', *ibid.*

20. *Ibid.*

21. Myers, Steve Lee: 'U.S. and Britain End Raids on Iraq, Calling Mission a Success', *New York Times*, online version, International Edition (20 December 1998).

22. Robinson: *loc. cit.* (note 2).

23. *Ibid.*

24. Sources: Defense Department, *BBC*, *Wire Reports*, *The Washington Post* (20 December 1998).

25. 'Saddam Claims Victory over "Enemies of God"', *Gulf News* (21 December 1998), quoting from Reuters.

26. Goldman, John J.: 'Annan: U.S. Deny Iraq Spy Accusations', *Los Angeles Times* (7 January 1999).

27. 'Iraq Condemns "Grave New Escalation"', *BBC Online* (25 February 1999).

28. 'Iraq: Efforts to Oust Saddam Hussein Doomed to Fail', *CNN Interactive* (1 February 1999).

29. Miller, Marjorie: 'Most in the Arab World View Punitive Strikes on Iraq as Doomed to Fail', *Los Angeles Times* (19 December 1998). The author is quoting from Ghassan Khatib, Palestinian political analyst in Jerusalem.

30. Robinson: *loc. cit.* (note 2).

31. Lynfield, Ben: 'US Strikes Spark Palestinian Anger', *The Jerusalem Post*, Internet edition, (18 December 1998).

32. *Ibid.*, quoting from Egyptian President Hosni Mubarak.

33. *Ibid.*, emphasis added.

34. Lynfield: *loc. cit.* (note 31).

35. *Ibid.*

36. Miller: *loc. cit.* (note 29).

37. 'Ecevit: Turkey Had Taken "Some Wrong Steps" over Iraq', *Iran Daily*, no. 499 (4 February 1999).

38. 'Turkish Parliament Chief Satisfied with Outcome of Iran Visit', *Ettela'at International Edition*, no. 1150 (4 February 1999).

39. 'Tehran-Ankara Cooperation to Promote Peace', *ibid.*, no. 1152 (8 February 1999).

40. 'Iraq Appreciates Iran stance', *Iran Daily*, no. 471 (31 December 1998).

41. 'Clinton to Explain his Iraq, Cuba Policies to Pope', *CNN Interactive* (26 January 1999).

42. Goshko, John M.: 'On Security Council, Mixed Views of Attack', *Washington Post* (17 December 1998).

43. *Ibid.*

44. Any attempt to increase fuel price in Iran produces a steep rise in the price of other commodities and foodstuffs. Recent debates about an increase in local fuel prices caused a record price rise of 0.2 percent, according to the Central Bank of Iran. See *Ettela'at International*, 23 December 1998.

45. Brown, Warren: 'U.S. to Transfer Oil to Bolster Prices', *The Washington Post* (12 February 1999).

46. Kemp, Geoffrey & Robert E. Harkavy: *Strategic Geography and the Changing Middle-East* (Washington, DC: Brookings Institution Press, 1997), p. 111.

47. Kemp, Geoffrey: 'The Persian Gulf Remains the Strategic Prize', *Survival*, vol. 40, no. 4 (Winter 1998-99), pp. 132-149.

48. For a better vision of the magnitude of the U.S. presence in the Persian Gulf, see for example 'U.S. Forces in Gulf by the Numbers', *New York Times* (17 December 1998); or 'World: Middle East Military Facts and Figures', *BBC Online* (13 November 1998).

49. Kemp: *loc. cit.* (note 47).

50. International Institute of Strategic Studies: *The Military Balance, 1998/99* (Oxford: Oxford University Press, 1998), p. 272.

10   IRAQ AND THE UNIPOLAR WORLD ORDER

Birthe Hansen

A Decade-long Stalemate

Ironically, Iraqi president Saddam Hussein may have been among the very first to recognize that a new world order had come into being at the end of the Cold War. So far, the new order has brought Iraq serious problems and in the period between 1990 and 1999 the relationship between Iraq and US has been a process of warfare and stand-offs, the subject of this chapter.[1]

Saddam Hussein pointed to the fact that there was now only one superpower present posing dangers to states like Iraq, as US-allies would progress at their expense. However, Iraq was also the first state to challenge an important dimension of the new order. The August 1990 invasion of Kuwait sent shock waves around the world. Was this what could be expected from the post-Cold War era, or was the Cold War still operative with new, aggressive expressions?

As a consequence of its aggression, however, Iraq was defeated in Operation Desert Storm. It subsequently lost control of its north-eastern part as a result of the UN-established 'safe haven' for the Iraqi Kurds; it became subject to sanctions; and, from the mid-1990s, it was subjected to series of air-strikes.[2] All this as a result of Iraq's refusal to fully comply with the UN demands stated in the 1991 cease-fire resolution. By mid-1999, more than eighth years after the end of the Gulf War, Iraq was still suffering from these problems. On the other hand, the United States, which led the 1990-91 coalition against Iraq, remained preoccupied with putting relentless pressure on Iraq. The US even increased its efforts in spite of declining international support and a preoccupation with other major tasks such as the stalled Middle East peace process (from the mid-1990s) and Yugoslavia (Serbia), including the Kosovo conflict in the spring of 1999.

This raises the question why both sides to the conflict were prepared to adhere to their positions through an almost decade-long stand-off. When considering and analysing Persian Gulf security, the policies of both Iraq and the United States are of great importance. Iraq is one of the regional great powers, and its long-lasting isolation has a

profound impact on the region. Likewise, the presence of the United States, as the only superpower, is of tremendous effect. The purpose of this article is to offer partial explanations of the behaviour of the two parties by means of propositions deduced and developed from the neorealist theory (according to Kenneth Waltz) with an emphasis on the concepts of 'peripheral loser' and 'rational management'.

Peripheral Losers and Rational Management

The concept of 'peripheral loser' refers to a state which is, on the one hand, not clearly or exclusively inside any of the bipolar rival networks of alignments but, on the other hand, is still encompassed by the rivalry, hence deeply influenced by the Cold War. Under unipolarity (defined as an international distribution of aggregate capabilities[3] identifying only one state as a superpower)[4] most states are expected to adjust to the unipolar dynamics and world order, but some might not do so. Why certain states fall out with the unipole is the problem.

A cautious hypothesis, based on empirical generalizations, leads to the statement that the risk of falling out with the unipole shortly after a systemic change (defined as a change in polarity, like the end of a hot or a cold war) is especially high if a state is a peripheral loser. However, why Iraq has been one of the most 'stubborn' of the peripheral losers, seen from the perspective of the unipole, probably requires additional explanations, referring to Iraq's special attributes and the specifics of the American world order. Having only military means and political manoeuvres left as means to improve its international position, the specific composition of Iraqi strength is likely to be an important factor.

The concept of 'rational management' refers to the unipole's (*in casu* the American) incentives to manage global affairs. Even though great and superpowers always have such incentives, according to Waltz, those of a unipole are even stronger, as it enjoys the preeminent position in the international system, hence has the greatest interest in managing world affairs. The assumption of 'rationality' is an analytical construct, implying that the unipole, everything else being equal, is expected to manage international affairs according to criteria of concern and prospects of success.[5]

In order to explain the Iraqi-US stand-off, a version of the neorealist theory is applied with an emphasis on systemic change, unipolarity and capability analysis, as well as on some specific, sub-theoretical considerations on peripheral losers and rational management.[6] It appears reasonable to include the following points:[7]

Iraq invaded Kuwait due to a misperception of the international

systemic change of 1989 and to a decline in relative capabilities. The United States was ready to respond with war, *in casu* Operation Desert Storm, due to the managerial incentives of the unipole and with a view to making an example of the Iraqi case in a time of international turbulence. Iraq was not willing to comply with the international demands because of its status as a so-called peripheral loser with bleak prospects for the future and a lack of political instruments. The United States was specifically tough on Iraq because of its incentive to manage world affairs, the Iraqi combination of being both defiant in the face of the American world order and a threshold state with regard to weapons of mass destruction (WMD).

Before applying them, the concepts need some elaboration, which is followed by the perspectives on the Gulf security in the American-led unipolar world order.

Unipolarity and Peripheral Losers
In general, neorealist theory implies a strong emphasis on the distribution of aggregate, relative capabilities, and on changes in these. There is also a focus on the policies of the great powers of the international system. As the distribution of capabilities indicates the relations of strength, changes in this consequently affect outcomes, and the great powers (poles) are by definition strong and important. Moreover, a strong analytical emphasis is usually placed on the number of poles, as specific international dynamics are believed to be associated with each number, i.e. each form of polarity. In the case of unipolarity, the specific dynamics are expected to be reflected in international politics, and the policy of the United States becomes the natural focus.

Attributing explanatory power to polarity means that we have to identify the specific dynamics of a given polarity. In the case of unipolarity, three dynamics relate specifically to the US-Iraqi stand-off:

The unipole will undertake managerial functions worldwide, as it has the greatest stakes in the world order and therefore an incentive to manage. This management will be determined mainly by the unipole's interests. The unipole holds a comparatively privileged position as it has no equal adversaries, but it faces the trap of possible exhaustion caused by over-management, and it risks falling out with many other states, as its pursuit of widespread interests cannot help antagonizing other states. Other states have an incentive to flock around the unipole, a pattern referred to as 'uni-polarization'. In cases of security threats, they have no other options as there are no alternative great power to rely on. Hence they have to work hard to obtain security guarantees.

Generally, states tend to adapt easily, also to new world orders. In principle, however, all states have two possible ways of responding: To adapt or not. While most do, some do not and these states create problems for themselves just as they pose challenges to the pole or poles in question. For adaptive states, the incentive to flock is highly dependent on the degree of the security threat.

Polarity notwithstanding, states in an international system always face the challenges posed by the balance of power, as well as what has been called 'the alliance security dilemma'. The latter entails a choice between, on the one hand, obtaining additional security by alignment and, on the other hand, retaining autonomy. The expectation is thus that the tendency to flock is directly proportional to the severity of security problems. One such security problem is that of invasion. Even when other states are invaded, many states will perceive this as a security problem, as they could be next in line if a green light is given for invasion.

Thanks to its privileged position, the unipole evidently enjoys a considerable freedom of action in the sense that it has many options of action, comparatively many resources, and the ability to balance any threats. On the other hand, however, unlike other types of poles the unipole needs to watch and manage the whole world rather than merely a part of it. Consequently, it is expected to make priorities in accordance with its general role.

These propositions are meant to cover the state of unipolarity, but need to be complemented with more dynamic ones pertaining to the period of concrete transformation of an international system. When do states react most strongly? When they are under most pressure or when world politics appears most insecure and unpredictable? It is perfectly compatible with the neorealist notion that change in the distribution of power creates a strong response. Systemic change thus produces expectations of remarkable outcomes in international politics, as the states are under heavy pressure while at the same time experiencing great difficulties with overlooking the context. Even if polarity had changed, states might still be in doubt about the change itself as well as its consequences. This leads to expectations based on the turbulence and lack of transparency, and with ample space for misperceptions and miscalculations about the consequences of the dramatic changes of power.

Systemic change increases the probability of the following outcomes due to the changed relations of power, including different options of alignment, and the increased risk of misperception and miscalculation:[8] Changes in the composition of the state system, e.g.

the rise of new states or the collapse of existing ones; the outbreak or end of conflicts; the outbreak or end of civil war; and instances of realignment.

Indeed, the Iraqi invasion of Kuwait took place during such a transitional phase between one world order and another, and there is ample historical evidence that such periods are marked by international turbulence, which may include wars and the outbreak of civil wars. Hence, the transformation perspective appears a proper one when trying to explain the Iraqi invasion as well as the US response in the form of Operation Desert Storm.

Iraq's Invasion of Kuwait

Iraq invaded Kuwait on 7 August 1990, following massive Iraqi troop concentrations on the Kuwaiti border. Almost everybody apparently saw these deployments as mere pressure on the Kuwaitis, following Iraqi-Kuwaiti disagreements on oil prices as well as, later, the al-Rumaylah oilfield.

In the spring of 1990 Saddam Hussein had revealed an increasingly aggressive Iraqi strategy for recovering and rebuilding the Iraqi state, which had suffered severely from the Iraq-Iran War and the political isolation in the Middle East. In 1989 Iraq had pursued an integrative strategy comprising cooperative steps such as the efforts to set up the Arab Cooperation Council (ACC). However, seen from an Iraqi perspective this integrative strategy proved to be a failure,[9] and at the ACC-meeting in Amman in February 1990, the first indication of a new Iraqi approach was revealed in the form of strong Iraqi attacks on the United States.

On 2 April 1990 Saddam Hussein made his famous speech, in which he warned Israel against any move and threatened retaliation.[10] One month later, in May 1990, Iraq hosted the Baghdad summit of the Arab League with the title *Threats to Arab National Security*. One of the main themes was the alleged Israeli threat; another was the West's threat to the Arab world; and a third was the development of the region. From the Iraqi point of view, this third theme covered the promotion of equality between the rich Southern Gulf States and less wealthy Arab states[11]. However, Iraq found itself rather isolated at the summit, where only the PLO and Jordan supported its positions. After the Baghdad summit Iraq completely abandoned the last vestiges of the integrative and cooperative strategy in favour of an offensive position. Throughout the transition, however, Iraq maintained the same understanding of the post-Cold War Middle Eastern situation.

Clear and explicit references were repeatedly made to the new

global situation and the changed relations of strength. The US was thus labelled the only superpower at the ACC Amman meeting in February 1990: 'The US has emerged in a superior position in international politics'.[12] This theme was elaborated upon at the Amman meeting and at the Baghdad summit.

The new US position allegedly had two main consequences for the Middle East, namely a 'US control of the oil market' (as it was stated at the Amman summit in February 1990)[13] and a strengthening of Western 'proxies'. The states which had once depended on Soviet support and guarantees were now weakened vis-à-vis the pro-Western states, and the most important obstacle to further US influence had vanished because of the Soviet decline. Saddam Hussein thus declared that Iraq was afraid US proxies might seek to benefit from this, pointing especially to Israel, but also to the oil-rich Gulf states.

Iraq further expressed the fear that the US would have a free reign in the absence of Soviet power which could inhibit Arab identity and integrity. Saddam Hussein thus concluded that Western progress represented a threat to Iraq, and warned that the US might use Israel to halt the Iraqi missile programme and damage Iraqi military capacity.[14] In April 1990 he warned Israel directly against any action.

The background against which Iraq feared that the emerging, post-Cold War order could imperil its prospects was serious. Iraq was facing a huge reconstructing project after the eight year-long war with Iran. Its position (measured in terms of relative, aggregate capabilities) in the region had declined due to the war, in the aftermath of which Iraq had become rather isolated politically. Its initial integrative strategic approach did not seem to redress this,[15] hence it was abandoned in favour of an offensive strategic approach.

All available evidence points to an Iraqi miscalculation of the likelihood as well as risk of foreign interference. When Iraq decided to send its troops across the Kuwaiti border, the decision was probably based on a conviction that the US would take a neutral stand and not interfere in internal Arab affairs. Saddam Hussein told Ambassador Glaspie during their talks in late July that the US would not accept the scale of losses (ten thousand men a day) that Iraq would in such a conflict. Proof of such Iraqi calculations and considerations can be found in the work by Freedman and Karsh.[16] As it was later revealed in the Congressional hearings on the talks between Ambassador Glaspie and Saddam Hussein the US had sent confusing signals during the crisis before the invasion, and had tried to combine appeasement with deterrence of Iraq.

Iraq had apparently counted on appeasement being the dominant

aspect of the American stand, also because the US had forwarded a 'no-position' stand on the Iraq-Kuwait dispute at the meeting between Saddam Hussein and Ambassador Glaspie on 25 July 1990 and had even expressed satisfaction with the preferred Iraqi oil price.[17] The assurances that were broadcast in July by Assistant Secretary of State for Middle East Affairs, John Kelly, to the effect that the Southern Gulf States and the US had no formal defence treaties, were also strong signals of appeasement to Iraq.[18] Furthermore, the US was heavily preoccupied with Eurasian developments such as German reunification and the adjustment of the nuclearized Soviet Union.

Before the 1990 invasion Iraq was in a situation in which dramatic outcomes was highly probable: The systemic change of 1989 had affected Iraq negatively by reducing its options of great power alignment and support. Iraq had suffered from a declining position in the region in terms of capabilities and was facing further decline. The international context was marked by confusion and risk of misperception following the shifting balance of power. Saddam Hussein failed to fully recognize the changes by projecting bipolar dynamics into the new situation and by miscalculating the US position towards an invasion.

When examining these findings, the Iraqi invasion of Kuwait can be explained by the systemic change of 1989, triggered by the prospects of further decline of Iraqi capabilities.

Operation Desert Storm

The United States reacted strongly to the Iraqi invasion, explicitly 'did not rule out any option' and began the build-up of forces in Saudi Arabia. By mid-January 1991 Operation Desert Storm was launched primarily in the form of air-strikes. One month later ground forces were brought into action. The operation was launched after diplomatic efforts, the implementation of sanctions, the formation of an international coalition against Iraq, and a military build-up throughout the autumn of 1990. The pressure failed to make Iraq withdraw from Kuwait and the war between Iraq and the coalition, led by the US and acting on a UN mandate, began and resulted in Iraqi defeat.

The vast majority of initiatives between the invasion and Operation Desert Storm was taken by the United States, which also provided the bulk of troops and military equipment as well as the leadership of the whole military operation. By means of diplomatic activity the US had also gathered a broad international coalition behind its actions, even though some states warned against the operation, advocating continued diplomatic pressure as their alternative.

The Coalition was put together during early autumn 1990 under clear and explicit US leadership. A total of at least 36 countries joined in,[19] including former Soviet allies and clients, pro-US states, and some former members of the Non-Aligned Movement. The Multilateral Force (MLF) assembled by the Coalition thus included democracies and dictatorships, rich and poor countries as well as representatives from all continents (even some volunteers from the Afghan Mujahedin movement). Amongst those aligned against Iraq were also a number of Arab states: Morocco, Egypt, Syria, Saudi Arabia, Oman, Bahrain, Qatar, the United Arab Emirates and, of course, Kuwait, represented by the exiled Al Sabah government.

The Arab participation was extensive and remarkable. The major Arab countries responded positively and publicly in spite of the presence of anti-imperialist and anti-American movements in their countries. There was an American fear that these governments might withdraw from the Coalition to avoid being overthrown for their stance alongside the US. Nevertheless, none of the Arab states left the Coalition and some of them even increased their contributions in the course of the conflict. Eventually, some even fought alongside the US, putting their reputations in the Arab brotherhood at risk and exposing themselves to internal critique. Most remarkable was the presence in the Coalition of the radical state and former loyal Soviet ally, Syria.

From a theoretical perspective the actions and behaviour of the United States are compatible with the expectations concerning a unipole, at least as far as the incentive to manage world affairs and the ability to set the international agenda are concerned.

A unipole is not expected to manage all kinds of problems which might arise globally. The Iraqi invasion, however, posed a serious challenge to the emerging world order, to the US and to other states. Interstate invasion threatens the order, especially if it improves the position of the aggressor substantially, as a successful Iraqi invasion might have done. Iraq might have risen to become the major regional power and might even have used the aggrandizement to gain further influence. Letting Iraq get away with the annexation of Kuwait would have been tantamount to sending the wrong message to other states with major problems at a critical juncture. This message would have been that invasion was a possible, perhaps even legitimate, way of solving their problems. A successful invasion might also have made US policy in the Middle East much more difficult, both in terms of security and oil supply, and it might have disturbed allied states' belief in the credibility of the US as a great power ally. To other states, especially small ones, interstate invasion is always frightening as they

might become victims themselves.

In this light the US response was almost inevitable, and the massive support from other states, in the international coalition and in the UN, could be seen as the consequence of the Iraqi challenge to the world order and interstate relations.

The next task, however, is to explain the ongoing US-Iraqi stand-off which was still not resolved in the spring of 1999, more than eight years after the unilateral cease-fire which ended the Gulf War in 1991.

The Conflict between 1991 and 1999

It is less obvious why the relationship between Iraq and the US developed so badly for the following eight years. During this period Iraq remained the subject of international sanctions, as well as the target of repeated US (and British) air-strikes. The US demanded full Iraqi compliance with UN Security Council Resolution 687 (henceforth SC687), which was passed in connection with the 1991 cease-fire. SC687 demanded (among other things) that Iraq destroyed it's WMD capacity in cooperation with the UN.

Iraq claimed to comply but did not allow the UN weapons inspectors free admission to examine whether or not the Iraqi capacity of mass destruction had been eliminated as demanded. Throughout the period, international support for the US pressure on Iraq declined. Mainly France and Russia advocated an relaxation or lifting of the sanctions, and only Great Britain participated fully in the military actions against Iraq. This development raises to at least three questions, pertaining to the US 'hard-line' policy, Iraqi non-compliance, and US leadership.

The US Hard-line Policy

Why did the US allocate so many resources to, and resorted to military means against, a state that was hardly a serious threat any longer? or alternatively: Why did the US, when pursuing the case, not overthrow the Iraqi leader?

The main reason why the US stuck to its 'hard-line' policy towards Iraq and refused to accept 'anything but everything' was probably its wish to make an example of the Iraqi case. To budge would have been tantamount to sending a strong signal to other potential aggressors that they would be able to evade international demands by standing firm and just accepting sanctions for a period. This might have invited calculations that were deeply problematic, seen from a US perspective. Another crucial factor seems to have been the fact that Iraq, in addition to challenging important dimensions of the

US world order, had a WMD capacity. States not accepting important elements in the prevailing order create managerial problems, but WMD states that do so hamper this management by limiting US options of response. It is much harder to put pressure on a WMD state, and the presence of WMD imposes self-restraint because of the risks entailed. The combinations are shown in Table 11, indicating the severity of managerial problems the combinations pose to the US unipole.

TABLE 11: SEVERITY OF PROBLEMS FOR US MANAGEMENT, CAUSED BY VARIOUS TYPES OF STATES	World order acceptance	World order defiance
WMD Capacity	Low	Very high
No WMD Capacity	Very low	High

States may change their policy and thereby be re-classified, e.g. a state may turn from defiance to acceptance, it may go nuclear, or join the Nonproliferation Treaty (NPT). For example, Brazil and South Africa signed the NPT, and Ukraine gave up nuclear weapons, whereas India and Pakistan conducted nuclear tests. Changes are important, and the US has a particular incentive to prevent states on the nuclear threshold from crossing that threshold.[20]

In brief, the US has an incentive to 'move' states into the 'right' categories and foremost, to prevent non-acceptance states from achieving WMD capacity. This would enhance their ability to contest the prevailing world order and limit US options of dealing with them. For states already possessing a WMD capacity (especially nuclearized states), the challenge facing the US is to sway them into world order acceptance or, at least, to reduce their non-acceptance. WMD states not only create problems, they are also in a better position to resist international pressure than non-WMD states. Consequently, if defiant towards the world order, states with a WMD capacity have a strong incentive to retain at least part of this.

The category 'WMD capacity/World order defiance' corresponds roughly to the American notion of so-called 'rogue states'. However, the categories in Table 11 are analytical categories, whereas 'rogue states' is a political notion that often includes an emphasis of the political nature of those states as being tyrannical or authoritarian. Furthermore, the notion and the specific category may not overlap over time. It almost did in the 1990s when the US announced its policy for major regional contingencies with as proclaimed focus on 'deterring

and, if necessary, fighting and defeating aggression by potentially hostile regional powers, such as North Korea, Iran or Iraq'. This objective was included in the 'Integrated Regional Approaches', and was formulated clearly in the 1994 *National Security Strategy of Engagement and Enlargement*.[21]

Finally, Table 11 also shows that the US has an incentive to develop anti-WMD measures, such as missile defense systems capable of intercepting hostile WMD missiles, regardless of whether they are targeted against US territory or merely have a regional reach.

Iraqi Defiance
Why did Iraq not fully comply and cooperate with the UN inspection team and bring an end to sanctions and isolation?

Table 12 indicates a strong Iraqi incentive to maintain a WMD capacity, and the Iraqi status as a peripheral loser explains the Iraqi need for action. Apparently, Iraq had not lost quite enough to gain attention from the US or to be deemed worth integrating, as were the real losers in the former Soviet 'empire'. This made Iraq's prospects rather bleak. There were neither any signs of aid or support, nor any prospects of such superpower guarantees as Iraq needed in order to compensate for the loss of the Soviet Union and rebuild itself and its position in the Middle East after the end of the war with Iran. In brief, Iraq had suffered losses from the end of the Cold War, but not enough to gain adequate attention, and it was facing a tough and protracted task of rebuilding, surrounded by neighbouring states that were still supported by the US.

Another important factor seems to have been the serious national crises suffered by Iraq in the 1990s. The aftermath of Iraq's 1991 defeat posed challenges to the very survival of the Iraqi state. Internal unrest or even civil war often follow defeat, and the Iraqi state is a fragile one. It comprises three major groups (Shi'ites, Sunnis, and Kurds), and nationalism remains weakly developed in the sense that many people's primary loyalty is to their families and clans rather than to the State or nation.

Furthermore, Iraqi capabilities have continuously declined throughout the 1990s. According to neorealism, capability analysis is a useful tool, implying that state security is a function of relative capabilities.[22] Declining relative capabilities implies a weakening of a state's strength and consequently of it's power. Other states can more easily disregard the ambitions of a another state weak in capabilities than a strong one.

A capability analysis requires measuring a state's capabilities at

a given time, comparing these with capabilities at another given time, measuring the differences (positive or negative), and comparing both measures with those of other states. Table 12 shows the development of Iraqi capabilities from 1990 to 1999 (actually, the trend dates back to the Iraq-Iran War which ended in 1988) with '-' indicating a decline of capabilities and '+' an increase. The table clearly tells a story of decline of the sort that often produces action.

TABLE 12: DEVELOPMENT OF IRAQI CAPABILITIES 1990-1999		
Parameter	Trend	Comments
Size of territory	-	Iraq was deprived sovereignty and control of its north-eastern part by Operation Provide Comfort and the Kurdish safe haven
Economic capacity	-	The Iraqi economy had seriously deteriorated due to the sanctions, the isolation and the war-related infra-structural damages
Size of population	-	Iraq was divided from its Kurdish population by the safe haven
Military capacity	-	Iraq had suffered war-related damages and has since had difficulties in reconstruction and maintenance due to the sanctions
Resource endowment	(-)	Iraq had been deprived the opportunity to exploit its oil wealth because of the sanctions, and some of it is placed in the safe haven. However, some 'saving of oil' has taken place
Political stability	-	Kurdish and Shi'ite unrest; power struggles in the elite (e.g., the episode of the sons-in-law 1995-96)
Political competence	?	Not assessed, but apparently very negative[23]

An examination of the above parameters clearly shows Iraq as having suffered a steady decline in capabilities, both in absolute and relative terms. Iraq has been considerably weakened vis-à-vis its neighbours, to the extent that it only has an edge in terms of military capability. In absolute terms, the military capability has seen a lesser decline, as Iraq devoted an increasing percentage of its ever-more limited resources to its military forces.

In addition, Iraq had a qualitative 'either/or' WMD capacity. According to Table 11, defiant states have a strong incentive to maintain such a capacity or parts of it. The Iraqi instruments were thus

limited with one exception, namely the military, which helps explain its choice of strategy in the face of external pressure. The only other capability which Iraq could rely on was political competence. This has not been thoroughly assessed, but it is evident that this was the easiest to manipulate by Iraq. It was 'easier' for the leadership of Saddam Hussein to affect international politics by means of their political actions than to improve, e.g., Iraq's economic performance (in the short term).

Iraq has, between 1990 and 1999 been close to face the threat of its very survival; it has been almost 'cornered'. The closer, the more desperate a state becomes. Considering the Iraqi situation, it is obvious that Iraq has few instruments left for improving its security. Only its military capacity and political competence seem available. During the period in question, Iraq used its military capacity for two purposes: to maintain internal order (contributing to turn Iraq into a 'garrison' state) and to deter—partly by means of its WMD capacity which shielded it against international pressure against the core of the state, partly by means of its re-organized conventional forces, deterring its minor neighbour states (especially Kuwait) from totally ignoring Iraq in the oil regime.

With respect to the capability of political competence, Saddam Hussein tried to make the best of the terrible situation (into which his former decisions had led Iraq). The Iraqi leadership worked to split the international Gulf War coalition, gave priority to diplomacy towards France and Russia (the 'soft' parties) and kept appealing to the Arab masses. Regarding the international inspectors, Iraq cooperated on-and-off and placed successive minor obstacles in the way of inspection. These obstacles apparently aimed at being too insignificant for the UN to fall out with Iraq, but too substantial to let inspection succeed.

The Iraqi policy between 1990 and 1999 could be described as acceptance of societal decay in order to maintain a small WMD-capacity, probably with the purpose of deterring international pressure on Iraq and securing the survival of the Iraqi state.

Decline in the US International Position?

Did the decreasing international support and growing critique of the US policy indicate a decline of the US international position and leadership? If the above framework of analysis is accepted, it did not.

Diminishing security concerns produce receding incentives to opt for alignment combined with a loss of autonomy. From this point of view, states with geographic proximity to a threat, or states which may profit from indirect action (i.e., obtaining necessary good-will in other

areas) are expected to 'flock' in such cases. On the other hand, the US determination to pursue a general objective almost unilaterally tends to confirm the notion of US unipolarity. Whether or not it will weaken the US position in the longer term is another matter, as it may conceivably lead to exhaustion and/or produce antagonisms and counter-alignment.

Probably, the effects will not be serious, as the actions are of comparatively low costs to the US which also has the ability to compensate in other areas. One manifestation thereof is the attempt to prevent possible clashes with the 'muslim world' by defending ex-Yugoslav Moslems, as has been the case in Bosnia-Herzegovina as well as in Kosovo. The effects were significant in the Arab world, where it served both to elicit leadership approval and to popularly legitimize the leadership's affiliation with the US.

Unipolarity and Persian Gulf Security: Perspectives

It is evident that the Iraqi-US stand-off is not the only Persian Gulf challenge created by unipolarity. Unipolarity generally tends to induce increased regional activity, both with respect to conflict and cooperation.[24] A higher degree of regional interaction is therefore a central expectation.

In the Middle East there have been some indicators of movement in this direction, such as the institutional build-up of the *Union Maghréb Arabe*, the Economic Cooperation Organization, and the Israeli-Arab peace process. However, in the Persian Gulf area increased interaction apparently has a tough time as long as Iraq remains isolated and Iran's relationship with the US remains unresolved. Even the name of the Gulf has been externalized; the US renamed it simply 'the Gulf'.

While many tensions between Iran and the US continue to exist in the 1990s, two things should not be overlooked. Firstly, Iran opted for a neutral stand during the Gulf conflict 1990-91 rather than aligning itself with Iraq, i.e. it did *not* exploit an obvious opportunity to challenge the US. Secondly, Iran has continuously sent signals (although typically counter-weighed by other signals) of a desire to improve relations with the US, most notably illustrated by president Khatami's visit to the US in the spring of 1999.

Saudi Arabia enjoyed the privileged position of a superpower ally through the 1990s. The US affiliation did, however, trigger opposition. One interpretation is that it was the alignment choice of the Fahd dynasty and its one-sided direction that caused dissatisfaction. It was perceived that Saudi Arabia simply committed itself too much, too unilaterally. It has been shown that political opposition in Saudi Arabia

is rising, and that some of the rise is connected with the US influence in the country.[25] With concepts from alliance theory, Saudi Arabia deposited its security in American hands and thereby ended up on the entrapment/chain-ganging horn of the alliance security dilemma, entailing a loss of autonomy.[26]

The two Yemens which united in May 1990 were peripheral losers in a situation similar to that of Iraq. Being primarily a Soviet ally, Iraq had enjoyed support from both bipolar superpowers during its war against Iran. Likewise, each of the Yemeni states had obtained support from one of the superpowers, as a counter-weight to the other superpower's support for the respective other. Four years after their unification into the Republic of Yemen (RoY), a bloody civil war broke out. It lasted from May to July 1994 and ended with a clarification of the internal power relations, and with the attempt to unify also *de facto* in vital areas, such as the military command structure. In contrast to Iraq, however, RoY neither attacked any other state, nor displayed any aggressive behaviour, or came close to achieving a WMD capacity. It had great difficulties in adapting, manifested by the bloody civil war, but the US did not intervene.

The evolving security framework in the Persian Gulf region, under the auspices of unipolarity, will depend, to a large extent, on the regional positions of Iran and Iraq, which will have to be redefined after so many years of isolation. This challenge will coincide with those produced by the development in the Arab-Israeli peace process.

Whatever unipolarity may bring in respect to 'narrow' security matters, it will definitely trigger tension. Not only are there many states that are poorly suited for coping with the competitive setting of the world market and which will defy various aspects of US foreign policy. Within all Middle Eastern states there are also groups of citizens who can hardly meet the demands of the world market or whose values will be severely challenged by the US 'style'.

The evolving American world order will thus meet different challenges from, particularly, the major states in the Persian Gulf region: Iraq, Iran, and Saudi Arabia; and it will trigger civil opposition, probably expressed in terms of islamic fundamentalism. However, unipolarity also creates strong longer-term incentives to flock and to adapt for lack of obvious alternatives. Only when a serious challenge to unipolarity arises will serious options of realignment become available. Until then, the concepts of *peripheral losers* and *rational management* will remain useful concepts for the analysis of the (unipolar) world order of the 1990s and well into the next millennium.

Solving the Problem?

When considering the opportunities for resolving the conflict between Iraq and the US, the above framework appears useful.

The US policy towards Iraq is part of a global project involving the setting of priorities. If more serious problems arise than that posed by Iraq (as seen from a US perspective) US priorities may change according to the laws of 'rational management'—also because the Iraqi WMD capabilities have been substantially reduced, probably as much as any external power might require. It is virtually impossible to ensure a complete absence of chemical and biological weapons (which Iraq in the spring of 1999 was still accused of maintaining); hence the only meaningful objective must be reduction. Consequently, if more serious problems arise, the US may opt for settling of the conflict.

From the Iraqi perspective the societal decay may prove so devastating that it threatens the very survival of the Iraqi state even more than does the loss of the WMD capacity and the ensuing ability to resist external pressure. Hence, the leadership may change its strategy according to a new set of priorities—or it may be toppled from the inside. A possible successor to Saddam Hussein may opt for a more defensive political strategy that may pave the way for a compromise with the US. Indeed, even small changes could conceivably break the deadlock, as both sides have probably reaped all the possible benefits from the present situation.

Notes

1. I want to thank Dr. Carsten Jensen and Dr. Bjørn Møller for useful comments, and Dr. Lars Bærentzen for inspiring discussions

2. Iraq was subject to air-strikes in 1994 and from 1998-99. This was after the UNSCOM report of October 1997 to the UN Security Council, in which the assessment was very critical and the implication was that the sanctions against Iraq would hardly be eased or lifted in the short term.

3. Capabilities encompass size of territory, population, resource endowment, economy, military, political stability and political competence. See Waltz, Kenneth N.: *Theory of International Politics* (New York: Random House, 1979). The scores cannot be considered in isolation in the sense that no state is able to become a superpower by holding one capability (as nuclear weapons), but losses or gains in any capability will, of course, produce a difference in the aggregate balance. See Hansen, Birthe: 'The Unipolar World Order and its Dynamics', *DUPI Working Paper*, no. 2 (Copenhagen: Danish Institute of International Affairs, 1998). The important thing, however, is that capabilities should be analyzed in a relative perspective: are they increasing or decreasing in relation to the aggregate capabilities of other states. See Waltz: *op. cit.*

4. Hansen, Birthe: 'Unipolarity—a Theoretical Model', *Arbejdspapir*, no. 10 (Copenhagen: Institute of Political Science, University of Copenhagen, 1993); idem: *op. cit.* 1998 (note 3); idem: *Unipolarity and the Middle East* (London: Curzon Press, 2000).

5. This should not be confused with 'rationality' which Kenneth Waltz argues is not a necessary assumption of neorealism. See *op. cit.* (note 3).

6. Waltz: *op. cit.* 1979 (note 3); Hansen: *op. cit.* 2000 (note 4).

7. There is always a problem when applying systemic-structural theory: it does not account for explanations of individual outcomes but for 'phenomena'. However, if an outcome that is part of a phenomenon it should be possible to provide at least part of the explanation of the individual outcome by means of the theory, as all outcomes in the group are influenced by the same variables.

8. Hansen: *op. cit.* 2000 (note 4).

9. Karsh, Efraim & Inari Rautsi: *Saddam Hussein. A Political Biography* (Aylesbury: Futura, 1991).

10. *FBIS-NES*, 3 April, 1990, pp. 32-35.

11. The Iraqi demands were also put forward at the preparatory meeting between foreign ministers; Iraq referred again to its war efforts against Iran.

12. Dannreuther, Roland: 'The Gulf Conflict: A Political and Strategic Analysis', *Adelphi Papers*, no. 264 (1992), p. 14.

13. Cooley, John K.: 'Pre-war Gulf Diplomacy', *Survival*, vol. 33, no. 2 (1991), p. 126.

14. Dannreuther: *op. cit.* (note 12), p. 13.

15. Karsh & Rautsi: *op. cit.* (note 9).

16. Freedman, Lawrence & Efraim Karsh: *The Gulf Conflict 1990-1991* (London: Faber and Faber, 1993), pp. 50-60.

17. Cooley: *op. cit.* (note 13), pp. 127-128.

18. *Ibid.*

19. For a survey of the participants, see Cooper, Andrew Fenton, Richard A. Higgot & Kim Richard Nossal: 'Bound to Follow? Leadership and Followership in the Gulf Conflict', *Political Science Quarterly*, no. 106 (1991), p. 392.

20. This might explain why the US in 1999 went so tough against Yugoslavia (Serbia) which was defiant and probably building up a substantial chemical capacity. By May 1999, Yugoslavia (Serbia) was not affiliated with any threatening WMD-capacity. It had had exchanges with China, but on the other hand the sanctions had proved more effective than against Iraq. In brief, a WMD-threat was not considered probable (US intelligence information was not available on this). However, even small chemical stockpiles combined with world order defiance was a problem, and the problem was put in a context of further consolidating the world order.

21. The White House: *A National Security Strategy of Engagement and Enlargement* (Washington, DC: GPO, 1994).

22. Hansen: *op. cit.* 1998 (note 3).

23. Iraq had carried out two unsuccessful invasions in ten years: Iran (1980) and Kuwait (1990). The invasions definitely have imposed severe damages and created huge problems for Iraq. Relatively speaking, Iraq has thus scored far worse than most other states in the Middle East regarding political competence. However, a full analysis should comprise a counter-factual analysis of Iraq's alternatives. Such an analysis has neither been available or carried out by me, therefore the capability has been given a 'not assessed' evaluation.

24. Hansen: *op. cit.* 2000 (note 4).

25. Dekmejian, Hrair R.: 'The Rise of Political Islamism in Saudi Arabia'. *Middle East Journal*, vol. 48, no. 4 (1994).

26. On entrapment see Snyder, Glenn H.: 'The Security Dilemma in Alliance Politics', *World Politics*, vol. 36, no. 4 (1984), pp. 461-495. On chain-ganging see Christensen, Thomas J. & Jack Snyder: 'Chain Gangs and Passed Bucks: Predicting Alliance Patterns in Multipolarity', *International Organization*, vol. 44, no. 2 (1990), pp. 137-168.

11   IRAN-EU-USA RELATIONS

Seen through the Rushdie Affair

Lars Erslev Andersen

> Let us remember that the book is actually not about Islam, but about
> migration, metamorphosis, split identities, love, death, London, and
> Bombay (Salman Rushdie to Indian Prime Minister Rajiv Gandhi,
> October 1988)[1]

Thaw and Power Struggle

It was a clearly relieved and elated Salman Rushdie who, in the fall of
1998, could tell the press that he was now able to take a walk or go to
a soccer game with his favourite team, the Tottenham Hotspurs,
without having to make arrangements with security guards several days
in advance.[2] Rushdie owed this new situation to a meeting between the
British and Iranian foreign ministers at the United Nations General
Assembly in New York in September 1998,   several days after
moderate Iranian President Khatami, in his speech to the assembly, had
declared the Rushdie affair to be over. The result of the meeting was
that Iranian Foreign Minister Kharazzi gave his assurance that his
government would do nothing to execute Ayatollah Khomeini's death
sentence against Salman Rushdie. However, it was not this statement
as such that gave Rushdie relief and convinced the British to reestablish
diplomatic ties with Iran at the ambassadorial level.

After all, closer inspection reveals that there was nothing new in
the Iranian foreign minister's assurances. While in Copenhagen back in
February of 1995, Iranian Deputy Foreign Minister Vaezi had given his
Danish counterpart Niels Helveg Petersen the same assurance, even
though the Iranian government refused to send it in writing to the EU
headquarters in Brussels. On several other occasions the Teheran
government had clearly indicated that it had no intention of
contributing to the execution of Khomeini's death sentence. Rather,
both Rushdie's joy and the British government's decision to send an
ambassador to Teheran (thereby normalizing relations, both politically
and economically), was due to the fact that the Iranian foreign minister
publicly renounced the US$2.5 million bounty which a foundation had
offered to Rushdie's assassin. After the meeting Dr. Kharazzi stated at
a press conference, with his British counterpart Robin Cook also in

attendance:[3]

> I explained to mr. Cook the offense and distress the book *The Satanic Verses* has caused to muslims throughout the world, and repeated that the government of the Islamic Republic of Iran has no intention, nor is it going to take any action whatsoever to threaten the life of the author of *The Satanic Verses* or anybody associated with his work, nor will it encourage or assist anybody to do so. Accordingly the government disassociates itself from any reward which has been offered in this regard and does not support it.

It was the fact that the Iranian government unambiguously distanced itself from this bounty, offered by the 15th Khordad Foundation as a reward to Rushdie's murderer, that gladdened Rushdie, led to renewed British-Iranian diplomatic relations, and prompted the EU Presidency to issue a statement on 28 September 1998 expressing satisfaction with Dr. Kharazzi's aforementioned statement. The EU statement continued:[4]

> It removes an obstacle for a better relationship between EU and Iran and increases the possibility that closer cooperation can be discussed in a renewed dialogue. The EU has noticed the suggestion made by president Khatami to the UN General Assembly to make year 2001 into 'a year for the dialogue among civilizations'.

Thus, the EU chose to draw foreign policy conclusions from the statements by President Khatami and Dr. Kharazzi at the UN General Assembly in New York. This was also true of Denmark, where on 25 September Foreign Minister Niels Helveg Petersen accepted an invitation to visit Iran[5]—even though, in a briefing to the Danish press on 28 September he modified somewhat his promise to travel to Iran.[6] This reorientation came about without the Iranian leaders having actually said anything new.

Not only did the EU Presidency choose to ignore the threats that were issued by influential Islamic scholars and more or less self-appointed groups in Pakistan and London in the wake of Kharazzi's statements. It also disregarded the immediate reaction from both prominent and powerful clerics and radical student groups in Iran. Such reactions could certainly be regarded as both inevitable and predictable. More serious was the fact that, as things stood in the fall of 1998, the government in Teheran was simply unable to prevent a foundation from offering a bounty, even though top Iranian politicians thought it was wrong—as Foreign Ministry spokesman Mohammad Mohammadi was

quick to point out.[7]

It stands to reason that the various foreign ministries in the EU capitals must have been aware of the balance of power and the political structures in the Islamic Republic. Hence, they must have known that the current government could do nothing about the infamous bounty as long as the relationship between the political leadership and the religious powers remained as it had been since the creation of the republic. In other words, they must have appreciated the Iranian foreign minister's statements solely because of its 'moral value'.

Should any Western political leader have harboured doubts concerning the actual power structures in Iran, these must have been erased when Ayatollah Hassan Saneil of the 15th Khordad Foundation, on 12 October, was quoted, in an editorial in the paper *Jomhun Islami*, as follows:[8]

> I, as leader of the Khordad Foundation, increase the bounty by US$300,000 for execution of the decree (Khomeini's death sentence) .... It has been a great honour for this foundation to offer a bounty for the killing of Salman Rushdie and we will continue to see it as an honour. We must not allow this matter to be forgotten.

In comparison it seems less significant that as early as 10 October a student group offered a bounty of US$333,000, or that on 18 October the people of the village Kiapey announced they were offering ten rugs plus land and a house near the Caspian Sea to anyone who could get away with murdering Rushdie.[9]

As Carmel Bedford, spokeswoman for the International Rushdie Committee in London, told the AP news bureau and others on 11 October, such reactions were to be expected, although they were obviously unpleasant. On the other hand, it was difficult to overlook the provocation in Ayatollah Saneil's raising the Khordad Foundation's bounty to US$2.8 million without the Iranian government's doing anything at all about it. Whether or not the Western governments have confidence in Kharazzi and Khatami, the Khordad leader's statements demonstrate that the popularly elected government in Teheran is not alone in determining Iran's policies, including its foreign policy. It seems unlikely that Kharazzi and Khatami should not have consulted, and received a green light from, the religious leader of Iran, Ayatollah Ali Khamenei, prior to the foreign minister publicly distancing the government from the bounty. In general, there are quite narrow limits to what the foreign minister can do on his own, which also applies to the Rushdie affair.

Since the surprising election, with great popular support, of Ayatollah Khatami as president in May 1997, a power struggle has continued between the supporters of the religious leader Khamenei and groups backing Khatami's reform policy. That is how it appears on the surface, but it is far more difficult to ascertain what goes on behind the scenes. A more complicated political game may be played, where Khamenei and Khatami have chosen—by mutual, albeit tacit, agreement—to play the roles of 'bad cop' and 'good cop', respective. If this should be the case, we cannot automatically assume that the game is being played exclusively to deceive the West. It may simply imply that the political situation in Iran is far more complex than a power struggle between relatively well-defined wings.

Khamenei has both de facto and formal responsibility for the Khordad Foundation. By tacitly accepting that Iran's *political* leader distances himself from the bounty, the *religious* leader becomes able to assess how far the system can depart from the Khomeini line. At the same time, Khamenei is able to slow down the dialogue with the West, which has become Khatami's trademark. In other words, a strategic understanding between the president and the religious leader would make it possible for Khatami to invite dialogue on the foreign policy level and carry out reforms on the domestic policy level, while Khamenei is able to keep the Islamic establishment in check by slowing Khatami's reform tempo. It must be admitted that this theory is based primarily on speculation. It does, however, help explain two questions raised by the aforementioned events in New York.

First of all, it explains why the EU chose to listen to Kharazzi and draw conclusions from his statements to British Foreign Minister Robin Cook. The European foreign ministers were fully aware of the tangled web of the power struggle in Teheran, but chose to clearly support the reform line by promising Iran improved relations with the West. The implied economic 'carrot' was a trump card which Khatami could play in his foreign policy power struggle. This was apparently the strategy which the EU opted for under the name 'critical dialogue' at the Edinburgh summit in 1992, but which was largely abandoned in 1997, having produced no results. However, with the election of Khatami for president and the ensuing power struggle, a resumption of the dialogue may have seemed worth another try, which could explain the EU declaration of 28 September 1998 that seemingly disregarded the obviously conflicting signals from Teheran on the Rushdie affair.

Secondly, the theory helps explain the peculiar struggle between conservatives and liberals over reform policies, which took place in Iran in 1997 and 1998. On the one hand, Khatami can meet the

people's demands for liberalization while, on the other hand, Khamenei can ensure that this liberalization does not proceed so fast as to cause a revolt by the Islamic forces which continue to dominate the state apparatus—a revolt that might take Iran back to the policies of Khomeini in the 1980s. The on-going power struggle is one between a conservative, self-elective and dictatorial state apparatus and an Iranian society longing for reforms, political influence, and improved standards of living. It is within the framework of this conflict that Iranian politicians must try to manoeuvre, and it is with respect to this conflict that Western governments must try to formulate a strategy.

Since 1992, with only a brief hiatus, the EU has opted for a strategy of 'critical dialogue' in the hope of strengthening the liberal forces, while the United States has employed political and economic sanctions combined with active support for subversive activities as means to isolate the government of Iran as a first step to its being overthrown. The Rushdie affair plays a key role in both strategies. To the EU, it represents the most important obstacle to normalizing relations with Iran, whereas to the United States it constitutes the most obvious evidence of Iran's failure to respect the human rights convention. Along with other factors, this is believed to legitimize the tough and uncompromising US stance toward Iran.[10]

The significance of the Rushdie affair thus goes far beyond what the question of freedom of speech and concern for the author's life would warrant. It has major political significance, even today. In the following, I shall present the domestic and foreign policy significance of the affair by focusing on Khomeini's *fatwa* as a political act. I shall therefore neither take any position on whether or not it meets the standards of a *fatwa* in the Islamic legal context, nor give any opinion on whether it may be legitimized and justified on constitutional grounds. Important though the questions surely are, Khomeini's sentence serves political purposes both in Iran and with regard to Iran's relations with the rest of the world. It is on these purposes that the rest of this chapter will concentrate.[11]

Khomeini's Testament

Khomeini pronounced his sentence on *The Satanic Verses* in February 1989, i.e. exactly ten years after his return from many years of exile and the beginning of his endeavour to fashion Iran into an Islamic state.

The pronunciation of the sentence coincided with some basic changes in Iran's ideology, constitution, and foreign policy. The previous year, Khomeini had accepted a cease-fire with Iraq based on

the UN Security Council resolution 598 of July 1987. At the same time, it was clear there was no real heir apparent to Khomeini, who at this point knew he was near death. Thus, Khomeini approved several proposed constitutional amendments which meant a de facto division of power between a political and a religious leader. The combination of the cease-fire (enforced by people such as Hashemi Rafsanjani, Iran's president from 1989 to 1993 and 1993 to 1997) with the negotiations over a new constitution, and accompanied by the political trickery resulting in the election of Ali Khamenei as the new religious leader after Khomeini's death, created quite a fierce political struggle. This produced, in its turn, an odd alliance of moderate conservatives and technocrats, which was unable to take action.[12] The hard-liners who, along with Khomeini, stubbornly insisted that Iran continue its war with Iraq to the bitter end, were thus sidetracked.

The result of this power struggle was, on the one hand, that the Islamic Republic was able to survive Khomeini's death; on the other hand, that Iran embarked upon a more pragmatic policy line, both with regard to the economy and foreign policy.[13] Economic reforms were to be implemented that would presumably attract foreign investors (which was, strictly speaking, a breach of the constitution) and enable the country to take foreign loans. The latter was in total conflict with the Islamic revolutionary dogma, according to which Iran should be completely independent of both the West and the East. With regard to foreign policy, the technocrats called for greater openness toward the financially strong nations which, at that time, were to be found either in Southeast Asia or the West.

In other words, the Iranians were about to abandon some of the most basic principles of Khomeini's political philosophy and, consequently, of the Islamic revolution itself. Managing to approve the constitutional amendments before his death, Khomeini was obviously aware of the new trends and admitted to their necessity, both with regard to the cease-fire and the new constitution, even though he certainly did not like them. In his own words, they were like swallowing poison.

Seen in this context, the judgment against Rushdie and the novel *The Satanic Verses* could be seen as an antidote which, ten years after the revolution, was intended to keep the Iranians on the true path of the Revolution. Once again, Khomeini knew how to exploit something that he had not himself started as a means of uniting the Iranian nation behind his policies. The death sentence against Rushdie had the same mobilizing effect that the war against Iraq and the occupation of the American Embassy had had at the beginning of his term in office.

Thus, apart from the religious questions and the blasphemous content of the book, the *fatwa* served the clear political purpose of mobilizing the Iranian people, once again for the cause of Islam.

It is difficult to tell whether Khomeini would have ruled differently if conditions in Iran had been different, but it is striking how relatively late in the course of events his reaction came, after the world had already witnessed violent demonstrations and reactions elsewhere on the globe. The book was published on 26 September 1988, just before elections in India. Rajiv Gandhi's Congress Party needed votes from Moslem voters and the book's condemnation in India as early as 5 October must be seen in this context. Rushdie himself reacted quickly in a letter to Gandhi, in which he said of the opposition leaders: 'You know, as I know, that Mr. Shahabuddin, Mr. Khursid Alam Khan, Mr. Suleiman Seit and their allies don't really care about my novel one way or the other. The real issue is, who is to get the Muslim vote?'[14]

Pakistan and South Africa quickly followed suit by banning the book, after Moslem demonstrations in the streets in both countries and violent ones in Pakistan. Thus, on 12 February 1989 (the day before the book appeared in the United States) six were killed and hundreds injured. Benazir Bhutto, hardly favourably disposed to Rushdie who had ridiculed her in his novel *Shame*, was pressured by Moslem fundamentalists to ban the book. As the leader of the first democratically elected government in ten years, it was obviously a dilemma for her, but there was no way out.

In England, relations between immigrant Moslems and the native English people had long been tense. Unemployment among Moslems was high; they were hard hit by a tax reform; unlike other minorities such as Jews and Catholics they received no public subsidies for the operation of their own schools; feminist criticism of Third World family patterns was aimed exclusively at Moslems; and the blasphemy paragraph in British law deals only with Christianity. Attempts by Moslems to make themselves heard by the politicians and other efforts to improve conditions not only failed, but were systematically ignored. As a result, dissatisfaction among Moslems was strong, particularly in areas such as Bradford with a large concentration of Moslems. Initially moderate protests soon developed into radical demands that the book be withdrawn and that economic compensation be paid to Islamic charities. On 14 January 1989 the world witnessed the burning of books in Bradford, and the media portrayed the violent protests as spontaneous actions by dogmatic Moslems. In reality, it was a carefully arranged course of events, in which the first pages of the book were

photocopied and distributed, followed by the calling of a demonstration, after the media had been briefed to ensure their presence. Financial backing came from Pakistan and Saudi Arabia, which were vying to gain influence among Moslem immigrants in England.[15] The event had an enormous impact around the world, but it probably rather reflected social indignation than any anger over a book which nobody had read.

Khomeini's *fatwa* was not issued until 14 February 1989, and the political content of this act was underlined by the fact that *The Satanic Verses* was initially reviewed in Iran without causing any great outcry. Moreover, Rushdie's earlier novels *Shame* and *Midnight's Children* were not only known and translated into Persian, but *Shame* had even won a prize for the best translation of a novel. The prize was awarded by no less a personage than then-President and now religious head Ali Khamenei, i.e. the person who succeeded Khomeini and whose views were quoted in the *Iran Times* on 10 March 1989. After the *fatwa*, whoever might intend to write a similar book, turn it into a film, display it in movie theatres, or publish it, would henceforth have to contend with mortal danger from Muslims.

Before the *fatwa* was issued, Khamenei had proposed a solution, whereby Rushdie would avoid further charges by admitting his guilt and withdrawing the book. This was flatly rejected by Khomeini, who had a different agenda. Considering the widespread and large demonstrations against Rushdie that had already taken place around the world, there was no reason to show any mercy. The affair had to be exploited politically, and so it was.

With his *fatwa*, Khomeini managed once more to place himself at the centre of events and draw renewed attention to his ideology, the foundation of the Islamic revolution. At the same time, however, he created a legacy that thoroughly destroyed the chances for new Iranian leaders to implement the political programme that had been the main rationale of the cease-fire with Iraq in 1988 and the constitutional changes in 1989. Ten years later, his *fatwa* remains one of the worst obstacles to normalized relations between Iran and the rest of the world, while domestically it has become a Gordian knot that can hardly be cut without extreme difficulty.

The Reaction

Notwithstanding the unanimous condemnation of the book in the Islamic world, it also showed the diversity of Islam. Thus, *The Satanic Verses* helped open the eyes of Westerners to the fact that Islam can

hardly be reduced to the stereotyped picture of Moslem fundamentalists. However, Khomeini's *fatwa* contravened this by seemingly confirming the worst prejudices against Islam that flourished in the Western world—thereby contributing to the West's view of Islam as a cultural, or even civilizational foe.[16] The *fatwa* thus strengthened the animosity that had built up against Islam during the 1990s, undoubtedly influencing political decision-makers in their attitudes toward Iran and the Middle East.[17]

The *fatwa*, of course, elicited sharp protests from the European nations. On 20 February, twelve EC foreign ministers met and agreed to a declaration that made 'normal, constructive relations with the Islamic Republic of Iran' contingent on Iran's withdrawal of its threats of violence.[18] The wording of the statement was clear: Unless the Iranian government unambiguously rejected Khomeini's *fatwa* (which the EC ministers saw as a violation of national sovereignty) there could be no normal relations with the Islamic Republic. However, just a month later these same ministers decided to send their ambassadors back to Teheran, even though there had been no concessions whatsoever from Iran which, on the contrary, had re-affirmed the *fatwa*. Iran, which reacted to the 20 February declaration by also recalling its ambassadors from the EC countries, now allowed them to return, while the foreign minister triumphantly stated that Islam had forced the EC back to reality.[19]

The true background to the EC's *de facto* capitulation to Iran is not easily determined. Some link it to the European countries' considerable economic interests in Iran, which is not unreasonable.[20] In any event, after the 1988 cease-fire Europe was clearly interested in improving relations with the Islamic Republic which constituted an attractive market, especially in view of the new, more pragmatic, Iranian policy orientation, and with the United States out of the picture. Thus, German Foreign Minister Hans-Dietrich Genscher visited Teheran as early as August 1988, his French counterpart Roland Dumas was there in February 1989, and both French President Mitterand and British Foreign Minister Douglas Hurd had planned visits.[21] Even though these efforts for economic inroads were thwarted by the *fatwa*, the fact that they were planned for shows that there was a genuine interest, which may explain why the EC ambassadors were back at their posts just one month after the harsh declaration by the foreign ministers. Financial interests may also explain why the EC countries continued vacillating in their Iran policy until the policy of critical dialogue was approved at the 1992 Edinburgh summit, even though Iran had actually persisted in its threats and even intensified them in

some respects. Indeed, the Rushdie affair had been linked to the Western hostages taken in Lebanon on 23 February (i.e. after the EC ministers' declaration, but before the return of the ambassadors to Teheran) when a group in Lebanon threatened to kill seventeen Western hostages if the West refused to condemn Rushdie and his book.[22]

However, the EC's lack of political consistency and its passive attitude until the start of the critical dialogue may also reflect a sort of confused bewilderment with regard to the *fatwa*. Both the *fatwa* itself and Iran's stubborn insistence on supporting it must have appeared to Western statesmen as fanatic. Hence, they probably could not bring themselves to believe the conflict would last, but many a politician may have thought that the whole thing would blow over with the passage of time. Apart from their rhetoric, the European countries took a rather passive stand, as Rushdie was quick to point out. While more or less actively pushing Rushdie aside several countries, including Denmark, soon took new steps towards an improvement of trade relations.

While Iran persevered in the Rushdie matter, continued to liquidate opposition politicians abroad, and was involved in various forms of terrorist activities, the country's government began conveying signals of greater openness and a more pragmatic policy. This was expressed in negotiations with the World Bank and the International Monetary Fund (IMF) concerning the establishment of free trade zones as well as in Iran's very pragmatic role in the UN's conflict with Iraq following the Iraqi occupation of Kuwait in August 1990.[23]

For obvious reasons this conflict, which totally captured the attention of the international community for more than half a year, completely pushed the Rushdie affair into the background. Moreover, Iran actually backed the UN resolutions condemning the Iraqi occupation and also recognized the emir family in Kuwait as the legitimate government. While Khomeini had been exporting the revolution, Iran had not recognized the government of Kuwait, but demanded its replacement with a Shi'ite leadership. Except for some attempts at mediation in the conflict, Iran kept a low profile, despite the massive US military presence in the Gulf in connection with the UN build-up of forces against Iraq. In comparison with the Khomeini period, Teheran was thus clearly playing a different tune, for which it was rewarded with improved relations with the Arab nations. In 1992, for example, Saudi Arabia resumed the diplomatic ties that had been severed in 1988.

The European countries had also noticed Iran's good behaviour in the Iraq-Kuwait conflict, and only revelations of Iranian espionage

in England for the purpose of killing Rushdie prevented Douglas Hurd from travelling to Iran in 1992.[24] Similarly, Germany attempted to unfreeze relations. Genscher thus travelled to Iran once again in 1991, and Iranian Foreign Minister Ali-Akbar Velayati visited Bonn that same year. As a result of this dialogue, two German hostages in Lebanon were freed in 1992. During 1992, however, relations between Teheran and Bonn were chilled once again, which was manifested in greater German support for Rushdie and a ban against Iranian publishers' participation in the major book fair in Frankfurt. The non-socialist government in Denmark was also eager to cultivate contacts with the government in Iran at that time, as Prime Minister Poul Nyrup Rasmussen hastened to point out when he was hit by a Rushdie affair of his own making in 1996.[25] He pointed to the fact that during the non-socialist government two Danish ministers had visited Tehran (1991 and 1992) and that two Iranian ministers had been invited and received in Copenhagen (1991).

During 1991 and the first half of 1992 the European countries thus heeded what they saw as positive signals from Iran, whilst ignoring the negative ones, with the result that the Rushdie affair was toned down completely. This alone illustrates how the Rushdie affair is not simply a matter of freedom of expression, of saving an author's life, of protecting fundamental principles of European culture, or of defending international law. Even though such considerations play a role, apparently they are only allowed to do so when it does not jeopardize more important economic and security interests. Both the German and Danish foreign policies in 1991 thus show how 'flexibly' the issue could be handled in the political discourse and how it could be toned down when overriding security issues so dictated, but brought to the forefront to justify a rejectionist policy towards Iran, when 'high politics' demanded it.

The stumbling course from 1989 to 1992 probably also reflected the fact that there were no real prospects of a coordinated Iran policy within the EC, but that individual countries acted solely out of concern for their national interests. This changed, however, when the EC became the European Union in 1992, entailing enhanced cooperation on foreign policy.[26] With respect to Iran, this meant that when the European Council met in Edinburgh in December 1992 it could decide to embark on the so-called policy of 'critical dialogue'.[27]

The dialogue was intended to take place between high-ranking officials in the EU troika and an Iranian deputy foreign minister. The first meeting took place under Danish chairmanship in June 1993. The dialogue was further intended to be conducted bilaterally between the

various EU countries and Iran. The content was to include topics such as human rights in Iran, Iran's involvement in international terrorism, and the country's attempts at interfering in regional conflicts, such as the peace process in the Middle East and the situation in the Balkans, arms control and, of course, the Rushdie affair. The idea was to reward progress in these areas with an increasing degree of normalization and improved economic cooperation. The intention was, furthermore, to support so-called 'moderate' groups and tendencies in Iran, improved relations for whom would presumably strengthen them politically, thereby promoting European interests.

Details about the content and results of this critical dialogue are hard to come by, probably because very little came out of it. Nevertheless, in a meeting with Iranian Deputy Foreign Minister Vaezi in 1995, Danish Foreign Minister Niels Helveg Petersen was given a number of oral declarations in which the Iranian government condemned international terrorism, pledged to respect international law, and promised that the government was not striving to take Rushdie's life, but that, on the contrary, it would in no way contribute to the execution of the *fatwa*. The Copenhagen Declaration, as it came to be called, was put on the agenda of the EU's critical dialogue, partly at Rushdie's urging, but when the Iranians refused to put in writing what they had orally promised Helveg Petersen, this initiative, too, came to naught. On 27 June 1995 the foreign minister stated that 'I find it difficult to see any reason to talk with Iran now, if they will not even repeat the declaration they made in Copenhagen. We must admit that the critical dialogue is in a crisis,' whereupon the government discontinued the dialogue.[28]

However, this did not close the book on relations with Iran and the Rushdie affair for the Nyrup government.[29] As we have seen, because of closer EU cooperation on the matter, the Social Democratic-led government actually implemented a more conservative Iran policy than that of the former, non-socialist government. Ironically, it was thus the Nyrup government which had to deal with a Rushdie affair of its own. The occasion for this was that the Prime Minister's Office, in an unusually clumsy manner, denied Salman Rushdie an entry visa, ostensibly because Denmark could not guarantee his safety. Rushdie was to have arrived on 14 October to receive the European Aristeion Prize for his novel *The Moor's Last Sigh*. The prize was to be awarded in Copenhagen, which had been designated the European City of Culture in 1996. At home, the affair created a violent storm of protest against the government, while in London Rushdie was furious, claiming that by refusing him entry, Denmark was supporting Iran.

In the end, the Danish government lost all the prestige it had accumulated for its policy regarding Rushdie, particularly through Helveg Petersen's efforts in connection with the above-mentioned Copenhagen declaration. The non-socialist parties wanted to throw the government out of office, but the left wing provided Nyrup Rasmussen with a safety net. The result was the approval by parliament of one of the most unusual foreign policy resolutions in recent history. Not only was the government to work on both the national and international levels to pressure Iran to develop democracy, show respect for human rights and international law, etc. (as it had been doing all along). It was also obliged to 'maintain a dialogue with groups working for democracy and respect for human rights in Iran.'[30] What the latter was supposed to mean, and how it was to be done, remained unclear, but it is difficult not to read it as requesting the Danish government to actively support opposition groups in Iran. Danish policy thereby became alarmingly similar to US policy. The whole affair ended with the sacking of a civil servant and Rushdie's visit to Copenhagen to receive his prize on 13 November.

While Denmark's efforts at critical dialogue thus came to naught, things went differently in Germany, where a different and more heavy-handed interpretation of the strategy prevailed. Here the dialogue was not intended to be conducted solely by high-ranking individuals, but also to take place between intelligence services.[31] Scandals erupted in which the German press revealed that there had been meetings and cooperation between Chancellor Kohl's special advisor on intelligence matters, Bernd Schmidbauer, and the Iranian Minister of Information and Security, Ali Fallahian, at that time was head of Iran's foreign intelligence service. In this capacity, Fallahian had been responsible for the murder of about sixty opposition politicians, and he had long been known by the German and American intelligence services as the architect behind several Iranian backed international terror groups. He was nevertheless received at the Chancellor's Office by Mr. Schmidbauer on 17 October 1993, where he was promised unspecified computer equipment to the value of US$70,000. He also visited the headquarters of the German intelligence service, as well as several large German firms, such as Siemens—all of which occurred, even though the German federal police had issued an arrest warrant for Fallahian, in connection with their investigation of the shooting of four members of the Kurdish Democratic Party of Iran at a restaurant called Mykenos in Berlin on 17 September 1992.

The affair created a strong political commotion in which the opposition criticized the government for allowing the intelligence

service, rather than the Foreign Ministry, to determine German policy toward Iran. This peculiar German form of critical dialogue also drew the wrath of Washington and strong criticism from Israel. Schmidbauer and the German government defended themselves by stating that their contacts with the Iranian intelligence service, also involving German training of Iranian intelligence personnel, were producing results. They pointed to Iran's softening on the Rushdie matter and the reduction in Iranian support for terrorism. They also pointed out that it had contributed to the release of two German hostages in Lebanon in 1992. The latter may be a coincidence, but neither with regard to the murder of Iranians abroad, the Rushdie affair, or terrorism, did the German effort produce any visible changes in Iranian practice.

When a German court determined in April 1997 that the murders at the Mykenos restaurant had been ordered by the highest levels in the Iranian leadership, and that both President Rafsanjani and Ali Fallahian were involved, both the German and the EU's critical dialogue with Iran was discontinued. There was a new diplomatic crisis, as the EU recalled its ambassadors for consultations. The crisis lasted until November 1997 when relations were resumed at the ambassadorial level, although it remains unclear what (presumably nothing) had been done in the meantime, or what the results had been.

The US Reaction

The United States was not just furious over Germany's Iran policy, but it was generally annoyed by Europe's dialogue with the Iranians.

Since 1993, the American strategy had been guided by the so-called 'dual containment' policy, which was intended to isolate Iraq and Iran in order to destabilize their governments. In 1995 American firms were banned from conducting business with Iran, even when mediated by companies in third countries. Thus, for example, American firms could not invest in projects by Canadian companies in Iran. In 1996 a law was passed applying American sanctions to foreign, including European, companies investing over US$20 million in Iran, and which also allocated funds to the CIA to attempt to overthrow the government in Teheran.

This 'tough' policy was justified by the American view that Iran was involved in international terrorism, that it was producing weapons of mass destruction, and that it opposed the Middle East peace process. To this were added serious violations of human rights and, of course, the Rushdie affair. These accusations against Iran can be found in the report on international terrorism which is published and updated annually by the American State Department.[32]

After Khatami's election for president and, in particular, his invitation to a dialogue between civilizations on CNN (7 January 1998), there have been signs of a softening in relations between the United States and Iran. At the same time, after a number of prominent American scholars criticized the containment policy for both being ineffective and costing American business huge sums of money,[33] politicians and officials have begun considering the possibility of a new American policy toward Iran that would be closer to the EU's policy.

Is the Future Bright for Rushdie?
Having sent out a number of probes in the spring and summer of 1998, the EU in September decided to resume the dialogue with Iran. The reason was the above-mentioned Iranian government's distanced itself from the bounty offered by the Khordad Foundation as a reward to the assassin of Rushdie. Even though this was certainly a very positive signal from Khatami and his foreign minister, as indicated above it is uncertain how much weight can be attributed to such Iranian declarations. In other words, the central question is how much power the political leadership in Teheran actually has.

Formally, according to the constitution, the president, the government, and the parliament (*Majlis*) have considerable powers. In reality, however, the freedom of action enjoyed by the political and democratically elected system is more narrowly circumscribed. The political system is encircled, so to speak, by a number of councils and committees the role of which is to insure that laws and reforms are implemented on an Islamic foundation. Moreover, in this context, 'Islam' means the interpretation championed by Ayatollah Khomeini and institutionalized during the 1980s.

These councils must approve all legislation passed by the parliament and all candidates who wish to run in presidential and parliamentary elections and for the important Assembly of Experts. The latter appoints Iran's most powerful person, the religious leader, who at any time can block initiatives taken from within the political system. In the most recent elections to the Assembly of Experts, which were held in October 1998, the approval process used to select candidates was roundly criticized. Several moderate politicians accused the Council of Guardians, which determine eligibility, of favouring conservative candidates and dropping Khatami's supporters.

The religious leader is also supreme commander of the armed forces, appoints the president of the supreme court, the chief of police, etc. Finally, Ayatollah Ali Khamenei, as the religious leader, is the supreme authority over the foundations (*bunyards*) that were established

after the revolution, including the aforementioned 15th Khordad Foundation.[34] Most of these foundations were established at the initiative of Ayatollah Khomeini and the funds were taken from the Shah's property, which was seized after he fled in January 1979. They have various purposes, but they generally include some sort of charity in their activities, i.e. social assistance, while some are primarily involved in propaganda, such as the dissemination of Khomeini's written works. They have in common the fact that they are free of government control and several of them are enormously wealthy. By their nature, it is impossible to determine how much wealth they have, but some sources say they control up to forty percent of the Iranian economy.

The 15th Khordad Foundation was established in 1979 on Khomeini's orders and it is the most secret of all. Its purpose is to support the poor and families affected by the war against Iraq, and it is claimed that it helped 471,886 families in 1991/92.[35] The very day after Khomeini's *fatwa* against Rushdie it offered a bounty of US$1 million, which was increased in the following days by voluntary contributions. Since then, the fund has increased the bounty several times, most recently on 12 October 1998, when it reached US$2.8 million. If the Khatami government wishes to live up to its assurances that it will oppose the foundation's bounty with a ban, there must be a change in the law. Such a change in legislation would require the approval of the entire religious apparatus, which is presently controlled by a majority of conservative *mullahs*. The signals coming from Iran in September and October 1998 did not indicate that Khatami's government would have much chance of producing a ban, if it even wants one.[36]

Conclusion

The pattern in the attitude of the West toward Iran seems to be the same in 1998 as it has been since 14 February 1979.

Throughout this period two different voices have been heard from Teheran, one speaking of dialogue, openness and pragmatism, the other clinging to the aggressive rhetoric of the Khomeini era. As we have seen, on several occasions the West has put its trust in the conciliatory voice, but has been deeply disappointed. In 1998 it has chosen once again to hear the conciliatory voice calling for dialogue between civilizations and proclaiming the Rushdie affair to be over, disregarding the fact that the conservative forces have a majority in the Assembly of Experts, the Khordad Foundation is raising the bounty, and the government-controlled media are saying it is impossible to abandon the

content of Khomeini's decree. Is this smart, one might ask?

In fact, there are many indications that the prospects of a critical dialogue are better today than ever before in the twenty years' history of the Islamic Republic. It does make a difference, even in Iran, when seventy percent of the voters reject the system's candidate for president in favour of one who campaigned with promises of political reform, and who has adhered to these promises in the face of opposition from the *mullah*-controlled state apparatus. Since Khatami took office as president, the political discussion has been more open, there is more freedom of expression, and the various political factions are actually functioning as political parties, to the extent that we have to acknowledge that there is some form of political pluralism. The opposition who wants reform enjoys greater leeway since Khatami came into office than ever before in the history of the republic. Hence, perhaps for the first time, there is a real possibility that critical dialogue may achieve the results that have been absent in the past.

There is hardly any doubt that Khatami enjoys considerable popular support, and it is neither wrong nor a slip of the tongue to say that his government is in the opposition. That is precisely what it is: the opposition to the system holding the reigns of real power, populated by conservative mullahs. In the presidential elections of May 1997 Iranians showed that they were utterly tired of this system.

Notes

1. Cited from Fischer, Michael M. J. & Mehdi Abedi: *Debating Muslims. Cultural Dialogues in Postmodernity and Tradition* (London: University of Wisconsin Press, 1990) p. 388.

2. Rose, Flemming: 'Rushdie ånder lettet op' [Rushdie Breathes a Sigh of Relief], *Berlingske Tidende* (25 September 1998).

3. *IRNA* (24 September 1998).

4. Declaration by the Presidency on behalf of the European Union on the issue of the author Salman Rushdie.

5. *Berlingske Tidende* (26 September 1998).

6. According to the official account, 'The foreign minister expressed his satisfaction with Iran's official withdrawal of the death sentence against Salman Rushdie. For practical reasons (full calendar), the foreign minister is unable to accept an invitation from the Iranian Foreign Ministry in the near future'. See *Account of Press Briefing* (28 September 1998), StF. 3 jr. no. 110.D. 10/5.

7. Mohammadi: 'The death sentence cannot be revoked,' *IRNA*, 28 September 1998. The conservative newspaper *Kayhan* wrote in its editorial of 27 September: 'The government and the Islamic Republic of Iran's statesmen are obligated to lay the groundwork for the execution of this decree and it is revealing that they cannot offer the least guarantee that this resolution will be

carried out.'

8. Cited from Valinejad, Afshin: 'Iran Group Raises Rushdie Bounty,' *AP* (12 October 1998).

9. *AP* (18 October 1998).

10. Concerning the United States' Middle East policy, see Andersen, Lars Erslev in *NATO Nyt* , no. 2 (Summer 1998).

11. In his book *Fatwa, Violence & Discourtesy* (Aarhus: Aarhus University Press, 1998) Mehdi Mozaffari discusses the religious and legal aspects of the fatwa. See also Petersen, E. Ladewig: 'Fatwa og jihad' [Fatwa and Jihad], *Historisk Tidsskrift*, vol. 97, no. 2 (Copenhagen, 1997).

12. See Halliday, Fred: 'Western Europe and the Iranian Revolution 1979-97', in B.A. Roberson (ed.): *The Middle East and Europe. The Power Deficit* (London: Routledge 1998), p. 140.

13. It has even been argued that, after Khomeini, Iran is entering a new phase in the country's history called the 'Second Republic'. See, for instance, Ehteshami, Anoushiravan: *After Khomeini. The Iranian Second Republic* (London: Routledge 1995).

14. Fischer & Abedi: *op. cit.* (note 1), p. 396.

15. *Ibid.*, pp. 389-391.

16. See Huntington, Samuel P.: 'The Clash of Civilizations,', *Foreign Affairs*, vol. 72, no. 3 (1993), pp. 22-49.

17. Eriksen, Thomas Hylland: *Det Nye Fiendebildet* [The New Enemy] (Oslo: Universitetsforlaget 1995).

18. Mozaffari: *op. cit.* (note 11).

19. See Halliday: *loc. cit.* (note 12), p. 131.

20. Andersen, Stefan Birkebjerg: *Avisårbogen 1989* [Newspaper Yearbook, 1989] (Odense: Odense Universitetsforlag, 1991), p. 117.

21. Ehteshani, Anoushiravan & Raymond A. Hinnebusch: *Syria and Iran. Middle Powers in a Penetrated Regional System* (London: Routledge 1997), pp. 46ff.

22. Halliday: *loc. cit.* (note 12), pp. 143-144.

23. 'Inquiry on Denmark's policy toward the reactionary Iranian theocracy. Prime Minister Poul Nyrup Rasmussen and Foreign Minister Niels Helveg Petersen's response on November 14, 1996 and the ensuing debate', cited here from Christensen, Svend Aage & Ole Wæver: *DUPIDOK 1996. Danish Foreign Policy Documentation* (Copenhagen: DUPI, 1997), p. 519.

24. *Ibid.*, p. 519.

25. *Ibid.*

26. See Laursen, Andreas: 'EU og Israel/Palestina' [The EU and Israel/Palestine] in Lars Erslev Andersen (ed.): *EU og Middelhavet* [The EU and the Mediterranean] (Odense: Odense Universitetsforlag, 1998) p. 57.

27. Presidency Conclusions, Edinburgh, 12 December 1992: 'Considering Iran's importance in the region, the European Council confirms its belief that a dialogue should be maintained with the Iranian government. This dialogue should be critical and reflect concern over Iran's actions and

demand improvements in a number of areas, particularly human rights, the death sentence pronounced in a fatwa by Ayatollah Khomeini against author Salman Rushdie in violation of international law, and terrorism. Improvements in these areas will determine the extent to which closer ties may be established and confidence created.' (SN 456/1/92).

28. Cited from Andersen, Stefan Birkebjerg & Lone Hollmann: *Avisårbogen 1995* [Newspaper Yearbook] (Odense: Odense Universitetsforlag, 1997), p. 48.

29. The Nyrup government was formed when the non-socialist government under Poul Schlüter was forced to step down in January 1993.

30. Inquiry, *loc. cit.* (note 23), p. 524.

31. Lan, Charles: 'Germany's New *Ostpolitik*', *Foreign Affairs*, vol. 75, no. 6 (1996), pp. 77-89; Halliday: *loc. cit.* (note 12), p. 145.

32. Available on-line from http://www.state.gov/www/global/terrorism/.

33. See the special section on 'Changing Course in the Persian Gulf', in the May/June 1997 issue of *Foreign Affairs*, containing contributions by Zbigniew Brzezinzki, Brent Scowcroft, Richard Murphy, Jahangir Amuzegar, Graham Fuller, and Ian Lesser.

34. The foundation's name refers to the revolt against the Shah's reforms, which began on June 5, 1963 and led to the arrest of Khomeini.

35. Cf. Schirazi, M.: *The Constitution of Iran. Politics and the State in the Islamic Republic* (London: I.B. Tauris 1998) p. 156. On *bunyads*, see Hooshang Amirahmadi's article in John L. Esposito: *The Oxford Encyclopedia of the Modern Islamic World*, vol. I, pp. 234-237.

36. It must be stressed that the Iranian government has never taken the initiative to pass a ban and it must be pointed out that the Iranian government has not withdrawn the death sentence—as maintained by Niels Helveg Petersen (note 6), but it has merely distanced itself from the bounty and given assurances that it would not contribute actively to an execution of the death sentence.

12   TROUBLED WATERS

Triple Track Diplomacy in the Persian Gulf

Majid Tehranian

Multi-Track Diplomacy

The role of multiple-track diplomacy in peace negotiations has received increasing attention in the post-Cold War era.[1]

It is generally recognized that the role of civil society in international relations is on the rise. Market forces from the top and civil society forces from the bottom have undermined the authority of the territorial state in a post-Westphalian world order. The boundaries between domestic and foreign policy also are increasingly blurred. While global market forces are imposing serious constraints on the power of the smaller and medium sized states, an international civil society is pressuring the states to observe the global norms in human rights and environmental protection. The role of non-governmental organizations (NGOs) in peacemaking and peacebuilding is of critical importance. Given the enormous sensitivity of the states to 'foreign' interference, this role would be more effective if mediated by independent agencies that enjoy the confidence of the contending governments. In contrast to dual track diplomacy that provides an NGO channel parallel to official diplomatic negotiations, triple track diplomacy attempts to build a bridge between NGOs and governments. This case study of a triple track diplomatic initiative presents the problems and prospects of such an approach.

In collaboration with several other non-governmental organizations (NGOs), in 1998, the Toda Institute for Global Peace and Policy Research initiated a project on Persian Gulf security. As part of its Human Security and Global Governance (HUGG) research program, the project is named HUGG West Asia. In its first phase, the project focuses on confidence building among the Gulf states by establishing an International Commission for Security and Cooperation in West Asia. The Commission consists of distinguished diplomats and scholars from the eight littoral states plus the five permanent member-states of the United Nations Security Council and a UN representative. The project will act as a second track diplomatic bridge between peace scholars and governments by opening up channels of communication,

massaging all submitted peace proposals to prepare them for the consideration of the relevant governments, and promoting a regional security regime for durable peace. The Commission met in Istanbul on 6-7 March, 1999, for the first time and unanimously recommended the establishment of a centre for the promotion of regional cooperation and confidence building in security, political, economic, social, and cultural arenas. The Commission also recommended that its next meeting should take place in one of the Gulf littoral states focusing on confidence building among the states.

This essay reviews the evolving security regimes in the Gulf region, provides a background to the HUGG West Asia project, reports on the substance of the discussions at the Istanbul conference, and concludes with the prospects for the establishment of an indigenous security regime in the Gulf region.

The Evolving Gulf Security Regimes
During the 20th century, the Persian Gulf seems to have gone through at least three distinctly different security regimes, including *Pax Britannica*, *Pax Saudi-Iranica*, and *Pax Americana*.[2]

Pax Britannica lasted from 1918, the conclusion of World War I, to 1971, which marked the withdrawal of British forces from the East of the Suez. The destruction of the Ottoman Empire and the transfer of Iraq, Trans-Jordan, and Palestine to Britain as League of Nations mandates, inaugurated this period. The Iranian Majlis turned down the proposed Anglo-Iranian Treaty of 1919. The treaty would have reduced Iran to the status of a protectorate like Egypt. Nevertheless, Britain exercised considerable influence in the political affairs of Iran. The *coup d'etat* of 1921 by Colonel Reza Khan, masterminded by the British, brought Iran for the next twenty years under a pro-British dictatorship. Although much less independent, the Gulf Arab emirates (Kuwait, Bahrain, Oman, and what now constitutes the United Arab Emirates, UAE) were at the same time carved out of the nominally Ottoman territories by the British. Like Iraq and Trans-Jordan, the borders of the emirates were drawn up to pay political debts while ensuring a system of divide and rule. Many of the current border disputes in the region stem from such colonial schemes (e. g. disputes between Iraq and Kuwait, Qatar and Bahrain, Iran and UAE).

The era of *Pax Britannica* came to an end with the postwar dismemberment of the British Empire and the rise of nationalist regimes in Iran, Iraq, Syria, Palestine/Israel, and Egypt. A new era emerged in 1971 when the British forces were withdrawn from the East of the Suez. Under the circumstances, *Pax Americana* could have

effectively replaced *Pax Britannica*. However, the United States defeat in Vietnam had led to the emergence of the Nixon Doctrine calling for the establishment of proxy powers in various regions of the world to act on behalf of the United States interests. In the Persian Gulf, the monarchist regimes of Saudi Arabia and Iran presented themselves as candidates for this role. The two regimes were thus bolstered by extensive US political and military aid. The emergence of a *Pax Saudi-Iranica* had anticipated and unanticipated consequences. It led to Saudi-Iranian rapprochement on the Shi'a-Sunni conflicts, the Organization of Islamic Conference, but also to a new unity in the Organization of Petroleum Exporting Countries (OPEC) that quadrupled the price of oil in 1973. Some boundary disputes were resolved, including the Iranian abandonment of sovereignty claims over Bahrain, an understanding between Iran and Sharjah on the Abu Musa island, and continental shelf agreements among the littoral states. In 1975, Iran and Iraq also reached an agreement in Algiers regarding their boundary dispute over Shatt-al-Arab and the withdrawal of Iranian support for the Kurdish rebellion in Iraq. As part of the new security regime, Iran also assisted the government of Oman to successfully defeat a Marxist rebellion in the Dhuffar Province.

The Islamic Revolution of 1979 in Iran brought *Pax Saudi-Iranica* to an end. With the tacit support of Saudi Arabia, Kuwait, as well as Western powers, Iraq invaded Iran in 1980. A historical pattern was repeating itself. As in the case of modern revolutions in France, Russia, China, and Cuba, the new revolutionary regime in Iran presented an ideological threat to its neighbouring conservative governments. Although the rhetoric far outweighed the power of a newly established and disorganized government, it was considered opportune by Iraq and its Arab and Western allies to nip the revolution in the bud. However, as in other historical instances, the Iraqi invasion had a counter-intuitive effect. It unified a divided revolutionary regime against the enemy in a patriotic war that 'imperialists and their lackeys had imposed on the country' (*jang-i-tahmili*). The consequence was an eight-year tug of war in which both sides suffered incalculable material and human costs. Initially, Iraq had the upper hand, but as the Iranians better organized themselves, the tide turned against Iraq around 1987. During a tanker war that threatened oil exports from the Gulf, Kuwait also requested the United States to protect its ships. These dual circumstances brought the United States with full force into the region.

A third period thus began under the aegis of *Pax Americana*. The approaching end of the Cold War had made it possible for the US and Soviet Union to jointly pressure Iran and Iraq to accept a cease-fire in

1988.[3] Under the threat of great power intervention, Ayatollah Khomeini had no choice but to drink the 'poisonous cup.' The invasion of Kuwait by Iraq on August 2, 1990 ensured that intervention.

Thanks to his Arab and Western allies, by 1990 Saddam Hussein had acquired a new powerful war machine and tested armed forces.[4] He therefore turned his attention to Iraq's old territorial ambition, Kuwait, which was now demanding repayments for its wartime loans. Iraq invaded and occupied Kuwait in August 1990 by a *blitzkrieg*. The United States response was a rapid deployment of forces to oppose the Iraqi invasion. It is not entirely certain if this turn of events was premeditated. On the one hand, the massive destruction of Saddam's war machine may be considered a calculated strategy by the United States to undo the Frankenstein monster that was created in the Iraqi war against Iran. This interpretation is supported by US Ambassador April Glaspie's assurances of neutrality between Iraq and Kuwait that must have encouraged Saddam to gamble at an invasion of Kuwait. It is further supported by the subsequent US refusal to allow Saddam a face-saving exit out of Kuwait. On the other hand, the US responses to the events could be considered to have been spontaneous and without premeditation.

At any rate, the events were unanticipated by Saddam. Coming at the heel of the end of the Cold War and the disappearance of the Soviet Union as a superpower, Saddam was gambling on an easy victory. During the Iran-Iraq war, he had assumed a new stature as a *Pan-Arab nationalist* and was hoping to cash in on his prestige by championing the cause of a united Arab world against all enemies. But he had miscalculated a second time. From the globalist perspective of the United States and its allies, the emergence of a hostile regional superpower in the Persian Gulf would have proved disastrous for Western oil and strategic interests. From a domestic perspective also, the Republican Party in power in Washington wished to exorcise the 'Vietnam syndrome' in the United States that had deterred it from playing a more active global, military role. The invasion of Kuwait assumed a symbolic significance in the post-Cold War era. Should a potentate be allowed to seize regional power by virtue of a Western default? President Bush quickly responded to that question by deploying the largest post-Cold War military force into Saudi Arabia. Following fruitless peace negotiations in which the United States was unwilling to allow Saddam even a face-saving withdrawal, the United Nations forces with the tacit approval of all five Great Powers, and led by the United States, re-conquered Kuwait and restored its monarchy to power. Iraq itself came under UN economic sanctions, and no-fly

zones in the north and the south were established in order to protect the dissident Kurds and Shi'ites. Following Egyptian President Nasser's challenges of the 1950s and 1960s, the colliding moral spaces of Western globalism and Pan-Arabism led in 1991 to a decisive defeat for the latter.

Although *Pax Americana* has been a fact of life in the Gulf during the 1990s, it has proved to be an unstable regional security regime. The failure of the US policy of dual containment of Iran and Iraq calls for a new design. Since 1996 under the leadership of President Khatami, Iran has regained the respect of the international community for its restrained foreign policies. Although Saddam Hussein is still in power and defiant in Iraq, France, Russia, and China have diverged from the United States and Britain in their recommendation for ending the isolation of the country. The time is thus ripe for inaugurating a new indigenous security regime under which Iran, Iraq, and GCC can settle their border disputes, guarantee non-interference in each other's internal affairs, and cooperate for a durable peace. The new regime, however, would be impossible without guarantees from the great powers.

Why HUGG West Asia?

The two Gulf wars (1980-1988 and 1990-1991) and the risks of an impending third one have created grave threats to international peace and security. As the source of some sixty percent of the world oil reserves and exports, the region has invited unprecedented numbers of foreign interventions and spiralling arms races that lead nowhere except to greater insecurity for the regional states and further threats to world peace.

The human costs during the two decades of warfare (1980-1999) in the region have been staggering. About one million people were killed and another one million were maimed in the Iran-Iraq War of 1980-1988. The invasion of Kuwait by Iraq on 2 August 1990 and the subsequent high technology war against Iraq by the UN forces involved fewer casualties, but it nonetheless entailed disastrous results. The breakdown of the Iraqi physical and social infrastructure as well as the continuing economic sanctions against Iraq have resulted in the premature death of about half a million Iraqi children each year due to malnutrition and infectious diseases. Under present circumstances, prospects for the normalization of relations among several of the contending states in this affair appear dim. Iran, Iraq, and the United States have severed their diplomatic relations. Similarly, Kuwait, Saudi Arabia, and Iraq continue to act as belligerents.

In the absence of diplomatic relations among the main parties to the regional disputes, prospects for peace are slim, unless international civil society assumes its responsibility by providing alternative channels of communication and negotiation. The role of NGOs in multiple-track diplomacy is thus indispensable. Although governments are often protective of their 'rights' to conduct foreign relations without interference from 'meddlers,' they would welcome the additional information and facilitation that may result from NGO involvement. For instance, the US Department of State has often treated the role of such figures as Jimmy Carter and Jesse Jackson in supervising elections and releasing hostages with disdain. However, it also has had to acknowledge the positive contributions they have made in the process. These include release of hostages, supervision of elections, and a general opening of channels of communication.

To initiate a peacebuilding effort, the design and preparation for the Toda Institute's initiative for security and cooperation in the West Asian region took place largely in 1998. In this process, three major obstacles had to be overcome. First, the conflict over the name of the project was resolved by changing it from HUGG Gulf to HUGG West Asia. The Arab participants would not take part in the project if the region was to be called by its historic name, the Persian Gulf. The Iranians would refuse participation if the project were to be called by the name the Arabs preferred, namely 'the Arab Gulf.' A compromise was reached by calling the project HUGG West Asia, a label that more accurately fits the region than its colonial label of 'the Middle East.' The latter is a strategic label devoid of any historical or cultural content. Captain Alfred Mahan, Theodore Roosevelt's close friend and colleague in the US Navy, coined the term 'the Middle East' in the late 19th century.[5] He argued that in order to have world domination, a state must have naval superiority through control of landmasses lying between the Near East and Far East, i. e. the Middle East. The control of this piece of real estate was therefore critical to Captain Mahan, who probably had no notion of its cultural and historical complexity.

A second obstacle to overcome was the traditional suspicions and conspiracy theories that characterize the colonial past of the region. Two bloody wars in the last two decades and a creeping third one have taken their toll on trust. We had a triple-T problem: Tehranian, Toda, and *Tudeh*. Initially some Arab colleagues suspected that the project was an Iranian government conspiracy because the director of the Toda Institute is Iranian-born. Once they were dissuaded from this thought, an imaginative colleague in the region suggested that Toda corresponded to *Tudeh*, the name of the Iranian Communist Party. The

project therefore must be a communist conspiracy! The Institute obviously had to explain that it had been named after Mr. Toda, the second President of Soka Gakkai, to honour his work for peace and global citizenship. Finally, someone suggested that since the first conference was held in Istanbul, it must be a Turkish-American-Israeli conspiracy against the rest of West Asia. Reasons for the choice of Istanbul, however, were convincing enough to dispel that suspicion: to avoid partiality, the first conference would not be held at any of the littoral states. Thus, Istanbul was the nearest major city to the region that could be found.

A third obstacle presented itself as the conference time approached. The capture of Öcalan, the Kurdish nationalist leader, and his dispatch to Turkey to stand trial created some security fears. In the light of worldwide Kurdish demonstrations against Öcalan's capture, we considered a postponement of the conference. But assurances by the Turkish government of the security of the participants and the determination to press on kept us on target.

Despite these difficulties, there were many good omens as well. Because the project was an independent initiative supported by several peace and policy research institutes from outside the region, fears of partiality and manipulation were allayed. The co-sponsoring organizations included the Toda Institute, Copenhagen Peace Research Institute, Norwegian Institute of International Affairs, and the Centre for Middle Eastern and Central Asian Studies of Australian National University. The distinguished diplomats and scholars who accepted our invitation to join the International Commission also helped to diminish the anxiety about 'conspiracies.'

To further allay any fears or suspicions, a letter of request was sent to all of the foreign ministers of the eight littoral states and the five permanent state-members of the UN Security Council. It listed the purpose of the project, and requested them to nominate someone from their own country for Commission membership. The letter emphasized that the Commission members should have the confidence of their own governments and civil societies without necessarily representing them. The objective was clearly to have a non-governmental commission whose members were participating in the security dialogue in their personal capacity rather than as officials of their governments. One foreign minister, that of Britain, responded negatively to our request. Russia, Iran, and Oman nominated representatives, while the remaining foreign ministers left our request unanswered. Informal contacts with non-responding government officials, however, indicated a bemused interest in the project. Selection of other representatives thus had to

employ the project's informal academic and governmental channels to identify those who might qualify as eminent citizens of their own countries, enjoying equal respect from their governments and civil societies.

The first meeting of the International Commission for Security and Cooperation in West Asia took place successfully on 6-7 March 1999, in Istanbul, Turkey. The fact that representatives of countries with broken diplomatic relations could meet in an atmosphere of friendship and cooperation helped build confidence among them as a prelude to serious discussions. This was a proof of Woody Allan's assertion that 'ninety percent of life is just being there!'.

On a sad note, however, *Tehran Times* of 6 March 6 1999 (Internet version), reported on the conference under the headline: 'Institute close to CIA hosts conference on Persian Gulf security in Turkey.' We immediately wrote to the editors to deplore their irresponsible and false reports while denying the allegations of any CIA connection and emphasizing the NGO nature of the project. However, the incident showed once again that the lot of peacemakers is not easy at all. The project was being abused as a pawn in the power struggles between the conservatives and the liberals in Tehran. As the mouthpiece of the conservatives, *Tehran Times* was thus trying to discredit the peacemaking initiatives of President Mohammad Khatami's government towards the Arab states and the West.

Regardless of the hurdles, what are the objectives and methods of the project? As a triple-track diplomatic initiative, the project consists of the government first track and an International Commission acting as a second track while a third track of peace scholars feed it with proposals to promote a regional non-aggression pact, an arms control agreement, and a regional cooperation organization.

The Istanbul Conference

Invitees to the Istanbul Conference consisted of representatives from the eight littoral states, the five permanent members of the UN Security Council, the UN Secretary-General's office, and a number of observers. The main themes that were discussed at the conference were the following:

Procedural Matters.

Conference participants agreed first and foremost that the Chatham House confidentiality rules must apply to discussions, i.e. conference reports must refrain from any direct attribution of comments. This rule provided a secure atmosphere for open and frank discussions. The

participants also agreed that Yemen should be added to the Commission. Yemen is expected to join GCC and its participation is vital to a viable security regime in the region. Most participants expressed a preference for soft rather than hard agenda items, as well as concrete rather than vague measures. They added that the language and framing of problems must be free of stereotypes and threats. The Commission should work first on confidence building measures and common grounds such as the price of Gulf oil.

Models of Regional Cooperation.
There are currently two good models for regional security regimes established by the Organization for Security and Cooperation in Europe (OSCE) and the Association of South East Asian Nations (ASEAN) in which arms control, transparency, and preventive diplomacy have been combined to provide enduring regional peace. Past security organizations in West Asia have been often prompted from the outside, e.g. the Baghdad Pact followed by the Central Treaty Organization. The Commission could learn from such examples. To succeed, however, the new regional organization must be initiated from within the region itself. Furthermore, participants felt the support and guarantees of the five permanent members of the UN Security Council were vital to regional security in the Gulf.

The experiences of other regional groupings are not, however, directly transferable to the Gulf. Despite this warning, there are three basic requirements for any successful regional formation: consensus, inclusiveness, and functionalism. Consensus building means regular visits by government officials to develop a common view on regional problems and possible solutions. Inclusiveness means to include all states of a given region regardless of their ideological or political orientations. Functionalism suggests that it is easier to achieve agreement on functional cooperation such as regional transportation and telecommunication than sensitive political and economic issues.

It takes a long time before the potential member-states of a regional organization can gain sufficient confidence and trust in each other to commit to long-term, cooperative relations. In the case of the Gulf states, the following confidence building measures will help:

Agreement on frontiers by peaceful negotiation for any needed adjustments; prior notification of military exercises; reciprocal observation of military exercises; reciprocal inspection of military facilities; transparency in arms production and imports; replacement of US with UN forces in the Gulf; great power guarantees of regional security through United Nations Security Council; preventive

diplomacy through regular exchange of views on outstanding problems; regional games in popular sports such as soccer; regional exchange of performing artists; regional research and training centre for security and cooperation; regional educational exchange programs; studies of security perceptions of the Gulf states; studies of mutual misperceptions and stereotypes in order to remove them; delinkage of Gulf issues from the Arab-Israeli disputes; focus on process rather than outcome; cultural exchange among non-governmental organizations; regional exchange among journalists; encouragement of European Union to get more involved in the Gulf security issues; starting perhaps with a single step such as the formation of a regional centre for security studies.

Major Security Concerns.
It is important to recognize the legitimate security concerns of the Gulf states before responding to them in a new regional security regime. While the Gulf region as a whole shares some common security concerns, each state in the region also has its own unique preoccupations. However, it can be safely said that stability in the flows and price of oil, non-interference in their internal affairs, and long-term economic development, are the common concerns of all of the Gulf petroleum exporting states.

At the crossroads of East and West, Iran is bordering twelve different sovereign states, all of which are characterized by internal and external insecurity. Iran's security anxieties are thus real. Witness the Iraqi invasion of 1980 and the skirmishes with Afghanistan in 1998. As the largest of the Gulf states in population, Iran views its role as the balancer of power. Although successive Iranian governments have consistently denied any hegemonic intentions, they are often accused of such designs. To assume domination, however, Iran faces competition with the outside powers. Under *Pax Saudi-Iranica*, for a short period, Iran assumed a proxy role for the United States. After the Iranian revolution, however, the United States has tried to isolate Iran.

The two Gulf wars and increasing political maturity have led the Iranian regime to make greater efforts toward confidence building with the Gulf states, except Iraq. Ever since the Iran-Iraq war, relations between the two countries have been tense. Each regime provides a base of operation for opposition groups to the other regime. War reparations, return of Iraqi jets that are claimed by Iran as part of war reparations, exchange of war prisoners, and ideological differences are the main issues at stake. However, both states wish for the United States to leave the Persian Gulf. Both desire higher prices for oil. And both consider themselves vanguards of the revolutionary movements in

the region. Iraq claims leadership of the secular nationalists and republicans while Iran champions the cause of the Islamic revolution.

Iraq's internal divisions sixty percent Shi'a, twenty percent Sunni, and twenty percent Kurdish) have shaped its security perceptions. With its historical memories of grandeur as the centre of the Abbasid Dynasty during the 9-13th centuries, Iraq has in modern times competed with Egypt and Syria for leadership in the Arab world. Following 1968, under the Ba'athist regime, this competition reached its peak during the Iraqi invasions of Iran and Kuwait. During the first Gulf war, Iraq enjoyed the support of Arab countries except Libya and Syria. In the second Gulf War, however, it was isolated except for Jordanian and Palestinian support. Having been subjected to nearly a decade of economic sanctions, the Iraqi regime suffers from intense insecurity. It views itself as the victim of Western imperialism, conservative Arab perfidy, and Iranian hostility. Dominated by Sunni Arab leadership, the Ba'athist regime's suspicion of its own Shi'a and Kurdish population adds to this sense of insecurity.

The GCC consists of six countries that vary in size and attitudes. Saudi Arabia has successfully served as the GCC leader shaping its policies in the Gulf. As a group, the GCC considers itself a balancing power vis-à-vis the two Gulf big boys, namely Iran and Iraq. As relatively rich but less populated countries, the GCC governments also look for protection from the United States against possible threats from Iran and Iraq. However, feelings about the presence of the US forces are mixed. Too close an identification with the US opens the GCC regimes to accusations of complicity with un-Islamic and imperialist powers. Although the recent rapprochement with Iran is not universal among the GCC members, Saudi Arabia has led the way. The United Arab Emirates continues to have a serious conflict with Iran on the issue of sovereignty over the three Gulf islands (Abu Musa, Greater and Smaller Tunbs). Bahrain has accused the Iranian regime of subversive activities within its borders. Oman and Qatar seem to enjoy the best relations with Iran. Expanding commercial relations between Iran and the southern Gulf states, however, are paving the way for greater common and enduring interests. Saudi Arabia and the UAE are currently at odds over the GCC opening to Iran. Symbolic issues such as the name of 'the Gulf' and practical issues such as the control of the three Gulf islands continue to divide the two sides of the Gulf.

Conclusion

This brief account of an effort at peacebuilding in a war-torn region of the world has reviewed the historical evolution of security regimes in

the Persian Gulf. It has argued that the current situation is both untenable and conducive to a new, indigenous security regime for long-term regional security and cooperation. The essay has provided the background to the HUGG West Asia Project, an NGO initiative aiming at the establishment of such a regime. In reporting the deliberations of the first meeting of the International Commission for Security and Cooperation in West Asia, held in Istanbul on 6-7 March 1999, the essay has also outlined the main obstacles to establishing regional cooperation for security as well as the opportunities that present circumstances can afford in that direction.[6]

As soon as the Gulf states adopt the Commission's recommendation for the establishment of a regional centre for security and cooperation, the task of the HUGG West Asia Project may be considered completed. However, until such a time, much needs to be done. Regular meetings of the Commission are planned for the next few years. [A second meeting was held in Cyprus in May 2000, and a third one in Qatar in January 2001, *The Editor*]. In preparation for these meetings, research projects are under way exploring the security perceptions of Iran, Iraq, and GCC and how a common ground can be developed among them. Other issues for research and policy development include arms control, border disputes, trade and development problems, oil production controls and prices, scientific, technological, and cultural cooperation, the role of great powers, the European Union, and the United Nations, the structure and program of a regional research centre, and the formation of a regional organization.

Notes

1. The literature on conflict management and the role of non-governmental organizations in international affairs is a growth industry. Some recent volumes include Väyrynen, Raimo (ed.): *New Directions in Conflict Theory: Conflict Resolution and Conflict Transformation* (London: Sage, 1991); Kriesberg, Louis: *Constructive Conflicts: From Escalation to Resolution* (London: Rowman & Littlefield, 1998); Folger, Joseph P. & Tricia S. Jones (eds.): *New Directions in Mediation: Communication, Research, and Perspectives* (Thousand Oaks, CA: Sage, 1994); Fisher, Julie: *Nongovernments: NGOs and the Political Development of the Third World* (West Hartford, CT: Kumarian Press, 1998); Carroll, Thomas F.: *Intermediary NGOs: The Supporting Link in Grassroots Development* (West Hartford, CT: Kumarian Press, 1992); Diamond, Louise & John McDonald: *Multi-track Diplomacy. A Systems Approach to Peace*. 3rd Edition (West Hartford, CT: Kumaranian Press, 1996); Lepgold, Joseph & Thomas G. Weiss: *Collective Conflict Management and Changing World Politics* (Albany, NY: State University of New York, 1998); Mayer, Richard J.: *Conflict Management: The Courage to*

Confront, 2nd ed. (Columbus: Battelle Press, 1995).

2. Without necessarily implicating him in my terminology and analysis, this part borrows from Mojtahed-Zadeh: 'Regional Alliance in the Persian Gulf: Past Trend and Future Prospects,' *The Iranian Journal of International Affairs*, vol. 10, no. 1-2 (Spring-Summer 1998), pp. 1-20.

3. Hume, Cameron R.: *The United Nations, Iran, and Iraq: How Peacemaking Changed* (Bloomington, IN: Indiana University Press, 1994).

4. Tehranian, Majid: *Global Communication and World Politics: Domination, Development, and Discourse* (Boulder, CO: Lynne Rienner, 1999).

5. Mahan, Alfred Thayer: *The Influence Of Sea Power Upon History, 1660-1783* (Boston: Little, Brown, 1894).

6. A source of inspiration has been Sick, Gary G. & Lawrence G. Potter (eds.): *The Persian Gulf at the Millennium: Essays in Politics, Economy, Security, and Religion* (New York: St. Martin's Press, 1997).

CONCLUSION

Alternatives to 'Dual Containment'

Bjørn Møller

The preceding chapters have, hopefully, shown the Persian Gulf region (or simply 'Gulf region' as the Arabs prefer) to be 'an interesting place'. The introductory chapter highlighted some of the regional dynamics and their complexities in what is an almost classical multipolar setting (albeit strongly penetrated by outside powers). The chapters by Gawdat Baghat, Wolfango Piccoli, and Dietrich Jung broadened the view by looking at the relations of the regional states with powers on its periphery, i.e. Israel and Turkey, while Jamal al-Suwaidi provided an insight into the perspective of a small GCC country. The chapter by Gulshan Dietl analyzed the region in the larger context of the 'Greater Middle East'.

Regardless of the perspective, one external actors stands out as decisive, namely the United States. Its shifting and ambivalent attitude to the region was analyzed by Lars Erslev Andersen, while Bjørn Møller, Anthony McDermott and Jalil Roshandel provided critical analyses of the US Persian Gulf policy in general, and its management of the Iraqi crisis in particular—which was countered by a somewhat more positive, albeit not uncritical, assessment in the chapter by Birthe Hansen.

Revision of Dual Containment?

The preferred term for the US policy has been 'dual containment', i.e. a simultaneous attempted isolation of both Iran and Iraq, combined with support for the members of the GCC.

Since late 1998 there have been signs of movement towards a revision of the dual containment strategy, at least with regard to Iran.[1] For instance, US Secretary of State, Madeleine Albright, in a speech, 17 June 1998,[2] struck a conciliatory cord with regard to Iran:

> We are ready to explore further ways to build mutual confidence and avoid misunderstandings. The Islamic Republic should consider parallel steps. If such a process can be initiated and sustained in a way that addresses the concerns of both sides, then we in the United States can see the prospect of a very different relationship. As the wall of mistrust

comes down, we can develop with the Islamic Republic, when it is ready, a road map leading to normal relations. Obviously, two decades of mistrust cannot be erased overnight. The gap between us remains wide. But it is time to test the possibilities for bridging this gap.

If it is true that this policy is approaching revision, an important question becomes what to put in its place. The chapter by Majid Tehranian provided some ideas to this effect, while others shall be advanced in this conclusion.

From Containment to Integration
As an escape from the present multipolar, 'pre- or early westphalian' and profoundly unstable regional setting, one could envision a four-stage process leading in the direction of a regional security community.[3]

The nucleus of this would be the GCC (Gulf Cooperation Council) which would be well-advised to emulate other regional organizations such as NATO, the European Union (EU) and the Association of South-East Asian Nations (ASEAN) by expanding in order to 'embrace' its former enemies.[4] The United States would have an important role to play in the process, even though its purpose would be to make the region self-contained and self-sustaining with regard to security. This would allow the US to disengage, in due course. The four stages of such a process are outlined in Table 13.

The rationale of this process is that the present roll-back strategy with regard to Iraq is both counter-productive, superfluous and a humanitarian disaster. It could safely be abandoned in favour of a simple military containment, which could be manifested in US security guarantees to, and some military support for, the GCC countries and a regulation of arms transfers to Iraq—for which the available arms control regimes for missiles and nuclear, chemical and biological weapons should suffice. If need be they might be supplemented with regional ('zone') arrangements, such as a 'WMD-free zone'.[5] With regard to their indigenous military efforts, it would be wiser for the present GCC states to place the emphasis on a strengthening of their defensive capabilities than to aim for all-purpose armed forces that could be perceived as threatening by their larger, but less prosperous, neighbours.

Iran simply no longer needs containing in the traditional sense, if ever it did.[6] While one cannot entirely discount the hypothesis of Iranian expansionist designs, the available facts about its military also lend themselves to a more 'innocent' interpretation. First of all, Iran

has not yet made up for its wartime losses, and its military strength thus remains inferior to what it was at a time when it was regarded (by the US at least) as a stabilizing factor. Secondly, the arms acquisitions of the Islamic Republic as well as its military expenditures remain well below those of the GCC. Thirdly, most of Iran's arms acquisitions have been entirely consistent with defensive intentions. In such an evaluation, one must, in all fairness, take into account that the country must remain fearful of an eventually resurgent Iraq; that it has long borders facing unstable countries such as Afghanistan and some former Soviet republics; that it borders on a South Asia that has always been very conflict-ridden and which is now openly nuclearized;[7] and that it must be worried about the new American assertiveness that might even lead to intervention (say, in the name of 'counter-proliferation').[8]

Table 13: ALTERNATIVES TO DUAL CONTAINMENT			
	IRAQ	**IRAN**	**GCC**
Dual Contain-ment	**Roll Back** (Militarily, economically)	**Contain** (Economically, militarily)	**Support** (Militarily)
Alternative Phase 1	**Contain** (Militarily)	**Normalize** (Integrate)	**Support** (Militarily, defensively)
Phase 2	**Normalize** (Integrate)	**Support** (Security guarantee)	**Support** (Security guarantees)
Phase 3	**Support** (Security guarantee)	**Support** (Security guarantee)	**Support** (Security guarantees)
Phase 4	**Disregard** (Security community, collective security, general security guarantees)		

With the possible partial exception of the (alleged) nuclear weapons programme and the ballistic missiles, the 'Iranian threat' is thus not so much a military threat[9] as something *sui generis*, namely a threat of terrorism (to which all countries are vulnerable) and one of 'ideological contagion'. However, there are many indications that Iranian foreign and defence policy has entered, since around 1988-89, a more pragmatic phase, that the terrorist element has been down-played considerably, and that further liberalization is underway after the

election of President Khatami.[10]

The most sensible course of action would thus be to integrate Iran into the GCC, under the auspices of which the remaining problems would be easier to solve that with the GCC countries forming a united front against Tehran. Support for the GCC countries may still be needed, but should be limited to strengthening their defensive military capabilities, underpinned by a security guarantee.

In due course, the region could proceed to Phase Two, where relations with Iraq will be normalized. Perhaps this will require a change of regime in Baghdad, but this should not be assumed to be a *sine qua non*. History has seen several dictatorial regimes whose international behaviour has been tempered by a skilful application of deterrence and containment strategies. In addition to containing Iraq militarily outside powers (and especially the United States) might extend security guarantees to Iran similar to those provided to (the rest of) the GCC, which would, at this stage, probably no longer need direct military assistance.

Gradually, Phase Two might evolve into Phase Three where even Iraq is integrated into the GCC, and where all could be the beneficiaries of security guarantees on the part of the United States and other external powers. At this stage, stability would be ensured, but it might not yet be so reliable (or believed to be so by the regional states) that the rest of the world, and the United States in particular could completely disengage. The required involvement would, however, be much less extensive and demanding that previously.

In the fullness of time, the region may reach Phase Four, where it comes to constitute a security community, implying that the risk of, and preparations for, war have receded into the background.[11] The GCC may thus establish a self-contained regional collective security arrangement. It would benefit from, but would no longer depend on, outside support. External powers could thus safely disengage, leaving behind merely a general security guarantee that would most likely never be needed.

Notes

1. Milward, William: 'Containing Iran', *Commentary. A Canadian Security Intelligence Service Publication*, no. 63 (November 1995), pp. 1-14; Sicherman, Harvey: 'America's Alliance Anxieties. The Strange Death of Dual Containment', *Orbis. A Journal of World Affairs*, vol. 41, no. 2 (Spring 1997), pp. 223-240; Sick, Gary: 'Rethinking Dual Containment', *Survival*, vol. 40, no. 1 (Spring 1998), pp. 5-32; Brzezinski, Zbigniew, Brent Scowcroft & Richard Murphy: 'Differentiated Containment', *Foreign Affairs*, vol. 76, no. 3 (May-

June 1997), pp. 20-30; Wright, Robin & Shaul Bakhash: 'The U.S. and Iran: An Offer They Can't Refuse?', *Foreign Policy*, vol. 108 (Fall 1997), pp. 124-137; Baghat, Gawdat: 'Beyond Containment: US-Iranian Relations at a Crossroads', *Security Dialogue*, vol. 28, no. 4 (December 1997), pp. 453-464.

2. http://secretary.state.gov/www/statements/1998/980617a.html.

3. On the notion of security communities, see Deutsch, Karl W. *et al.*: *Political Community and the North Atlantic Area. International Organization in the Light of Historical Experience* (Princeton, NJ: Princeton University Press, 1957); and Adler, Emmanuel & Michael Barnett (eds.): *Security Communities* (Cambridge: Cambridge University Press, 1998).

4. On NATO enlargement see Haglund, David G. (ed.): *Will NATO Go East? The Debate Over Enlarging the Atlantic Alliance* (Kingston: Centre for International Relations, Queen's University, 1996); idem, S. Neil MacFarlane & Joel S. Sokolsky (eds.): *NATO's Eastern Dilemmas* (Boulder, CO: Westview, 1994); Solomon, Gerald B.: *The NATO Enlargement Debate, 1990-1997* (Westport, CT: Praeger, 1998). On the EU see Bonvicini, Gianni, Murizio Cremasco, Reinhardt Rummel & Peter Schmidt (eds.): *A Renewed Partnership for Europe. Tackling European Security Challenges by EU-NATO Interaction* (Baden-Baden: Nomos Verlagsgesellschaft, 1996). On ASEAN see Cunha, Derek da (ed.): *The Evolving Pacific Power Structure* (Singapore: Institute of Southeast Asian Studies, 1996). For an application to the Gulf see Balakrishnan, K.S.: 'Asian-Pacific Security and the ASEAN Regional Forum: Lessons for the GCC', *The Emirates Occasional Papers*, no. 25 (1998).

5. Prawitz, Jan & Jim Leonard: *A Zone Free of Weapons of Mass Destruction in the Middle East* (Geneva: UNIDIR, 1996).

6. Gerges, Fawaz A.: 'Washington's Misguided Iran Policy', *Survival*, vol. 38, no. 4 (Winter 1996-97), pp. 5-15; Chubin, Sharam: 'US Policy Towards Iran Should Change—But It Probably Won't', *ibid.*, pp. 16-19; al-Suwaidi, Jamal S.: 'Gulf Security and the Iranian Challenge', *Security Dialogue*, vol. 27, no. 3 (September 1996), pp. 277-294.

7. See, for instance, Harrison, Selig, Paul H. Kreisberg & Dennis Kux (eds.): *India and Pakistan. The First Fifty Years* (Cambridge: Cambridge University Press, 1999); Hagerty, Devin T.: *The Consequences of Nuclear Proliferation. Lessons from South Asia* (Cambridge, MA: MIT Press, 1998); Chellany, Brahma: 'After the Tests: India's Options', *Survival*, vol. 40, no. 4 (Winter 1998-99), pp. 93-111; Singh, Jasjit (ed.): *Nuclear India* (New Delhi: Knowledge World and Institute for Defence Studies and Analyses, 1998).

8. Arnett, Eric: 'Beyond Threat Perception: Assessing Military Capability and Reducing the Risk of War in Southern Asia', in idem (ed.): *Military Capacity and the Risk of War. China, India, Pakistan and Iran* (Oxford: Oxford University Press, 1997), pp. 1-24, especially pp. 5-6 and 16-20; Loftian, Saideh: 'Threat Perception and Military Planning in Iran: Credible Scenarios of Conflict and Opportunities for Confidence Building', *ibid.*, pp. 195-222; Chubin, Sharam: *Iran's National Security Policy. Capabilities, Intentions and Impact* (Washington, DC: The Carnegie Endowment for

International Peace, 1994).

9. For a much more alarmist analysis, based partly on questionable sources (which the author does not question) see also Ritcheson, Philip L.: 'Iranian Military Resurgence: Scope, Motivations, and Implications for Regional Security', *Armed Forces and Society*, vol. 21, no. 4 (Summer 1995), pp. 573-592. See also Katzman, Kenneth: 'The Politico-Military Threat from Iran', in Jamal S. al-Suwaidi (ed.): *Iran and the Gulf. A Search for Stability* (Abu Dhabi, UAE: Emirates Centre for Strategic Studies and Research and London: I.B. Tauris, 1996), pp. 195-210; Cordesman, Anthony H.: 'Threats and Non-Threats from Iran', *ibid.*, pp. 211-286; Arnett, Eric: 'Iran is not Iraq', *Bulletin of the Atomic Scientists*, vol. 64, no. 1 (January 1998), pp. 12-14.

10. Hunter, Shireen T.: 'Iran after Khomeini', *The Washington Papers*, no. 156 (Washington, DC: CSIS, 1992); Clawson, Patrick: 'Iran after Khomeini: Weakened and Weary', in Daniel Pipes (ed.): *Sandstorm. Middle East Conflicts and America* (Lanham: University Press of America, 1993), pp. 269-276; Kupchan, Charles A.: 'Iran after Khomeini: Ready to Talk', *ibid.*, pp. 277-284; Rundle, Christopher: 'Iran: Continuity and Change since the Revolution—Carrying Water in a Sieve?', in M. Jane Davis (ed.): *Politics and International Relations in the Middle East. Continuity and Change* (Aldershot: Edward Elgar, 1995), pp. 105-117; Mahtasham, Elahe: 'An Iranian Perspective', in James Gow (ed.): *Iraq, the Gulf Conflict and the World Community* (London: Brassey's/Centre for Defence Studies, 1993), pp. 107-120; Al-Suwaidi, Jamal S.: 'Gulf Security and the Iranian Challenge', *Security Dialogue*, vol. 27, no. 3 (September 1996), pp. 277-294. See also Kazemi, Farhad: 'Review Article: Models of Iranian Politics, the Road to the Islamic Revolution, and the Challenge of Civil Society', *World Politics*, vol. 47, no. 4 (July 1995), pp. 555-574. For an excellent analysis of Iran's evolution from a revolutionary to a 'normal' state, see Walt, Stephen M.: *Revolution and War* (Ithaca: Cornell University Press, 1996), pp. 210-268.

11. For a rather pessimistic view see Barnett, Michael & F. Gregory Gause III: 'Caravans in Opposite Directions: Society, State and the Development of a Community in the Gulf Cooperation Council', in Adler & Barnett (eds.): *op. cit.* (note 4), pp. 161-197.

CONTRIBUTORS

Lars Erslev Andersen is associate professor and former director of the Centre for Middle Eastern Studies, University of Odense, Denmark. His book include, among others, *Middle East Studies in Denmark* (1994), *EU and the Mediterranean* (1998, in Danish), *Yemen: Between Tribe and Modernity* (1994, in Danish), *Iran from Revolution to Reform* (1999, in Danish), and *Satanic, Divine—and All Too Human. The Rushdie Case Ten Years after Khomeini's Death Sentence* (1999, in Danish).

Gawdat Bahgat is Director of the Centre for Middle Eastern Studies at Indiana University of Pennsylvania, the United States. In the last few years he has published three books and more than forty articles in English and Arabic on the Persian Gulf. His books are *The Gulf Monarchies: New Economic and Political Realities*, *The Future of the Gulf* and *The Persian Gulf at the Dawn of the New Millennium*. His articles have appeared in international journals in the United States, the United Kingdom, Canada, Norway, Germany, Austria, Italy, Lebanon, Iran, and India.

Gulshan Dietl is a professor and chairperson, Centre for West Asian and African Studies, School of International Studies, Jawaharlal Nehru University, New Delhi. She has also served as the Director, Gulf Studies Programme; and held visiting appointments as the Fulbright Scholar-in-Residence and Research Fellow, Copenhagen Peace Research Institute. Her publications include *The Dulles Era: America Enters West Asia* (New Delhi: Lancer International, 1985), *Through Two Wars and Beyond: A Study of the Gulf Cooperation Council* (New Delhi: Lancer Books, 1991) and nearly eighty papers and articles on political, foreign policy and security issues in the Gulf and West Asia.

Birthe Hansen, Ph.D., is associate professor at the Institute of Political Science, University of Copenhagen, senior advisor to the Danish Institute of International Affairs, and a former member of the Danish Defence Commission. Her most recent book is *Unipolarity and the Middle East* (2000).

Dietrich Jung holds degrees in political science and Islamic studies and a Ph.D. in Political Science from the University of Hamburg.

Formerly a research fellow at the Unit for the Study of Wars, Armaments and Development, University of Hamburg, and visiting assistant professor at Bilkent University in Ankara, he is presently a research fellow at the Copenhagen Peace Research Institute. He has published extensively on Middle Eastern issues in *Iranian Journal of International Studies, Orient, Politische Vierteljahresschrift, Blätter für deutsche und internationale Politik, Zeitschrift für Internationale Beziehungen*. He is also the author of *Tradition, Modernity, War. The Foundations of a Methodology for Research on the Causes of War in the Context of Globalization* (1995, in German).

Anthony L. McDermott has been a senior researcher at the International Peace Research Institute, Oslo (PRIO) and co-editor of *Security Dialogue*, the international affairs quarterly, since the beginning of 1997. He has an MA in Arabic and Turkish from Oxford University, UK and held a fellowship at the American University in Cairo in Arabic Studies. For twenty years he worked for the *Financial Times* (London) in the foreign department. A sabbatical was spent at Brown University, Rhode Island in the US in 1992. He has written extensively in international journals on the Middle East and the UN system, finances, reform, and peace-keeping operations; and humanitarian intervention in modern conflicts. Recent publications have included: *Humanitarian Force* and *Sovereign Intervention* (both PRIO Reports, 1997 and 1999 respectively). He is the author of the following books: *Egypt from Nasser to Mubarak: A Flawed Revolution* and *The Multinational Force in Beirut 1982-84*. Macmillan is due to publish in 1999 *The New Politics of Financing the UN*.

Bjørn Møller, Ph.D. in Political Science and M.A. in History, is a senior research fellow and programme director at the Copenhagen Peace Research Institute COPRI. He has served as editor of the international research newsletter *NOD & Conversion* (1986-2000), as project director of the Global Non-Offensive Defence Network project (1993-2000), and as Secretary General of the International Peace Research Association, IPRA (1997-2000). He is the author of the following books: *Resolving the Security Dilemma in Europe. The German Debate on Non-Offensive Defence* (1991), *Common Security and Nonoffensive Defense. A Neorealist Perspective* (1992), *Dictionary of Alternative Defence* (1995); and editor or co-editor of the following books: *Non-Offensive Defence for the Twenty-First Century* (1994), *Defence Doctrines and Conversion* (1996), *Defensive Restructuring of*

the Armed Forces in Southern Africa (1997); and *Security, Arms Control and Defence Restructuring in East Asia* (1998).

Wolfango Piccoli is an Italian citizen, resident in Turkey. He has a degree in Political Science/International Relations from the University of Bologna, and an MA in International Relations from the Bilkent University in Ankara. In September 1999 he joined the European University Institute. He is the author of several articles on Turkey.

Jalil Roshandel holds an MA and a Ph.D. in Political Science, both from *Université Des Sciences Sociales, Toulouse-I*. He started his academic career in 1989 as Assistant Professor and later as the Vice-Dean of the Faculty of Law and Political Science at the University of Tehran. Since 1993 he has been working as a senior research fellow at the Institute for Political and International Studies (IPIS) in Tehran. In 1998/99 he was a guest senior research fellow at the Copenhagen Peace Research Institute (COPRI). He is the author of over thirty books and papers on strategic and security issues, Persian Gulf security and confidence-building, Iranian nuclear program and international security, and some others focused on the Central Asia and the Caucasus.

Jamal S. al-Suwaidi, Ph.D., is Director of the Emirates Centre for Strategic Studies and Research in Abu Dhabi, United Arab Emirates. He also teaches at the UAS University in Al Ain. Among his recent books are *Iran and the Gulf. A Search for Stability* (1996) and *The Yemini War: Causes and Consequences*.

Majid Tehranian is professor of international communication at the University of Hawaii and director of the Toda Institute for Global Peace and Policy Research. His latest books include *Technologies of Power: Information Machines and Democratic Prospects* (1990), *Restructuring for World Peace: At the Threshold of the 21st Century* (1992), *Global Communication and World Politics: Domination, Development, and Discourse* (1999), *Worlds Apart: Human Security and Global Governance* (1999), and *Asian Peace: Security and Regional Governance in Asia Pacific* (1999).

BIBLIOGRAPHY

Recent Books on the Persian Gulf Region

Bjørn Møller

Agha, Hussein & Ahmed Khalidi: *Syria and Iran. Rivalry and Coope-*
ration (London: Royal Institute of International Affairs, 1995).

al-Suwaidi, Jamal S. (ed.): *Iran and the Gulf. A Search for Stability*
(Abu Dhabi: The Emirates Centre for Strategic Studies and
Research and London: I.B. Tauris, 1996).

AlFaraj, Sami & Laith Kubba, with Mohammad K. Shiyyab & Dov S.
Zakheim (Edited by Brent Thomson): *Common Ground on Iraq-*
Kuwait Reconciliation (Washington, DC: Search for Common
Ground, 1998).

Anon. (ed.): *Caspian Sea Energy Resources* (Abu Dhabi: The Emirates
Centre for Strategic Studies and Research, 2000).

Anon. (ed.): *The Gulf: Future Security and British Policy* (Abu Dhabi:
The Emirates Centre for Strategic Studies and Research, 2000).

Arnett, Eric (ed.): *Military Capacity and the Risk of War. China, India,*
Pakistan and Iran (Oxford: Oxford University Press/SIPRI,
1997).

Arnove, Anthony (ed.): *Iraq under Siege. The Deadly Impact of*
Sanctions and War (London: Pluto, 2000).

Aspin, Les & William Dickinson: *Defense for a New Era. Lessons of*
the Persian Gulf War (Washington, DC: Brassey's US, 1992).

Barkey, Henri J.: *Reluctant Neighbour. Turkey's Role in the Middle*
East (Washington, DC: United States Institute of Peace Press,
1996).

Barnett, Michael N.: *Dialogues in Arab Politics: Negotiations in*
Regional Order (New York: Columbia University Press, 1998).

Baudrillard, Jean: *The Gulf War Did Not Take Place* (Bloomington:
Indiana University Press, 1995).

Bengio, Ofra: *Saddam's Word. The Political Discourse in Iraq*
(Oxford: Oxford University Press, 1998).

Birand, Mehmet Ali: *Shirts of Steel. An Anatomy of the Turkish Armed*
Forces (London: I.B. Tauris, 1991).

Brom, Schlomo & Yiftah Shapir (eds.): *The Middle East Military*
Balance 1999-2000 (Cambridge, MA: The MIT Press, 2000).

Bruinessen, Martin van: *Agha, Shaikh and State. The Social and Political Structures of Kurdistan* (London: Zed Books, 1992).

Campbell, David: *Politics Without Principle. Sovereignty, Ethics, and the Narratives of the Gulf War* (Boulder, CO: Lynne Rienner, 1994).

Chubin, Sharam: *Iran's National Security Policy. Capabilities, Intentions and Impact* (Washington, DC: The Carnegie Endowment for International Peace, 1994).

Clark, Ramsey: *The Fire This Time. U.S. War Crimes in the Gulf* (New York: Thunder's Mouth Press, 1992).

Cordesman, Anthony D.: *Iran's Military Forces in Transition. Conventional Threats and Weapons of Mass Destruction* (Westport, CT: Praeger Press, 1999).

Cordesman, Anthony H.: *After the Storm. The Changing Military Balance in the Middle East* (Boulder, CO: Westview, 1993).

Cordesman, Anthony & Abraham R. Wagner: *The Lessons of Modern War, Vol. 4: The Gulf War* (Boulder: Westview, 1996).

Ederington, L. Benjamin & Michael J. Mazarr (eds.): *Turning Point. The Gulf War and U.S. Military Strategy* (Boulder, CO: Westview Press, 1994).

Ehteshami, Anoushiravan & Raymond A. Hinnebusch: *Syria and Iran. Middle Powers in a Penetrated Regional System* (London: Routledge, 1997).

Entessar, Nader: *Kurdish Ethnonationalism* (Boulder, CO: Lynne Rienner, 1992).

Ertürk, Korkut A. (ed.): *Rethinking Central Asia. Non-Eurocentric Studies in History, Social Structure and Identity* (Reading: Ithaca Press, 1999).

Faour, Muhammad: *The Arab World After Desert Storm* (Washington, DC: United States Institute for Peace, 1993).

Feldman, Shai & Abdullah Toukan: *Bridging the Gap: A Future Security Architecture for the Middle East* (Lanham: Rowman & Littlefield, 1997).

Francona, Rick: *Ally to Adversary. An Eyewitness Account of Iraq's Fall from Grace* (Annapolis: Naval Institute Press, 1999).

Freedman, Lawrence & Efraim Karsh: *The Gulf Conflict 1990-1991. Diplomacy and War in the New World Order* (Princeton, N.J.: Princeton University Press, 1993).

Freedman, Robert O. & Peggy Meyerhoff Pearlstone (eds.): *The Middle East After Iraq's Invasion of Kuwait* (Gainesville, FL: University Press of Florida, 1993).

Friedman, Norman: *Desert Victory. The War for Kuwait* (Annapolis, ML: Naval Institute Press, 1991).

Fuller, Graham E. & Ian O. Lessler: *A Sense of Siege. The Geopolitics of Islam and the West* (Boulder, CO: Westview, 1995).

Gieling, Saskia: *Religion and War in Revolutionary Iran* (London: I.B. Tauris, 1999).

Gow, James (ed.): *Iraq, the Gulf Conflict and the World Community* (London: Brassey's/Centre for Defence Studies, 1993).

Graham-Brown, Sarah: *Sanctioning Saddam. The Politics of Intervention in Iraq* (London: I.B. Tauris, 1999).

Guazzone, Laura (ed.): *The Islamist Dilemma. The Political Role of Islamist Movements in the Contemporary Arab World* (Reading: Ithaca Press, 1995).

Halliday, Fred: *Islam and the Myth of Confrontation* (London: I.B. Tauris, 1996).

Hassan, Hamdi A.: *The Iraqi Invasion of Kuwait. Religion, Identity and Otherness in the Analysis of War and Conflict* (London: Pluto Press, 1999).

Heper, Metin, Öncü, Ayshe & Heinz Kramer (eds.): *Turkey and the West. Changing Political and Cultural Identities* (London: I.B. Tauris, 1993).

Hibbard, Scott W. & David Little: *Islamic Activism and U.S. Foreign Policy* (Washington, DC: United States Institute of Peace, 1997).

Hobwood, Derek, Habib Ishow & Thomas Koszinowski (eds.): *Iraq. Power and Society* (Reading: Ithaca Press, 1993).

Hoveyda, Fereydoun: *The Broken Crescent. The 'Threat' of Militant Islamic Fundamentalism* (Westport, CT: Praeger Press, 1998).

Huband, Mark: *Warriors of the Prophet. The Struggle for Islam* (Boulder, CO: Westview, 1999).

Hudson, Michael C.: *The Middle East Dilemma. The Politics and Economics of Arab Integration* (New York: Columbia University Press, 1999).

Hume, Cameron R.: *The United Nations, Iran, and Iraq. How Peacemaking Changed* (Bloomington: Indiana University Press, 1994).

Hunter, Shireen T.: *The Future of Islam and the West. Clash of Civilizations or Peaceful Coexistence* (Westport, CT: Praeger Press, 1998).

Ismael, Tareq Y. & Jacqueline S. Ismael (eds.): *The Gulf War and the New World Order: International Relations in the Middle East* (Gainesville, FL: University Press of Florida, 1994).

Janning, Josef & Dirk Rumberg (eds.): *Peace and Stability in the*

Middle East and North Africa (Gütersloh: Bertelsmann Foundation Publishers, 1996).

Jones, Peter: *Towards a Regional Security Regime for the Middle East: Issues and Options* (Stockholm: SIPRI, 1998).

Keaney, Thomas A. & Eliot A. Cohen: *Revolution in Warfare? Air Power in the Persian Gulf* (Annapolis, ML: Naval Institute Press, 1995).

Kechichian, Joseph A.: *Oman and the World. The Emergence of an Independent Foreign* Policy (Santa Monica: RAND, 1995).

Kemp, Geoffrey & Janice Gross Stein: *Powder Keg in the Middle East. The Struggle for Gulf Security* (Lanham, ML: Rowman & Littlefield, 1995).

Kemp, Geoffrey & Jeremy Pressman: *Point of No Return. The Deadly Struggle for Middle East Peace* (Washington, DC: Carnegie Endowment for International Peace/Brookings Institution Press, 1997).

Kemp, Geoffrey & Robert E. Harkavy: *Strategic Geography and the Changing Middle East* (Washington, DC: Carnegie Endowment for International Peace/Brookings Institution Press, 1997).

Kramer, Heinz: *A Changing Turkey. The Challenge to Europe and the United States* (Washington, DC: Brookings Institution Press, 2000).

Lauterpacht, E., C.J. Greenwood, Marc Weller & Daniel Bethelheim (eds.): *The Kuwait Crisis: Basic Documents* (Cambridge: Grotius Publications, 1991).

Levran, Aharon: *Israeli Strategy After Desert Storm. Lessons of the Second Gulf War* (London: Frank Cass, 1997).

Long, David E. & Christian Koch (eds.): *Gulf Security in the Twenty-First Century* (Abu Dhabi: The Emirates Centre for Strategic Studies and Research, 1997).

Makiya, Kanan: *Republic of Fear. The Politics of Modern Iraq* (Berkeley, CA: University of California Press, 1998).

Mallat, Chibli: *The Middle East into the 21st Century* (Reading: Ithaca Press, 1996).

Mastiny, Vojzech & R. Craig Nation (eds.): *Turkey Between East and West: New Challenges for a Rising Regional Power* (Boulder, CO: Westview, 1996).

Moore, John Morton: *Crisis in the Gulf: Enforcing the Rule of Law* (New York: Oceana Publications, 1992).

Munro, Alan: *An Arabian Affairs. Politics and Diplomacy behind the Gulf War* (London: Brassey's, 1996).

Murden, Simon: *Emergent Regional Powers and International Relations in the Gulf: 1988-1991* (Reading: Ithaca Press, 1995).

Olcott, Martha Brill: *Central Asia's New States. Independence, Foreign Policy, and Regional Security* (Washington, DC: United States Institute for Peace, 1996).

Peimani, Hooman: *Iran and the United States* (Westport, CT: Praeger Press, 1999).

Pokrant, Marvin: *Desert Shield at Sea. What the Navy Really Did* (Westport, CT: Greenwood Press, 1999).

Rahman, H.: *The Making of the Gulf War. Origin's of Kuwait's Longstanding Territorial Dispute with Iraq* (Reading: Ithaca Press, 1997).

Rajae, Farhand (ed.): *Iranian Perspectives on the Iran-Iraq War* (Gainsville, FL: University Press of Florida, 1997).

Record, Jeffrey: *Hollow Victory. A Contrary View of the Gulf War* (Washington, DC: Brassey's, US, 1993).

Renshon, Stanley A. (ed.): *The Political Psychology of the Gulf War. Leaders, Publics, and the Process of Conflict* (Pittsburgh: University of Pittsburgh Press, 1993).

Ritter, William Scott: *Endgame. Solving the Iraq Problem—Once and for All* (New York: Simon & Schuster, 1999).

Robins, Philip: *Turkey and the Middle East* (London: Royal Institute of International Affairs, 1991).

Sadri, Hounan A.: *Revolutionary States, Leaders, and Foreign Relations. A Comparative Study of China, Cuba and Iran* (Westport, CT: Praeger Press, 1997).

Salem, Paul (ed.): *Conflict Resolution in the Arab World: Selected Essays* (Beirut: American University of Beirut, 1997).

Sayigh, Yesid: *Arab Military Industry. Capability, Performance and Impact* (London: Brassey's Defence Publishers, 1992).

Sayigh, Yesid & Avi Shlaim: *The Cold War and the Middle East* (Oxford: Clarendon Press, 1997).

Scales, Robert S. Jr.: *Certain Victory: The U.S. Army in the Gulf War* (Washington, DC: Brassey's, US, 1994).

Sela, Avraham (ed.): *Political Encyclopedia of the Middle East* (New York: Continuum Publishing Co., 1999).

Sela, Avraham: *The Decline of the Arab-Israeli Conflict: Middle East Politics and the Quest for Regional Order* (Albany, NY: State University of New York Press, 1997).

Sick, Gary G. & Lawrence Potter (eds.): *The Persian Gulf at the Millennium. Essays in Politics, Economy, Security, and Religion*

(New York: St. Martin's Press, 1997)

Simons, Geoff: *Imposing Economic Sanctions. Legal Remedy or Genocidal Tool?* (London: Pluto Press, 1999).

Tanter, Raymond: *Rogue Regimes. Terrorism and Proliferation* (New York: St. Martin's Press, 1998).

Taylor, Philip M.: *War and the Media. Propaganda and Persuasion in the Gulf War*. 2nd edition (Manchester: Manchester University Press, 1998).

Weller, M. (ed.): *Iraq and Kuwait: The Hostilities and their Aftermath.* Cambridge International Documents, vol. 3 (Cambridge: Grotius Publications, 1993).

Wright, J.W. Jr.: *The Political Economy of Middle East Peace* (London: Routledge, 1999).

Zahlan, Rosemary Said: *The Making of the Modern Gulf States.* Revised and Updated Edition (Reading: Ithaca Press, 1998).

INDEX

Persons, Countries, International Organizations